ENDOMETRIOSIS: EMERGING RESEARCH AND INTERVENTION STRATEGIES

ANNALS OF THE NEW YORK ACADEMY OF SCIENCES
Volume 955

ENDOMETRIOSIS: EMERGING RESEARCH AND INTERVENTION STRATEGIES

Edited by Koji Yoshinaga and Estella C. Parrott

The New York Academy of Sciences
New York, New York
2002

♾ The paper used in this publication meets the minimum requirements of the American National Standard for Information Sciences—Permanence of Paper for Printed Library Materials, ANSI Z39.48-1984.

Library of Congress Cataloging-in-Publication Data

Endometriosis: emerging research and intervention strategies / edited by Koji Yoshinaga and Estella C. Parrott.
p. cm. — (Annals of the New York Academy of Sciences, ISSN 0077-8923; v. 955)
Includes bibliographical references and index.
ISBN 1-57331-380-7 (cloth: alk. paper) — ISBN 1-57331-381-5 (paper: alk. paper)
1. Endometriosis—Congresses.
[DNLM: 1. Endometriosis—therapy—Congresses. 2. Research—Congresses.
WP 390 E566 2002] I. Yoshinaga, Koji, 1932– . II. Parrott, Estella C. III. Series.
Q11.N5 vol. 955
[RG483.E53]
500 s—dc21
[618] 2002000878

GYAT/PCP
Printed in the United States of America
ISBN 1-57331-380-7 (cloth)
ISBN 1-57331-381-5 (paper)
ISSN 0077-8923

ANNALS OF THE NEW YORK ACADEMY OF SCIENCES

Volume 955
March 2002

ENDOMETRIOSIS: EMERGING RESEARCH AND INTERVENTION STRATEGIES

Editors
KOJI YOSHINAGA AND ESTELLA C. PARROTT

Conference Organizers
ESTELLA C. PARROTT, KOJI YOSHINAGA, LINDA C. GIUDICE, KEVIN G. OSTEEN, AND JERROLD HEINDEL

[This volume is the result of the NIH workshop entitled "Endometriosis: Emerging Research and Intervention Strategies" held at NIH on April 9–10, 2001, in Bethesda, Maryland, and sponsored by the National Institute of Child Health and Human Development, the National Institute of Environmental Health Sciences, and the Office of Research on Women's Health.]

CONTENTS

Financial assistance was received from:

- NATIONAL INSTITUTE OF CHILD HEALTH AND HUMAN DEVELOPMENT, NIH
- NATIONAL INSTITUTE OF ENVIRONMENTAL HEALTH SCIENCES, NIH
- OFFICE OF RESEARCH ON WOMEN'S HEALTH, NIH
- PHARMACIA CORPORATION
- SERONO SYMPOSIA USA, INCORPORATED
- TAP PHARMACEUTICAL PRODUCTS, INCORPORATED
- WYETH-AYERST RESEARCH

Foreword

In 1995, the National Institute of Child Health and Human Development (NICHD) held a meeting on endometriosis entitled "Conference on Endometriosis 2000". Since then, six years have passed. During these intervening years, what progress has been made in the research on endometriosis? What new therapies have become available? What kind of research is needed to improve diagnosis, treatment, and development of new drugs? To answer these questions and to plan future research support, we decided to hold a workshop entitled "Endometriosis: Emerging Research and Intervention Strategies". The Organizing Committee comprised Linda C. Giudice (Stanford University), Kevin G. Osteen (Vanderbilt University), Jerrold Heindel (NIEHS, NIH), Estella C. Parrott (NICHD, NIH), and Koji Yoshinaga (NICHD, NIH), who selected important topics and appropriate speakers. The objectives of this workshop were (1) to familiarize participants with the state of the science and key issues related to the basic biology, epidemiology, growth and development, environmental influences, and genetic expression that characterize endometriosis, (2) to review current intervention strategies and explore the development of novel therapeutic agents important in optimizing clinical outcomes, and (3) to present potential areas of future research directions and propose opportunities for research in epidemiology, basic science, and clinical research.

This volume contains presentations made at this workshop. The presentations are divided into nine sessions and each session is followed by a panel discussion. During the final session of the workshop, the participants condensed the presented ideas and pointed out important research opportunities to facilitate our understanding of endometriosis and to assist in the development of new and appropriate diagnostic methods and treatment of modalities.

It is hoped that the information presented here will not only serve to update our knowledge of endometriosis, but also increase our knowledge about the etiology of this disease, to devise novel methods for treatment and for noninvasive diagnosis. It is also intended that the information will be fully utilized to plan research support in this field that will ultimately alleviate the suffering from this disease and improve women's reproductive health.

The National Institute of Child Health and Human Development, the National Institute of Environmental Health Sciences, and the Office of Research on Women's Health, NIH, sponsored this conference. These units of NIH support research on endometriosis and will continue to promote improvement of women's health. The Organizing Committee expresses its appreciation for the generous unrestricted educational grants from the pharmaceutical companies listed in the acknowledgment of financial assistance.

— Koji Yoshinaga
— Estella C. Parrott

Clinical Aspects of Endometriosis

ANA A. MURPHY

Emory University School of Medicine, Atlanta, Georgia, USA

ABSTRACT: Endometriosis is one of the most commonly encountered gynecologic diseases requiring medical and/or surgical therapy. It is a leading cause of hysterectomy in the United States and has significant associated morbidity. The most frequent symptoms of genital tract endometriosis are dysmenorrhea, dyspareunia, chronic pelvic pain, and infertility. Endometriosis occurs in the pelvis, most commonly the ovaries and the dependent areas covered with peritoneum. Diagnosis requires surgical intervention and is usually made by laparoscopy. In women being evaluated for pelvic pain, the diagnosis of endometriosis is made frequently (40–60%) and varies with the population being studied. Infertility and endometriosis have long been associated. Although women with infertility may have pelvic pain, subfertility (20–30%) can be the only presenting symptom. In asymptomatic women, the diagnosis of endometriosis ranges from 2% to 22% of reproductive-age women. Its true incidence and natural history remain to be clarified. Endometriosis is a significant public health issue because of the large number of women it affects and the significant morbidity associated with this disease.

KEYWORDS: pelvic pain; infertility; diagnosis; natural history; extrapelvic; location; histogenesis; staging

INTRODUCTION

Endometriosis is one of the most commonly encountered gynecologic diseases, yet it is still an enigmatic disease. The etiology of this disease is still to be elucidated. The two most common widely held theories involve menstrual regurgitation and metaplasia of the mesothelium or peritoneum. It is likely that both may play a role. However, this still does not explain extrapelvic endometriosis such as that found in the chest wall and lung. Indeed, endometriosis is probably not a homogeneous disease process. The natural history is very poorly understood. Although it is widely held to be a progressive disease, the data are fraught with problems. Risk factors or facilitating factors for the disease(s) are not well understood. Nevertheless, there has been an explosion in clinical and basic science information in the last 5 years.

This is an exciting time for those involved in elucidating this enigmatic disease. Endometriosis is a disease that requires a multidisciplinary approach and this workshop is a perfect example. As we begin to put the basic science and clinical information together, the sum will be greater than the parts. Translational research is dependent on collaboration of basic scientists and clinicians. Endometriosis is a

Address for correspondence: Ana A. Murphy, M.D., Emory Center for Reproductive Medicine and Fertility, 20 Linden Avenue, Suite 4701, Atlanta, GA 30308. Voice: 404-686-1843; fax: 404-686-4956.

amurphy@emory.edu

significant public health issue because of the large number of women it affects and the significant morbidity associated with this disease. Translational research on endometriosis can have a major impact on women's reproductive health and can lead to strategies for prevention and more effective, targeted therapies for patients with pelvic pain and infertility.

The major objective of this paper is to acquaint nonclinicians with the clinical presentation of this disease. The secondary objective is to present information on the heterogeneity of the disease process that will be helpful in designing studies.

SIGNS AND SYMPTOMS OF PELVIC ENDOMETRIOSIS

Endometriosis occurs in the pelvis, most commonly the ovaries and the dependent areas covered with peritoneum such as the pouch of Douglas and the uterosacral ligaments. The most frequent symptoms of genital tract endometriosis are dysmenorrhea, dyspareunia, chronic pelvic pain, and infertility. In women being evaluated for pelvic pain, the diagnosis of endometriosis is made frequently (40–60%) and varies with the population being studied.[1,2] Dysmenorrhea is most often associated with endometriosis if it is severe and unresponsive to nonsteroidal anti-inflammatory agents and/or oral contraceptives. The pain may progress and begin prior to the onset of menses or become chronic and be noted throughout most of the menstrual cycle. When rectovaginal or uterosacral ligament involvement is noted, the pain is often referred to the rectum or lower back. Pain radiating down the leg(s) may also be seen.

Multiple studies have looked at the possible association of pelvic pain with either location or type of implant. Perper noted that the total number of implants was associated directly with the intensity of dysmenorrhea experienced in the last 60 days prior to laparoscopy, although lesion morphology (atypical vs. classic) was not associated.[3] In a large study by Koninckx,[4] subtle/atypical lesions were not associated with pelvic pain. In this study, location and depth (deep retroperitoneal disease) was significantly associated with pain. Muzii did not find an association of atypical lesions with pain.[5] Linear analogue score for dysmenorrhea correlated significantly with the total endometriosis score, the partial score for deep (ovarian) endometriosis, and the partial score for adhesions. There was no correlation with the score for superficial implants, the total number of implants, or the number of typical or atypical implants. Fedele[6] found that dysmenorrhea, pelvic pain, and deep dyspareunia did not correlate with location when lesion sites were evaluated as ovary, peritoneum, and both ovary and peritoneum. However, depth of peritoneal penetration was not studied. The interpretation of the data available is hampered by the significant variation among these studies in the scope of anatomic information provided and the mode of evaluation of pelvic pain.

Dyspareunia is frequently associated with rectovaginal and uterosacral ligament disease. Fixation of the uterus or ovary by adhesions, especially if an endometrioma is noted, is also associated with dyspareunia. Chronic, recurrent pelvic pain associated with endometriosis is often a disabling disease. However, Koninckx *et al.*[4] suggest that deeply infiltrating endometriosis is strongly associated with pelvic pain and that the association with endometriomas and adhesions is no longer significant if depth is taken into account. In another paper, they suggest that the diagnosis of deep disease is enhanced by examination during menstruation.[7] CA-125 may be a useful adjunct if drawn in the menstrual phase. However, it is important to understand the wide spectrum seen in patients with endometriosis. Women with extensive endometriosis may have little or no pain symptoms and come to the attention of physicians because of associated infertility or as an incidental finding. Conversely, women with only minimal or mild involvement may manifest with disabling pelvic pain.

Menstrual outflow obstruction is associated with endometriosis in young adolescents.[8] In these patients, pain and/or abdomino/pelvic mass is the presenting symptom. It has been hypothesized that endometriosis associated with outflow tract obstruction may be very different from that seen in women without obstruction.[9] Endometriosis is a common diagnosis (45–65%) in adolescents without outflow obstruction, but with significant pelvic pain.[10,11] Adolescents without outflow obstruction tend to be older and to present with dysmenorrhea or acute pain. One of the first reports of atypical endometriosis (20%) was in adolescents.[11]

Infertility and endometriosis have long been associated and thought to have an incidence of 20–30% in women with subfertility.[12] Although women with infertility may have pelvic pain, infertility can be the only presenting symptom. Interestingly, Koninckx[4] noted that women with pain and infertility had more severe disease, as classified by the revised American Fertility Society (rAFS), than women with infertility or pain alone. The association of infertility/subfertility to endometriosis is the subject of a separate article in this workshop.

Although relatively rare, endometriosis occurs in the menopause and may be more common in women taking hormone replacement therapy.[13] However, it may not only occur in the absence of hormone replacement therapy, but it may also occur *de novo* in the menopause.[14,15] Although rare in men, endometriosis is frequently associated with hormonal therapy.[16] The epidemiology of endometriosis is the subject of a separate article in these proceedings.

EXTRAPELVIC ENDOMETRIOSIS

While genital tract involvement is the rule, endometriosis is also seen in the gastrointestinal tract, the urinary tract, lungs, scars, and nerves. Extrapelvic endometriosis is not as well understood as pelvic endometriosis. It is not clear whether endometriosis occurring outside the reproductive organs is the same disease as pelvic endometriosis. Extrapelvic endometriosis is defined as endometriotic lesions found outside the pelvis and includes cervix, vagina, vulva, intestinal tract, urinary tract, abdominal wall, thoracic cage and lungs, extremities, and the central nervous system. In a study done at Johns Hopkins, pathologic review found endometriosis in all organs, except the spleen.[17] The diagnosis of extrapelvic endometriosis is commonly made during examination of the abdominal cavity and may be asymptomatic or exhibit symptoms based on the organ system.

The gastrointestinal tract is the most common site of extrapelvic endometriosis, with the sigmoid colon, descending colon, and rectum representing the areas most commonly involved.[18] The rectovaginal septum with rectosigmoid involvement is thought to be the most common form of extrapelvic endometriosis. These lesions may present with intestinal obstruction or symptoms such as pain, distension, diarrhea, constipation, and rectal bleeding. It may also be an incidental finding at the time of laparoscopy. Its treatment is dependent on symptoms, extent of disease, location, and degree of bowel dysfunction. Neoplastic changes in bowel endometriosis are very infrequent.[19]

Endometriotic implants on the anterior cul-de-sac or bladder flap are relatively common. These may give rise to urinary symptoms such as dysuria, urgency, frequency, suprapubic pain, and dyspareunia. These symptoms are noted to be similar to the symptoms of interstitial cystitis.[15] Hematuria is a late sign and often denotes invasion through the bladder wall. Ureteral endometriosis is almost always asymptomatic unless obstruction with hydronephrosis occurs. Characteristically, the symptoms may occur cyclicly, with the symptoms noted above as well as hematuria, flank pain, and urinary track infection.[20] Involvement of the ureter is frequently unilateral, although bilateral involvement may occur with and without obstruction. Obstruction can lead to loss of a kidney.

Lung and chest wall endometriosis usually presents with symptoms such as pneumothorax, hemothorax, or hemoptysis associated with menses.[21] The diagnosis is often made with video-assisted thoracic surgery. Less frequently, it presents as an asymptomatic pulmonary nodule. A significant number (33%) of women have no pelvic disease.

DIAGNOSIS

Endometriosis can be suspected from the history, pelvic examination, and ancillary tests such as ultrasound, MRI, and CA-125. However, its diagnosis requires visualization of the pelvis with surgical intervention (laparoscopy or laparotomy) unless extrapelvic endometriosis can be visualized and biopsied. Endometriosis occurs most frequently in the pelvis, commonly the ovaries, uterosacral ligaments, pouch of Douglas, and rectovaginal septum. Endometriomas, or deep disease of the ovary, are cysts of endometriosis within the ovary. Deep disease or invasion of endometriosis most commonly occurs in the uterosacral ligaments, rectovaginal septum, rectum/sigmoid colon, ureters, bladder, and appendix. Deep retroperitoneal disease is often associated with pelvic pain, the most common symptom of endometriosis.[4]

Endometriosis is classically defined as the presence of endometrial tissue (specifically, endometrial glands and stroma) outside the uterine cavity. Pathologic diagnosis of endometriosis demands endometrial glands and stroma; however, hemosiderin deposition and fibromuscular metaplasia are also frequently seen in association with endometriosis. The histologic diagnosis is often "suspected" or "compatible with endometriosis" when either stroma or glands are found in conjunction with hemosiderin deposition and/or fibromuscular metaplasia. It is still argued that the diagnosis can be made visually and does not need pathologic confirmation. Obviously, studies that incorporate histologic diagnosis into the diagnosis are more rigorous and carry more weight.

The phenotypic appearance of endometriosis implants now includes adhesions, superficial pigmented lesions (red, brown, black), superficial nonpigmented lesions (clear vesicles), white lesions, peritoneal pockets, nodular deep lesions, and deep cystic lesions (endometrioma).[22] The pathologic diagnosis in these types of lesions is made between 60% and 80% of the time.[23] There are a number of other lesions that mimic the classic black implants and the nonclassic or atypical lesions. Other diseases that can be confused with endometriosis include psammoma bodies, endosalpingiosis, mesothelial cancers, granulation tissue, old suture remnants, splenosis, Walthard rest, inflammatory cystic inclusions, CO_2 laser char, and hemangiomas.[24]

Different morphologic appearances may represent different stages of the disease. Koninckx[4] prospectively examined the type, pelvic area, depth of infiltration, and volume of lesions of endometriosis in 643 laparoscopies for infertility, pelvic pain, or both. The incidence, area, and volume of atypical or nonclassic lesions decreased with age when compared to black/classic lesions. Increasing age was associated with increasing incidence, area, and volume of classic lesions and increased depth of infiltration. It is now relatively well accepted that the classic dark lesions are probably a later stage of disease.

NATURAL HISTORY

The natural history of this disease is poorly understood. Multiple studies have attempted to infer it from studies that have a control arm that includes laparoscopic visualization of the disease at two different intervals (TABLE 1). Thomas and Cooke studied 26 women with endometriosis whose "disease did not impede collection of oocytes by the fimbria" and who had a median rAFS score of 2.[25] Four of the 17 patients on placebo had complete remission of disease by laparoscopy. No mention is made of progression. The study by Mahmood and Templeton noted a 27% spontaneous regression of visible lesions.[26] Telimaa reported 17 women with minimal disease treated with placebo.[27] Of this group, 2 had no visible disease on repeat laparoscopy. In a Japanese study, 7 untreated patients underwent second and third laparoscopies.[28] The endometriosis score increased gradually in 4 of the 7 and was unchanged or decreased in 3 over an 8-month period. In the latter group, 1 patient with severe disease was again examined at 16 months with significant, rapid progression of disease. A recent study performed second-look laparoscopy at 3 months in 43 women in the placebo group of a drug study.[29] In this group, 37 women were stage I and II in the rAFS classification. Twenty-one in that group had a decrease in rAFS stage and 27 in rAFS score. A randomized, controlled laser laparoscopy study of pelvic pain associated with minimal to moderate endometriosis studied 24 of 31 control patients with continuing pain at 6 months.[30] Although untreated painful endometriosis progresses (7/24) or remains static (10/24) in the majority of patients, this study suggests that it spontaneously improves in 29% (7/24).

TABLE 1. Placebo-controlled studies with second-look laparoscopy

Change in rAFS score	Thomas[25] (n = 17)	Mahmood[26] (n = 11)	Telimaa[27] (n = 17)	Sutton[30] (n = 24)	Hoshiai[28] (n = 7)	Harrison[29] (n = 43)
Progressed	47%	64%	24%	29%	57%	5%
Unchanged	24%	9%	59%	42%	14%	46%
Regressed	29%	27%	17%	29%	29%	49%

NOTE: Adapted from reference 30.

Overall, these studies are problematic since such a small number of patients have been studied. Additionally, these studies generally included women with minimal and mild stages of disease. Nevertheless, the data in this select group of patients suggest that endometriosis is not a predictably progressive disease, especially in women with minimal or mild disease. To more objectively validate these conclusions, a significant number of women at all stages of disease, both symptomatic (pain/infertility) and asymptomatic (true controls), need to be prospectively followed serially with laparoscopy over time. Given that an invasive test such as laparoscopy is required, such studies are exceedingly difficult to accomplish.

Others[4,31] have suggested a cross-sectional design to study the manifestation of disease progression. A very large population of women with endometriosis that encompass the entire age range from adolescents to older age groups is studied. Obviously, the questions that can be asked with this type of study differ from the laparoscoped control arm of drug studies examined above. Redwine[31] prospectively looked at the distribution of endometriosis by age groups and fertility in 132 consecutive patients primarily with pelvic pain. His results suggest that endometriosis is a positionally static disease, not spreading in the pelvis with advancing age. In fact, there was an apparent decrease in disease with age when examining frequency of areas involved. The endometriosis was not staged, but mapped by area. Exposure to pregnancy resulted in a small decrease in pelvic involvement. As noted above, Koninckx[4] showed that the incidence, area, and volume of atypical/nonclassic lesions decreased with age when compared to black/classic lesions. Increasing age was associated with increasing incidence, area, and volume of classic lesions and increased depth of infiltration. Redwine noted in a cross-sectional study that the incidence of subtle endometriosis, which is widely accepted as an early stage of endometriosis, decreases with age.[32] Their combined data were taken as suggestive evidence of endometriosis as a progressive disease. The data obtained from the control arm of laparoscopy studies and the cross-sectional data are not necessarily incompatible as the populations studied varied widely in terms of disease severity. The more recent cross-sectional studies are more likely to have patients with more extensive disease, as would be expected, in the practice of investigators well known for their surgical skills.

PROPOSED HYPOTHESIS FOR HISTOGENESIS BASED ON LOCATION OF ENDOMETRIOTIC DISEASE

Nisolle and Donnez[33] recently proposed that peritoneal endometriosis, ovarian endometriosis, and adenomyotic nodules of the rectovaginal septum are three different disease entities. They provide evidence to support significant morphologic and morphometric similarity between eutopic endometrium and red peritoneal lesions to suggest that red lesions are the first manifestation of implanted regurgitated endometrium. Growth and progression are manifested by shedding/bleeding that leads to inflammation and scarring, producing the black lesion. Subsequent fibrosis results in an opacified white lesion.

Ovarian endometriomas have been hypothesized to result from invagination of the cortex and its mesothelium/peritoneum after the accumulation of menstrual debris from superficial implants.[34,35] This would imply that shedding and bleeding progressively cause invagination and that the histogenesis is similar to the peritoneal implant. Others have suggested that endometriomas result from coelomic metaplasia of invaginated epithelial inclusion cysts.[36] The peritoneum or mesothelium is thought to have the capacity to differentiate into tissues of Müllerian origin. This implies that regurgitation of menstrual blood into the peritoneal cavity is not necessary for the histogenesis of endometriosis.

Müllerian remnants or rests have recently been proposed as the tissue of origin of deep infiltrating endometriosis of the rectovaginal septum. Nisolle and Donnez[33] suggest that this entity corresponds to an adenomyotic nodule that is characterized by extensive smooth muscle proliferation. Evidence to support this hypothesis consists of immunocytochemical results showing poor differentiation and hormonal independence of these lesions. Alternatively, Koninckx and Martin[37] proposed adenomyotic nodules to be the consequence of deep infiltrating endometriosis. Thus, they believe that this deep form of endometriosis with its significant smooth muscle cell proliferation is the natural evolution of peritoneal endometriosis in some women. Their data do not support the contention that adenomyosis is responsive to physiologic levels of progesterone.[38]

The proposed hypotheses for the histogenesis of endometriosis are controversial. Why is the above information of clinical importance? The different theories of histogenesis proposed for the different forms of endometriosis based on location add another layer of heterogeneity and complexity to the populations being studied if location is not specified or taken into account. Studies that use only peritoneal implants or only endometriomas as a source of endometriosis cells are more likely to be homogeneous than studies that examine these tissues as if they were interchangeable. Unfortunately, it is unclear whether they are or not.

STAGING OF ENDOMETRIOSIS

The rAFS classification is based on the location, bulk of disease, and amount and severity of adhesions.[39] Few studies demonstrate any correlation between staging of endometriosis and pain, lesion morphology, volume of disease, or response to therapy.[4,6,38] The exception is the strong association of deep infiltrating lesions and pain.[4,38] This classification system does not take deep peritoneal disease into account; it only takes deep ovarian disease into account (endometrioma). Unfortunately, the use of an arbitrary weighted system for assigning scores to individual categories of disease or for computing a total score has severely limited the rAFS classification system to predict infertility as well.[40] There is no differentiation between classic and nonclassic lesions. By convention, its users do not distinguish between classic and nonclassic lesions and just add them together to assign the score. Extrapelvic sites are not accounted. Obviously, it is important to understand the classification system because the vast majority of studies to be presented will use it.

CONCLUSIONS

Endometriosis was first described by Rokitansky in 1860 and yet it still remains an enigmatic disease. The complexity of its clinical presentation, its natural history, the variation in anatomic/morphologic presentation, the possible different etiologies for endometriosis based on location, and the lack of a staging classification that reflects clinical outcome result in very heterogeneous populations for translational and clinical studies. This implies that populations studied must be rigorously defined and very large so that subpopulations can be examined.

A unifying hypothesis must address at least some of the following issues. How does endometriosis survive, attach, and invade the peritoneum? What characteristics of the mesothelium in women with endometriosis facilitate or promote adhesion or implantation? What differentiates the endometrium of women with endometriosis from that of normal women and how does it promote/facilitate adhesion and implantation of endometriosis? The cellular and soluble portions of the peritoneal fluid are an integral part of the disease process. What is their role in the initiation, maintenance, and growth of the disease? What is the role of the systemic and local immune system? The lack of a unifying hypothesis for the pathophysiology of endometriosis hinders our understanding and our ability to formulate meaningful hypotheses to test in the laboratory and/or the bedside.

There is growing evidence to suggest that endometriosis is associated with a significant inflammatory response that may be mediated by activated macrophages and lymphocytes and increased levels of cytokines, chemokines, and growth factors.[41] The result is an environment that promotes implantation and proliferation. Our laboratory has proposed the first unifying hypothesis that suggests that endometriosis is a disease of oxidative stress.[42] Only by hypothesis testing can we begin to understand the mechanisms involved in the pathogenesis of endometriosis. Correlation of basic science with a well-defined clinical population is the key to successful translational research that will lead to the development of new diagnostic and targeted therapeutic approaches.

REFERENCES

1. GRUPPO ITALIANO PER LO STUDIO DELL'ENDOMETRIOSI. 1994. Prevalence and anatomical distribution of endometriosis in women with selected gynecological conditions: results from a multicentric Italian study. Hum. Reprod. **9:** 1158–1162.
2. ESKENAZI, B. & M. WARNER. 1997. Epidemiology of endometriosis. Obstet. Gynecol. Clin. North Am. **24:** 235–258.
3. PERPER, M.M. *et al.* 1995. Dysmenorrhea is related to the number of implants in endometriosis patients. Fertil. Steril. **63:** 500–503.
4. KONINCKX, P.R. *et al.* 1991. Suggestive evidence that pelvic endometriosis is a progressive disease, whereas deeply infiltrating endometriosis is associated with pelvic pain. Fertil. Steril. **55:** 759–765.
5. MUZII, L. *et al.* 1997. Correlation between endometriosis-associated dysmenorrhea and the presence of typical or atypical lesions. Fertil. Steril. **68:** 19–22.
6. FEDELE, L. *et al.* 1990. Stage and localization of pelvic endometriosis and pain. Fertil. Steril. **53:** 155–158.
7. KONINCKX, P.R. *et al.* 1996. Diagnosis of deep endometriosis by clinical examination during menstruation and plasma CA-125. Fertil. Steril. **65:** 280–287.
8. OLIVE, D.L. & D. HENDERSON. 1987. Endometriosis and mullerian anomalies. Obstet. Gynecol. **69:** 412–415.
9. SANFILIPPO, J.S. *et al.* 1986. Endometriosis in association with uterine anomaly. Am. J. Obstet. Gynecol. **154:** 39–43.
10. CHATMAN, D. & A. WARD. 1982. Endometriosis in adolescents. J. Reprod. Med. **27:** 156–159.

11. GOLDSTEIN, D., C. DE CHOLNOKY & S. EMANS. 1980. Adolescent endometriosis. J. Adolesc. Health Care **1:** 37–41.
12. WALKER, K.G. *et al.* 1993. The prevalence of endometriosis in women with infertile partners. Eur. J. Obstet. Gynecol. Reprod. Biol. **21:** 195–197.
13. LAM, A., M. FRENCH & F. CHARNOCK. 1992. Bilateral ureteric obstruction due to recurrent endometriosis associated with hormone replacement therapy. Aust. N.Z. J. Obstet. Gynaecol. **32:** 83–85.
14. CHINEGWUNDOH, F.I. *et al.* 1995. Renal and diaphragmatic endometriosis *de novo* associated with hormone replacement therapy. J. Urol. **153:** 380–381.
15. WESTNEY, O.L., C.L. AMUNDSEN & E. MCGUIRE. 2000. Bladder endometriosis: conservative management. J. Urol. **163:** 1814–1817.
16. MARTIN, J. & A. HAUCK. 1985. Endometriosis in the male. Am. Surg. **51:** 426–429.
17. MARKHAM, S.M., S.E. CARPENTER & J.A. ROCK. 1989. Extrapelvic endometriosis. *In* Obstetrics and Gynecology Clinics of North America, pp. 193–219. Saunders. Philadelphia.
18. ROCK, J.A. & S.M. MARKHAM. 1987. Extrapelvic endometriosis. *In* Endometriosis, pp. 185–192. Alan R. Liss. New York.
19. YANTISS, R., P. CLEMENT & Y. YOUNG. 2000. Neoplastic and pre-neoplastic changes in gastrointestinal endometriosis: a study of seventeen cases. Am. J. Surg. Urol. **24:** 513–524.
20. SALEH, N. & E. DAW. 1980. Endometriosis in non-gynecological sites. Practitioner **224:** 1189–1201.
21. JOSEPH, J. & S.A. SAHN. 1996. Thoracic endometriosis syndrome: new observations from an analysis of 110 cases. Am. J. Med. **100:** 164–170.
22. JANSEN, R.P. & P. RUSSELL. 1985. Nonpigmented endometriosis: clinical, laparoscopic, and pathologic definition. Am. J. Obstet. Gynecol. **153:** 31.
23. MARTIN, D.C. *et al.* 1989. Laparoscopic appearances of peritoneal endometriosis. Fertil. Steril. **51:** 63–67.
24. MARTIN, D. & F. LING. 1999. Endometriosis and pain. Clin. Obstet. Gynecol. **42:** 664–697.
25. THOMAS, E.J. & I.D. COOKE. 1987. Successful treatment of asymptomatic endometriosis: does it benefit infertile women? Br. Med J. **294:** 1117–1119.
26. MAHMOOD, T.A. & A. TEMPLETON. 1990. The impact of treatment on the natural history of endometriosis. Hum. Reprod. **5:** 965–970.
27. TELIMAA, S. *et al.* 1987. Placebo controlled comparison of danazol and high-dose medroxyprogesterone acetate in the treatment of endometriosis. Gynecol. Endocrinol. **1:** 13–23.
28. HOSHIAI, H. *et al.* 1993. Old problems, potential explanations, and solutions: laparoscopic evaluation of the onset and progression of endometriosis. Am. J. Obstet. Gynecol. **169:** 714–719.
29. HARRISON, R.F. & C. BARRY-KINSELLA. 2000. Efficacy of medroxyprogesterone treatment in infertile women with endometriosis: a prospective, randomized, placebo-controlled study. Fertil. Steril. **74:** 24–30.
30. SUTTON, J.G. *et al.* 1997. Follow-up report on a randomized controlled trial of laser laparoscopy in the treatment of pelvic pain associated with minimal to moderate endometriosis. Fertl. Steril. **68:** 1070–1074.
31. REDWINE, D.B. 1987. The distribution of endometriosis in the pelvis by age groups and fertility. Fertil. Steril. **47:** 173–180.
32. REDWINE, D. 1987. Age-related evolution in color appearance of endometriosis. Fertil. Steril. **48:** 1062–1063.
33. NISOLLE, M. & J. DONNEZ. 1997. Peritoneal endometriosis, ovarian endometriosis, and adenomyotic nodules of the rectovaginal septum are three different entities. Fertil. Steril. **68:** 585–596.
34. BROSENS, I.A., P. PUTTEMANS & J. DEPREST. 1994. The endoscopic localization of endometrial implants in the ovarian chocolate cyst. Fertil. Steril. **61:** 1034–1038.
35. HUGHESDON, P.E. 1957. The structure of endometrial cysts of the ovary. J. Obstet. Gynaecol. Br. Emp. **44:** 69–84.
36. DONNEZ, J.M. *et al.* 1996. Large ovarian endometriomas. Hum. Reprod. **11:** 641–646.

37. KONINCKX, P.R. & D.C. MARTIN. 1992. Deep endometriosis: a consequence of infiltration or retraction or possible adenomyosis externa? Fertil. Steril. **58:** 924–928.
38. CORNILLIE, F.J. *et al.* 1990. Deeply infiltrating pelvic endometriosis: histology and clinical significance. Fertil. Steril. **53:** 978–983.
39. THE AMERICAN FERTILITY SOCIETY. 1985. Revised American Fertility Society classification of endometriosis. Fertil. Steril. **43:** 351–352.
40. GUZICK, D.S. *et al.* 1997. Prediction of pregnancy in infertile women based on American Society for Reproductive Medicine's revised classification of endometriosis. Fertil. Steril. **67:** 822–829.
41. LEBOVIC, D.I., M. MUELLER & R. TAYLOR. 2001. Immunobiology of endometriosis. Fertil. Steril. **75:** 1–10.
42. MURPHY, A.A. *et al.* 1998. Endometriosis: a disease of oxidative stress? Semin. Reprod. Endocrinol. **16:** 263–273.

The Epidemiology of Endometriosis

DANIEL W. CRAMER[a] AND STACEY A. MISSMER[b]

[a]*Department of Obstetrics, Gynecology, and Reproductive Biology, Brigham and Women's Hospital, Harvard Medical School, Boston, Massachusetts, USA*

[b]*Department of Epidemiology, Harvard School of Public Health, Boston, Massachusetts, USA*

ABSTRACT: Advances in understanding the epidemiology of endometriosis have lagged behind other diseases because of methodologic problems related to disease definition and control selection. Nevertheless, a better picture of the epidemiology of endometriosis has emerged over the past few decades. Prevalence estimates of the disease in clinic populations vary from about a 4% occurrence of largely asymptomatic endometriosis found in women undergoing tubal ligation to 50% of teenagers with intractable dysmenorrhea. General population incidence during the 1970s in this country has been suggested to be 1.6 per 1000 white females aged 15–49, while a more current study based upon hospital discharges finds endometriosis as a first listed diagnosis in 1.3 per 1000 discharges in women aged 15–44. There is a clinical impression that blacks have lower rates of endometriosis and Orientals have higher rates than whites. A variety of personal risk factors for endometriosis have also been described. Women with endometriosis may be taller and thinner. Menstrual factors reported to increase risk include dysmenorrhea, early menarche, and shorter cycle lengths. There is support for the idea that lifestyle exposures that might raise or lower estrogen levels could affect risk, including a decreased risk associated with smoking and exercise and an increased risk associated with caffeine or alcohol use. These risk factors appear to be compatible with the central importance of retrograde menstruation influenced by outflow obstruction that might affect its amount, immune factors that might affect its ability to be cleared, or hormonal stimuli that might affect its growth. In this model, dysmenorrhea could be either a disease symptom or a manifestation of outflow obstruction. Nulliparity could be either a consequence of disease or a cause since nulliparous women would not have the benefit of cervical dilation associated with labor and delivery. Since there is evidence that family history is a risk factor for disease, a challenge is how to integrate genetic factors into the model. The genetics of endometriosis might be advanced if we could identify an "endometriosis phenotype". We propose that this may consist of early menarche, short cycles, painful periods, subfertility, and possibly tall stature that could be explained by genetic factors that predispose to poor endowment of germ cells and canalization defects of the cervix. The value of establishing an "endometriosis phenotype" is that, as candidates for genetic markers are identified, particular genotypes can be correlated with these factors even if a formal diagnosis of endometriosis has not been made. Additional well-designed case-control and cohort studies will be necessary to test theories related to patho-

Address for correspondence: Daniel W. Cramer, Department of Obstetrics, Gynecology, and Reproductive Biology, Brigham and Women's Hospital, Harvard Medical School, Boston, MA 02115. Voice: 617-732-4895; fax: 617-732-4899.

dcramer@partners.org

genesis, establish the precise relationship between reproductive morbidity and endometriosis, identify specific genetic factors, and establish long-term risks.

Keywords: prevalence; menses; alcohol; caffeine; smoking

INTRODUCTION

We are pleased that the organizers of this NICHD workshop included a section on the "Epidemiology of Endometriosis" since it provides recognition that epidemiologic studies can contribute to the scientific investigation of this disease. We think it is fair to say there have been few NIH studies of the epidemiology of endometriosis in major part because it was perceived that there were unique problems in studying this disease from an epidemiologic standpoint. While these problems need to be considered, they should not be viewed as "fatal flaws" of proposals for epidemiologic studies of endometriosis. Indeed, despite a relative paucity of studies and diverse designs, some fairly consistent observations have emerged from studies completed to date—findings that we believe have led to a better understanding of the pathogenesis of endometriosis. In this monograph, we will review methodologic issues, summarize the epidemiologic findings as they fit with pathogenetic models, suggest hypotheses that may be tested in future epidemiologic studies, and make some recommendations about the design of those studies. We will also present some original data from our own studies of women undergoing *in vitro* fertilization (IVF), some of whom carry a diagnosis of endometriosis. We hope to convince the reader that epidemiology can play an important role in helping to devise strategies for the primary or secondary prevention of the disease.

METHODOLOGIC ISSUES

There are two major methodologic issues, which have been problematic for epidemiologic studies of endometriosis, especially case-control studies. The first is that the current clinical definition of the disease includes a wide spectrum of symptoms and pathologic findings. A second problem is that no strategy for control selection appears entirely satisfactory to deal with factors that might influence who comes to a diagnosis of endometriosis and that could be related to exposures of interest.

Traditionally, endometriosis has been defined as the presence of functional endometrial glands and stroma outside of the uterus (ectopic endometrium), but in the pelvic cavity. This definition allows women found to have asymptomatic disease at the time of unrelated surgery (e.g., tubal ligation) to be included as cases. However, from a public health standpoint, we are interested in disease, which produces symptoms or causes hospitalization. Thus, some gynecologists have suggested that endometriosis be defined not only by the presence of ectopic endometrium, but also by evidence that the lesions are active cellularly or have affected normal physiology.[1] Examples of cellular activity or physiologic effect might include evidence that the lesions are deep (>5 mm), manifest as ovarian endometriomas, or are associated with pelvic adhesions not attributable to other causes.

Holt and Weiss have encouraged epidemiologists to operationalize these definitions in case selection.[2] At the very least, it would seem that asymptomatic endometriosis found at tubal ligation should not be included in studies where most cases were symptomatic. We believe this would obviate the common criticism that methods for control selection should take care to rule out asymptomatic disease, for example, requiring all controls to have had laparotomy or laparoscopy. Alternatively, there seems to be good agreement that ovarian endometriomas represent an important form of endometriotic disease. Since follow-up studies suggest these women may be at risk for ovarian cancer,[3] it would seem that this would be one group that both clinicians and epidemiologists could agree should be a high priority for epidemiologic study.

Regardless of the case definition that the epidemiologist ultimately decides upon for his or her study, it is necessary to address what factors allowed the cases to come to diagnosis and whether these factors should be matched in selecting controls. To be sure, this argument can be carried to the extreme. To require that a control be matched to a case on the basis of both symptoms and diagnostic procedures would lead to a highly selected control group that would not allow many factors of potential interest to be studied due to overmatching. However, it does seem reasonable to match on factors influencing the likelihood of receiving medical attention such as availability of medical insurance and accessibility to gynecologic services. Cohort studies or case-control studies conducted within health maintenance organizations (HMOs) or in countries where there is universal health care may be valuable in this respect, but should not be made a prerequisite. While it is fair to say that the ideal epidemiologic study has not yet been performed, it is worthwhile to review the picture that has developed to date.

EPIDEMIOLOGIC FINDINGS

Under this topic, we consider demographic factors such as age and race, which influence risk of endometriosis, as well as personal risk factors (TABLE 1), which distinguish individuals with similar demographic backgrounds.

Demographic Factors

Prevalence estimates of endometriosis in clinic populations vary by diagnosis. In four of the largest studies completed to date,[4–7] the prevalence of largely asymptomatic endometriosis found in women undergoing tubal ligation was about 4%, ranging from 1% to 7%. In a multicenter study of infertility, endometriosis was the diagnosis in 17% of women with primary infertility,[8] but in other series the prevalence varied from about 9% to 50%.[9,10] Among women with pelvic pain, the prevalence of endometriosis ranged from about 5% to 21%,[9,11–13] with the larger studies suggesting about 8%. A group that appears to be at considerable risk for endometriosis are adolescents with intractable dysmenorrhea or pelvic pain, where about 50% are found to have the diagnosis.[14,15] This observation suggests that adolescents with severe dysmenorrhea (generally defined as requiring analgesics and bed rest) have a high likelihood of having endometriosis and require particular attention for efforts at early detection or prevention. A suggestion that we would offer is that such

TABLE 1. Summary of risk factors for endometriosis

Variable	Description of association	References
Age at menarche	Early age at menarche fairly consistently found to increase risk	8, 19–23
Cycle length	Shorter, more regular cycles fairly consistently increase risk	7, 8, 20, 22–24
Dysmenorrhea	Strong predictor, but assumed to be a symptom of existing disease	8, 18, 19
Parity	Decreasing risk with higher parity	7
Weight, BMI	Weak inverse association	8, 18, 19
Height	Taller height increases risk	8, 19
Exercise	Regular exercise may decrease risk	8, 19, 23
Smoking	Smoking may decrease risk	8, 18, 22
Alcohol	Use may increase risk	19, 36
Caffeine	Use may increase risk	37, 38
Family history	Good evidence that family history increases risk	27–31
PCB, dioxin exposure	Good primate data, but inconsistent data in women	41–43

women be considered for continuous regimens of a progesterone-dominant birth control pill.

Incidence data in the general population are less readily available. A population-based study during the 1970s using medical records[16] suggested an incidence of surgically or pathologically confirmed disease of 1.6 per 1000 white females aged 15–49. A more recent study based upon hospital discharges finds endometriosis as a first listed diagnosis in 1.3 per 1000 discharges in women aged 15–44.[17] Thus, endometriosis appears confined to the childbearing and immediate postmenopausal years, providing demographic support for the idea that pathogenesis involves the estrogen milieu. Two clinical studies have suggested that, compared to whites, blacks may have a lower risk and Orientals may have a higher risk for disease.[7,11]

Menstrual and Reproductive Factors

Dysmenorrhea is strongly associated with risk for endometriosis, but has generally been interpreted as a symptom of disease.[8,18,19] Other menstrual risk factors related to endometriosis are age at menarche and cycle length. Most epidemiologic studies addressing the topic have found that an early menarche, often defined as ≤ age 11, increases the risk for endometriosis.[8,19–23] Most of these same studies and others have found that risk is also increased with a shorter cycle length, often defined as ≤27 days.[7,8,20,22–24] There is less consistent evidence related to duration and heaviness of menstrual flow. Because early menarche and short cycles appear to be such consistent risk factors for endometriosis, it seems reasonable to predict that, if we better understood their physiologic determinants, then we might better understand the pathophysiology of endometriosis.

Because infertility may be a consequence of the disease and may also be part of case definition in any particular study, it can be problematic to study pregnancy history as a risk factor for endometriosis. A study based on endometriosis found at tubal ligation, despite our previous comment about its general lack of value, did suggest that higher parity is associated with a lower risk for observing endometriosis.[7]

Constitutional and Genetic Risk Factors

Regarding body habitus, weak inverse associations with weight and BMI have been found[8,18,19] and an increased risk with taller height has been reported for endometriosis.[8,19] Of interest regarding the latter association, taller women may have higher follicular-phase estradiol levels.[25] Conversely, regular exercise, which may lower estrogen levels,[26] has been associated with a reduced risk for endometriosis.[8,19,23]

There appears to be good evidence that women with endometriosis are more likely to have a mother or sister with the disease than control subjects.[27–29] There is also a high concordance of endometriosis among identical twins.[30,31] A number of genetic polymorphisms have been investigated, including those related to the detoxification enzyme glutathione-S-transferase,[32] esterase D,[33] the estrogen receptor gene,[34] and the N314D polymorphism of galactose transferase that is associated with decreased galactose metabolism.[35]

Exposures

Both alcohol use and caffeine use have been reported to increase risk of endometriosis[19,36–38] and, at least for alcohol, there is evidence that this substance may increase estrogen levels.[39] Conversely, a factor believed to lower estrogen levels is smoking, which has been associated with a decreased risk for endometriosis.[8,18,22] For these lifestyle exposures, there is the possibility that confounding factors such as menstrual symptoms or socioeconomic status might be operating. However, because of the importance of these exposures, they should continue to be examined in epidemiologic and experimental studies.

The association between oral contraceptives and endometriosis has been a difficult one to sort out because menstrual symptoms that are either risk factors for or markers of early endometriosis might also be indications for oral contraceptive use. One of the better studies addressing the topic was a cohort study of women attending a family planning clinic, which found a decreased risk for endometriosis associated with current use, but a slightly increased risk associated with former use.[40] Concern has been raised about whether women who have had hysterectomy and oophorectomy for endometriosis should receive unopposed estrogen therapy, but definitive studies are lacking.

Lastly, under this category we mention environmental exposures such as polychlorinated biphenyl (PCB) or dioxin. Based on animal studies suggesting that PCB or dioxin exposure might relate to endometriosis, possibly through their effects on the immune system,[41] there has been considerable interest in this exposure as a risk factor in women. However, results of two studies completed to date, based on serum levels of dioxin or PCB, have been contradictory.[42,43]

TABLE 2. Risk factors for endometriosis from the logistic model applied in an IVF population

Parameter	Estimate (p value)	Interpretation
Cycle length	–0.0634 (0.03)	Longer cycle decreases risk
Pain	0.9732 (<0.0001)	Moderate to severe dysmenorrhea increase
Weight (kg)	–0.0085 (0.03)	Heavier weight decreases risk

Risk Factors for Endometriosis in an IVF Population

In our ongoing study of women coming to IVF in several Boston clinics, we examined what factors were associated with a diagnosis of endometriosis as recorded by both the physician's review and the patient's perception of the nature of their infertility problem. In 179 cases, both agreed that endometriosis was the problem; in 294 cases, there was no diagnosis or disagreement about the diagnosis; and the remaining 906 subjects with definite cause(s) for their infertility other than endometriosis were the control group. In a logistic model comparing cases to controls and excluding the idiopathic group, the three significant predictors of endometriosis were menstrual pain, shorter cycle length, and weight (with heavier women having decreased risk) (TABLE 2). Restricted to those subjects who were tested for N314D, 31 (20.8%) out of 149 endometriosis cases either carried or were homozygous for N314D; compared to 113 (15.0%) out of 755 controls ($p = 0.06$), this was a finding of borderline significance. Forty-five (17.8%) of the 253 women with "idiopathic" infertility were carriers or homozygotes, which was higher, but not significantly different, compared to controls.

INTERPRETATION

FIGURE 1 illustrates one model for the pathogenesis of endometriosis, which attempts to integrate the diverse risk factors discussed above. This model emphasizes the importance of retrograde menstruation as a key factor in disease pathogenesis. In some cases, retrograde menstruation might alone be sufficient to cause disease such as when it is excessive—say, because of outflow obstruction, for example, vaginal or cervical stenosis or a noncommunicating uterine horn. In other cases, a "normal degree" of retrograde menstruation might operate in conjunction with immune factors that might affect its ability to be cleared from the pelvis or with hormonal stimuli that might affect its growth. We must also consider the possibility that there are other pathways such as coelomic metaplasia that we don't yet fully understand or know what the epidemiologic correlates might be.

With this model as perspective, there are two questions that we would like to discuss: (1) how can we distinguish whether some of the risk factors described are causes or consequences of the disease?; (2) how can we integrate genetic factors into the model? Because endometriosis could be asymptomatic for many years, it is arguable that many of the risk factors discussed could be either causes or consequences of the disease. We believe three are of particular interest: dysmenorrhea, infertility or subfertility, and immune function.

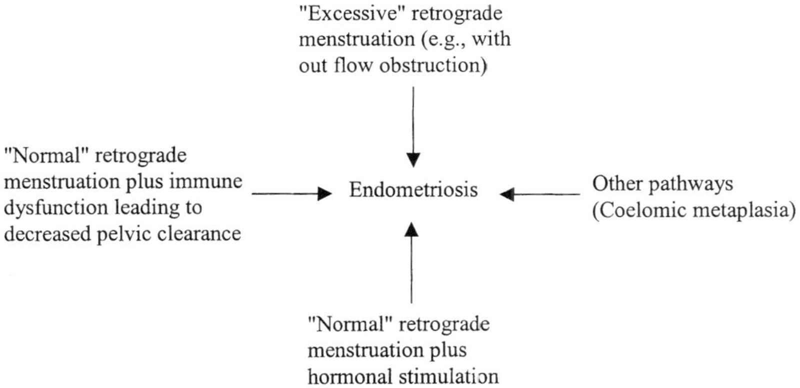

FIGURE 1. Model for pathogenesis of endometriosis involving retrograde menstruation.

Dysmenorrhea is a strong risk factor for endometriosis, but has generally been considered simply to represent a symptom of existing disease since it is easy to imagine that monthly bleeding from pelvic lesions is painful. However, since dysmenorrhea may correlate with stronger uterine contractility,[44] an alternate interpretation is that dysmenorrhea is associated with some degree of outflow obstruction, stronger uterine cramping, and increased propensity to retrograde menstruation. Taking a careful menstrual history and recording changes in dysmenorrhea over time with events like childbearing or operative dilation of the cervix might help sort out the sequence.

There is similar difficulty in sorting out the relationship between childbearing and endometriosis. While disruption of pelvic anatomy and ovarian function leading to infertility may clearly be a consequence of endometriosis, it is also reasonable to propose that delayed childbearing could also be a cause of endometriosis. Although avoided menstruation is one explanation for a protective effect of childbearing, it should be appreciated that permanent cervical dilation occurs with labor and delivery, possibly reducing the resistance to menstrual flow and decreasing the likelihood of retrograde menstruation. In addition, the decidual reaction that occurs on the ovarian and pelvic surface during pregnancy attributed to high hormone levels might make this tissue less susceptible to endometriosis implantation or growth. Clearly, we can't study the association between childbearing and endometriosis in those studies where cases are defined on the basis of a presenting complaint of infertility; however, the question can be addressed where pelvic pain or mass is the complaint.

It has been proposed that retrograde menstruation occurs to some degree in all women; however, it is only those who are unable to clear the menstrual debris because of immune dysfunction that will go on to develop disease.[45] This has been the mechanism suggested to explain the possible link with PCB or dioxin exposure—substances that might damage the immune system. Alternatively, immune dysfunction might also be a consequence of the disease. Women with endometriosis might develop antibodies against their endometrium and go on to develop autoimmune disorders. The latter issue can be addressed by careful follow-up studies of women diagnosed with endometriosis.

TABLE 3. Generalized linear model for predictors of cycle length in an IVF population

Parameter	Estimate (p value)	Interpretation
Age	–0.1991 (<0.0001)	Older women have shorter cycles
Endo. case	–1.1668 (0.01)	Endometriosis cases have shorter cycles
Height (cm)	–0.0870 (0.002)	Taller women have shorter cycles
Weight (kg)	0.0260 (<0.0001)	Heavier women have longer cycles
Age at menarche	0.2325 (0.06)	Earlier menarche associated with shorter cycles
N314D	0.6060 (0.19)	No significant association

A second important question for epidemiologists is as follows: how can genetic factors be integrated into the model depicted in FIGURE 1. A hypothesis that we would like to propose is that there may be an "endometriosis phenotype" defined by early menarche, short cycles, painful periods, subfertility, and (possibly) tall stature. This phenotype might be explained by a variety of genetic factors that may predispose to a poor endowment of germ cells and canalization defects of the cervix. An association between early menarche and short cycles would explain the consistency of these events as risk factors for endometriosis. A link between poor endowment of germ cells and canalization defects would explain dysmenorrhea and subfertility as apparent hallmarks of endometriosis. The potential value of establishing an "endometriosis phenotype" is that, as candidates for genetic markers are identified, a particular genotype can be correlated with these factors regardless of whether a formal diagnosis of endometriosis has been made.

Several premises involved in this hypothesis require elaboration. The first premise is that cycle length during early reproductive life and age at menarche are positively correlated. TABLE 3 shows the results of a general linear model applied to our IVF data in which we have made cycle length the dependent variable. In this model, the significant predictors were found to be current age (cycles shorten as women age), case status (endometriosis cases have shorter cycles), height (taller women have shorter cycles), weight (heavier women have longer cycles), and age at first period (women with an earlier menarche have shorter cycles). Using the same variables in a logistic model to determine predictors of moderate or severe dysmenorrhea, we found age (older women have less painful periods), case status (endometriosis cases have more painful periods), weight (heavier women have more painful periods), and N314D (carriers or homozygotes have more painful periods) (TABLE 4).

The second premise is that a shorter cycle length and early menarche may indicate a reduced germ cell endowment. As we saw in TABLE 3 and has previously been reported,[46] cycle length decreases as women get older. This appears to correlate with a decreasing number of germ cells. Thus, it seems reasonable to speculate that a short cycle length at an early age may indicate a smaller germ cell endowment. Indeed, follicle counts performed at autopsy in a classic study ranged between 85,000 and 684,000 in girls and women less than 20, suggesting that varying germ cell endowments must occur.[47] We have also observed that an earlier age at menarche and shorter cycles are two major components of a model predicting early menopause.[48]

TABLE 4. Logistic model for predictors of dysmenorrhea in an IVF population

Parameter	Estimate (*p* value)	Interpretation
Age	−0.0705 (<0.0001)	Older women have less painful periods
Endo. case	1.2712 (<0.0001)	Endometriosis cases have more painful periods
Weight (kg)	0.0053 (0.04)	Heavier women have more painful periods
N314D	0.3646 (0.05)	Carriers or homozygotes have more painful periods

The third and fourth premises are that canalization defects of the female tract may accompany a decreased germ cell endowment and may have genetic determinants. Case report suggests an association between vaginal agenesis and premature menopause.[49] Vaginal agenesis has also been associated with Turner's mosaicism known to cause oocyte deficiency.[50] Turning to the animal literature, strains of mice have been described that are born with a depleted number of oocytes, and these animals also have immature genital tracts as well as a predisposition to develop ovarian neoplasms.[51] In another interesting mouse model, fetuses exposed to high levels of galactose through maternal consumption were born with oocyte depletion and delayed vaginal opening.[52] This has been our basis for arguing that some cases of vaginal agenesis might relate to errors of galactose metabolism, including the N314D variant of galactose transferase.[52] Bringing relevance of these observations to endometriosis, we have reported that mothers of women with vaginal agenesis more frequently reported a personal history of endometriosis, especially if they carried the N314D variant of galactose transferase.[35,53] Clearly, the search for genetic factors in endometriosis is just beginning. We would argue that the scope of this investigation should be broadened to include the possibility that maternal genotype and intrauterine exposures may need to be considered.

RECOMMENDATIONS

Based on our review of the epidemiology of endometriosis and its interpretation, we think the following recommendations are reasonable:

(1) Epidemiologic studies of endometriosis should focus on active rather than asymptomatic disease.
(2) Criteria for control selection should include an attempt to match on factors that could have affected the likelihood that a case came to diagnosis, such as availability of medical insurance and access to gynecologic services.
(3) "Core" exposures to be studied should at least include menstrual factors, reproductive history, body habitus, lifestyle factors (e.g., exercise, smoking, caffeine use, or alcohol use), environmental exposures, and family history.
(4) Because risk factors suggest the importance of retrograde menstruation, an avenue for prevention to explore is the use of continuous regimens of oral contraceptives to reduce menstruation.
(5) In searching for genetic factors, the possibility should be considered that there is an "endometriosis phenotype" consisting of early menarche, short

cycle lengths, decreased germ cell endowment, and canalization defects of the cervix that predispose to subfertility, dysmenorrhea, and retrograde menstruation.

(6) Long-term follow-up studies on women with existing endometriosis are warranted to confirm previously identified risks for certain cancers as well as to examine potential links with autoimmune disorders.

REFERENCES

1. AUDEBERT, A., T. BACKSTROM, D.H. BARLOW *et al.* 1992. Endometriosis 1991: a discussion document. Hum. Reprod. **7:** 432–435.
2. HOLT, V.L. & N.S. WEISS. 2000. Recommendations for the design of epidemiologic studies of endometriosis. Epidemiology **11:** 654–659.
3. BRINTON, L.A., G. GRIDLEY, I. PERSSON *et al.* 1997. Cancer risk after a hospital discharge diagnosis of endometriosis. Am. J. Obstet. Gynecol. **176:** 572–579.
4. KIRSHON, B. & A.N. POINDEXTER. 1988. Contraception: a risk factor for endometriosis. Obstet. Gynecol. **71:** 829–831.
5. STRATHY, J.H., C.A. MOLGAARD, C.B. COULAM & L.J. MELTON. 1982. Endometriosis and infertility: a laparoscopic study of endometriosis among fertile and infertile women. Fertil. Steril. **38:** 667–672.
6. MAHMOOD, T.A. & A. TEMPLETON. 1991. Prevalence and genesis of endometriosis. Hum. Reprod. **6:** 544–549.
7. SANGI-HAGHPEYKAR, H. & A.N. POINDEXTER. 1995. Epidemiology of endometriosis among parous women. Obstet. Gynecol. **85:** 983–992.
8. CRAMER, D.W., E. WILSON, R.J. STILLMAN *et al.* 1986. The relation of endometriosis to menstrual characteristics, smoking, and exercise. JAMA **255:** 1904–1908.
9. DUIGNAN, N.H., J.A. JORDAN, B.M. COUGHLAN & R. LOGAN-EDWARDS. 1972. One thousand consecutive cases of diagnostic laparoscopy. J. Obstet. Gynaecol. Br. Commonw. **79:** 1016–1020.
10. WILLIAMS, T.J. & J.R. PRATT. 1977. Endometriosis in 1000 consecutive celiotomies: incidence and management. Am. J. Obstet. Gynecol. **129:** 245–250.
11. HASSON, H.M. 1976. Incidence of endometriosis in diagnostic laparoscopy. J. Reprod. Med. **16:** 135–140.
12. KLEPPINGER, R.K. 1976. One thousand laparoscopies at a community hospital. J. Reprod. Med. **13:** 13–17.
13. LISTON, W.A., W.P. BRADFORD, J. DOWNIE & M.G. KERR. 1972. Laparoscopy in a general gynecologic unit. Am. J. Obstet. Gynecol. **113:** 672–675.
14. BULLOCK, J.L., F.M. MASSEY & R.D. GAMBRELL. 1974. Symptomatic endometriosis in teen-agers: a reappraisal. Obstet. Gynecol. **43:** 896.
15. GOLDSTEIN, D.P., C. DECHOLNOKY, S.J. EMANS *et al.* 1980. Laparoscopy on the diagnosis and management of pelvic pain in adolescents. J. Reprod. Med. **24:** 251.
16. HOUSTON, D.E., K.L. NOLLER *et al.* 1987. Incidence of pelvic endometriosis in Rochester, Minnesota, 1970–1979. Am. J. Epidemiol. **125:** 959–969.
17. NATIONAL CENTER FOR HEALTH STATISTICS. 1997. Ambulatory and inpatient procedures in the United States, 1994. Vital Health Stat. **132:** 1–113.
18. DARROW, S.L., J.E. VENA, R.E. BATT *et al.* 1993. Menstrual cycle characteristics and the risk of endometriosis. Epidemiology **4:** 135–142.
19. SIGNORELLO, L.B., B.L. HARLOW, D.W. CRAMER *et al.* 1997. Epidemiologic determinants of endometriosis: a hospital-based case-control study. Ann. Epidemiol. **7:** 267–274.
20. PARAZZINI, F., C. LA VECCHIA, S. FRANESCHI *et al.* 1989. Risk factors for endometrioid, mucinous, and serous benign ovarian cysts. Int. J. Epidemiol. **18:** 108–112.
21. PARAZZINI, F., M. FERRARONI, L. FEDELE *et al.* 1995. Pelvic endometriosis: reproductive and menstrual risk factors at different stages in Lombardy, northern Italy. J. Epidemiol. Community Health **49:** 61–64.

22. MATORRAS, R., F. RODIQUEZ, J.I. PIUOAN *et al.* 1995. Epidemiology of endometriosis in infertile women. Fertil. Steril. **63:** 34–38.
23. MOEN, M.H. & B. SCHEI. 1997. Epidemiology of endometriosis in a Norwegian county. Acta Obstet. Gynecol. Scand. **76:** 559–562.
24. ARUMUGAM, K. & J.M. LIM. 1997. Menstrual characteristics associated with endometriosis. Br. J. Obstet. Gynaecol. **104:** 948–950.
25. DORGAN, J.F., M.E. REICHMAN, J.T. JUDD & C. BROWN. 1995. The relationship of body size to plasma levels of estrogens and androgens in premenopausal women. Cancer Causes Control **6:** 3–8.
26. BAKER, E.R., R.S. MATHUR, R.F. KIRK *et al.* 1981. Female runners and secondary amenorrhea: correlation with age, parity mileage, and plasma hormonal and sex-hormone-binding globulin concentrations. Fertil. Steril. **36:** 183–187.
27. SIMPSON, J.L., S. ELIAS, L.R. MALINAK & V.C. BUTTRAM. 1980. Heritable aspects of endometriosis. I. Genetic studies. Am. J. Obstet. Gynecol. **137:** 327–331.
28. COXHEAD, D. & E.J. THOMAS. 1993. Familial inheritance of endometriosis in a British population: a case control study. J. Obstet. Gynecol. **13:** 42–44.
29. MOEN, M.H. & P. MAGNUS. 1993. The familial risk of endometriosis. Acta Obstet. Gynecol. Scand. **72:** 560–564.
30. MOEN, M.H. 1994. Endometriosis in monozygotic twins. Acta Obstet. Gynecol. Scand. **73:** 59–62.
31. HADFIELD, R.M., H.J. MARDON, D.H. BARLOW & S.H. KENNEDY. 1997. Endometriosis in monozygotic twins. Fertil. Steril. **68:** 941–942.
32. BARANOVA, H., R. BOTHORISHVILLI, M. CANIS *et al.* 1997. Glutathione-S-transferase M1 gene polymorphism and susceptibility to endometriosis in a French population. Mol. Hum. Reprod. **3:** 775–780.
33. SPITSYN, V.A., E.N. ANDREEVA, L.V. ADAMIAN *et al.* 1996. Genetic aspects of endometriosis: features of the distribution of polymorphic gene frequencies. Genetika **32:** 1693–1699.
34. GEORGIOU, I., M. SYRROU, I. BOUBA *et al.* 1999. Association of estrogen receptor gene polymorphisms with endometriosis. Fertil. Steril. **72:** 164–166.
35. CRAMER, D.W., M.D. HORNSTEIN, W.G. NG & R.L. BARBIERI. 1996. Endometriosis associated with the N314D mutation of galactose-1-phosphate uridyl transferase (GALT). Mol. Hum. Reprod. **2:** 149–152.
36. GRODSTEIN, F., M.B. GOLDMAN & D.W. CRAMER. 1994. Infertility in women and moderate alcohol use. Am. J. Public Health **84:** 1429–1432.
37. GRODSTEIN, F., M.B. GOLDMAN, L. RYAN & D.W. CRAMER. 1993. Relation of female and infertility to consumption of caffeinated beverages. Am. J. Epidemiol. **137:** 133–136.
38. BERUBE, S., S. MARCOUX, R. MAHEUX *et al.* 1998. Characteristics related to the prevalence of minimal or mild endometriosis in infertile women. Epidemiology **9:** 504–510.
39. REICHMAN, M.E., J.T. JUDD, C. LONGSCOPE *et al.* 1993. Effects of alcohol consumption on plasma and urinary hormone concentration in premenopausal women. J. Natl. Cancer Inst. **85:** 722–727.
40. VESSEY, M.P., L. VILLARD-MACKINTOSH & R. PAINTER. 1993. Epidemiology of endometriosis in women attending family planning clinics. Br. Med. J. **306:** 182–184.
41. RIER, S.E., D.C. MARTIN, R.E. BOWMAN *et al.* 1993. Endometriosis in rhesus monkeys (*Macaca mulatta*) following chronic exposure to 2,3,7,8-tetrachlorodibenzo-*p*-dioxin. Fundam. Appl. Toxicol. **21:** 433–441.
42. MAYANI, A., S. BAREL, S. SOBACK & M. ALMAGOR. 1997. Dioxin concentrations in women with endometriosis. Hum. Reprod. **12:** 373–375.
43. LEBEL, G., S. DODIN & E. DEWAILLY. 1998. Organochlorine exposure and the risk of endometriosis. Fertil. Steril. **69:** 221–228.
44. SCHULMAN, H., R. DUVIVERR & M.S. BLATTNER. 1983. The uterine contractility index: a research and diagnostic tool in dysmenorrhea. Am. J. Obstet. Gynecol. **45:** 1049–1058.
45. OLIVE, D.L. & C.B. HAMMOND. 1985. Endometriosis: pathogenesis and mechanisms of infertility. Postgrad. Obstet. Gynecol. **5:** 1.
46. TRELOAR, A.D., R.E. BOYNTON, B.G. BENN *et al.* 1967. Variation of the human menstrual cycle through reproductive life. Int. J. Fertil. **12:** 77–126.

47. Block, E. 1952. Quantitative morphological investigations of the follicular system in women: variations at different ages. Acta Anat. **14:** 108–123.
48. Cramer, D.W. & H. Xu. 1996. Predicting age at menopause. Maturitas **23:** 319–326.
49. Cramer, D.W., V.A. Ravnikar, M. Craighill *et al.* 1987. Müllerian aplasia associated with maternal deficiency of galactose-1-phosphate uridyl transferase. Fertil. Steril. **47:** 930–934.
50. Gardo, S., Z. Papp & J. Gaal. 1971. XO-XX mosaicism in the Rokitansky-Küster-Hauser syndrome. Lancet **2:** 1380–1381.
51. Murphy, E.D. & E.S. Russell. 1963. Ovarian tumorigenesis following genic deletion of germ cells in hybrid mice. Acta Unio Int. Cancer **19:** 779–782.
52. Chen, V.T., D.R. Mattison, L. Feienbaum *et al.* 1981. Reduction in oocyte number following prenatal exposure to a diet high in galactose. Science **214:** 1145–1147.
53. Cramer, D.W., D.P. Goldstein, C. Fraer & J.K.V. Reichardt. 1996. Vaginal agenesis (Mayer-Rokitansky-Küster-Hauser syndrome) associated with the N314D mutation of galactose-1-phosphate uridyl transferase (GALT). Mol. Hum. Reprod. **2:** 144–148.

Endometriosis and Infertility

A Cause-Effect Relationship?

ROBERT L. BARBIERI AND STACEY MISSMER

Department of Obstetrics, Gynecology, and Reproductive Biology, Brigham and Women's Hospital, Harvard Medical School, and Department of Epidemiology, Harvard School of Public Health, Boston, Massachusetts, USA

ABSTRACT: Two major methodological problems that impact clinical research in endometriosis are the absence of a low-cost, highly reliable method for diagnosing endometriosis and the possibility that endometriosis is actually multiple different diseases that we have not yet been able to differentiate. Animal models of endometriosis clearly demonstrate that advanced endometriosis causes reduced fertility. In humans, endometriosis and infertility are commonly associated. However, few data from high-quality clinical trials demonstrate that endometriosis causes infertility in humans. Future research should focus on the implications of the observation that, in ovarian endometriosis cysts, the epithelium is monoclonal. This observation suggests that nonrandom somatic mutations cause ovarian endometriosis cysts. If somatic mutations cause ovarian endometriosis cysts, it is likely that a small number of genes can be identified that play a central role in pathogenesis of this disease.

KEYWORDS: endometriosis; infertility; CA-125; hMG-IUI; cervical stenosis; lateral cervical displacement

INTRODUCTION

Endometriosis is the presence of endometrial glands and/or stroma outside of the uterus. Many women with endometriosis are asymptomatic. Women with endometriosis and symptoms typically present for clinical care because of pelvic pain, infertility, and/or an endometrioma (an ovarian endometriosis cyst). Numerous studies report that endometriosis can cause pelvic pain and that effective treatment of endometriosis decreases pelvic pain. These studies indicate that there is a cause-effect relationship between pelvic pain and endometriosis for some women. Many studies suggest that endometriosis is associated with infertility. However, the scientific evidence that links endometriosis and infertility in a cause-effect relationship is weak. Issues that will be reviewed in this paper include discussions of (1) the "gold" standard for the diagnosis of endometriosis, (2) methodological problems in the study of endometriosis, (3) animal models that report a cause-effect relationship between endometriosis and reduced fertility, and (4) human studies that investigate the possible cause-effect relationship between endometriosis and infertility.

Address for correspondence: Robert L. Barbieri, Department of Obstetrics, Gynecology, and Reproductive Biology, Brigham and Women's Hospital, Harvard Medical School, Boston, MA 02115. Voice: 617-732-4265; fax: 617-277-1440.
rbarbieri@partners.org

THE DIAGNOSIS OF ENDOMETRIOSIS: SEARCH FOR A GOLD STANDARD

Endometriosis is defined as the presence of endometrial glands and stroma outside the uterus.[1] From a theoretical perspective, the diagnosis of endometriosis can be made by four approaches: (1) clinical diagnosis based on history, physical examination, and noninvasive laboratory tests,[2] (2) surgical visualization of endometriosis lesions,[3] (3) surgical biopsy of suspected endometriosis lesions with histological confirmation, and (4) use of biochemical markers, such as serum CA-125.[4] Each approach to the diagnosis of endometriosis has advantages and disadvantages.

Clinical suspicion of endometriosis may arise when a patient presents with symptoms such as dysmenorrhea, noncyclic abdominal pain, dyspareunia, pain on defecation, premenstrual spotting, and/or infertility. Physical examination findings suggestive of endometriosis include cul-de-sac tenderness and nodularity,[5] uterosacral thickening, presence of a fixed adnexal mass, cervical stenosis,[6] and lateral displacement of the cervix.[7] A response of symptoms to treatment with gonadotropin-releasing hormone agonists supports the clinical diagnosis of endometriosis. Diagnosis based on the preceding findings offers the clinician a noninvasive, nonsurgical method of diagnosing endometriosis and identifies most cases of the disease in a clinical population of women with severe pelvic pain and a high prevalence of endometriosis. One study demonstrated that the clinical diagnosis of endometriosis had a specificity of 87% when surgical visualization of lesions and adhesions was used as the gold standard.[2] A limitation to the clinical diagnosis of endometriosis is that many other diseases, such as chronic pelvic inflammatory disease, adenomyosis, and ovarian pathology, can present with similar clinical findings. Surgical visualization helps to avoid misdiagnosis and ensures that serious pelvic pathological processes, such as ovarian cancer, that can mimic the presentation of endometriosis will not be missed.

Currently, most authorities contend that the gold standard for the diagnosis of endometriosis is the surgical visualization of endometriosis lesions[8,9] and that surgical biopsy with histopathologic confirmation is not necessary. A major disadvantage of this approach is that it requires an expensive surgical procedure to make the diagnosis of endometriosis. Another disadvantage of surgical visualization for the diagnosis of endometriosis is that the accuracy of the method is dependent on the skill and experience of the surgeon. One study of intersurgeon variability in the diagnosis of endometriosis reported that the rate of pathological confirmation of visually diagnosed endometriosis was 42%, 65%, and 76% for three different surgeons.[3] Studies of inter- and intrasurgeon variability in the diagnosis of endometriosis report low reproducibility and a kappa coefficient in the range of 0.28.[10] These findings suggest that, in clinical practice, the diagnosis of endometriosis with surgical visualization is associated with a high degree of variability. In addition to inter- and intrasurgeon variability, the diagnosis of endometriosis through surgical visualization of endometriosis lesions may be impaired by the location and volume of endometriosis lesions. Subperitoneal and deeply invasive lesions in the cul-de-sac of Douglas may be difficult to detect with standard laparoscopy procedures. Small lesions and lesions with atypical presentations may also be difficult to detect. Nevertheless, surgical visualization is currently the gold standard for the diagnosis of endometriosis.

Biopsy and histological diagnosis may be a superior surgical method to reliably diagnose endometriosis. The criteria for histological diagnosis of endometriosis include the presence of one of the following components: (1) both endometrial glands and stroma, (2) glandular epithelium with hemosiderin, or (3) endometrial stroma-like tissue with hemosiderin. One weakness of using surgical biopsy and histological diagnosis for diagnosing endometriosis is that diagnostic criteria vary among pathologists[11–13] and no study has demonstrated high interobserver reproducibility in the histological diagnosis of this disorder.

In 1986, we reported that CA-125 was elevated in the serum of women with stage III and IV endometriosis (FIG. 1).[4] This was the first report of a possible "blood test" for the diagnosis of endometriosis. Many investigators have subsequently replicated this finding.[14–16] In our study, preoperative CA-125 levels were measured in 147 women undergoing diagnostic laparoscopy or laparotomy. Serum CA-125 levels were elevated in women with stage III or IV endometriosis compared to control women with normal surgical laparoscopy results [66.5 (14.5) vs. 8.2 (0.6) U/mL, mean (SEM), $p < 0.001$]. Fifty-four percent of women with stage III or IV endometriosis and 0% of the control women had serum CA-125 measurements > 35 U/mL. Some women with stage II endometriosis (13%), uterine leiomyomata (14%), and chronic pelvic inflammatory disease (5%) also had serum CA-125 measurements > 35 U/mL. This study also demonstrated that endometriosis lesions overexpressed CA-125 using immunocytochemistry techniques. Other biochemical markers have been hypothesized to be helpful in the diagnosis of endometriosis, including (1) endometrial integrin levels, (2) antiendometrial autoantibodies, and (3) eutopic endometrial expression of P450-CYP19 (aromatase).[17]

METHODOLOGICAL PROBLEMS: DISEASE ASCERTAINMENT AND HETEROGENEITY

Valid ascertainment of endometriosis may be difficult, both in case-control studies and in population-based studies. Diseases that are diagnosed by expensive and invasive procedures may be subject to significant underascertainment of cases.[18] This problem is especially significant in population-based studies of endometriosis in which an important validity issue is the complete identification of all subjects with the disease. If only the subset of women with the disease who are symptomatic, have adequate access to health care, and seek treatment undergo the requisite surgical diagnostic procedure, then it is likely that some women in the control group will have undiagnosed disease.

A major concern in research involving endometriosis is the possibility that the disease as we currently define it actually represents a constellation of many unique diseases that we cannot currently differentiate. Many diseases that are initially thought to be a single homogenous disorder are eventually proven to be multiple unique diseases, each with a unique molecular pathophysiology. For example, advances in our understanding of hypertension have revealed many unique molecular causes of hypertension (primary aldosteronism, renal artery stenosis, glucocorticoid remediable hyperaldosteronism, Liddle syndrome, and others) and the role of the environment (salt intake, body mass index, alcohol, stress) in influencing the phenotype. These research discoveries have greatly advanced our ability to understand, diagnose, and treat hypertension. It is likely that endometriosis is not a single unique disorder, but represents a constellation of many diseases.

A number of authorities have proposed that endometriosis is actually two or more distinct diseases with unique pathogenesis. The best molecular evidence for unique pathogenesis of different forms of endometriosis is the observation that ovarian endometriosis cysts are typically *monoclonal*, whereas superficial peritoneal implants of endometriosis appear to be *polyclonal*. Using the human androgen receptor gene (HUMARA) as an X-linked polymorphic marker, Jimbo and colleagues[19] examined the clonal status of epithelial cells in endometrial cysts. In 11 ovarian endometriosis cysts, the investigators observed that all were monoclonal in the methylation pattern of the HUMARA alleles. Similar observations have been reported by other investigators.[20,21] These observations indicate that ovarian endometriosis cysts are monoclonal and probably arise from a somatic mutation.

Since ovarian endometriosis cysts are monoclonal tumors, it is likely that a somatic mutation in a progenitor cell is a primary initiating event in the pathophysiology of these lesions. If a somatic mutation is the initiating step, it is likely that the mutations affect a small number of genes (nonrandom mutations) and that these genes can be identified using modern molecular biology techniques.

ANIMAL MODELS OF ENDOMETRIOSIS AND REDUCED FERTILITY

Laboratory results from studies in rabbits, rats, and monkeys indicate that experimentally induced, "advanced-stage" (American Society of Reproductive Medicine stage III and IV disease) endometriosis causes a decrease in fecundability. These studies have been reviewed in a previous publication.[22] In laboratory animals, endometriosis is surgically induced by suturing small squares of endometrium on pelvic peritoneal surfaces and bowel mesentery. In experiments in rabbits, Schenken and Asch[23] removed the right uterine horn from New Zealand white rabbits and sutured 25-mm^2 endometrial squares onto pelvic peritoneal surfaces. Control animals had adipose tissue sutured onto their peritoneal surfaces. Twenty-five days after the initial surgery, a staging procedure was performed. In the group that received the endometrial implants, the majority of animals were observed to have significant adhesions from bowel and pelvic organs to the implants. Only 13% of the animals in the control group developed major pelvic adhesions. Fourteen days after the surgical staging procedure, the animals received a dose of chorionic gonadotropin and were inseminated with sperm from bucks with proven fertility. In the control group, 75% of the animals became pregnant. In the experimental group, only 25% of the animals became pregnant. Hahn and colleagues[24] have reported similar results.

Schenken and colleagues[25] studied the effects of experimentally induced endometriosis on fertility in monkeys. Animals with surgically induced endometriosis and control animals with adipose tissue autografts were mated. In control animals and animals with minimal endometriosis, the pregnancy rate per cycle was 42% and 35%, respectively. In the animals with advanced endometriosis, the cycle pregnancy rate was reduced to 12%. The presence of ovarian adhesions was associated with a 0% pregnancy rate. These studies support the hypothesis that advanced endometriosis is associated with a reduction in fecundability in laboratory animals. The major pelvic adhesions associated with advanced endometriosis may contribute to reduced fecundability by impairing egg release from the ovary, blocking sperm entry into the peritoneal cavity, and inhibiting tubal pickup of the oocyte.

ENDOMETRIOSIS AND INFERTILITY IN HUMANS

The hypothesis that endometriosis causes a decrease in fecundability in women has not been definitively proven by consistent data from studies with a rigorous scientific design. Many possible mechanisms may explain an association between endometriosis and infertility in women. For women with advanced-stage endometriosis (stage III and IV), adhesions may impair proper egg release from the ovary and inhibit tubal pickup of the oocyte. Women with early-stage endometriosis (stage I and II) often have reduced fecundability, but it is not clear if the endometriosis is causally linked to the infertility. For women with endometriosis, especially those with early-stage disease, functional abnormalities in peritoneal, tubal, and endometrial function may inhibit fertility. These factors have been reviewed in a previous publication.[26] Numerous investigators have reported that women with endometriosis have an increased volume of peritoneal fluid,[27] increased peritoneal concentration of activated macrophages,[28] and increased peritoneal fluid concentration of prostaglandin, interleukin-1, tumor necrosis factor, and proteases.[29] Peritoneal fluid from women with advanced endometriosis appears to inhibit sperm function, thereby possibly reducing fertility.[30] These functional alterations in the peritoneal environment may impair gamete, embryo, fallopian tube function.

A few investigators have reported that antiendometrial antibodies are increased in women with endometriosis and that these antibodies may impair endometrial function.[31,32] Some women with early-stage endometriosis have luteal phase dysfunction,[33] abnormal follicle growth,[34] multiple premature LH surges,[35] and luteinized unruptured follicle syndrome.

A recently evolving concept is that eutopic endometrium may be abnormal in women with endometriosis. This suggests that a Müllerian tract "field defect" may be present in women with endometriosis. Lessey and colleagues[36] reported that the endometrial expression of β_3 integrin is significantly suppressed in women with stage I and II endometriosis. It is possible that a decrease in β_3 integrin expression is associated with an impaired interaction of the embryo with the endometrium. McBean and Brumsted reported that, in women with endometriosis, the eutopic endometrium abnormally expresses the Müllerian antigen, CA-125.[37] These investigators obtained endometrial biopsies in the luteal phase of the menstrual cycle from women with advanced endometriosis and women with surgically documented normal anatomy. The eutopic endometrial tissue was cultured and the spent media was assayed for CA-125. The eutopic endometrial tissue from women with advanced endometriosis demonstrated two to four times more CA-125 secretion than endometrial tissue from women with a normal pelvis. This study demonstrates that CA-125 expression may be altered in the eutopic endometrium of women with advanced endometriosis. These findings are supported by the *in vivo* observation that CA-125 concentrations are elevated in the menstrual discharge of women with endometriosis.[38]

Many therapeutic interventions have been proposed to increase fecundability in women with endometriosis. In this chapter, only prospective, randomized, controlled trials will be reviewed. Interventions that have been proposed to increase fecundabil-

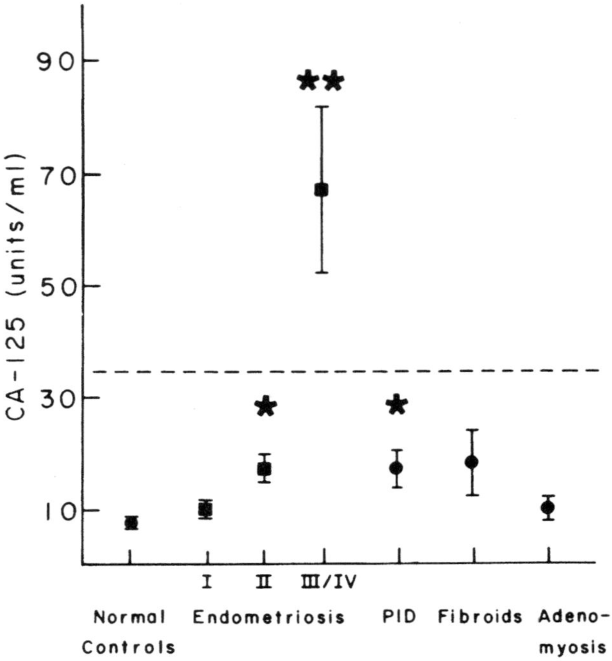

FIGURE 1. CA-125 concentrations in 146 women undergoing diagnostic laparoscopy or laparotomy. Mean (SEM). $*p < 0.05$, $**p < 0.001$, compared with controls. Normal control women had a surgically documented normal pelvis. Reprinted by permission from the American Society for Reproductive Medicine (1986. *Fertil. Steril.* **45:** 630-634).[4]

ity in women with endometriosis include (1) hormone suppression of ovarian function to suppress the activity of the endometriosis implants with drugs such as leuprolide, buserelin, and danazol, (2) surgical treatment of endometriosis lesions and adhesions, (3) empirical ovarian hyperstimulation (with clomiphene or gonadotropins, with or without intrauterine insemination), and (4) assisted reproductive technologies.

Most clinical trials report that hormone therapy of endometriosis lesions does not improve fecundability in infertile women with endometriosis.[39] In one representative study, women with stage I or II endometriosis were randomized to receive hormone treatment with the GnRH agonist analogue, buserelin, for 6 months or to a no-treatment group. Median follow-up was approximately 18 months in both groups.[40] The 1-year actuarial pregnancy rate was 30% in the women treated with buserelin and 37% in the control women. The 2-year actuarial pregnancy rate was 61% in the buserelin group and 60% in the control group. Using the 2-year actuarial pregnancy rates to calculate fecundability, both groups had a pregnancy rate per cycle of 4%. The available data suggest[41] that, in women with early-stage endometriosis and infertility, hormone therapy of endometriosis lesions does not improve fecundability.

A number of observational studies suggest that advanced endometriosis is more commonly associated with infertility than early-stage endometriosis.[42] In addition, a number of observational studies suggest that surgical treatment can improve fertility in women with advanced endometriosis.[43]

The effect of surgical treatment of endometriosis lesions on fecundability in women with infertility and early-stage endometriosis is controversial. Marcoux and colleagues[44] reported that surgical treatment (electrosurgical ablation or excision) of stage I and II endometriosis improves fecundability in infertile women. The investigators randomized 341 women with stage I or II endometriosis to a diagnostic laparoscopy only or to a diagnostic laparoscopy combined with surgical resection and/or ablation of endometriosis lesions. During 36 weeks of postoperative follow-up, the fecundability was 2.4% per cycle in the diagnostic laparoscopy group and 4.7% per cycle in the surgical resection/ablation of endometriosis lesions group ($p < 0.006$). The cumulative pregnancy rate was 18% in the diagnostic laparoscopy group and 31% in the surgical resection/ablation of endometriosis lesions group. This report suggests that surgical treatment of early-stage endometriosis improves fertility. However, another small-scale prospective controlled trial was unable to confirm these findings.[45]

Multiple studies suggest that, in women with endometriosis, empirical ovarian stimulation increases fecundability. Fedele and colleagues[46] randomized 40 women with stage I or II endometriosis to three cycles of hMG ovarian stimulation plus intrauterine insemination (IUI) or no treatment. The pregnancy rate per cycle was 4.5% in the no-treatment group. The pregnancy rate per cycle was 15% in the group that received hMG-IUI ($p < 0.05$), suggesting that fecundability can be increased in women with infertility and early-stage endometriosis using ovarian stimulation. Similar results were observed in a large-scale trial sponsored by the National Institute of Child Health and Human Development[47] and other randomized studies.[48] An unfortunate consequence of this treatment approach is a relatively high rate of twin and triplet pregnancy. IVF-ET may be a better treatment method because it allows for a theoretically greater degree of control over the rate of twin and triplet pregnancy.

In one small randomized study of the impact of IVF-ET on infertility in women with endometriosis, 20 women with endometriosis were randomized to undergo IVF-ET or expectant management.[49] None of the women in the expectant management group became pregnant. Five of the 15 women in the IVF-ET treatment group became pregnant (not statistically significant). Because of the small sample size, this study did not have the statistical power to detect clinically relevant differences in pregnancy rate between the two groups. Although high-quality clinical trials do not definitively demonstrate that endometriosis causes infertility, clinicians are regularly challenged to provide therapy for women with both infertility and endometriosis. Empirical treatment strategies for approaching women with infertility and endometriosis are presented in TABLES 1 and 2. These tables provide guidelines for the treatment of women with infertility and early-stage or advanced-stage endometriosis.

FUTURE RESEARCH DIRECTIONS

Three important long-term research goals are to (1) understand the molecular pathogenesis of the monoclonal ovarian endometriosis lesions of the ovary, (2) under-

TABLE 1. Treatment of infertility in women with early-stage endometriosis

- Step 1: Identify and treat all reversible causes of infertility in the couple. Determine if a male factor is contributing to the infertility.
- Step 2: If the woman is younger than 32 years, consider expectant management or timed intercourse by monitoring of urine LH or use of basal body temperature charts. If the woman is older than 32 years, consider expectant management, timed intercourse, or immediate progression to Step 3.
- Step 3: Consider empirical treatment with clomiphene with or without intrauterine insemination.
- Step 4: Consider empirical treatment with gonadotropins with or without intrauterine insemination.
- Step 5: Consider *in vitro* fertilization–embryo transfer or gamete intrafallopian tube transfer.

TABLE 2. Treatment of infertility in women with advanced endometriosis

- Step 1: Identify and treat all reversible causes of infertility.
- Step 2: If an endometrioma is diagnosed, consider surgical resection.
- Step 3: If major pelvic adhesions are present and the patient has had no previous fertility surgery, consider a conservative surgical procedure to resect adhesions and endometriosis implants and to restore pelvic anatomy to normal.
- Step 4: Consider empirical clomiphene treatment with or without intrauterine insemination.
- Step 5: Consider empirical gonadotropin treatment with or without intrauterine insemination.
- Step 6: Consider *in vitro* fertilization–embryo transfer.

stand more clearly the potential variations in the pathophysiology of endometriosis-varying pathologies that may be associated with varying risk factor profiles, and (3) develop nonsurgical methods of diagnosing endometriosis. Discovery of the molecular pathogenesis of endometriosis will help focus our future research and treatment efforts. Development of nonsurgical methods of diagnosing endometriosis will help us execute valid prospective population-based studies to understand the impact of endometriosis on fertility and quality of life.

The discovery that ovarian endometriosis cysts are monoclonal provides a clear path for future research into the molecular pathogenesis of ovarian endometriosis cysts. It is likely that the following research efforts need to be supported: (1) utilize high-resolution karyotyping of ovarian endometriosis cyst epithelium (obtained by laser dissection of small groups of cells) to identify nonrandom genetic rearrangements, (2) determine if peritoneal endometriosis lesions are monoclonal or polyclonal, (3) identify the genes involved in the somatic mutations in ovarian endometriosis epithelium, (4) perform transcript profiling between ovarian endometriosis, peritoneal endometriosis, and eutopic endometrium at different stages of the menstrual cycle, (5) develop cell lines from ovarian endometriosis epithelium for gene expression and protein synthesis experiments, and (6) identify genes based on the above projects to develop animal models of endometriosis. In preliminary investigations, nonrandom chromosomal loss and additions have already been reported in endometriosis lesions.[50]

The development of nonsurgical methods of diagnosing endometriosis is likely to be challenging. To date, no nonsurgical method of diagnosing endometriosis has achieved the sensitivity and specificity necessary to achieve Food and Drug Administration approval of a diagnostic test. In most cases, the sensitivity and specificity of the tests developed are in the range of 0.6 and 0.9, respectively, for the diagnosis of advanced disease. The sensitivity and specificity of the tests developed to date tend to be lower for the diagnosis of early-stage disease. In many cases of endometriosis, the total tissue mass of diseased tissue is less than 100 mg. The experience from cancer detection research is that it is difficult to develop successful tests to detect cancer if the mass of disease is less than 100 mg of diseased tissue.

Endometriosis is a ubiquitous and enigmatic disease process. In the postgenome era, molecular tools are now available to truly understand the initiating factors for this disease. Advances in our understanding of the pathophysiology of endometriosis will guide our future diagnostic and treatment efforts.

REFERENCES

1. Hornstein, M.D. & R.L. Barbieri. 1999. Endometriosis. *In* Kistner's Gynecology and Women's Health, pp. 492–518. Mosby. St. Louis.
2. Ling, F.W. 1999. Randomized controlled trial of depot leuprolide in patients with chronic pelvic pain and clinically suspected endometriosis. Obstet. Gynecol. **93:** 51–58.
3. Pardanani, S. & R.L. Barbieri. 1998. The gold standard for the surgical diagnosis of endometriosis: visual findings or biopsy results. J. Gynecol. Tech. **4:** 121–124.
4. Barbieri, R.L., J.M. Niloff, R.C. Bast *et al.* 1986. Elevated serum concentrations of CA-125 in patients with advanced endometriosis. Fertil. Steril. **45:** 630–634.
5. Barbieri, R.L. & A.M. Propst. 1999. Physical examination findings in endometriosis: uterosacral ligament abnormalities, lateral cervical displacement, and cervical stenosis. J. Gynecol. Tech. **5:** 157–159.
6. Barbieri, R.L. 1998. Stenosis of the external cervical os: an association with endometriosis in women with chronic pelvic pain. Fertil. Steril. **70:** 571–573.
7. Propst, A.M., K. Storti & R.L. Barbieri. 1998. Lateral cervical displacement: an association with endometriosis. Fertil. Steril. **70:** 568–569.
8. Martin, D.C., G.D. Hubert, R.V. Zwaag & W.M. Poston. 1993. Subtle appearances of peritoneal endometriosis. Fertil. Steril. **59:** 759–765.
9. Ueki, M., M. Seki, T. Tsurunaga *et al.* 1995. Visual findings and histological diagnosis of pelvic endometriosis under laparoscopy and laparotomy. Int. J. Fertil. **40:** 248–253.
10. Hornstein, M.D., A.J. Friedman, R.E. Gleason *et al.* 1993. The reproducibility of the revised American Fertility Society classification of endometriosis. Fertil. Steril. **59:** 1015–1021.
11. Jansen, R.P.S. & P. Russell. 1986. Non-pigmented endometriosis: clinical, laparoscopic, and pathologic definitions. Am. J. Obstet. Gynecol. **155:** 1154–1159.
12. Blaustein, A. 1982. Pelvic endometriosis. *In* Blaustein's Pathology of the Genital Tract. Second edition, pp. 464–478. Springer-Verlag. New York/Berlin.
13. Olive, D.L. & K.M. Silverberg. 1993. Endometriosis and adenomyosis. *In* Textbook of Gynecology, pp. 481–504. Saunders. Philadelphia.
14. Hornstein, M.D., P.P. Thomas, R.E. Gleason & R.L. Barbieri. 1992. Menstrual cyclicity of CA-125 in patients with endometriosis. Fertil. Steril. **58:** 279–283.
15. Giudice, L.C., A. Jacobs, J. Pineda *et al.* 1986. Serum levels of CA-125 in patients with endometriosis: a preliminary report. Fertil. Steril. **45:** 876–878.
16. Pittaway, D.E. & J.A. Fayez. 1986. The use of CA-125 in the diagnosis and management of endometriosis. Fertil. Steril. **46:** 790–795.

17. KITAWAKI, J., I. KUSUKI, H. KOSHIBA *et al.* 1999. Expression of aromatase cytochrome P450 in eutopic endometrium. Gynecol. Obstet. Invest. **48:** 21–28.
18. HOLT, V.L. & N.S. WEISS. 2000. Recommendations for the design of epidemiologic studies of endometriosis. Epidemiology **11:** 654–659.
19. JIMBO, J., Y. HITAMI, H. YOSHIKAA *et al.* 1997. Evidence for monoclonal expansion of epithelial cells in ovarian endometrial cysts. Am. J. Pathol. **150:** 1173–1178.
20. FUJIMOTO, J., R. HIROSE, H. SAKAGUCHI & T. TAMAYA. 1999. Expression of size-polymorphic androgen receptor gene in ovarian endometriosis. Steroids **64:** 526–529.
21. TAMURA, M., T. FUYAKA, T. MURAKAMI *et al.* 1998. Analysis of clonality in human endometriotic cysts based on evaluation of X-chromosome inactivation in archival formalin-fixed paraffin-embedded tissue. Lab. Invest. **78:** 213–218.
22. BARBIERI, R.L. 1999. Infertility. *In* Reproductive Endocrinology: Physiology, Pathophysiology, and Management. Fourth edition, pp. 562–593. Saunders. Philadelphia.
23. SCHENKEN, R.S. & R.H. ASCH. 1980. Surgical induction of endometriosis in the rabbit; effect on fertility and concentration of peritoneal fluid prostaglandins. Fertil. Steril. **34:** 581–587.
24. HAHN, D.W., R. CARRAHER & R. FOLDSEY. 1984. Studies on the mechanism of infertility associated with endometriosis and the effect of LHRH agonist in an animal model of endometriosis. *In* LHRH and Its Analogues, p. 203. Elsevier. Amsterdam/New York.
25. SCHENKEN, R.S., R.H. ASCH, R.F. WILLIAMS & G.D. HODGEN. 1984. Etiology of infertility in monkeys with endometriosis: luteinized unruptured follicles, luteal phase defects, pelvic adhesions, and spontaneous abortions. Fertil. Steril. **41:** 122–130.
26. BARBIERI, R.L. 1996. Infertility aspects of endometriosis. *In* Gynecology and Obstetrics, pp. 1–18. Lippincott–Raven. Philadelphia/New York.
27. HANEY, A.F., J.J. MUSCATO & J.B. WEINBERG. 1981. Peritoneal fluid cell populations in infertility patients. Fertil. Steril. **35:** 696–698.
28. HALME, J., S. BECKER & S. HASKILL. 1987. Altered maturation and function of peritoneal macrophages: possible role in the pathogenesis of endometriosis. Am. J. Obstet. Gynecol. **156:** 783–789.
29. FAKIH, H., B. BAGGETT & G. HOLTZ. 1987. Interleukin-1: a possible role in the infertility associated with endometriosis. Fertil. Steril. **47:** 213–218.
30. ORAL, E., A. ARICI, D.L. OLIVE & G. HUSZAR. 1996. Peritoneal fluid from women with moderate or severe endometriosis inhibits sperm motility: the role of seminal fluid components. Fertil. Steril. **66:** 787–792.
31. BADAWY, S.Z., V. CUENCA & A. STITZEL. 1984. Autoimmune phenomena in infertile patients with endometriosis. Obstet. Gynecol. **63:** 271–276.
32. WEED, J.C. & P.C. AQUEMBOURG. 1980. Endometriosis: can it produce an autoimmune response resulting in infertility. Clin. Obstet. Gynecol. **23:** 885–891.
33. CHEESMAN, K.L., S.D. CHEESMAN & R.T. CHATTERTON. 1978. Alterations in progesterone metabolism and luteal function in infertile women with endometriosis. Fertil. Steril. **29:** 270–275.
34. WARDLE, P.G., E.A. MCLAUGHLIN & A. MCDERMOTT. 1985. Endometriosis and ovulatory disorder: reduced fertilization *in vitro* compared with tubal and unexplained infertility. Lancet **2:** 236–242.
35. POLAN, M.L., M. TOTORA, B.V. CALDWELL *et al.* 1982. Abnormal ovarian cycles as diagnosed by ultrasound and serum estradiol levels. Fertil. Steril. **37:** 342–347.
36. LESSEY, B.A., A.J. CASTLEBAUM, S.W. SAWIN *et al.* 1994. Aberrant integrin expression in the endometrium of women with endometriosis. J. Clin. Endocrinol. Metab. **79:** 643.
37. MCBEAN, J.H. & J.R. BRUMSTED. 1993. *In vitro* CA-125 secretion from women with advanced endometriosis. Fertil. Steril. **59:** 89.
38. TAKAHASHI, K., H. NAGATA, A.A. MUSA *et al.* 1990. Clinical usefulness of CA-125 levels in the menstrual discharge of women with endometriosis. Fertil. Steril. **54:** 360.
39. HUGHES, E.G., D.M. FEDEROKOW & J.A. COLLINS. 1993. A quantitative overview of controlled trials in endometriosis-associated infertility. Fertil. Steril. **59:** 963–970.
40. FEDELE, L., F. PARAZZINI & E. RADICI. 1992. Buserelin acetate versus expectant management in the treatment of infertility associated with minimal or mild endometriosis. Am. J. Obstet. Gynecol. **166:** 1345–1350.

41. BARBIERI, R.L. 1996. Medical treatment of infertility associated with minimal to mild endometriosis. Int. J. Fertil. **41:** 276–278.
42. THORNTON, J.G., S. MORLEY, J. LILLEYMAN *et al.* 1997. The relationship between laparoscopic disease, pelvic pain, and infertility: an unbiased assessment. Eur. J. Obstet. Gynecol. **74:** 57–62.
43. ADAMSON, G.D. & D.J. PASTA. 1994. Surgical treatment of endometriosis associated infertility: meta-analysis compared with survival analysis. Am. J. Obstet. Gynecol. **171:** 1404–1405.
44. MARCOUX, S., R. MAHEUX & S. BERUBE. 1997. The Canadian Collaborative Group on Endometriosis: laparoscopic surgery in infertile women with minimal or mild endometriosis. N. Engl. J. Med. **337:** 217–222.
45. PARAZZINI, F. 1999. Ablation of lesions or no treatment in minimal-mild endometriosis in infertile women: a randomized trial. Hum. Reprod. **14:** 1332–1334.
46. FEDELE, L., S. BIANCHI, M. MARCHINI *et al.* 1992. Superovulation with human menopausal gonadotropins in the treatment of infertility associated with minimal or mild endometriosis. Fertil. Steril. **58:** 28–31.
47. GUZICK, D.S., S.A. CARSON, C. COUTIFARIS *et al.* 1999. Efficacy of superovulation and intrauterine insemination in the treatment of infertility. N. Engl. J. Med. **340:** 177–183.
48. TUMMON, I.S., L.J. ASHER, J.S. MARTIN & T. TULANDI. 1997. Randomized controlled trial of superovulation and insemination for infertility associated with minimal or mild endometriosis. Fertil. Steril. **68:** 8–12.
49. SOLIMAN, S., S. DAYA & J. COLLINS. 1993. A randomized trial of *in vitro* fertilization versus conventional treatment of infertility. Fertil. Steril. **59:** 1239–1245.
50. GOGUSEV, J., J. BOUGQUET DE JOLINIERE, L. TELVI *et al.* 1999. Detection of DNA copy number changes in human endometriosis by comparative genomic hybridization. Hum. Genet. **105:** 444–451.

Panel Discussion (Part I)

L.C. GIUDICE (*Stanford University, Stanford, CA*): Dr. Cramer, is there any epidemiologic evidence for premature menopause or an earlier age of menopause, or an earlier age for decreased ovarian reserve, in women with endometriosis?

D.W. CRAMER (*Brigham and Women's Hospital, Boston, MA*): I am aware of no data that would suggest this connection other than the fact that women with endometriosis appear to have fertility problems out of proportion to the severity of their disease. An epidemiologic study addressing a possible connection between early menopause and endometriosis would be very important, but complicated by the hormonal and surgical therapy that patients receive.

J.L. SIMPSON (*Baylor College of Medicine, Houston, TX*): My question concerns your statement about tall women—there being a correlation with endometriosis. Have you decided whether or not that is distinct from ethnic distributions?

CRAMER: In our original study describing this association, most of our cases and controls were white, so we did not adjust for race; however, it would be important to see whether this association holds in other ethnic groups. A biological explanation perhaps worth pursuing is whether an estrogen receptor polymorphism reported to influence height could also influence risk for endometriosis.

SIMPSON: Dr. Barbieri, I like (as you might gather) the hypothesis that endometriosis is monoclonal and genetic, but I am puzzled as to why you believe that you would need to hypothesize that the peritoneal implants are polyclonal. For example, by analogy with myomas where there are multiple myomas, all of which are still monoclonal, I would have hypothesized that they are all monoclonal, but it is just a different initiating mutation in the peritoneal versus ovarian lesions.

R.L. BARBIERI (*Harvard Medical School, Boston, MA*): I made that hypothesis to try to stimulate discussion in part. I would like to explore this with you, but I think that there would be more evidence that these are heterogeneous processes, different diseases. If we could show that the deep endometriosis lesions of the ovary are monoclonal and if we definitively demonstrated that all of the superficial peritoneal lesions are polyclonal, we would have different molecular pathways to get to different phenotypes. Superficial, always polyclonal; deep ovarian, always monoclonal. I would think that would suggest that there are different pathways for those two disease processes.

SIMPSON: Just as a follow-up, I think there could be different diseases, but are they going to all be monoclonal of the different diseases?

BARBIERI: Yes, an alternative is that they are different diseases and they are all monoclonal, but I think people have been unable to definitively demonstrate that potential lesions are monoclonal. People have tried pretty hard, in some initial attempts, to demonstrate that the superficial peritoneal lesions are monoclonal and have not been able to do it. Now, it is a challenging technical issue, probably needing something like laser microdissection of small nests of cells, but to date I think that the people who have tried it have come up with the fact that the superficial peritoneal lesions are polyclonal.

S. PARTHASARATHY (*Emory University, Atlanta, GA*): We recently made a very interesting observation that women with coronary artery disease in the later years had about four times the incidence of endometriosis during their younger years.

Would treatment to lower estrogen levels in the younger years for endometriosis have greater consequences when these women became older? Is there any epidemiological basis for that?

BARBIERI: I think some individuals at this conference are going to talk about manipulating estrogen levels and looking at the impact on disease, but I am not sure I have a specific answer.

PARTHASARATHY: Epidemiologically, is there any evidence to suggest that those who are deprived of estrogen would later tend to develop coronary artery disease?

BARBIERI: And higher estrogen levels in people who develop endometriosis?

CRAMER: Your observations regarding risk for coronary artery disease in women with endometriosis would be extremely important to confirm. If the association is present, it could be due either to hormonal or surgical treatment for endometriosis or to the possible link between endometriosis and early menopause that I mentioned.

B.A. LESSEY (*University of North Carolina, Chapel Hill, NC*): In a recent review in *Modern Trends*, we raised the possibility that, because of the heterogeneity, all women are not created equal in terms of their infertility, and medical management might in fact impede pregnancy in half the group and speed another 50% to getting pregnant. If you do the analysis, it turns out that an infinite number of patients, including both groups, would never be able to prove that medical management works. However, if you could use biomarkers to select out those patients who are most affected, you might have a possibility of proving it.

J. ROCK (*Emory University, Atlanta, GA*): One of the things that obviously is of importance is to determine the longitudinal progression of developmental disease. One of the things that we found in studying congenital anomalies is that there is a cohort of patients—Rokitansky's, uterine malformations, a variety of different groups that have associated ovarian malposition—where there are abnormalities in the dextral rotation of the ducts as they descend. Virtually every one of those patients has deep retroperitoneal disease. In talking with our colleagues in other children's hospitals, we do not appreciate it, but the incidence of endometriosis is really significant. They are seen in pelvic abnormalities where there are abnormalities in the development of the bladder and duplication of the bladder, and particularly in abnormalities in sacral development of the posterior pelvis where you have endometriosis actually extending way down into the faucet. Thus, in looking at your heterogeneity issue and truly identifying those patients who have the disease, it is really problematic because many of these patients have very deep disease that may be missed and not readily visible or biopsiable or palpable that manifest themselves with continual chronic pelvic pain. In terms of looking at a marker, a biochemical marker, something that allows us to detect the presence of some secretory product, this seems to be the most reliable way of looking at the disease before we see the end stage because clearly there is a whole cohort of women that have early disease who are never identified, who we only see way down the road.

N. VLAHOS (*The Johns Hopkins University, Baltimore, MD*): Recently, there have been several publications about the association of endometriosis and ovarian cancer, specifically clear cell carcinoma. I think the most recent report was on the green. Do you have any comments about that?

CRAMER: It is well known among pathologists that both clear cell and endometrioid types of ovarian cancer can be seen to arise within areas of endometriosis; the association has only been established from recent follow-up studies of women with endometriosis. Interestingly, these studies showed an increase in risk not only for ovarian cancer, but also for breast cancer and non-Hodgkin's lymphoma.

A. AKHMEDKMANOV (*New York University, New York, NY*): In your presentation, you suggested that as high as 50% of teenagers requiring laparoscopy for intractable dysmenorrhea may have endometriosis. How often is this condition and are there any biochemical markers associated with this condition?

CRAMER: That prevalence estimate comes from two case series of teenagers with intractable dysmenorrhea who came to surgery. These reports made no attempt to estimate the frequency of severe dysmenorrhea requiring surgical exploration in the general population. You are correct in speculating that teenagers with severe dysmenorrhea would be an important group to target for endometriosis. However, I don't believe any current markers, such as CA-125, are specific enough.

A.A. MURPHY (*Emory University, Atlanta, GA*): I would like to add that most of those adolescents all had the red lesions and they seem to be very secretorially active, so they may be a good group to study to find biomarkers for some of these early lesions.

O. MUNEYYIRCI-DELALE (*SUNY Downstate Medical Center, Brooklyn, NY*): I have done limited interviews with my patients and their mothers and grandmothers. When I interviewed the mothers, some of them had dysmenorrhea; however, when I interviewed the grandmothers, most of them did not have dysmenorrhea. When I tried to explain this, I found that most of the mothers had limited pregnancies and some had lactation amenorrhea. When I went to the grandmothers, most of them had more pregnancies and prolonged lactation amenorrhea. We really should look at this group and see what is going on—it might answer some of the questions we have.

CRAMER: I think those are very useful observations. It is possible that the memory of menstrual events does fade with time in the grandmothers. However, as I speculated in my talk, it is possible that an early delivery that dilated the cervix or multiple pregnancies and lactation that reduced the number of periods may have also contributed to the infrequent reports of dysmenorrhea and presumably the lower risk for endometriosis in the grandmothers.

Progesterone-Mediated Endometrial Maturation Limits Matrix Metalloproteinase (MMP) Expression in an Inflammatory-like Environment

A Regulatory System Altered in Endometriosis

KEVIN G. OSTEEN, KAYLON L. BRUNER-TRAN, NANCY R. KELLER, AND ESTHER EISENBERG

Women's Reproductive Health Research Center, Department of Obstetrics and Gynecology, Vanderbilt University School of Medicine, Nashville, Tennessee, USA

ABSTRACT: The human endometrium exhibits regular cycles of growth, differentiation, and breakdown in response to changing levels of ovarian steroids. Following the tissue loss and repair processes of menstruation, rising levels of estradiol initiate a development-like process leading to a complete restructuring of the endometrial surface. In contrast, while under the predominate influence of progesterone, proliferation declines as cell-specific differentiation prepares the endometrium for pregnancy over a 5- to 6-day period. In the absence of nidation, steroid support is lost; the endometrial surface begins a complex process of tissue breakdown and bleeding, producing a viscous mixture of cellular debris within a bloody menstrual effluent. Although most of the menstrual fluid exits the body, reflux of some material occurs in most women, providing a poorly understood opportunity for ectopic endometrial growth and establishment of the disease endometriosis. The cyclic restructuring of the endometrium requires numerous matrix metalloproteinases (MMPs) that mediate normal and pathological tissue turnover throughout the reproductive tract. The expression of multiple MMPs facilitates degradation of extracellular matrix during growth-related remodeling as well as tissue breakdown at the time of menstruation. However, these enzymes are absent during the early and mid-secretory phase and the suppression of endometrial MMPs remains important to maintaining the integrity of the endometrium during the highly invasive events required to establish a normal hemochorial placenta. Several research groups have suggested that steroid-mediated expression and action of MMPs during the menstrual cycle may provide a key mechanistic link between endometrial turnover and the invasive processes necessary for establishment of endometriosis.

KEYWORDS: endometrium; menstruation; interleukin-1; TNF-α

Address for correspondence: Kevin G. Osteen, Ph.D., Director, Women's Reproductive Health Research Center, B-1100 Medical Center North, Department of Obstetrics and Gynecology, Vanderbilt University School of Medicine, Nashville, TN 37232. Voice: 615-322-4196; fax: 615-343-7913.

kevin.osteen@mcmail.vanderbilt.edu

INTRODUCTION

Over some 35 years of reproductive life, cyclical production of ovarian estradiol and progesterone directs a predictable pattern of growth and functional maturation in the human endometrium. Although fundamental to reproductive success, without ovarian support the endometrium exhibits little morphological change and fails to exhibit the biochemical activity necessary for establishment or support of pregnancy.[1] Prior to sexual maturity or after the menopause, the endometrium appears as a low columnar or cuboidal epithelium with little associated stromal matrix. In contrast, during the reproductive years, the endometrium develops extensive surface and glandular epithelium with a rich stroma consisting of pluripotent mesenchymal cells, vascular elements, and a diverse, cycle-specific population of invasive cells of hemopoietic origin.[2,3] Pathologists generally divide the adult endometrium into three morphologically and functionally distinct layers: the *stratum basalis* that lies adjacent to the myometrium, the *stratum spongiosum* or intermediate layer, and the *stratum compactum*. It is from the *stratum basalis* that the endometrium regenerates after each menstrual shedding, while the two uppermost layers, referred to jointly as the *stratum functionalis*, undergo coordinated histologic and cytologic changes throughout the menstrual cycle.[4] The cyclic loss of tissue from the endometrial lining of the human and primate uterus represents a unique phenotype within mammalian evolution that is often linked to reproductive dysfunction. For example, the process of menstrual tissue loss and regrowth has been recognized for nearly 75 years as being associated with the risk of ectopic attachment of endometrial fragments leading to endometriosis.[5] Endometriosis is an enigmatic disease that naturally occurs only in association with the complex reproductive physiology of menstruating species. This disease is clearly linked to the steroid dependency of the endometrium and appears to be related to a woman's immune status as well as exposure to environmental factors. Once established, endometriosis can be difficult to treat effectively, although some success has been obtained with medical regimens that block endogenous steroid production or action. However, this medical approach is not appropriate for the long-term management of endometriosis since steroids support other aspects of a woman's overall health needs.

Among reproductive tract tissues, the endometrium is perhaps the most steroid-sensitive, and rising levels of ovarian estradiol rapidly initiate a wave of cellular mitosis in concert with menstrual repair processes and morphological restructuring. During the variable proliferative phase, which is rarely the idealized length of 14 days, the human endometrium exhibits extensive remodeling of the extracellular matrix, completely rebuilding the *stratum functionalis*. Endometrial restructuring and repair require the cooperative actions of numerous matrix metalloproteinases (MMPs), a family of secreted, locally active enzymes that are involved in multiple processes within the ovarian and endometrial cycles.[6] The MMPs are infrequently expressed in healthy adult tissues and have been studied most extensively for their actions in association with disease, including numerous pathologies of the female reproductive tract.[7] Since the actions of MMPs are potentially destructive, their expression and activation at both the cellular and tissue level are highly regulated within all normal organ systems.[8] For example, the MMPs can be regulated transcriptionally by numerous growth factors and cytokines as well as within the intercellular space, requiring posttranslational activation of the pro-form by proteolytic cleavage. Additionally, the enzymatic activity of activated MMPs is often limited or completely blocked by specific tissue inhibitors of MMPs (TIMPs), plasminogen activator inhibitor (PAI-1), and general protease inhibitors such as α-2 macroglobulin and α-1 antitrypsin.[6,7] Within the unique environment of the female reproductive tract, various steroids, growth factors, cytokines, and tissue inhibitors act cooperatively to regulate the focal and highly regional expression and action of MMPs during the endometrial cycle.

Recent MMP-related research has suggested that the cellular mechanisms of ectopic endometrial growth in endometriosis involve invasive events similar to metastatic neoplasms, requiring extracellular matrix degradation during penetration of the peritoneal mesothelium.[9,10] Additionally, steroid-mediated control of these enzymes in the endometrium provides a key connection between the normal function of this organ system and the basic pathophysiology of endometriosis. For example, in an experimental model of endometriosis, we have demonstrated that the establishment of ectopic human endometrium in nude mice can be blocked by inhibiting MMP expression or action in the human tissue. More specifically, we found that experimental endometriosis does not develop in mice receiving human tissues treated with progesterone *in vitro* or intraperitoneal TIMP injections.[11] This experimental endometriosis model suggested that exploring steroid-mediated regulation of members of the MMP family in the endometrium may provide new clues important for both understanding endometriosis and developing more effective treatment strategies for this disease.

MENSTRUATION

In spite of the enigmatic nature of endometriosis, including potential associations with environmental endocrine disrupters, the disease may essentially represent an untoward consequence of menstruation. The biological purpose of menstruation among primates and humans remains obscure, but cyclic sloughing of the endometrial surface may simply represent the need to discard terminally differentiated tissue no longer capable of initiating and supporting nidation. The process of menstruation is recognized as the beginning of each reproductive cycle, although the loss of endometrial tissue and associated bleeding actually represent a failure to conceive. Numerous theories have been proposed to explain the initial cellular mechanisms leading to menstruation, largely based on vascular tissue instability following the withdrawal of ovarian steroid support.[12] However, an *in situ* hybridization localization study detected focal expression of MMP-7 mRNA among glandular epithelium prior to any overt sign of tissue instability or breakdown.[13] Recent studies provide evidence that numerous members of the MMP family are expressed during menstruation and may play an important role in both tissue breakdown and repair processes.[13–16] Although MMP-7 expression represents an early endometrial reaction to progesterone withdrawal, *in vitro* studies using isolated cell types show that regulation of MMP-7 expression involves stromal-epithelial communication via the action of transforming growth factor-β.[17,18] Additionally, the expression of focal epithelial-specific MMP-7 and stromal-specific MMP-3 mRNA can be observed

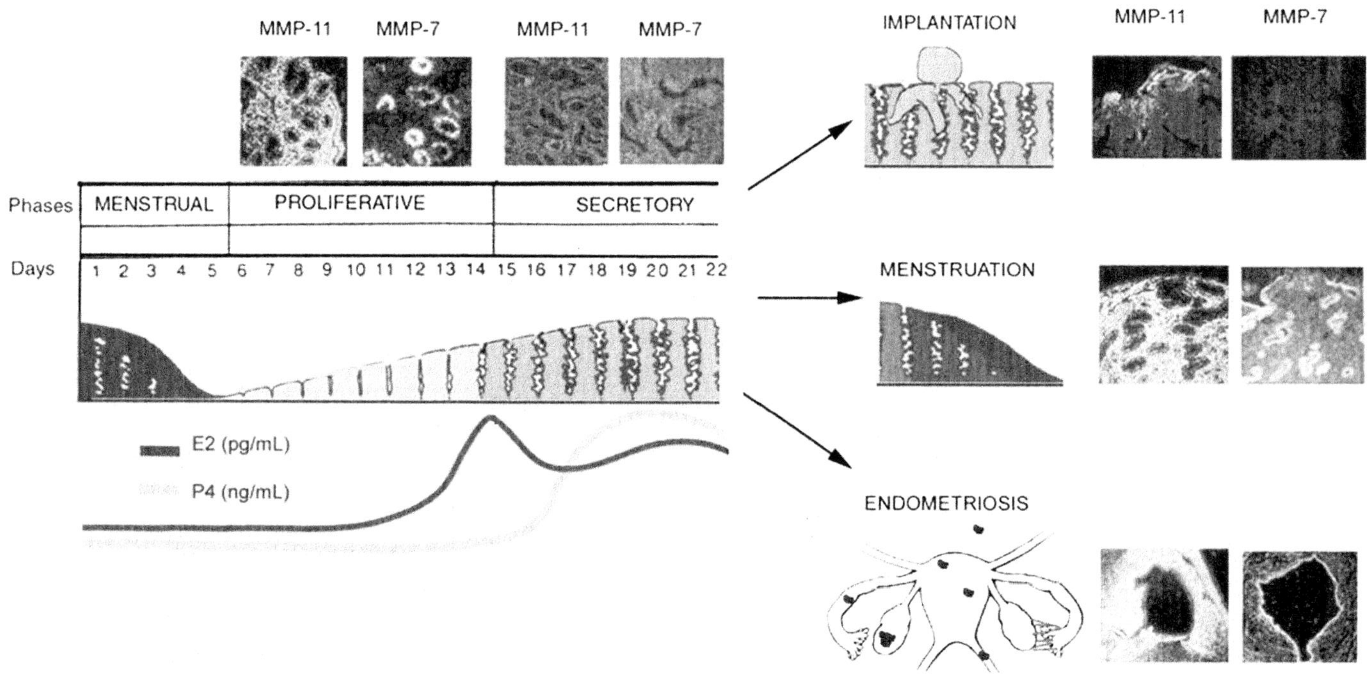

FIGURE 1. Schematic representation of endometrial events during the menstrual cycle and potential outcomes. Shown in adjacent photomicrographs are *in situ* hybridization analysis of expression of MMP-11 and MMP-7 mRNA during the proliferative, secretory, and menstrual phases of the cycle, as well as during pregnancy establishment and endometriosis. (Magnification: ×200.)

during *in vitro* repair processes that do not appear sensitive to steroidal regulation.[19] Although steroid-mediated MMP expression may link the process of menstruation to the pathophysiology of endometriosis, such observations indicate that the expression of these enzymes is also regulated by local cell-cell communication mechanisms. Therefore, it is important to examine how estrogen priming and subsequent estrogen and progesterone exposure act to stabilize the endometrium by regulating cell-specific MMP expression.

It is clear that estrogen is a positive risk factor for the development of endometriosis, while progesterone exposure during pregnancy both is a negative risk factor for disease development and represents a potential therapeutic strategy. Following ovulation, postovulatory increases in serum progesterone mediate a unique and highly localized tissue environment within the fundus of the endometrium that serves to protect maternal tissue integrity during the highly invasive establishment of the hemochorial placenta. Providing an environment receptive to invasion by cytotrophoblasts while maintaining endometrial tissue stability presents a significant biological challenge that is absolutely dependent on progesterone support. Numerous studies have shown that endometrial MMP expression can be stimulated by the inflammatory cytokines associated with both menstruation[16,20] and pregnancy establishment.[21,22] However, in the United States, where it is not possible to examine early human pregnancy, investigating the eutopic endometrium from patients with ectopic tubal pregnancies can offer valuable insight in the events surrounding nidation. We have found that MMP-7 mRNA is virtually absent in the eutopic endometrium of women with an ectopic pregnancy, but is highly elevated in association with interleukin-1α (IL-1α) expression near the ectopic pregnancy site.[23] Additionally, we have recently demonstrated that the ability of IL-1α to stimulate MMP-3 expression by endometrial stromal cells is blocked *in vivo* and *in vitro* by progesterone exposure.[22] The ability of progesterone to inhibit either stromal or epithelial expression of MMPs in an inflammatory environment may represent a key finding relative to the expression of these enzymes in the disease endometriosis. As shown in FIGURE 1, the cell-specific expression of MMP-11 by endometrial stromal cells and MMP-7 by epithelial cells does not occur in the eutopic endometrium of a patient with an ectopic pregnancy, even though these MMPs are broadly expressed in the absence of progesterone support during menstruation. The expression of MMP-11 and MMP-7 at ectopic sites of endometriosis during the secretory phase (FIG. 1) suggests that a defect(s) in progesterone-mediated MMP suppression may be associated with this disease process. Developing a mechanistic understanding of progesterone-mediated prevention of MMP expression within the inflammatory-like environment of early pregnancy should provide insights into the apparent overexpression of these enzymes associated with endometriosis.

STEROID-DIRECTED ENDOMETRIAL TISSUE TURNOVER

Following the onset of menstruation, it takes approximately 3 weeks of steroid support for the endometrium to prepare for the successful establishment of pregnancy. The predictable and precisely controlled response of endometrial tissue to changing levels of circulating steroids is related to changing patterns of steroid receptor

TABLE 1. Summary of the expression patterns of the MMP system in the human endometrium throughout the menstrual cycle

Proliferative	Secretory	Menstrual
MMP-1 +	MMP-1 –	MMP-1 +
MMP-2 ++	MMP-2 ++	MMP-2 ++
MMP-3 +	MMP-3 –	MMP-3 ++
MMP-7 ++	MMP-7 –	MMP-7 +++
MMP-9 –	MMP-9 –	MMP-9 +
MMP-10 –	MMP-10 –	MMP-10 ++
MMP-11 ++	MMP-11 –	MMP-11 +++
TIMP-1 +	TIMP-1 +	TIMP-1 +++
TIMP-2 +	TIMP-2 +	TIMP-2 ++
TIMP-3 +/–	TIMP-3 +	TIMP-3 +

NOTE: Relative levels of mRNA are expressed as – (absent), + (focal), ++ (moderate), or +++ (intense).

expression in stromal and epithelial elements across the menstrual cycle. Using classical biochemical analysis of changing tissue receptor concentrations, Lessey *et al.*[24] demonstrated that the highest levels of total tissue estrogen receptor (ER) were detected during the late proliferative to early secretory transition of the menstrual cycle, while levels of progesterone receptor (PR) peaked later in the cycle during the early to mid-secretory period. More recently, molecular analysis has revealed two isoforms of the estrogen receptor (ER-α and ER-β), each of which can be detected in stromal and epithelial cells of the human endometrium. Similar analysis has found that the progesterone receptor also occurs as two distinct isoforms in humans, PR-A and PR-B, derived from a single gene as a consequence of alternate initiation of transcription from distinct promoters.[25] Although ER-α and PR-B each appear to be the predominant steroid isotype expressed in the normal endometrium, changes in ER-α/ER-β and PR-A/PR-B expression ratios have been noted in tissues or cells isolated from women with endometriosis.[26,27] In general, changes in steroid receptor expression associated with endometriosis tend to increase tissue exposure to estrogens, while reducing tissue sensitivity to progestins.

In concert with the steroid-induced tissue restructuring that is the hallmark of the endometrium, numerous MMPs exhibit both cell-specific and cycle-dependent expression during the menstrual cycle (TABLE 1). *In situ* hybridization localization and *in vitro* analysis of secreted proteins have localized expression of MMP-1, MMP-2, MMP-3, MMP-7, MMP-9, MMP-10, and MMP-11 in the cycling human endometrium.[6] As noted previously in regard to estrogen-mediated cell growth, this steroid does not appear to directly affect MMP mRNA or protein expression in the cycling endometrium.[17,28] Nevertheless, many of the estrogen-associated growth factors known to impact uterine growth, such as members of the EGF superfamily, are known to impact the expression of the MMPs associated with tissue remodeling.[6,7] In contrast to the focal expression patterns of several MMPs associated with endometrial growth, under the dominance of progesterone, the cell-type expression of mRNA for MMPs is no longer detectable by *in situ* hybridization *in vivo* in normal endometrium.[13,14] *In vitro* studies from a number of laboratories using both short-term organ culture and monolayer cultures of isolated cell types have confirmed the ability of progesterone exposure to directly and indirectly suppress MMP gene and protein secretion.[17,18,20,22,28]

Because of the intimate relationship between a woman's steroid status and development or progression of endometriosis, physicians often utilize natural or bioactive steroidal compounds as a method of therapeutic intervention in the treatment of this disease. Unfortunately, it is also well established that ectopic endometriotic tissues often do not respond in a predictable fashion to medical therapies based solely on steroid-dependent endometrial tissue behavior. Numerous laboratories have identified profound differences in levels of steroid receptors, changes in specific receptor isotype expression, as well as alterations in important modifiers of nuclear steroid action such as retinoid receptors.[26,27,29] Certainly, it is tempting to explore the ability of progestins to suppress MMPs as a potential therapeutic strategy based on targeting this important class of biologic molecules. However, we have recently shown that natural progesterone exposure either *in vivo* or *in vitro* fails to suppress MMP-3 or MMP-7 expression in the eutopic or ectopic endometrium of some women with endometriosis.[30] Although an altered expression of MMPs has been previously associated with the ectopic growth of endometriosis,[31] the lack of progesterone-mediated MMP suppression in the eutopic endometrium was unexpected. As we develop a more complete understanding of steroid-mediated control of endometrial MMP expression, we may be able to anticipate the impact of advertent steroid exposures and perhaps inadvertent environmental exposures on MMP expression related to endometriosis. Modern analysis of steroid receptor function continues to reveal new concepts in our understanding of the molecular basis of steroid hormone action, allowing the targeting of specific tissues and possibly specific cell types as new concepts continue to emerge. For example, the identification of selective estrogen receptor modulators (SERMs) and our emerging view of selective progesterone receptor modulators (SPRMs) have already created new therapeutic options for protecting steroid-sensitive organ systems as well as treating disease. Although steroids are essential for endometrial dynamics, the action of local paracrine factors is equally critical for normal endometrial responses to either estrogen[32,33] or progesterone.[18,34] Thus, it will be equally important to incorporate key elements of steroid-directed cell-cell communication into any new therapeutic strategies aimed at treating endometriosis by modifying tissue MMP expression or action.

PROGESTERONE-DIRECTED ENDOMETRIAL STABILITY

The complex and interactive nature of MMP regulation by steroids, growth factors, and cytokines in the human endometrium provides for a remarkably complex biological system. At the time of pregnancy establishment, the maternal-fetal interface represents a unique site requiring multiple pathways of cell-cell communication involving cells of diverse origin. As noted above, early pregnancy is a fragile period during the establishment of pregnancy in terms of endometrial stability, which requires both progesterone support as well as the action of progesterone-related paracrine factors. Inflammatory cytokines have been associated with mediating

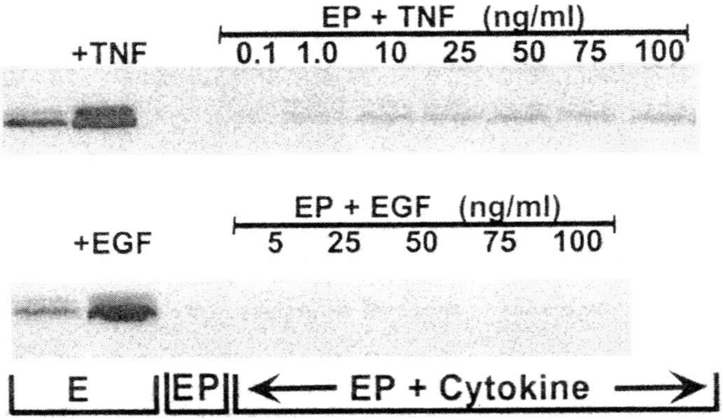

FIGURE 2. Western analysis of expression and regulation of MMP-3 protein in isolated endometrial stromal cells. Cells were isolated from proliferative-phase endometrium and grown as monolayers on type IV collagen. Cells were maintained in the presence of estradiol (E; 10^{-9} M) or estradiol plus progesterone (EP; E = 10^{-9} M; P = 5×10^{-7} M) in the presence or absence of TNF-α and EGF.

overexpression of MMPs associated with ectopic pregnancy,[23] endometriosis,[19] as well as other pathologies of reproductive tissues.[7] Our current understanding of the epidemiology of endometriosis dictates that a woman's exposure to endogenous or exogenous steroids is closely linked to her overall risk of developing endometriosis. During the normal secretory phase of the menstrual cycle, progesterone is a potent inhibitor of the focal expression of endometrial MMPs observed during proliferation-related tissue remodeling.[13,14] Although the mechanism of progesterone action on endometrial MMP expression appears to be complex,[6,7] progesterone acts broadly not only to inhibit estrogen action in the endometrium, but also to reduce the impact of other paracrine communication pathways. For example, our research group demonstrated that progesterone is not only critical for MMP-3 suppression during the secretory phase of the menstrual cycle,[17] but it can also prevent expression of this MMP in response to a potent inflammatory cytokine present during normal pregnancy establishment.[22] More recently, we have demonstrated that progesterone acts to restrict the actions of other cytokines known to impact MMP expression in the endometrium. As shown in FIGURE 2, in isolated human endometrial stromal cells, the expression of MMP-3 cannot be induced *in vitro* by a broad range of EGF or TNF-α exposure levels following 2 days of progesterone treatment. These new data further suggest that the altered expression patterns of MMPs in eutopic or ectopic tissues from women with endometriosis[30,31] may be a result of a resistance to normal progesterone action. It remains to be more clearly demonstrated whether defects in specific progesterone-mediated paracrine factors may impact the control of MMP expression or action in association with endometriosis. However, it is not difficult to visualize the potential negative impact that a lack of normal progesterone-mediated regulation of MMPs could have on the sequelae of events necessary for establishment or progression of this complex disease.

SUMMARY

Although the dynamics of endometrial tissue turnover during the menstrual cycle is complex, the regulation of MMP expression would, at present, appear to be under the interactive control of both steroids and locally produced factors. Cell-cell communication can occur through a number of mechanisms that involve direct cell-cell contact or paracrine signals. Additionally, since the extracellular matrix is not merely a supporting structure, but rather a dynamic component of the tissue's communication network, MMP-mediated changes in the composition of the matrix may also play a role in cell-cell signaling. During each menstrual cycle, the degree of tissue turnover that occurs in the human endometrium is extensive and, by most measures, rivals the dynamic events of organ formation during fetal development. While MMPs have been identified in numerous tissues, endometrial MMP expression appears to follow a pattern that is largely dependent upon the dynamic response of this tissue to changing patterns of ovarian steroids. Exploring the regulatory actions of locally produced growth factors and cytokines on members of the MMP family and their inhibitors will allow a better understanding of the normal steroid physiology of the human endometrium. Our emerging understanding of the role of MMPs in the inflammatory environment associated with the complex pathophysiology of endometriosis will provide new treatment options for women who suffer from the numerous consequences of this often debilitating disease.

ACKNOWLEDGMENTS

This work was supported in part through a cooperative agreement (No. U54-HD-37321) as part of the Specialized Cooperative Centers Program in Reproduction Research. Additional funding was provided by grants from the U.S. Environmental Protection Agency (No. R826300) and The Endometriosis Association.

REFERENCES

1. Osteen, K.G. 1998. The endocrinology of uterine decidualization. *In* The Endocrinology of Pregnancy, pp. 541–553. Humana Press. Totowa, NJ.
2. Healy, D. & G. Hodgen. 1989. The endocrinology of the human endometrium. Obstet. Gynecol. Surv. **38:** 509–530.
3. Tabibzadeh, S. 1991. The human endometrium: an active site of cytokine production and action. Endocr. Rev. **12:** 272–290.
4. Noyes, R.A., A.T. Hertig & J. Rock. 1950. Dating the endometrial biopsy. Fertil. Steril. **1:** 3–25.
5. Sampson, J.A. 1927. Peritoneal endometriosis due to menstrual dissemination of endometrial tissue into the peritoneal cavity. Am. J. Obstet. Gynecol. **14:** 422–469.
6. Curry, T.E. & K.G. Osteen. 2001. Cyclic changes in the matrix metalloproteinase system in the ovary and uterus. Biol. Reprod. **64:** 1285–1296.
7. Hulboy, D.L., L.A. Rudolph & L.M. Matrisian. 1997. Matrix metalloproteinases as mediators of reproductive function. Mol. Hum. Reprod. **3:** 27–45.
8. Matrisian, L.M. 1994. Matrix metalloproteinase gene expression. Ann. N.Y. Acad. Sci. **732:** 42–50.
9. Spuijbroek, M.D.E.H., G.A.J. Dunselman, P.P.C.A. Menheere & J.L.H. Evers. 1992. Early endometriosis invades the extracellular matrix. Fertil. Steril. **58:** 929–933.

10. KOKS, C.A., P.G. GROOTHUIS, G.A. DUNSELMAN *et al.* 2000. Adhesion of menstrual endometrium to extracellular matrix: the possible role of integrin alpha(6)-beta(1) and laminin interaction. Mol. Hum. Reprod. **6:** 170–177.
11. BRUNER, K.L., L.M. MATRISIAN, W.H. RODGERS *et al.* 1997. Suppression of matrix metalloproteinases inhibits establishment of ectopic lesions by human tissue in nude mice. J. Clin. Invest. **99:** 2851–2857.
12. SPEROFF, L., R.H. GLASS & N.G. KASE. 1998. Clinical Gynecologic Endocrinology and Infertility. Fifth edition, pp. 132–134. Williams & Wilkins. Baltimore.
13. RODGERS, W.H., K.G. OSTEEN, L.M. MATRISIAN *et al.* 1993. Expression and localization of matrilysin (Pump-1, MMP-7), a matrix metalloproteinase in the human endometrium. Am. J. Obstet. Gynecol. **168:** 253–260.
14. RODGERS, W.H., L.M. MATRISIAN, L.C. GIUDICE *et al.* 1994. Patterns of matrix metalloproteinase expression in cycling endometrium imply differential functions and regulation by steroids. J. Clin. Invest. **94:** 946–953.
15. MARBAIX, E., I. KOKORINE, P. MOULIN *et al.* 1996. Menstrual breakdown of human endometrium can be mimicked *in vitro* and is selectively and reversibly blocked by inhibitors of matrix metalloproteinases. Proc. Natl. Acad. Sci. U.S.A. **93:** 9120–9125.
16. SALAMONSEN, L.A. & D.E. WOOLLEY. 1999. Menstruation: induction by matrix metalloproteinases and inflammatory cells. J. Reprod. Immunol. **44:** 1–27.
17. OSTEEN, K.G., W.H. RODGERS, M. GAIRE *et al.* 1994. Stromal-epithelial interaction mediates steroidal regulation of metalloproteinase expression in human endometrium. Proc. Natl. Acad. Sci. U.S.A. **91:** 10129–10133.
18. BRUNER, K.L., W.H. RODGERS, M. KOR *et al.* 1995. Transforming growth factor-β mediates the progesterone suppression of an epithelial metalloproteinase by adjacent stroma. Proc. Natl. Acad. Sci. U.S.A. **92:** 7362–7366.
19. BRUNER, K.L., N.R. KELLER & K.G. OSTEEN. 1999. Interleukin-1α opposes suppression of human endometrial matrix metalloproteinases by progesterone in a model of experimental endometriosis. *In* Understanding and Managing Endometriosis: Advances in Research and Practice. Parthenon Pub. New York.
20. SINGER, C.F., E. MARBAIX, I. KOKORINE *et al.* 1997. Paracrine stimulation of interstitial collagenase (MMP-1) in the human endometrium by interleukin 1 alpha and its dual block by ovarian steroids. Proc. Natl. Acad. Sci. U.S.A. **94:** 10341–10345.
21. SIMON, C., A. MERCADER, M.J. GIMENO & A. PELLICER. 1997. The interleukin-1 system and human implantation. Am. J. Reprod. Med. **37:** 64–72.
22. KELLER, N.R., E. SIERRA-RIVERA, E. EISENBERG & K.G. OSTEEN. 2000. Progesterone exposure prevents matrix metalloproteinase-3 (MMP-3) stimulation by interleukin-1α in human endometrial stromal cells. J. Clin. Endocrinol. Metab. **85:** 1611–1619.
23. OSTEEN, K.G., E. SIERRA-RIVERA, N.R. KELLER & D.B. FOX. 1997. Interleukin-1 alpha opposes progesterone-mediated suppression of MMP-7: a possible role of this cytokine during human implantation. Ann. N.Y. Acad. Sci. **828:** 137–145.
24. LESSEY, B.A., A.P. KILLAM, D.A. METZGER *et al.* 1988. Immunohistochemical analysis of human uterine estrogen and progesterone receptors in the normal human uterus throughout the menstrual cycle. J. Clin. Endocrinol. Metab. **67:** 334–340.
25. MCDONNELL, D.P. 1995. Unraveling the human progesterone receptor signal transduction pathway: insights into antiprogestin action. TEM **6:** 133–138.
26. BRANDENBERGER, A.W., D.I. LEBOVIC, M.K. TEE *et al.* 1999. Oestrogen receptor (ER)–alpha and ER-beta isoforms in normal endometrial and endometriosis-derived stromal cells. Mol. Hum. Reprod. **5:** 651–655.
27. ATTIA, G.R., K. ZEITOUN, D. EDWARDS *et al.* 2000. Progesterone receptor isoform A, but not B is expressed in endometriosis. J. Clin. Endocrinol. Metab. **85:** 2897–2902.
28. SCHATZ, F., C. PAPP, E. TOTH-PAL & C. LOCKWOOD. 1994. Ovarian-steroid modulation of stromelysin-1 expression in human endometrial stroma and decidual cells. J. Clin. Endocrinol. Metab. **78:** 1467–1472.
29. SEGARS, J.H. 1997. Endometriosis and nuclear hormone receptors. *In* Endometrium and Endometriosis, pp. 321–332. Blackwell Science. Malden, MA.
30. BRUNER-TRAN, K.L., E. EISENBERG & K.G. OSTEEN. 2000. Establishment of experimental endometriosis by eutopic or ectopic endometrial tissue acquired from women with endometriosis cannot be prevented by progesterone treatments [abstract]. Presented

at the Fifty-sixth Annual Meeting of the American Society for Reproductive Medicine, October 2000, San Diego.
31. OSTEEN, K.G., K.L. BRUNER & K.L. SHARPE-TIMMS. 1996. Steroid and growth factors regulation of matrix metalloproteinase expression and endometriosis. Semin. Reprod. Endocrinol. **14:** 247–255.
32. COOKE, P.S., F.D. UCHIMA, D.K. FUJII *et al.* 1986. Restoration of normal morphology and estrogen responsiveness in cultured vaginal and uterine epithelia transplanted with stroma. Proc. Natl. Acad. Sci. U.S.A. **83:** 2109–2113.
33. PIERRO, E., F. MINICI, O. ALESIANI *et al.* 2001. Stromal-epithelial interactions modulate estrogen responsiveness in normal human endometrium. Biol. Reprod. **64:** 831–838.
34. KURITA, T., P. YOUNG, J.R. BRODY *et al.* 1998. Stromal progesterone receptors mediate the inhibitory effects of progesterone on estrogen-induced uterine epithelial cell deoxyribonucleic acid synthesis. Endocrinology **139:** 4708–4713.

Mechanisms of Action of Estrogen and Progesterone

FRANCESCO J. DEMAYO, BIHONG ZHAO, NORIO TAKAMOTO, AND SOPHIA Y. TSAI

Department of Molecular and Cell Biology, Baylor College of Medicine, Houston, Texas 77030, USA

ABSTRACT: Estrogen and progesterone are steroid hormones that play a pivotal role in the regulation of mammalian reproduction. One primary action of these hormones is to regulate the development and function of the uterus. These hormones act by regulating the transcription of specific genes in the uterus. The actions of these hormones are mediated by their specific hormone receptors. These receptors are nuclear transcription factors, whose transcriptional regulatory activity is mediated by the binding of the specific steroid to these molecules. Once these receptors bind hormone, they can bind to specific *cis*-acting sequences in the promoter region of responsive genes and regulate transcription of these genes. In the regulation of transcription, these receptors interact with specific cofactors to activate the transcriptional machinery. A second gene family, the Steroid Receptor Coactivator (SRC) family, has been identified that serves to modulate the transcriptional activity of the hormone receptors. To date, three members of the SRC family have been identified. During the last decade, gene targeting technology has been used to identify the role of these receptors in the regulation of reproduction and uterine biology.

KEYWORDS: nuclear receptors; uterus; mouse

INTRODUCTION

The ovarian steroids, estrogen and progesterone, regulate all aspects of female reproduction from sexual behavior through pregnancy and lactation. These hormones act primarily by regulating transcription of specific hormone–responsive, target genes. The transcriptional regulatory activities of these hormones are mediated by specific nuclear receptors (reviewed in reference 1). These nuclear receptors are transcription factors whose activity is regulated by binding the specific steroid. Estrogen signaling is mediated by one of two receptors, estrogen receptor alpha, ERα, and estrogen receptor beta, ERβ (reviewed in reference 2). Progesterone signaling is mediated by the progesterone receptor, PR, of which two isoforms, PRA and PRB, have been identified (reviewed in reference 3). These isoforms result from alternative translation of the mRNA.[4] Knockout mice have been generated for both ERs[5–7] and PR,[8] specifically for PRA.[9] These animals have been used to define the

Address for correspondence: Francesco J. DeMayo, Ph.D., Department of Molecular and Cell Biology, Baylor College of Medicine, Houston, TX 77030. Voice: 713-798-6241; fax: 713-790-1275.
fdemayo@bcm.tmc.edu

mechanisms by which these hormones regulate uterine gene expression and function. Here, we will review the molecular biology of the nuclear receptors and how gene ablation of these receptors and associated cofactors have shed light on the role of these receptors in uterine biology.

NUCLEAR RECEPTORS

The nuclear receptors represent the largest family of transcription factors. These are transcription factors that share a similar structure homology (reviewed in references 10–15). The structure of these receptors is shown in FIGURE 1. As shown in FIGURE 1, these receptors contain six regions of homology that contribute to the functional domains of the receptors. Of the functional domains of the receptors, the three major domains are the ligand binding domain (LBD), the DNA binding domain (DBD), and the activation domain (AF). The LBD is located at the carboxyl terminus of the molecule, region E. The LBD gives the receptor specificity for the specific hormone or molecule that regulates the transcriptional activity of the receptor. The DBD is located in the central portion of the molecule, region C. The DBD gives the receptor specificity for the target genes that the receptor will regulate. This specificity is determined by which DNA sequences the DBD will recognize. These sequences or hormone response elements, HREs, are located in enhancer/promoter regions of the target genes. The AFs are located throughout the molecule, regions A/B and E.[14] These domains are responsible for linking the receptors to the cellular transcriptional machinery and regulated transcription of target genes. The nuclear receptor family includes the receptors for the steroid hormones, thyroid hormone, and retinoids, as well as the orphan nuclear receptors. The latter group is named orphan nuclear receptors because this group consists of receptors for which a specific ligand has yet to be identified. The identification of ligands that regulate the orphan nuclear receptors is an active area of research.

The molecular mechanisms by which the ovarian steroid hormones regulate the transcription of target genes through their receptors have been actively investigated over the last 30 years (reviewed in references 1, 10, and 14). FIGURE 2 summarizes the current model for the activation of gene transcription by the steroid hormone receptors. In the absence of ligand, the receptors are associated with chaperone proteins and are transcriptionally inactive. The steroid hormone receptors can be activated by two mechanisms. The first, traditional ligand-dependent, mechanism by

A/B (Activation Domain)	**C (DNA Binding Domain)**	**D**	**E Ligand Binding and Activation Domain**	**F**

FIGURE 1. The schematic structure of the domains of the nuclear receptors.[10]

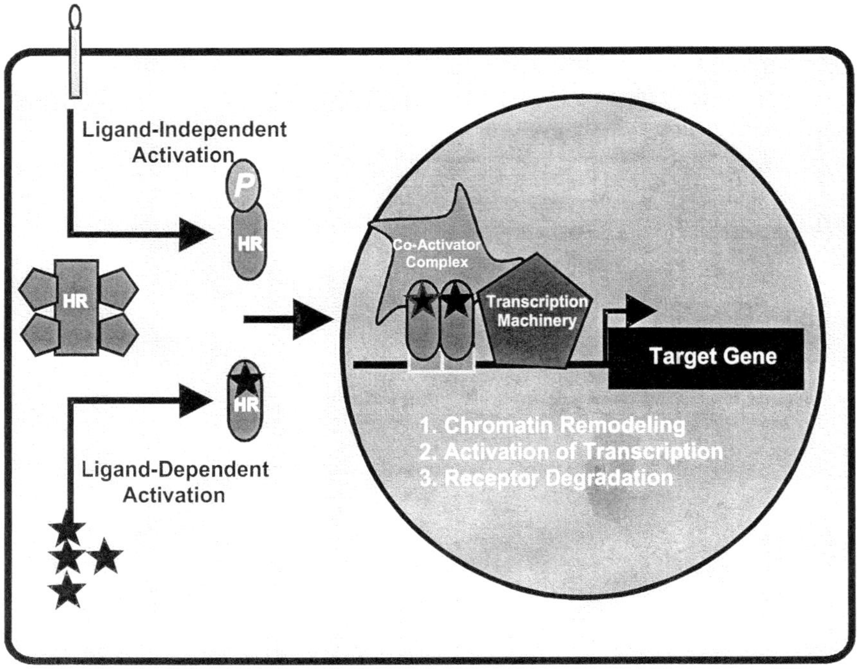

FIGURE 2. An overall schematic of the mechanism of action of nuclear receptor regulation of gene transcription. Unactivated receptor (*rectangle*) is surrounded by chaperone proteins (*pentangles*) and located in the cytoplasm or nucleus of the cell, depending upon the receptor. Upon activation, by either binding ligand (*stars*) or phosphorylation via signaling of membrane receptor, the receptor changes conformation (*oval*) and binds the hormone response element in the promoter/enhancer region of the target gene. Upon binding of DNA, the activated receptor recruits cofactors, the chromatin is modified, and the transcription machinery is activated. The receptor is then subject to degradation by ubiquitination.

which receptors can be activated is by the binding of the hormone to the LBD ligand. The second mechanism by which the receptors can be activated is through a ligand-independent mechanism.[16,17] The ligand-independent activation of the receptor is a result of the integration of other signaling pathways, usually membrane receptor signaling that results in the activation of kinases and ultimately the phosphorylation of the receptor. The activated receptor then undergoes conformational change that results in the dimerization of the receptors. In turn, these receptors attain the ability to bind the specific DNA HRE in the enhancer/promoter of the target gene. Upon the binding of the receptor to the HRE, the activated receptor then interacts with co-activators, which will link the steroid hormone receptor to the basal transcriptional machinery of the cell. The coactivators not only link the receptor to the transcription machinery, but also facilitate transcription by covalently modifying chromatin structure. These coactivators have histone acetyl transferase activity that functions to acetylate histone proteins, allowing the DNA to achieve a conformation that increases the accessibility of the promoter of the target gene to the activated receptor, and basal transcriptional machinery. This remodeling of the chromatin serves to facilitate the transcription of specific genes. These coactivators include members of the Steroid Receptor Coactivator (SRC) family, CREB binding protein and related p300 protein (CBP/p300), High Mobility Group proteins (HMGs), and E3 ubiquitin-protein ligases (E6-AP and RPF-1) (reviewed in references 18 and 19). The latter group of coactivators function to direct the activated steroid hormone receptor to the proteosome complex for the degradation of the receptor.[20] Thus, the entire process of steroid hormone receptor activation results in the enhanced transcription of specific target genes, as well as the degradation of the activated steroid hormone receptor.

As described above, *in vitro* analyses of the molecular biology of the steroid hormone receptors have defined the mechanism by which the steroid hormone receptors regulate the transcription of specific target genes. Important to the understanding of the role of the steroid hormone receptors in regulating uterine physiology is the identification of the specific target genes that are regulated by the steroid hormone receptors. Over the last decade, the mouse has emerged as a model system to investigate the ovarian hormone receptors in uterine biology *in vivo*. This is due to the use of homologous recombination in ES cells that affords the ability to ablate knockout genes in the murine genome.[21] Thus, the mouse has been used to understand how the expression of the steroid hormone receptors is regulated in the uterus during pregnancy and the function of these receptors in regulating uterine biology.

EXPRESSION AND REGULATION OF THE STEROID HORMONE RECEPTORS IN THE MURINE UTERUS

The uterus is one of the major target organs for steroid hormone action. The uterus consists of multiple cell types including two layers of smooth muscle tissue, myometrium, surrounding the glandular endometrium. The endometrium can be further divided into the stromal layer, the luminal epithelium, and the glandular epithelium. The mouse uterus contains both estrogen receptors, ERα and ERβ,[22,23] as well as both isoforms of the progesterone receptor, PRA and PRB.[9,24] Initial investigations of the distribution and regulation of these receptors in the uterus consisted of measuring radiolabeled hormone to uterine sections.[25] Recent investigations have demonstrated that the expression and regulation of the levels of the ERs and PR are dependent upon the compartment of the uterus in which the receptor is expressed.[23,26] Therefore, the level and regulation of the ER and PR expression can vary through pregnancy depending on the compartment in which these receptors are expressed.

Tan and coworkers have described the expression of ERα, ERβ, and PR in the murine endometrium through the preimplantation and implantation period.[23] ERα was the predominant ER expressed in the murine uterus.[22,23] In early pregnancy, ERα is primarily expressed in the luminal epithelium. During the peri-implantation period, ERα expression increases in the uterine stromal compartment. During implantation, ERα levels decreased in the stroma at the sites of implantation. In postimplantation, ERα levels were highest in the secondary decidual zone surrounding the implanted fetus. The expression of PR also varied during this period. PR levels were low in early implantation. However, PR levels increased in epithelium and stroma during the implantation period. In postimplantation, PR levels were restricted to the stromal compartment of the endometrium.[23] The differential expression of ER and PR in the uterus during the implantation period in the mouse can be partially explained by investigating the mechanisms by which the expression of these receptors is regulated.

ERα and PR levels are regulated in part by their ligands. Furthermore, these receptors serve to regulate the expression of each other.[27–29] In general, ERα positively regulates the expression of itself, as well as PR. On the other hand, PR serves to repress its own expression and the expression of ERα. However, *in vivo* analyses of the regulation of ERα and PR levels reveal a more complex hierarchy of regulation that demonstrates a compartmental specific level of regulation of these receptors by each other. Tibbetts and coworkers investigated the effects of exogenous estrogen and progesterone on the expression of ERα and PR in the compartments of the uterus of ovariectomized mice.[26] They demonstrated that exogenous estrogen decreases levels of ERα in endometrial stroma and glandular epithelium, while increasing the levels of ERα in luminal epithelium and myometrium. Estrogen also differentially regulated the expression of PR. Exogenous estrogen decreased PR levels in luminal epithelium, while increasing levels of PR in the stroma and myometrium. When estrogen administration was supplemented with progesterone, progesterone repressed expression of ERα in the myometrium, while increasing expression of ERα in the glandular epithelium. In general, progesterone repressed PR expression in all compartments.

The direct versus indirect effects can in part explain the differential expression of ERα and PR in the different uterine compartments that the receptors may exert on each other. Tissue reconstitution experiments using wild-type and ERα knockout stroma and epithelium have demonstrated that estrogen regulation of uterine epithelial gene expression is dependent upon both stromal and epithelial ERα.[30] However, uterine epithelial cell proliferation[31] and repression of the uterine epithelial PR[32] are mediated by stroma ERα. Therefore, estrogen regulates the expression of growth factor(s) that can coordinate the expression of genes in the uterine epithelium.[33,34] This would explain how ERα can stimulate the expression of PR in the uterine stroma and, by an indirect pathway, inhibit PR levels in the epithelium. A summary of the compartmentalization of ERα signaling is shown in FIGURE 3. The generation of mice with the ablation of the steroid hormone receptors has aided the above investigation. These animals have served to define the role of the receptors in uterine biology and will serve as tools to identify the pathways by which these receptors regulate uterine biology.

αERKO AND βERKO MICE

The genes for both the ERα and ERβ have been ablated in mice using ES cell technology.[5–7] The mice resulting from these ablations are called the αERKO and βERKO mice, respectively. The analysis of the uterine phenotype in these mice has confirmed the expression analysis that ERα is the dominant ER in the uterus. ERα is expressed at significantly higher levels in the mouse uterus and the phenotype of

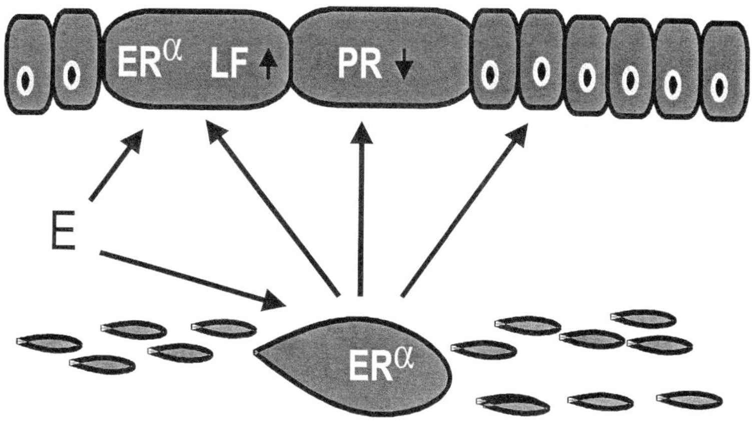

FIGURE 3. Mechanism of action of estrogen in the uterus. Estrogen regulates uterine gene expression (LF, for lactoferrin) in the epithelium directly through stimulation of the uterine epithelial ER as well as indirectly by the ER in the stroma regulating growth factor production, which activates epithelial gene expression. Estrogen, through stromal ER, stimulates growth factor(s) that can regulate repression of PR and uterine epithelial cell hyperplasia.

the αERKO mouse was a hypoplastic uterus with decreased expression of estrogen-regulated genes.[5,7] The αERKO mouse showed a decrease in uterine proliferative response,[31] regulation of estrogen-responsive genes,[30,35] uterine response to growth factors,[33,36] and repression of PR in response to estrogen stimulation.[32] The role of ERα in implantation was studied by investigating the induction of the decidualization reaction in these mice. The induction of decidualization of the uterine stroma has been shown to be dependent upon progesterone and not estrogen.[37] Since PR levels are regulated by ERα, a role for ER regulation of decidualization via the regulation of PR was possible. However, although ER regulated PR expression in the mouse uterus, analysis of the decidual reaction in these mice demonstrated that it was not required for PR regulation of gene expression[38] or decidualization expression.[38,39]

Ablation of the ERβ showed no obvious alteration in uterine morphology, although the mice demonstrated reduced fertility.[6,7] ERβ and ERα differ most in their amino terminus, which is responsible for activation of target gene transcription.[40] ERβ has less of an ability to activate gene expression and may play a role in dampening the response of ER target genes to ERα regulation.[41] Analysis of estrogen-responsive genes in the βERKO mouse showed that these mice had an increased response in uterine hyperplasia and gene expression in response to estrogen stimulation.[42] Thus, ERβ may play a role in antagonizing the effect of ERα stimulation of gene expression.[43] However, analysis of compound βERKO and αERKO mice indicate that ERβ acts as a partial agonist of ERα activity since the combined αERKO and βERKO mouse showed an increased hypoplasia of the mouse uterus.[7] Therefore, levels of ERα and ERβ may act coordinately to ensure the appropriate regulation of uterine growth and gene expression in response to estrogen stimulation.

PRKO MOUSE

PR signaling is required for embryonic implantation and antagonizes the hyperplasia and inflammatory response induced by estrogen stimulation. The mouse PR consists of two isoforms, PRA and PRB. PRB consists of an additional 160 amino acids on the amino terminus of PRA. The two isoforms are a result of differential usage of two in-frame translation initiation sites.[4] Both isoforms of the murine PR gene have been ablated[8] and, using site-directed mutagenesis in ES cells, the PRA isoform has been specifically ablated.[9] These mice have been termed PRKO and PRAKO, respectively. The PRKO mouse demonstrated that PR regulates all aspects of female reproduction. In the uterus, ablation of PR rendered the uterus incapable of undergoing a decidual reaction. When the PRKO mice were placed under chronic estrogen stimulation, increased hyperplasia and an inflammatory response were observed.[43] Ablation of PR validated the antiestrogen effects of PR signaling. The PRAKO mice were also incapable of eliciting a decidual response to steroid stimulation, demonstrating that the PRA isoform was responsible for the regulation of uterine stroma differentiation during implantation. Hence, the PRKO and PRAKO have been useful tools in validating the role of PR in the mouse uterus.[9]

THE SRC FAMILY OF COACTIVATORS

Steroid hormone regulation of uterine gene expression is also modulated by the interaction of coactivators with steroid hormone receptors. A family of steroid hormone receptor coactivators, SRCs, have been identified, consisting of three members to date. The first member of the SRC family to be identified was SRC-1. SRC-1 was identified by a yeast two-hybrid screen for interactions with the LBD of the PR.[44] Two other members of this family have been identified: SRC-2/GRIP-1/TIF-2[45,46] and SRC-3/pCIP/ACTR/RAC-3/AIB-1/TRAM-1.[47–51] These coactivators share a 40% sequence homology and contain a common motif, the nuclear receptor box that mediates the binding of these coactivators to the ligand-bound nuclear hormone receptor. The coactivators mediate the link between the nuclear receptors and the transcriptional machinery, and also have histone acetylase activity, which acts to remodel the chromatin for enhanced gene expression.[19] Functional significance for these coactivators is seen in human diseases and *in vivo* analysis of the function of these molecules. As with the steroid hormone receptors, *in vitro* analyses of these coactivators have defined their functional domains and the potential functions of these proteins. *In vivo* ablation of these genes through homologous recombination in embryonic stem cells has allowed establishment of animal models for the investigation of this family of proteins in a developmental and physiologically regulated system. Mice homozygous for the ablation of SRC-1 were fertile and viable. This was not surprising, considering the overlap in function and expression patterns among these coactivators. However, the SRC-1-null mice did manifest a uterine phenotype. The SRC-1 –/– mouse uterus showed a decreased growth in response to decidual stimuli when stimulated with estrogen and progesterone.[52] Thus, this coactivator is responsible for modulating the actions of PR in the mouse uterus.

FUTURE RESEARCH IN THE INVESTIGATION OF STEROID HORMONE REGULATION OF UTERINE PHYSIOLOGY

The various knockout mouse models for the steroid hormone receptors have served as valuable reagents for the investigation of uterine biology. However, there is a significant limitation to these models. First, the ablation of the steroid hormone receptors by current conventional gene targeting technology ablates the expression of these genes in all tissues. The phenotype of the αERKO, βERKO, PRKO, and PRAKO is not specific to the uterus. These animals show defects in neuronal, endocrine, ovarian, immunologic, as well as uterine physiology. Second, as discussed earlier, it has been demonstrated that uterine function of these receptors is dependent upon the uterine compartment in which these receptors are expressed. Therefore, to fully investigate the role of these receptors in uterine biology, ablation of the steroid hormone receptors in specific compartments of the uterus would help define the role of these receptors in uterine epithelial, stromal, and myometrial function without disrupting the endocrine milieu of the animal. Current technology using Cre recombinase allows for the cell-specific ablation of genes.[53,54] In this system, specific loxP, DNA sequences, which are recognized by these recombinases, are inserted around regulatory regions of the PR and ER genes using site-directed mutagenesis and homologous recombination in ES cells. Genes in which these sites have been inserted are termed floxed, flanked by lox P, genes. Mice with these floxed genes are then bred to transgenic mice expressing the recombinases under the control of a tissue-specific promoter. The sequences surrounded by the loxP are then edited by the activity of the respective recombinase. Establishment of such a system would facilitate the definition of the role of these receptors in the uterus. The limiting factor in this research is not the ability to generate floxed genes. This technology is relatively straightforward. The limiting factor in this research is the identification of promoters that will direct Cre expression in a uterine compartmental specific fashion with sufficient level of expression to induce recombination. To date, no such transgenic system exists. This factor has limited the use of transgenic technology to investigate the role of regulator proteins in regulating uterine biology.

HIGH-DENSITY MICROARRAY EXPRESSION ANALYSIS

The generation of knockout mouse models for the steroid hormone receptors allows the opportunity to investigate the molecular mechanisms that are regulated by these proteins in a genetically uniform and physiologically regulated system. Limited information is available describing the target genes and pathways regulated by the steroid hormone receptors. Identification of how the steroid hormone receptors alter gene expression in specific hormone target tissues is the first step in defining the molecular pathways regulated by these proteins. These animals can now be used to identify which physiological pathways these proteins regulate. Over the last decade, quantum leaps have been made in the techniques available to detect differential gene expression. The field has progressed from simple blot hybridization analysis,[55] subtractive hybridization library screening,[56] and differential display PCR,[57] allowing for the identification of a limited number of target genes. Currently, technologies such as serial amplification of gene expression, SAGE analysis,[58] and high-density microarray or "chip" analysis[59] allow for the identification of a large number of target genes for a given pathway. The high-density microarray technology has benefited from coevolution of the technology to spot, hybridize, and assay thousands of clones on a small glass slide with the ability to sequence whole genomes. High-density microarray analyses have already been used to identify differential gene expression in *Arabidopsis*,[60] *Saccharomyces*,[61] *Drosophila*,[62] mice,[63–67] and humans.[68–74] This technology has been used to identify differential gene expression in response to serum,[68] oncogene expression,[70] and hormone stimulation.[66] Microarray technology has been applied to the investigation of the processes of development,[63,64] aging,[65] and cancer.[72,73,75] The advantage of this technology is that large numbers of candidate target genes can be assayed to determine patterns of differential gene expression. Further, by the use of appropriate statistical analysis, the differentially expressed genes can be grouped according to function. Thus, expression patterns for a given cluster of genes can associate these genes with regulatory functions, even though the biochemical activity of the protein encoded for the gene has not yet been identified.[76] The field of high-density microarray analysis is relatively new and rapidly evolving. This approach will allow for the identification of the pathways regulated by the steroid hormones. Also, this approach may allow for the identification of genes that are expressed in specific compartments of the uterus and facilitate the establishment of transgenic models for the investigation of uterine biology.

ACKNOWLEDGMENTS

This research was supported by the NICHD/NIH through cooperative agreement [No. U54 HD07495-26/30] as part of the Specialized Cooperative Centers Program in Reproduction Research. We would also like to acknowledge the assistance of Janet DeMayo and John Ellsworth in preparation of this manuscript.

REFERENCES

1. O'Malley, B.W. & M.J. Tsai. 1992. Molecular pathways of steroid receptor action. Biol. Reprod. **46:** 163–167.
2. Enmark, E. & J.A. Gustafsson. 1999. Oestrogen receptors—an overview. J. Intern. Med. **246:** 133–138.
3. Lydon, J.P. *et al.* 1996. Reproductive phenotypes of the progesterone receptor null mutant mouse. J. Steroid Biochem. Mol. Biol. **56:** 67–77.
4. Conneely, O.M. *et al.* 1989. The chicken progesterone receptor A and B isoforms are products of an alternate translation initiation event. J. Biol. Chem. **264:** 14062–14064.
5. Lubahn, D.B. *et al.* 1993. Alteration of reproductive function, but not prenatal sexual development after insertional disruption of the mouse estrogen receptor gene. Proc. Natl. Acad. Sci. U.S.A. **90:** 11162–11166.
6. Krege, J.H. *et al.* 1998. Generation and reproductive phenotypes of mice lacking estrogen receptor beta. Proc. Natl. Acad. Sci. U.S.A. **95:** 15677–15684.
7. Dupont, S. *et al.* 2000. Effect of single and compound knockouts of estrogen receptors alpha (ERα) and beta (ERβ) on mouse reproductive phenotypes. Development **127:** 4277–4291.
8. Lydon, J.P. *et al.* 1995. Mice lacking progesterone receptor exhibit pleiotropic reproductive abnormalities. Genes Dev. **9:** 2266–2278.

9. MULAC-JERICEVIC, B. *et al.* 2000. Subgroup of reproductive functions of progesterone mediated by progesterone receptor-B isoform. Science **289:** 1751–1754.
10. TSAI, M.J. & B.W. O'MALLEY. 1994. Molecular mechanisms of action of steroid/thyroid receptor superfamily members. Annu. Rev. Biochem. **63:** 451–486.
11. EVANS, R.M. 1988. The steroid and thyroid hormone receptor superfamily. Science **240:** 889–895.
12. MANGELSDORF, D.J. *et al.* 1995. The nuclear receptor superfamily: the second decade. Cell **83:** 835–839.
13. PERLMANN, T. & R.M. EVANS. 1997. Nuclear receptors in Sicily: all in the famiglia. Cell **90:** 391–397.
14. PARKER, M.G. 1998. Transcriptional activation by oestrogen receptors. Biochem. Soc. Symp. **63:** 45–50.
15. RIBEIRO, R.C., P.J. KUSHNER & J.D. BAXTER. 1995. The nuclear hormone receptor gene superfamily. Annu. Rev. Med. **46:** 443–453.
16. POWER, R.F. *et al.* 1991. Dopamine activation of an orphan of the steroid receptor superfamily. Science **252:** 1546–1548.
17. POWER, R.F., O.M. CONNEELY & B.W. O'MALLEY. 1992. New insights into activation of the steroid hormone receptor superfamily. Trends Pharmacol. Sci. **13:** 318–323.
18. MCKENNA, N.J., R.B. LANZ & B.W. O'MALLEY. 1999. Nuclear receptor coregulators: cellular and molecular biology. Endocr. Rev. **20:** 321–344.
19. MCKENNA, N.J. *et al.* 1999. Nuclear receptor coactivators: multiple enzymes, multiple complexes, multiple functions. J. Steroid Biochem. Mol. Biol. **69:** 3–12.
20. NAWAZ, Z. *et al.* 1999. The Angelman syndrome–associated protein, E6-AP, is a coactivator for the nuclear hormone receptor superfamily. Mol. Cell. Biol. **19:** 1182–1189.
21. CAPECCHI, M.R. 1989. Altering the genome by homologous recombination. Science **244:** 1288–1292.
22. COUSE, J.F. *et al.* 1997. Tissue distribution and quantitative analysis of estrogen receptor-alpha (ERα) and estrogen receptor-beta (ERβ) messenger ribonucleic acid in the wild-type and ERα-knockout mouse. Endocrinology **138:** 4613–4621.
23. TAN, J. *et al.* 1999. Differential uterine expression of estrogen and progesterone receptors correlates with uterine preparation for implantation and decidualization in the mouse. Endocrinology **140:** 5310–5321.
24. SHYAMALA, G., W. SCHNEIDER & D. SCHOTT. 1990. Developmental regulation of murine mammary progesterone receptor gene expression. Endocrinology **126:** 2882–2889.
25. MURAKAMI, R. *et al.* 1990. Distribution of progestin-binding cells in estrogen-treated and untreated neonatal mouse uterus and oviduct: autoradiographic study with [^{125}I]progestin. Histochemistry **94:** 155–159.
26. TIBBETTS, T.A. *et al.* 1998. Mutual and intercompartmental regulation of estrogen receptor and progesterone receptor expression in the mouse uterus. Biol. Reprod. **59:** 1143–1152.
27. VERHAGE, H.G. *et al.* 1983. Subcellular compartmentalization of the progesterone receptor in cat uteri following the acute administration of progesterone. Biol. Reprod. **28:** 545–550.
28. WEST, N.B., H.G. VERHAGE & R.M. BRENNER. 1977. Changes in nuclear estradiol receptor and cell structure during estrous cycles and pregnancy in the oviduct and uterus of cats. Biol. Reprod. **17:** 138–143.
29. WEST, N.B. & R.M. BRENNER. 1985. Progesterone-mediated suppression of estradiol receptors in cynomolgus macaque cervix, endometrium, and oviduct during sequential estradiol-progesterone treatment. J. Steroid Biochem. **22:** 29–37.
30. BUCHANAN, D.L. *et al.* 1999. Tissue compartment–specific estrogen receptor-alpha participation in the mouse uterine epithelial secretory response. Endocrinology **140:** 484–491.
31. COOKE, P.S. *et al.* 1997. Stromal estrogen receptors mediate mitogenic effects of estradiol on uterine epithelium. Proc. Natl. Acad. Sci. U.S.A. **94:** 6535–6540.
32. KURITA, T. *et al.* 2001. Regulation of progesterone receptors and decidualization in uterine stroma of the estrogen receptor-alpha knockout mouse. Biol. Reprod. **64:** 272–283.
33. HOM, Y.K. *et al.* 1998. Uterine and vaginal organ growth requires epidermal growth factor receptor signaling from stroma. Endocrinology **139:** 913–921.

34. BUCHANAN, D.L. *et al.* 1998. Role of stromal and epithelial estrogen receptors in vaginal epithelial proliferation, stratification, and cornification. Endocrinology **139:** 4345–4352.
35. DAS, S.K. *et al.* 1997. Estrogenic responses in estrogen receptor-alpha deficient mice reveal a distinct estrogen signaling pathway. Proc. Natl. Acad. Sci. U.S.A. **94:** 12786–12791.
36. CURTIS, S.W. *et al.* 1996. Physiological coupling of growth factor and steroid receptor signaling pathways: estrogen receptor knockout mice lack estrogen-like response to epidermal growth factor. Proc. Natl. Acad. Sci. U.S.A. **93:** 12626–12634.
37. FINN, C.A. 1966. Endocrine control of endometrial sensitivity during the induction of the decidual cell reaction in the mouse. J. Endocrinol. **36:** 239–248.
38. CURTIS, S.W. *et al.* 1999. Disruption of estrogen signaling does not prevent progesterone action in the estrogen receptor alpha knockout mouse uterus. Proc. Natl. Acad. Sci. U.S.A. **96:** 3646–3651.
39. PARIA, B.C. *et al.* 1999. Uterine decidual response occurs in estrogen receptor-alpha-deficient mice. Endocrinology **140:** 2704–2710.
40. DELAUNAY, F. *et al.* 2000. Functional differences between the amino-terminal domains of estrogen receptors alpha and beta. Mol. Pharmacol. **58:** 584–590.
41. BARKHEM, T. *et al.* 1998. Differential response of estrogen receptor alpha and estrogen receptor beta to partial estrogen agonists/antagonists. Mol. Pharmacol. **54:** 105–112.
42. WEIHUA, Z. *et al.* 2000. Estrogen receptor (ER) β, a modulator of ERα in the uterus. Proc. Natl. Acad. Sci. U.S.A. **97:** 5936–5951.
43. TIBBETTS, T.A., O.M. CONNEELY & B.W. O'MALLEY. 1999. Progesterone via its receptor antagonizes the pro-inflammatory activity of estrogen in the mouse uterus. Biol. Reprod. **60:** 1158–1165.
44. ONATE, S.A. *et al.* 1995. Sequence and characterization of a coactivator for the steroid hormone receptor superfamily. Science **270:** 1354–1357.
45. HONG, H. *et al.* 1997. GRIP1, a transcriptional coactivator for the AF-2 transactivation domain of steroid, thyroid, retinoid, and vitamin D receptors. Mol. Cell. Biol. **17:** 2735–2744.
46. HONG, H. *et al.* 1996. GRIP1, a novel mouse protein that serves as a transcriptional coactivator in yeast for the hormone binding domains of steroid receptors. Proc. Natl. Acad. Sci. U.S.A. **93:** 4948–4952.
47. CHEN, H. *et al.* 1997. Nuclear receptor coactivator ACTR is a novel histone acetyltransferase and forms a multimeric activation complex with P/CAF and CBP/p300. Cell **90:** 569–580.
48. LI, H., P.J. GOMES & J.D. CHEN. 1997. RAC3, a steroid/nuclear receptor–associated coactivator that is related to SRC-1 and TIF2. Proc. Natl. Acad. Sci. U.S.A. **94:** 8479–8484.
49. ANZICK, S.L. *et al.* 1997. AIB1, a steroid receptor coactivator amplified in breast and ovarian cancer. Science **277:** 965–968.
50. TAKESHITA, A. *et al.* 1997. TRAM-1, a novel 160-kDa thyroid hormone receptor activator molecule, exhibits distinct properties from steroid receptor coactivator-1. J. Biol. Chem. **272:** 27629–27634.
51. SUEN, C.S. *et al.* 1998. A transcriptional coactivator, steroid receptor coactivator-3, selectively augments steroid receptor transcriptional activity. J. Biol. Chem. **273:** 27645–27653.
52. XU, J. *et al.* 1998. Partial hormone resistance in mice with disruption of the steroid receptor coactivator-1 (SRC-1) gene. Science **279:** 1922–1925.
53. O'GORMAN, S., D.T. FOX & G.M. WAHL. 1991. Recombinase-mediated gene activation and site-specific integration in mammalian cells. Science **251:** 1351–1355.
54. GU, H. *et al.* 1994. Deletion of a DNA polymerase beta gene segment in T cells using cell type–specific gene targeting. Science **265:** 103–106.
55. THOMAS, P.S. 1980. Hybridization of denatured RNA and small DNA fragments transferred to nitrocellulose. Proc. Natl. Acad. Sci. U.S.A. **77:** 5201–5205.
56. SCHWEINFEST, C.W. *et al.* 1990. Subtraction hybridization cDNA libraries from colon carcinoma and hepatic cancer. Genet. Anal. Tech. Appl. **7:** 64–70.
57. LIANG, P. & A.B. PARDEE. 1992. Differential display of eukaryotic messenger RNA by means of the polymerase chain reaction. Science **257:** 967–971.

58. VELCULESCU, V.E. *et al.* 1995. Serial analysis of gene expression. Science **270:** 484–487.
59. WATSON, S.J. & H. AKIL. 1999. Gene chips and arrays revealed: a primer on their power and their uses. Biol. Psychiatry **45:** 533–543.
60. SCHENA, M. 1996. Genome analysis with gene expression microarrays. Bioessays **18:** 427–431.
61. SPELLMAN, P.T. *et al.* 1998. Comprehensive identification of cell cycle–regulated genes of the yeast *Saccharomyces cerevisiae* by microarray hybridization. Mol. Biol. Cell **9:** 3273–3297.
62. BRYANT, Z. *et al.* 1999. Characterization of differentially expressed genes in purified *Drosophila* follicle cells: toward a general strategy for cell type–specific developmental analysis. Proc. Natl. Acad. Sci. U.S.A. **96:** 5559–5564.
63. TANAKA, T.S. *et al.* 2000. Genome-wide expression profiling of mid-gestation placenta and embryo using a 15,000 mouse developmental cDNA microarray. Proc. Natl. Acad. Sci. U.S.A. **97:** 9127–9132.
64. GRIMMOND, S. *et al.* 2000. Sexually dimorphic expression of protease nexin-1 and vanin-1 in the developing mouse gonad prior to overt differentiation suggests a role in mammalian sexual development. Hum. Mol. Genet. **9:** 1553–1560.
65. LEE, C.K. *et al.* 1999. Gene expression profile of aging and its retardation by caloric restriction. Science **285:** 1390–1393.
66. FENG, X. *et al.* 2000. Thyroid hormone regulation of hepatic genes *in vivo* detected by complementary DNA microarray. Mol. Endocrinol. **14:** 947–955.
67. WEBB, G.C. *et al.* 2000. Expression profiling of pancreatic beta cells: glucose regulation of secretory and metabolic pathway genes. Proc. Natl. Acad. Sci. U.S.A. **97:** 5773–5778.
68. IYER, V.R. *et al.* 1999. The transcriptional program in the response of human fibroblasts to serum. Science **283:** 83–87.
69. ICHIKAWA, J.K. *et al.* 2000. Interaction of *Pseudomonas aeruginosa* with epithelial cells: identification of differentially regulated genes by expression microarray analysis of human cDNAs. Proc. Natl. Acad. Sci. U.S.A. **97:** 9659–9664.
70. COLLER, H.A. *et al.* 2000. Expression analysis with oligonucleotide microarrays reveals that MYC regulates genes involved in growth, cell cycle, signaling, and adhesion. Proc. Natl. Acad. Sci. U.S.A. **97:** 3260–3265.
71. COLANTUONI, C. *et al.* 2000. High throughput analysis of gene expression in the human brain. J. Neurosci. Res. **59:** 1–10.
72. PEROU, C.M. *et al.* 1999. Distinctive gene expression patterns in human mammary epithelial cells and breast cancers. Proc. Natl. Acad. Sci. U.S.A. **96:** 9212–9217.
73. PEROU, C.M. *et al.* 2000. Molecular portraits of human breast tumours. Nature **406:** 747–752.
74. WANG, Y. *et al.* 1999. Identification of the genes responsive to etoposide-induced apoptosis: application of DNA chip technology. FEBS Lett. **26:** 445.
75. MOCH, H. *et al.* 1999. Identification of prognostic parameters for renal cell carcinoma by cDNA arrays and cell chips. Verh. Dtsch. Ges. Pathol. **83:** 225–232.
76. EISEN, M.B. *et al.* 1998. Cluster analysis and display of genome-wide expression patterns. Proc. Natl. Acad. Sci. U.S.A. **95:** 14863–14868.

Premenstrual and Menstrual Changes in the Macaque and Human Endometrium

Relevance to Endometriosis

ROBERT M. BRENNER,[a] NIHAR R. NAYAK,[a] OV D. SLAYDEN,[a] HILARY O. D. CRITCHLEY,[b] AND RODNEY W. KELLY[b]

[a]*Oregon Regional Primate Research Center, Oregon Health Sciences University, Beaverton, Oregon 97006, USA*

[b]*Centre for Reproductive Biology, University of Edinburgh, Edinburgh, EH3 9ET United Kingdom*

Abstract: According to current theory, endometriosis is initiated during retrograde menstruation when menstrual fragments flow out of the fimbriated end of the fallopian tubes and become established on the ovarian surface or other sites in the peritoneal cavity. In recent years, new data have accumulated on the properties of menstruating tissue itself, and several laboratories agree that this tissue is rich in matrix metalloproteinases (MMPs) that may facilitate endometriotic implantation. Recently, we found that vascular endothelial growth factor (VEGF) and its receptor VEGFR-2 (KDR) were dramatically upregulated in the stromal cells of the superficial endometrial zones by progesterone (P) withdrawal during the premenstrual phase. A unique role of VEGF at this stage of the cycle may be to stimulate MMP expression in stromal cells because VEGF, KDR, and MMPs were all coordinately induced in these cells in the superficial zone of the primate endometrium by P withdrawal. The rich content of MMPs and VEGF in the menstrual fragments could facilitate attachment and angiogenesis of menstrual fragments in ectopic sites. In addition, a variety of chemokines, cytokines, and cellular regulators are induced by P withdrawal in the premenstrual human endometrium. These include NFκB, prostaglandins, interleukin-8 (IL-8), cyclooxygenase-2 (COX-2), and monocyte chemotactic peptide-1 (MCP-1), among others. The perivascular expression of several of these factors may facilitate the rapid invasion of leukocytes into the endometrium, especially in the superficial zones. Consequently, menstrual fragments may be rich in IL-8 and MCP-1, both of which would add to the angiogenic potential of such fragments in ectopic sites. In sum, menstrual tissue is rich in VEGF, KDR, MMPs, leukocytes, chemokines, cytokines, and prostaglandins, all factors that may facilitate attachment and angiogenesis when menstrual fragments exit from the tubes and implant on pelvic sites. Additional research on these and other factors in premenstrual and menstrual endometrium may deepen our understanding of both the establishment and progression of this debilitating disease.

Keywords: endometrium; menstruation; progesterone withdrawal; VEGF; KDR; MMPs; prostaglandins; angiogenesis

Address for correspondence: Robert M. Brenner, Oregon Regional Primate Research Center, 505 NW 185th Avenue, Beaverton, OR 97006. Voice: 503-690-5331; fax: 503-690-5563.
BrennerR@OHSU.edu

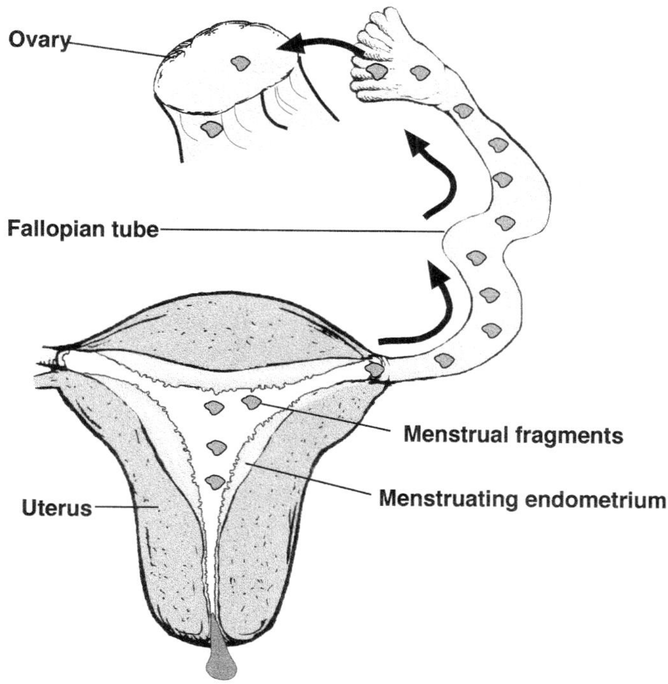

FIGURE 1. Initiation of endometriosis. This schematic drawing, based on the Sampson hypothesis of retrograde menstruation, shows fragments of menstruating endometrium flowing through the fallopian tubes and implanting on the ovary or other pelvic viscera. Drawing by Joel Ito and Robert M. Brenner (ORPRC).

INTRODUCTION

According to the Sampson hypothesis,[1] endometriosis is established during retrograde menstruation, when menstrual fragments flow out of the fimbriated end of the fallopian tubes and implant on the ovary and other peritoneal sites. This process is illustrated schematically in FIGURE 1. Internal bleeding in ovarian lesions can result in large ovarian cysts filled with trapped blood, so-called chocolate cysts, and repeated retrograde menstruation can lead to the spread of numerous endometriotic implants throughout the pelvic cavity. Endometriotic lesions are presumed to bleed periodically and stimulate inflammatory processes that lead to adhesions between the uterus, the ovary, and the pelvic viscera. The lesions regress during menopause and the condition is generally considered to be an estrogen-dependent disease. GnRH agonists are currently used[2] to block ovulation and suppress systemic estrogen levels, and this suppresses the growth of lesions and the associated pain. However, the suppression of estrogen by GnRH treatment leads to side effects resembling menopausal symptoms, such as vaginal atrophy, hot flushes, and bone loss. Add-back treatment with low-dose estrogen is used to ameliorate some of these symptoms,[3] but lesions often reoccur once GnRH therapy is stopped. Clearly, improved therapies are needed. Because endometriosis is presumed to originate from menstrual fragments, an increased understanding of the properties of premenstrual and menstrual tissues could lead to improvements in the treatment of this disease. This review focuses on our current understanding of premenstrual-menstrual processes in the human and nonhuman primate endometrium, and highlights their relevance to the establishment and development of endometriosis.

As is well known, the endometrium proliferates during the follicular phase under the influence of estradiol (E) and is prepared for implantation by the action of progesterone (P) during the luteal phase. By mid-luteal phase, the endometrium is fully primed for implantation. However, if pregnancy fails and the corpus luteum regresses, both P and E levels fall precipitously. It is the decline in P, though, not the decline in E, that is the physiological signal for menstruation: treatment with E at the end of the cycle cannot block menses.[4,5] The first few days after P withdrawal comprise the premenstrual phase, and the tissue that is sloughed off during the succeeding menstrual phase consists typically of just the superficial endometrial zones. The proliferative phase begins when the surface of the remaining endometrium heals and the surviving glands and stroma begin a new cycle of E-dependent, mitotic activity.[5–7]

The cyclic changes in estrogen receptor (ER) and progestin receptor (PR) levels in the human and nonhuman primate endometrium have been fully described elsewhere.[8–14] During the late secretory phase, in the superficial zones, the only steroid receptor that is strongly detected by immunocytochemistry is PR, and its expression is confined to the stromal cells, including the perivascular stromal cells associated with the spiral arterioles. The glands are essentially negative for ER and PR, except in the basalis zone, which continues to show strong expression of both ER and PR.[14] Thus, when the luteal phase ends and P levels fall, the only cells in the superficial zones that could "sense" this decline and respond to it directly are the PR-positive stromal and perivascular cells. Without doubt, these are the cells that initiate the menstrual cascade.

THE MENSTRUAL CASCADE

Premenstrual Increases in Vascular Endothelial Growth Factor (VEGF) and Its Receptor VEGFR-2 (KDR)

The menstrual cascade is a series of biochemical and cellular changes occurring primarily within the superficial zones. An early event is vasoconstriction of the spiral arterioles,[15] probably induced by increased expression of prostaglandins,[16] which is presumed to induce ischemic hypoxia in the superficial zones. This induced hypoxia leads to a marked upregulation of vascular endothelial growth factor (VEGF) in women.[17] VEGF is also dramatically upregulated premenstrually in the glands and stroma of the macaque endometrium.[18] VEGF may be expressed by various cell types and generally interacts with several receptors, including KDR and VEGFR-1 (FLT-1), which are located on the membranes of endothelial cells.[19,20] Of great interest, fibroblasts and smooth muscle cells can also express VEGF receptors.[21–23]

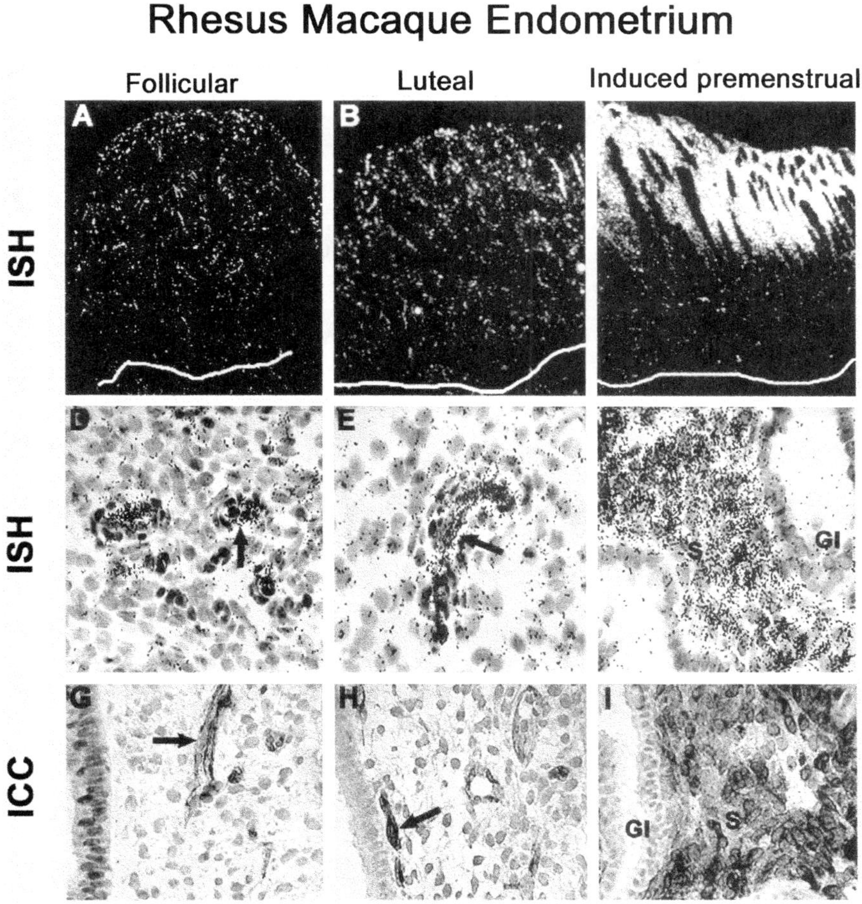

FIGURE 2. Rhesus macaque endometrium: expression of KDR. All magnifications are originals. Modified from Nayak *et al.*[24] Upper row: Dark field images of *in situ* hybridization of KDR (×25). Middle row: Bright field images of *in situ* hybridization of KDR (×312). Bottom row: Bright field images of immunocytochemistry for KDR (×312). First column: Induced follicular phase—KDR is only expressed in vascular endothelium. Second column: Induced luteal phase—KDR is only expressed in endothelium. Third column: Two days after P withdrawal—KDR is dramatically upregulated in the stroma of the superficial zone.

In a recent study, we examined the regulation of endometrial KDR at key times during the cycle in both women and macaques.[24] The human subjects in this study were fertile women with regular cycles undergoing hysterectomy for benign indications during the proliferative phase ($n = 4$), secretory phase ($n = 5$), and premenstrual phase ($n = 3$). Full-thickness endometrial samples were obtained that included superficial and basal endometrium plus the endometrial-myometrial junction. Tissues were cryosectioned and processed for immunocytochemistry (ICC), used for *in situ*

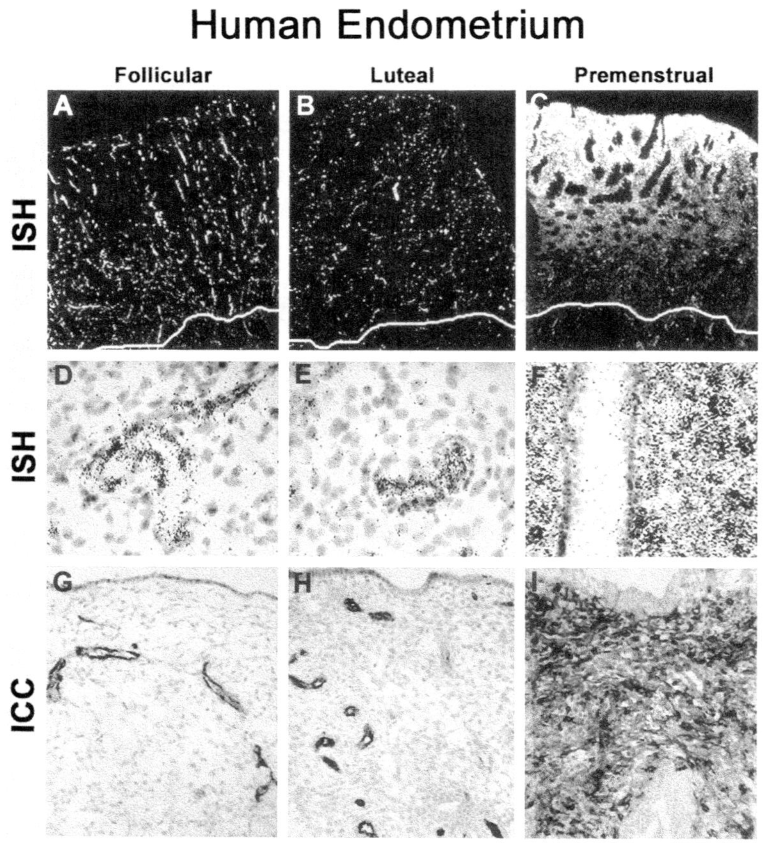

FIGURE 3. Human endometrium: expression of KDR. Modified from Nayak *et al.*[24] Upper row: Dark field images of *in situ* hybridization of KDR (×25). Middle row: Bright field images of *in situ* hybridization of KDR (×312). Bottom row: Bright field images of immunocytochemistry for KDR (×312). First column: Follicular phase—KDR is only expressed in vascular endothelium. Second column: Luteal phase—KDR is only expressed in endothelium. Third column: Premenstrual—KDR is dramatically upregulated in the stroma of the superficial zone.

hybridization (ISH), saved for biochemical studies, or fixed and embedded for identification of leukocyte subpopulations by ICC.

The experimental animals were adult female rhesus macaques (*Macaca mulatta*) under the care of the Division of Animal Resources of the Oregon Regional Primate Research Center (ORPRC). Animals were ovariectomized and treated sequentially with E and P Silastic implants to create artificial menstrual cycles as described previously.[25] To induce menstruation, P was removed and the E implant was left in place. Endometrial tissue samples were collected by hysterectomy at 2 days after P withdrawal and processed for ICC, ISH, or Northern blot analysis.[24]

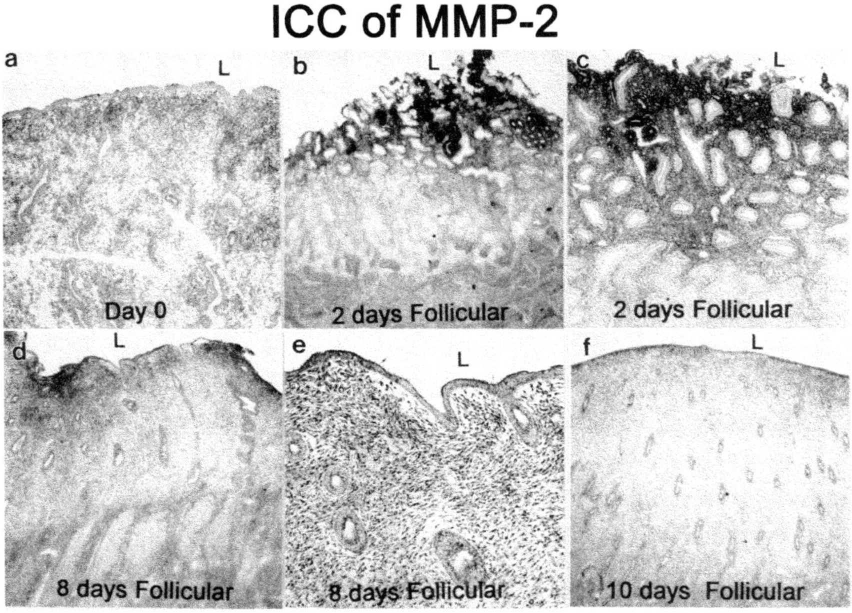

FIGURE 4. MMP-2 immunostaining in endometrium during an induced menstrual cycle. L = lumen. All magnifications are originals. Modified from Rudolph-Owen *et al.*[25] **(a)** Day 0. At the end of the luteal phase, MMP-2 staining is low (×25). **(b)** Two days follicular. Two days after P is withdrawn, MMP-2 staining intensity increases dramatically in the superficial zone stroma of the endometrium. The glands are negative (×25). **(c)** Two days follicular. At a higher magnification, variations in staining intensity are evident in the superficial zone, but the glands are negative and the deeper layers of the endometrium are unstained. Spiral arteries are intensely stained (see FIG. 8) (×50). **(d)** Eight days follicular. During the proliferative phase, only low levels of MMP-2 staining remain (×25). **(e)** Eight days follicular. At a higher magnification, the MMP-2 staining is evident only in the stroma (×50). **(f)** Ten days follicular. In the late follicular phase, MMP-2 staining is very low.

KDR was dramatically increased in the *stromal cells* of the superficial endometrial zones during the premenstrual phase in both the human and macaque endometrium. At all other times in the cycle, KDR expression was confined to the vascular endothelium. The increase in stromal cell KDR was detectable by Northern blot analysis, ISH, and ICC, and was cell-specific, zone-specific, cycle-phase-specific, and VEGF-receptor-type-specific—that is, it only occurred during the premenstrual/menstrual phase; did not occur in glandular epithelium, endothelium, or stromal cells of the deepest endometrial zones; and was not observed for VEGF-receptor type 1. As noted above, we have shown that the ligand, VEGF, is also dramatically upregulated premenstrually in the macaque endometrium in both the glands and the stroma. The above ICC and ISH findings are illustrated in FIGURES 2 and 3.

In the macaque[26] and human endometrium,[27] various matrix metalloproteinases (MMPs) are also transiently induced in the same superficial zone stromal cells by P

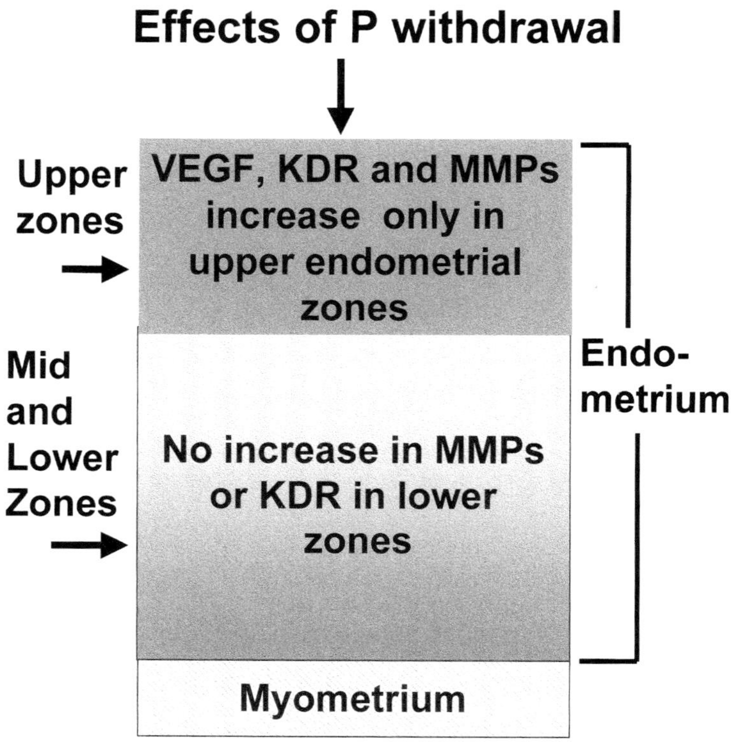

FIGURE 5. Effects of P withdrawal. Diagram illustrating that P withdrawal increases VEGF, KDR, and MMP expression dramatically in the superficial endometrial zones.

withdrawal (see FIG. 4). Once activated, various MMPs can destroy the extracellular matrix that holds the stromal and glandular cells together. Of great interest, VEGF has been reported to upregulate MMP expression in various cell types.[21,28] Consequently, we hypothesize that VEGF-KDR interactions play some role in endometrial MMP expression because the same cells express VEGF, KDR, and MMPs all at the same time in the superficial zones of the primate endometrium. In this instance, the physiological role of VEGF, acting through stromal cell KDR to elevate stromal MMPs, would be a nonangiogenic one as the tissue expressing these factors is eventually sloughed. FIGURE 5 illustrates this hypothesis.

If the Sampson hypothesis is correct,[1] the fragments that flow out of the fallopian tubes and implant on pelvic sites would be rich in MMPs and VEGF, and MMPs could act to facilitate attachment of the menstrual fragments, while VEGF could act to induce angiogenesis in these new ectopic sites. Evidence has already been presented that MMP inhibitors can block establishment of endometrial grafts in nude mice.[29] Thus, the role of VEGF and MMPs in the establishment of endometriotic implants deserves further investigation.

Our experiments in ovariectomized, artificially cycled macaques indicate that the premenstrual upregulation of VEGF, KDR, and MMPs in the superficial zones of the endometrium is estrogen-independent. For example, the same increases in KDR and MMPs occurred whether E remained or was withdrawn during P withdrawal.[24] Moreover, the postmenstrual repair phase is also estrogen-independent. For example, when macaques are ovariectomized at the end of the cycle, the subsequent menstruation is followed by a healing phase of the endometrial surface that occurs in the absence of E. The latter has been noted previously for the human endometrium.[30] However, E is essential for the subsequent growth that occurs after the endometrial surface has healed. Because menstrual fragments have little or no ER, E is unlikely to be important in the *establishment phase of endometriosis.* In fully established endometriotic lesions, though, ER and PR are detectable[31] and E undoubtedly acts through ER in these lesions to stimulate growth.

Regarding PR, new interesting data by Attia *et al.* indicate that only PR-A, not PR-B, is present in such lesions.[32] According to these authors, endometriotic lesions exhibit P resistance, as marked by an inability to induce 17β-hydroxysteroid dehydrogenase type 2, the enzyme that converts estradiol to estrone. Because estrone dominance is associated with a retardation of endometrial proliferation, these authors suggest that the lack of the stimulatory isoform, PR-B, explains the resistance of these lesions to suppression by P.[32]

A Two-Phase Mechanism of Menstrual Induction

Kelly *et al.*[33] proposed that menstrual induction occurs in two phases: the first phase reversible by P and the second phase irreversible. This hypothesis is based on the following: P normally suppresses the NFκB transcription factor in PR-positive, endometrial stromal cells, in part by elevating its inhibitor, IκB, which keeps NFκB sequestered in the cytoplasm in an inactive state. When P levels fall at the end of the cycle, intracellular IκB levels fall and NFκB translocates into the nucleus and activates transcription of various cytokine genes. These events occur first in PR-positive cells and lead, probably indirectly, to a distinct upregulation in cyclooxygenase-2 (COX-2) in the glandular epithelium, which results in increased synthesis of prostaglandins. Also, during the luteal phase, P increases the levels of prostaglandin dehydrogenase, which acts to lower prostaglandin levels.[34] When P levels decline, prostaglandin dehydrogenase activity decreases. Therefore, when P levels fall during the premenstrual phase, the combined effects of the increase in COX-2 and the decrease in prostaglandin dehydrogenase lead to elevated prostaglandins—molecules that are potent vasoconstrictors. As a consequence, ischemia, hypoxia, and reperfusion injury are all likely to occur in the upper superficial zones. As previously indicated, VEGF, KDR, and several MMPs are also elevated in PR-positive stromal cells by P withdrawal. NFκB signaling can induce KDR in endothelial cells in culture[35,36] and could play a similar role during P withdrawal in endometrial stromal cells, although the latter remains to be determined. Because the above intracellular events all occur in PR-positive cells, this early phase of menstrual induction should be reversible by P.

With time, activated NFκB enhances the secretion of a variety of cytokines that affect vascular permeability, induce leukocyte invasion, and further stimulate the secretion of prostaglandins and endothelins. Many leukocytic cell types secrete

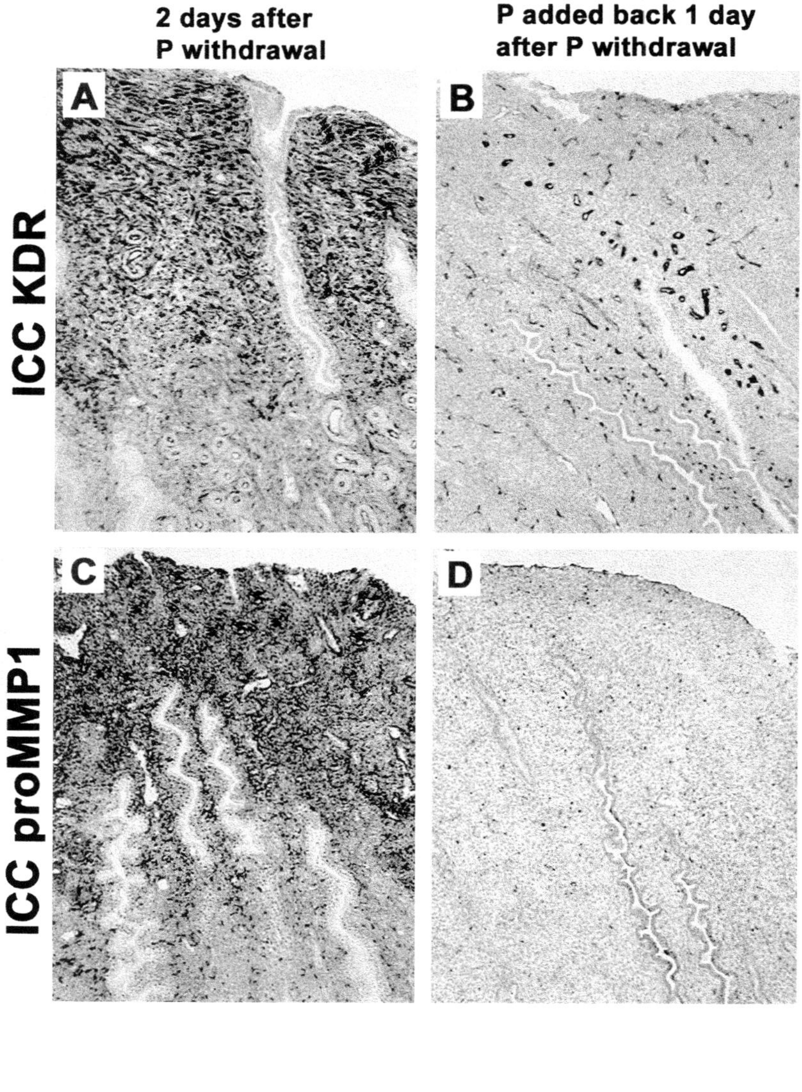

FIGURE 6. Macaque endometrium. Effects of P add-back on ICC of KDR and pro-MMP-1. Modified from Nayak *et al.*[24] At 2 days after P withdrawal, KDR (**A**) and pro-MMP-1 (**C**) are intensely stained in the superficial zones of the endometrium. When P is added back at 1 day after P withdrawal and the endometrium removed 1 day later, KDR (**B**) and pro-MMP-1 (**D**) are nondetectable by ICC. Of considerable interest, the KDR signal in the endothelium of the spiral arteries was not suppressed by P add-back. Endothelial cell and stromal cell KDR are apparently regulated by different mechanisms. All magnifications: ×50 (original).

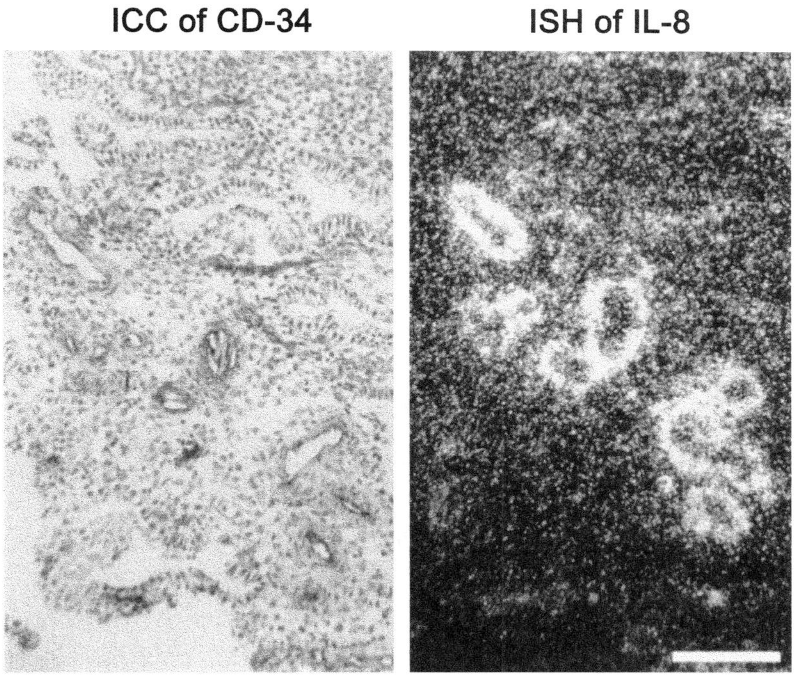

FIGURE 7. Human endometrium sampled at 2 days after P withdrawal. **(Left)** CC for the CD-34 marker for blood vessels. **(Right)** *In situ* hybridization for IL-8. Comparison of the two panels shows that IL-8 mRNA expression is localized in the perivascular regions of spiral arterioles. Magnification: Bar = 100 μm. Reproduced with permission from The Endocrine Society.[39]

MMPs and other lytic enzymes that facilitate tissue breakdown and bleeding. Because endometrial leukocytes and macrophages appear to be PR-negative, adding back P would not directly affect their synthetic activities. Endothelial cells, which are PR-negative, synthesize and release endothelins, and the invading leukocytes contribute their lytic effects to the menstrual cascade. Elevated prostaglandins eventually induce myometrial contractions strong enough to expel the menstrual slough and, by the time this occurs, the menstrual process is irreversible.

In a study designed to determine the effects of adding back P on menstruation, we treated ovariectomized macaques with E and P for 28 days to induce an artificial cycle. On day 28, we withdrew P to induce menstruation and then added P back at 12-h intervals to determine the times at which menstruation could be blocked. Adding back P up to 36 h after P withdrawal reliably blocked menstruation, but adding P back after 36 h did not.[37] In a follow-up study, we withdrew P for 24 h, then added it back, and sampled the endometrium at 24 h later. Controls were sampled at 48 h after P withdrawal. Adding back P not only blocked menstruation, but completely blocked upregulation of stromal KDR and MMP-1, as compared to controls[24] (see

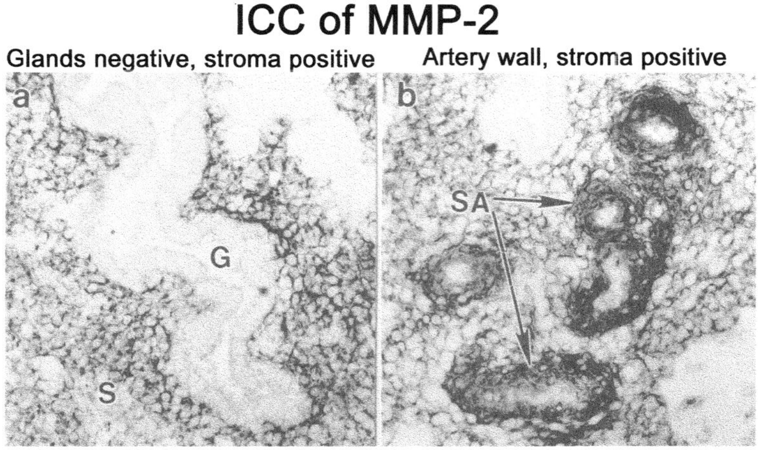

FIGURE 8. Macaque endometrium sampled at 2 days after P withdrawal. ICC of MMP-2. Modified from Rudolph-Owen *et al.*[25] **(a)** Region showing glands and stroma. MMP-2 staining is restricted to the stromal fibroblasts. The glands are negative. **(b)** Region showing spiral arterioles (SA) and stroma. The perivascular walls of the arterioles are intensely stained (×300).

FIG. 6). These new data support Kelly's hypothesis[33] of a two-stage development of the menstrual cascade and provide further evidence that VEGF-KDR interactions are components of that cascade.

The Perivascular Expression of Cytokines and MMPs

The PR-positive perivascular cells that surround and support the spiral arterioles play important roles in the menstrual cascade. Two cytokines of interest that are generated specifically within the perivascular stroma are IL-8 and MCP-1. These are among the cytokines that attract multiple leukocytic cell types into the endometrium. By utilizing an experimental model of P withdrawal in women, Critchley *et al.*[38] demonstrated that IL-8 and COX-2 mRNA and protein were substantially upregulated by 48 h after P withdrawal. Furthermore, ISH revealed that IL-8 was primarily expressed by the perivascular cells in late secretory endometrium.[39] This perivascular locus of IL-8 expression (FIG. 7) is likely to facilitate the attraction and migration of leukocytes into the endometrium.

In studies with tissues obtained from rhesus macaques after P withdrawal, we[25] noted that several MMPs, including MMP-2, were also strongly expressed by the perivascular walls of the spiral arterioles as well as the stroma (FIG. 8). These perivascular MMPs are presumed to weaken the vascular walls and precipitate menstrual bleeding. As Markee[15] noted, pieces of spiral arterioles may break off and become part of the menstrual slough. These vascular elements could act as intense foci of IL-8 and MMP expression and play a role in the attachment and establishment of endometriotic implants.

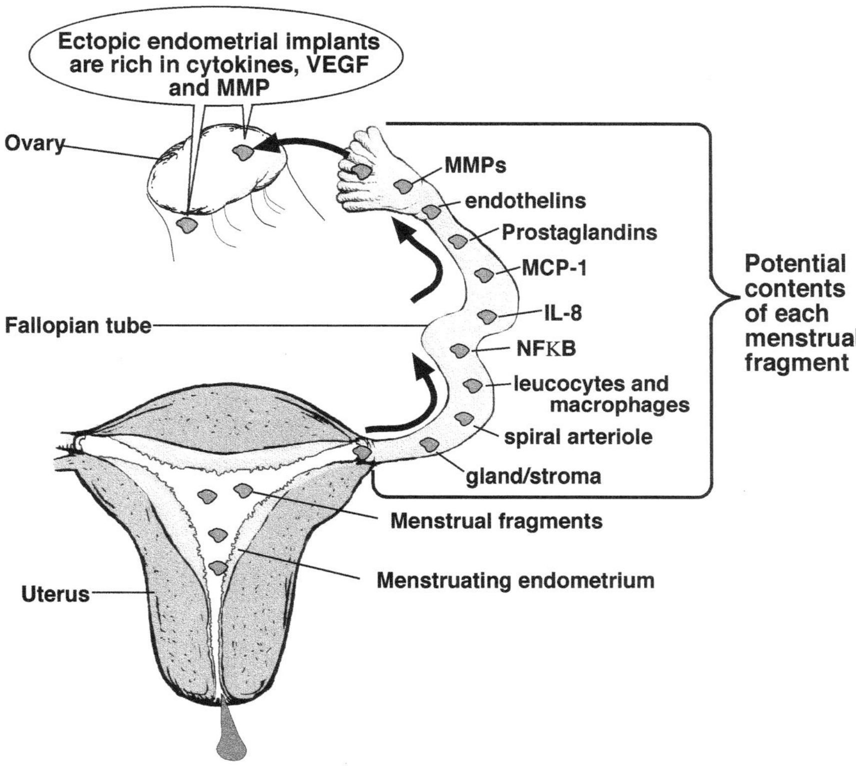

FIGURE 9. Initiation of endometriosis. A reprise of FIGURE 1 in which, for didactic purposes, each fragment is labeled with one of the many factors likely to be present in the retrograde menstrual slough. Drawing by Joel Ito and Robert M. Brenner (ORPRC).

SUMMARY

When the luteal phase ends and P levels fall, PR-positive stromal cells in the superficial zones of the primate endometrium respond to this decline and initiate the menstrual cascade. The early part of the cascade involves increased production of prostaglandins that induce vasoconstriction and hypoxia. Subsequently, there is increased expression of VEGF and stromal KDR, elevations in stromal MMPs, a leukocytic invasion, and perivascular expression of cytokines and MMPs. The later phases of this cascade become insensitive to P and irreversible, probably because PR-negative cellular elements become heavily involved and the tissue dissolution effects of MMPs reach an irreversible state. The sloughed tissue fragments are rich in VEGF and MMPs, and include large numbers of leukocytes that express MMPs, proteases, and various cytokines. Vascular segments rich in IL-8, other cytokines, and MMPs may also be present. When these tissue fragments flow out of the tubes and into the pelvic cavity, the various factors that they express probably facilitate their establishment as endometriotic implants. The peritoneal environment, which derives from ovarian exudates, plasma transudate, tubal fluid, macrophage secretions, and retrograde menstruation,[40] is also likely to play an as yet undefined role in the establishment of endometriosis. For example, macrophages in the peritoneal cavity release prostaglandins,[41] IL-8,[42] and VEGF.[43] The stimulus for the increase in MCP-1 observed in peritoneal fluid of women with endometriosis has not yet been determined.[44] All these factors may be involved in any reseeding process that spreads the lesions through the pelvic cavity. FIGURE 9 is a reprise of FIGURE 1 that illustrates this general hypothesis.

Although the retrograde flow of the menstrual slough through the tubes occurs in most women,[45,46] not all women develop endometriosis. Recent data suggest that the eutopic endometrium of women with endometriosis has higher endogenous aromatase levels[47] than are found in the endometrium of disease-free women. There may be other differences between the eutopic endometrium of normal and endometriosis-prone women, perhaps in the expression of many of the factors described above. This possibility deserves further research. The mechanisms underlying the establishment and pelvic spread of this debilitating disease are still unknown, and a deeper understanding may develop from new studies of the properties of the premenstrual and menstrual endometrium of women with and without endometriosis.

REFERENCES

1. SAMPSON, J.A. 1940. The development of the implantation theory for the origin of peritoneal endometriosis. Am. J. Obstet. Gynecol. **40:** 549–557.
2. BARBIERI, R.L. 1988. New therapy for endometriosis. N. Engl. J. Med. **318:** 512–513.
3. BARBIERI, R.L. 1992. Hormone treatment of endometriosis: the estrogen threshold hypothesis. Am. J. Obstet. Gynecol. **166:** 740–745.
4. HISAW, F.L. & F.L. HISAW, JR. 1961. Action of estrogen and progesterone on the reproductive tract of lower primates. *In* Sex and Internal Secretions, pp. 556–589. Williams & Wilkins. Baltimore.
5. CORNER, G.W. 1963. The Hormones in Human Reproduction. Atheneum. New York.
6. BARTELMEZ, G.W. 1933. Histological studies on the menstruating mucous membrane of the human uterus. Contrib. Embryol. **142:** 142–186.
7. NOYES, R.W., A.T. HERTIG & J. ROCK. 1950. Dating the endometrial biopsy. Fertil. Steril. **1:** 3–25.
8. CRITCHLEY, H.O.D., D.A. BAILEY, C.L. AU *et al.* 1993. Immunohistochemical sex steroid receptor distribution in endometrium from long-term subdermal levonorgestrel users and during the normal menstrual cycle. Hum. Reprod. **8:** 1632–1639.
9. GARCIA, E., P. BOUCHARD, J. DE BRUX *et al.* 1988. Use of immunocytochemistry of progesterone and estrogen receptors for endometrial dating. J. Clin. Endocrinol. Metab. **67:** 80–87.
10. LESSEY, B.A., A.P. KILLAM, D.A. METZGER *et al.* 1988. Immunohistochemical analysis of human uterine estrogen and progesterone receptors throughout the menstrual cycle. J. Clin. Endocrinol. Metab. **67:** 334–340.
11. BRENNER, R.M., N.B. WEST & M.C. MCCLELLAN. 1990. Estrogen and progestin receptors in the reproductive tract of male and female primates. Biol. Reprod. **42:** 11–19.
12. OKULICZ, W.C., A.M. SAVASTA, L.M. HOBERG & C. LONGCOPE. 1990. Biochemical and immunohistochemical analyses of estrogen and progesterone receptors in the rhesus monkey uterus during the proliferative and secretory phases of artificial menstrual cycles. Fertil. Steril. **53:** 913–920.
13. PRESS, M.F. & G.L. GREENE. 1984. An immunocytochemical method for demonstrating estrogen receptor in human uterus using monoclonal antibodies to human estrophilin. Lab. Invest. **50:** 480–486.

14. SNIJDERS, M.P.M.L., A.F.P.M. DE GOEIJ, M.J.C. DEBETS–TE BAERTS *et al.* 1992. Immunocytochemical analysis of oestrogen receptors and progesterone receptors in the human uterus throughout the menstrual cycle and after the menopause. J. Reprod. Fertil. **94:** 363–371.
15. MARKEE, J.E. 1940. Menstruation in intraocular endometrial transplants in the rhesus monkey. Contrib. Embryol. **28:** 219–308.
16. BAIRD, D.T., S.T. CAMERON, H.O.D. CRITCHLEY *et al.* 1996. Prostaglandins and menstruation. Eur. J. Obstet. Gynecol. **70:** 15–17.
17. SHARKEY, A.M., K. DAY, A. MCPHERSON *et al.* 2000. Vascular endothelial growth factor expression in human endometrium is regulated by hypoxia. J. Clin. Endocrinol. Metab. **85:** 402–409.
18. NAYAK, N.R. & R.M. BRENNER. 2001. Expression of endometrial VEGF and its receptors in the postmenstrual repair phase and throughout the cycle in rhesus macaques [abstract]. J. Soc. Gynecol. Invest. **8:** 76.
19. FERRARA, N. & T. DAVIS-SMYTH. 1997. The biology of vascular endothelial growth factor. Endocr. Rev. **18:** 4–25.
20. KLAGSBRUN, M. & P.A. D'AMORE. 1996. Vascular endothelial growth factor and its receptors. Cytokine Growth Factor Rev. **7:** 259–270.
21. WANG, H. & J.A. KEISER. 1998. Vascular endothelial growth factor upregulates the expression of matrix metalloproteinases in vascular smooth muscle cells: role of flt-1. Circ. Res. **83:** 832–840.
22. BROWN, L.F., K. TOGNAZZI, H.F. DVORAK & T.J. HARRIST. 1996. Strong expression of kinase insert domain–containing receptor, a vascular permeability factor/vascular endothelial growth factor receptor in AIDS-associated Kaposi's sarcoma and cutaneous angiosarcoma [short communication]. Am. J. Pathol. **148:** 1065–1074.
23. BOOCOCK, C.A., D.S. CHARNOCK-JONES, A. SHARKEY *et al.* 1995. Expression of vascular endothelial growth factor and its receptors flt and KDR in ovarian carcinoma. J. Soc. Gynecol. Invest. **87:** 506–516.
24. NAYAK, N.R., H.O.D. CRITCHLEY, O.D. SLAYDEN *et al.* 2000. Progesterone withdrawal up-regulates vascular endothelial growth factor receptor type 2 in the superficial zone stroma of the human and macaque endometrium: potential relevance to menstruation. J. Clin. Endocrinol. Metab. **85:** 3442–3452.
25. RUDOLPH-OWEN, L.A., O.D. SLAYDEN, L.M. MATRISIAN & R.M. BRENNER. 1998. Matrix metalloproteinase expression in *Macaca mulatta* endometrium: evidence for zone-specific regulatory tissue gradients. Biol. Reprod. **59:** 1349–1359.
26. BRENNER, R.M., L. RUDOLPH, L. MATRISIAN & O.D. SLAYDEN. 1996. Non-human primate models: artificial menstrual cycles, endometrial matrix metalloproteinases, and s.c. endometrial grafts. Hum. Reprod. **11:** 150–164.
27. SALAMONSEN, L.A. 1994. Matrix metalloproteinases and endometrial remodeling. Cell Biol. Int. **18:** 1139–1144.
28. UNEMORI, E.N., N. FERRARA, E.A. BAUER & E.P. AMENTO. 1992. Vascular endothelial growth factor induces interstitial collagenase expression in human endothelial cells. J. Cell. Physiol. **153:** 557–562.
29. BRUNER, K.L., L.M. MATRISIAN, W.H. RODGERS *et al.* 1997. Suppression of matrix metalloproteinases inhibits establishment of ectopic lesions by human endometrium in nude mice. J. Clin. Invest. **99:** 2851–2857.
30. FERENCZY, A., G. BERTRAND & M.M. GELFAND. 1979. Proliferation kinetics of human endometrium during the normal menstrual cycle. Am. J. Obstet. Gynecol. **133:** 859–867.
31. BERGQVIST, A., O.L. LJUNGBERG & L. SKOOG. 1993. Immunohistochemical analysis of oestrogen and progesterone receptors in endometriotic tissue and endometrium. Hum. Reprod. **8:** 1915–1922.
32. ATTIA, G.R., K. ZEITOUN, D. EDWARDS *et al.* 2000. Progesterone receptor isoform A, but not B is expressed in endometriosis. J. Clin. Endocrinol. Metab. **85:** 2897–2902.
33. KELLY, R.W., A.E. KING & H.O.D. CRITCHLEY. 2001. Cytokine control in human endometrium [abstract]. Reproduction **121:** 3–19.
34. CASEY, M.L., D.L. HEMSELL, P.C. MACDONALD & J.M. JOHNSTON. 1980. NAD+-dependent 15-hydroxyprostaglandin dehydrogenase activity in human endometrium. Prostaglandins **19:** 115–122.

35. PATTERSON, C., M.A. PERRELLA, C.M. HSIEH *et al.* 1995. Cloning and functional analysis of the promoter for KDR/flk-1, a receptor for vascular endothelial growth factor. J. Biol. Chem. **270:** 23111–23118.
36. ILLI, B., P. PURI, L. MORGANTE *et al.* 2000. Nuclear factor-kappaB and cAMP response element binding protein mediate opposite transcriptional effects on the Flk-1/KDR gene promoter. Circ. Res. **86:** E110–E117.
37. SLAYDEN, O.D., K. MAH & R.M. BRENNER. 1999. A critical period of progesterone withdrawal exists for endometrial MMPs and menstruation in macaques [abstract]. Biol. Reprod. **60**.
38. CRITCHLEY, H.O.D., R.L. JONES, R.G. LEA *et al.* 1999. Role of inflammatory mediators in human endometrium during progesterone withdrawal and early pregnancy. J. Clin. Endocrinol. Metab. **84:** 240–248.
39. MILNE, S.A., H.O.D. CRITCHLEY, T.A. DRUDY *et al.* 1999. Perivascular interleukin-8 messenger ribonucleic acid expression in human endometrium varies across the menstrual cycle and in early pregnancy deciduas. J. Clin. Endocrinol Metab. **84:** 2563–2567.
40. ORAL, E., D. OLIVE & A. ARICI. 1996. The peritoneal environment in endometriosis. Hum. Reprod. Update **2:** 385–398.
41. KARCK, U., F. REISTER, W. SCHAFER *et al.* 1996. PGE2 and PGF2alpha release by human peritoneal macrophages in endometriosis. Prostaglandins **51:** 49–60.
42. RANA, N., D.P. BRAUN, R. HOUSE *et al.* 1996. Basal and stimulated secretion of cytokines by peritoneal macrophages in women with endometriosis. Fertil. Steril. **65:** 925–930.
43. MCLAREN, J., A. PRENTICE, D.S. CHARNOCK-JONES & S.K. SMITH. 1996. Vascular endothelial growth factor (VEGF) concentrations are elevated in peritoneal fluid of women with endometriosis. Hum. Reprod. **11:** 220–223.
44. ARICI, A., E. ORAL, S. TAZUKE & D. OLIVE. 1997. Monocyte chemotactic protein-1 concentration in peritoneal fluid in patients with endometriosis and its modulation in human mesothelial cells. Fertil. Steril. **67:** 1065–1072.
45. BARTOSIK, D., S. JACOBBS & L. KELLY. 1986. Endometrial tissue in peritoneal fluid. Fertil. Steril. **46:** 800.
46. HALME, J., M.G. HAMMOND, J.F. HULKA *et al.* 1984. Retrograde menstruation in healthy women and in patients with endometriosis. Obstet. Gynecol. **64:** 151–154.
47. NOBLE, L.S., E.R. SIMPSON, A. JOHNS & S.E. BULUN. 1996. Aromatase expression in endometriosis. J. Clin. Endocrinol. Metab. **81:** 174–179.

Estrogen Production and Metabolism in Endometriosis

SERDAR E. BULUN, SIJUN YANG, ZHOJUAN FANG, BILGIN GURATES, MITSUTOSHI TAMURA, AND SIBY SEBASTIAN

Departments of Obstetrics and Gynecology and Molecular Genetics, University of Illinois at Chicago, Chicago, Illinois 60612, USA

ABSTRACT: Aromatase activity is absent in normal endometrium. In contrast, aromatase is expressed aberrantly in endometriosis, which gives rise to strikingly high levels of aromatase activity in this tissue. Both aromatase expression and activity are stimulated by PGE_2. This results in local production of estrogen, which induces PGE_2 formation and establishes a positive feedback cycle. Another abnormality in endometriosis, that is, deficient 17β-HSD type 2 expression, impairs the inactivation of estradiol to estrone. These molecular aberrations collectively favor accumulation of increasing quantities of estradiol and PGE_2 in endometriosis. The clinical relevance of these findings was exemplified by the successful treatment of an unusually aggressive case of postmenopausal endometriosis using an aromatase inhibitor.

KEYWORDS: aromatase; aromatase inhibitor; endometriosis; estrogen; estrogen biosynthesis; estrogen metabolism; 17β-hydroxysteroid dehydrogenase type 2; steroidogenesis; osteoporosis; progesterone

INTRODUCTION

Endometriosis is defined as the presence of endometrial glands and stroma within the pelvic peritoneum and other extrauterine sites and is linked to pelvic pain and infertility. It is estimated to affect 2% to 10% of women in the reproductive age group.[1,2] Endometriosis is viewed to be a polygenically inherited disease of complex multifactorial etiology.[3] Sampson's theory of transplantation of endometrial tissue on the pelvic peritoneum via retrograde menstruation is the most widely accepted explanation for the development of pelvic endometriosis because of convincing circumstantial and experimental evidence.[4] Since retrograde menstruation is observed in almost all cycling women, endometriosis is postulated to develop as a result of the coexistence of a defect in clearance of the menstrual efflux from pelvic peritoneal surfaces, possibly involving the immune system.[5] Alternatively, intrinsic molecular aberrations in pelvic endometriotic implants were proposed to significantly contribute to development of endometriosis. Aberrant expression of aromatase, certain cytokines, and tissue metalloproteinases; deficiency of 17β-hydroxysteroid dehydrogenase (17β-HSD) type 2; and resistance to the protective action of proges-

Address for correspondence: Serdar E. Bulun, M.D., Department of Obstetrics-Gynecology, University of Illinois at Chicago, 820 South Wood Street, M/C 808, Chicago, IL 60612. Voice: 312-996-8197; fax: 312-996-4238.
sbulun@uic.edu

terone are some of these molecular abnormalities.[6–12] Since endometriosis is an estrogen-dependent disorder, aromatase expression and 17β-HSD type 2 deficiency are of paramount importance in the pathophysiology of endometriosis. In this article, aberrant mechanisms of estrogen biosynthesis and metabolism in women with endometriosis are reviewed with emphasis on identifying targets for new treatment strategies.

DISCUSSION

Estrogen Biosynthesis and Metabolism in Humans

The conversion of androstenedione and testosterone to estrone and estradiol is catalyzed by aromatase, which is expressed in a number of human tissues and cells such as ovarian granulosa cells, placental syncytiotrophoblast, adipose tissue and skin fibroblasts, and the brain. In the reproductive-age woman, the ovary is the most important site of estrogen biosynthesis, and this takes place in a cyclic fashion. Upon binding of FSH to its G-protein-coupled receptor in the granulosa cell membrane, intracellular cAMP levels rise and enhance binding of two critical transcription factors, that is, steroidogenic factor-1 (SF-1) and cAMP response element binding protein (CREB), to the classically located proximal promoter II of the aromatase gene.[13,14] This, in turn, activates aromatase expression and consequently estrogen secretion from the preovulatory follicle.[14,15]

On the other hand, in postmenopausal women, estrogen formation takes place in extraglandular tissues such as the adipose tissue and skin[16–18] (FIG. 1). In contrast to cAMP regulation of aromatase expression in the ovary, this is controlled primarily by cytokines (IL-6, IL-11, TNFα) and glucocorticoids via the alternative use of promoter I.4 in adipose tissue and skin fibroblasts.[15] The major substrate for aromatase in adipose tissue and skin is androstenedione of adrenal origin. In postmenopausal women, approximately 2% of circulating androstenedione is converted to estrone, which is further converted to estradiol in these peripheral tissues. This may give rise to significant serum levels of estradiol capable of causing endometrial hyperplasia or even carcinoma.[17,18]

Aromatase Expression in Müllerian-Derived Tissues

Müllerian tissues are known targets of estrogen action. Until recently, estrogen action has been classically viewed to occur only via an "endocrine" mechanism: in other words, it was thought that only circulating estradiol, whether secreted by the ovary or formed in the adipose tissue, could exert an estrogenic effect after delivery to target tissues via the bloodstream. Studies on aromatase expression in breast cancer demonstrated that paracrine mechanisms play an important role in estrogen action in this tissue.[19] Estrogen produced by aromatase activity in breast adipose tissue fibroblasts was demonstrated to promote the growth of adjacent malignant breast epithelial cells.[20] Finally, we demonstrated an "intracrine" effect of estrogen in uterine leiomyomas and endometriosis: Estrogen produced by aromatase activity in the cytoplasm of leiomyoma smooth muscle cells or endometriotic stromal cells can exert its effects by readily binding to its nuclear receptor within the same

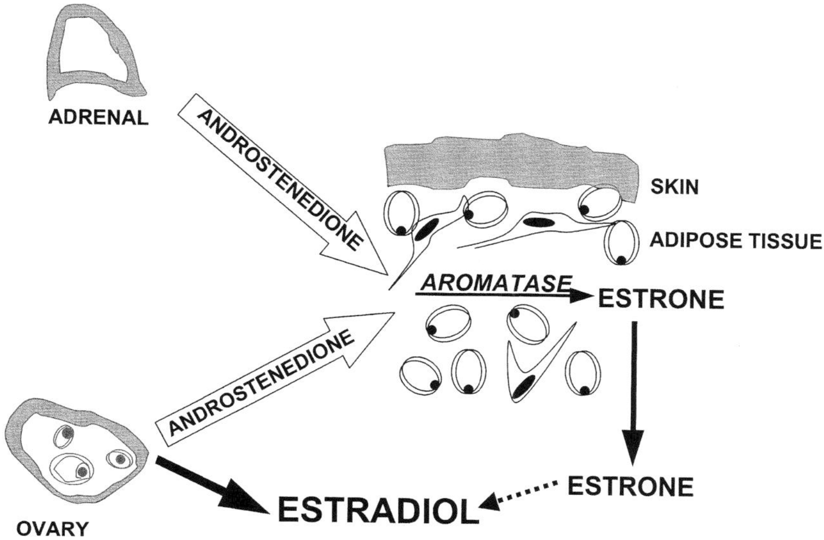

FIGURE 1. Extraovarian estrogen synthesis in women. Estradiol in women is either directly secreted by the ovary or produced in extraglandular sites (adipose tissue and skin). The principal substrate for extraglandular aromatase activity in ovulatory women is androstenedione of adrenal and ovarian origins. In women receiving GnRH agonists or postmenopausal women, however, the adrenal remains as the primary source of androstenedione. Androstenedione is converted by aromatase to estrone in adipose tissue and skin fibroblasts. Estrone is further converted to estradiol by 17β-HSD type 1 activity in these peripheral tissues. Thus, peripheral aromatization is the major source for circulating estradiol in the postmenopausal period or during ovarian suppression.

cell.[6,21,22] Disease-free endometrium and myometrium, on the other hand, lack aromatase expression.[21,22]

The Significance of Aromatase Expression in Endometriosis

Among estrogen-responsive pelvic disorders, aromatase expression was studied in greatest detail in endometriosis.[6,7,22,23] First, extremely high levels of aromatase mRNA were found in extraovarian endometriotic implants and endometriomas. Second, endometriosis-derived stromal cells in culture incubated with a cAMP analog displayed extraordinarily high levels of aromatase activity comparable to that in placental syncytiotrophoblast.[22] These exciting findings led us to test a battery of growth factors, cytokines, and other substances that might induce aromatase activity via a cAMP-dependent pathway in endometriosis. PGE_2 was found to be the most potent known inducer of aromatase activity in endometriotic stromal cells.[22] In fact, this PGE_2 effect was found to be mediated via the cAMP-inducing EP_2 receptor subtype (our unpublished observations). Moreover, estrogen was reported to increase PGE_2 formation by stimulating cyclooxygenase type 2 (COX-2) enzyme in endometrial stromal cells in culture.[24] Thus, a positive feedback loop for continuous local

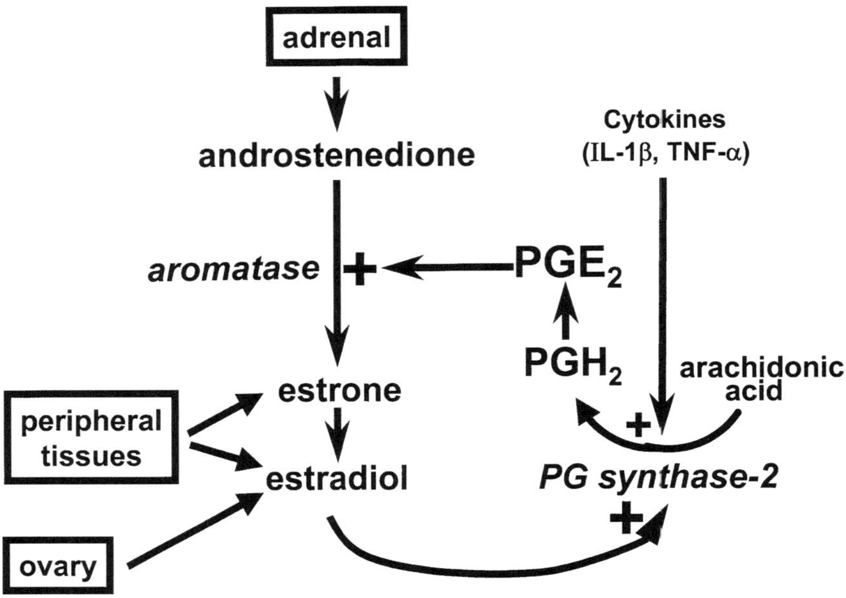

FIGURE 2. Origin of estrogen in endometriotic lesions. Estradiol in an endometriotic lesion arises from several body sites. In an ovulatory woman, estradiol is secreted directly from the ovary in a cyclic fashion. In the early follicular phase and after menopause, peripheral tissues (adipose and skin) are the most important sources to account for the circulating estradiol. Estradiol is also produced locally in the endometriotic implant itself in both ovulatory and postmenopausal women. The most important precursor, androstenedione of adrenal origin, becomes converted to estrone, which in turn is reduced to estradiol in the peripheral tissues and endometriotic implants. We demonstrated significant levels of 17β-HSD type 1 expression in endometriosis, which catalyzes the conversion of estrone to estradiol.[12] Estradiol both directly and indirectly (through cytokines) induces prostaglandin synthase-2 (cyclooxygenase-2), which gives rise to elevated concentrations of PGE_2 in endometriosis.[24] PGE_2, in turn, is the most potent known stimulator of aromatase in endometriotic stromal cells.[22] This establishes a positive feedback loop in favor of continuous estrogen formation in endometriosis.

productions of estrogen and PGs is established, favoring the proliferative and inflammatory characteristics of endometriosis (FIG. 2). Additionally, aromatase mRNA was detected in the eutopic endometrial samples of women with moderate to severe endometriosis (but not in those of disease-free women), albeit in much smaller quantities compared with endometriotic implants.[6] This may be suggestive of a genetic defect in women with endometriosis, which is manifested by this subtle finding in the eutopic endometrium. We propose that when defective endometrium with low levels of aberrant aromatase expression reaches the pelvic peritoneum by retrograde menstruation, it causes an inflammatory reaction that exponentially increases local aromatase activity, that is, estrogen formation, induced directly or indirectly by PGs and cytokines.[22] It would be rather naive to propose that aberrant aromatase expression is the only important molecular mechanism in the development and growth of pelvic endometriosis. There may be many other molecular mechanisms that favor the development of endometriosis: for example, abnormal expression of proteinase-type enzymes that remodel tissues or their inhibitors (matrix metalloproteinases, tissue inhibitor of metalloproteinase-1), certain cytokines (IL-6, RANTES), and growth factors (EGF).[8–11] Alternatively, a defective immune system that fails to clear peritoneal surfaces of the retrograde menstrual efflux has been proposed in the development of endometriosis.[5,25] The development of endometriosis in an individual woman probably requires the coexistence of a threshold number of these aberrations. Nonetheless, aberrant aromatase expression is clinically relevant since aromatase inhibitors suppress postmenopausal endometriosis.[26]

Regulation of Aromatase Expression in Endometriotic Stromal Cells

As emphasized earlier, PGE_2 was found to be the most potent known inducer of aromatase activity by increasing cAMP levels in endometriotic stromal cells.[22] On the other hand, neither cAMP analogs nor PGE_2 was capable of stimulating any detectable aromatase activity in eutopic endometrial stromal cells in culture. The obvious question became what are the molecular differences that give rise to aromatase expression in endometriosis and its inhibition in eutopic endometrium. To address this, we first determined that the cAMP-inducible promoter II was used for *in vivo* aromatase expression in endometriotic tissue.[7] Then, a stimulatory transcription factor, SF-1, and an inhibitory factor, chicken ovalbumin upstream promoter transcription factor (COUP-TF), were found to compete for the same binding site in aromatase promoter II. COUP-TF was ubiquitously expressed in both eutopic endometrium and endometriosis, whereas SF-1 was expressed specifically in endometriosis, but not in eutopic endometrium, and binds to aromatase promoter more avidly than COUP-TF.[7] Thus, SF-1 and other transcription factors (e.g., CREB) activate transcription in endometriosis, whereas COUP-TF, which occupies the same DNA site in eutopic endometrium, inhibits this process[7] (FIG. 3). In summary, one of the molecular alterations leading to local aromatase expression in endometriosis, but not in normal endometrium, is the aberrant production of SF-1 in endometriotic stromal cells, which overcomes the protective inhibition maintained normally by COUP-TF in the eutopic endometrium.

Interconversions of Estrone and Estradiol in Endometriosis

The primary substrate for aromatase activity in endometriosis is androstenedione of adrenal and ovarian origins in premenopausal women and adrenal androstenedione in postmenopausal women. The major product of aromatase activity in endometriosis, namely estrone, is only weakly estrogenic and must be converted to the potent estrogen estradiol to exert a full estrogenic effect. We demonstrated that the enzyme 17β-HSD type 1, which catalyzes the conversion of estrone to estradiol, is expressed in endometriosis.[12,27] In contrast, the enzyme 17β-HSD type 2 (encoded by a separate gene) inactivates estradiol by catalyzing its conversion to estrone in eutopic endometrial glandular cells during the luteal phase.[27] Progesterone actually induces the activity of this enzyme in endometrial glandular cells in culture, making inactivation of estradiol to estrone one of the antiestrogenic properties of progesterone.[28] The expression of 17β-HSD type 2 is absent from endometriotic glandular

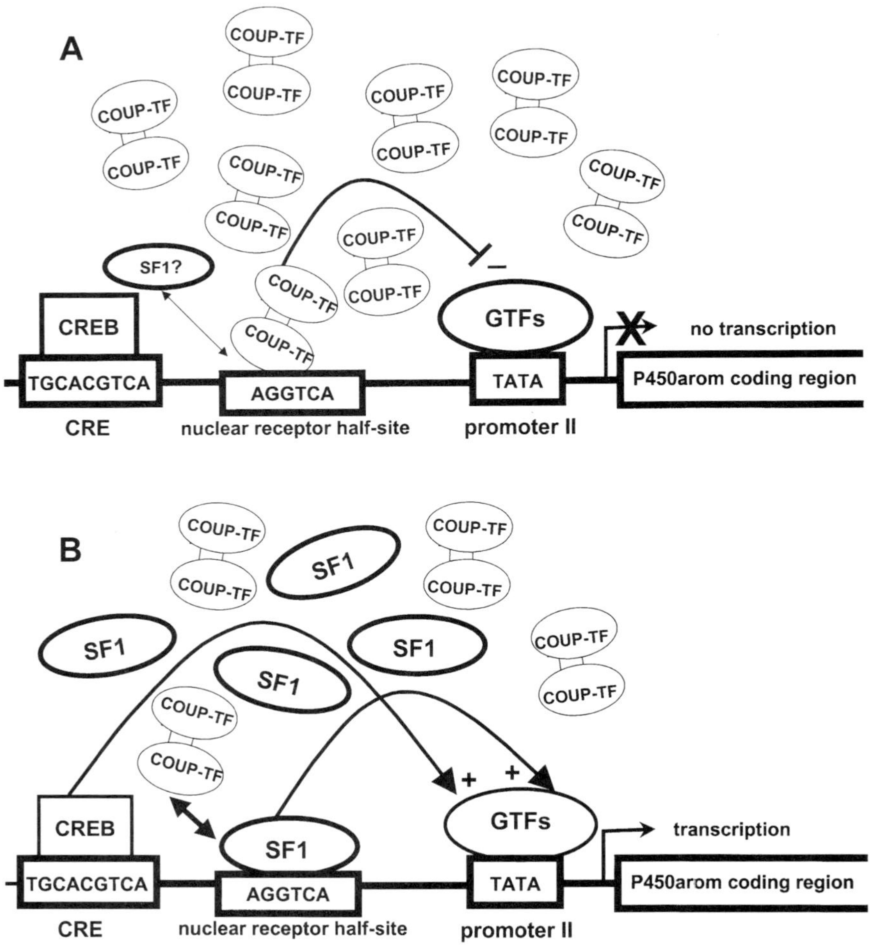

FIGURE 3. Proposed mechanism of regulation of aromatase (P450arom) expression by SF-1 and COUP-TF in eutopic endometrium and endometriosis. **(Top)** Panel A: Binding of COUP-TF (dimer) to a specific DNA site (nuclear receptor half-site) upstream of aromatase promoter II in eutopic endometrial stromal cells. In the eutopic endometrium, COUP-TF binds to the nuclear receptor half-site practically in the absence of any competition by SF-1 since SF-1 expression is not detected in the majority of eutopic endometrial samples. Thus, COUP-TF exerts its inhibitory effect on the complex of general transcription factors (GTFs) that bind to the TATA box. **(Bottom)** Panel B: In the endometriotic stromal cell, where SF-1 is also present, SF-1 binds as a monomer to the nuclear receptor half-site with a higher affinity compared with that of COUP-TF, which binds to this site relatively loosely as a dimer. Upon replacing COUP-TF, SF-1 synergizes with cAMP response element binding protein (CREB, bound to upstream CRE) and other factors to activate transcription of the aromatase gene in response to cAMP.[7]

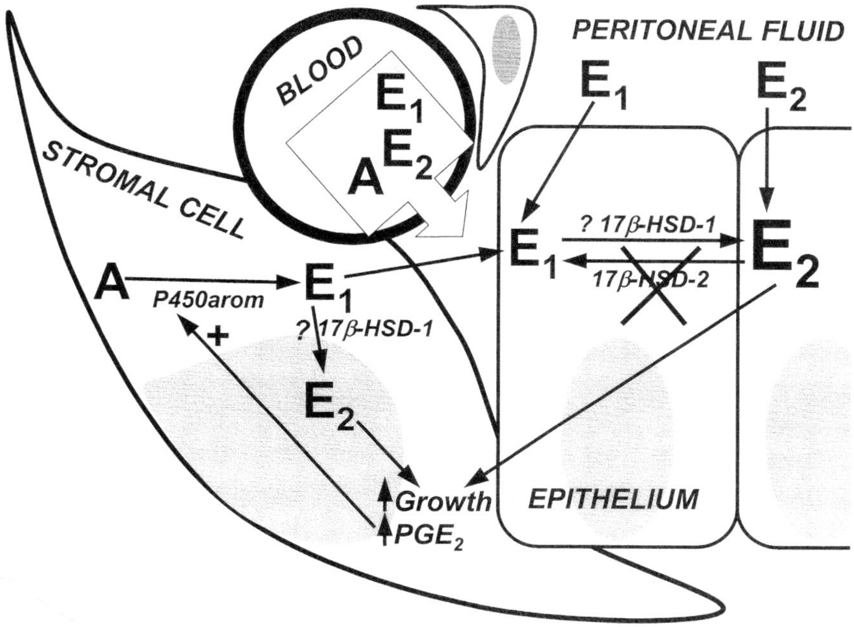

FIGURE 4. Defective inactivation of estradiol in endometriosis. Estradiol (E_2) reaches the endometriotic lesions via the bloodstream (and possibly peritoneal fluid). Additionally, aromatase (P450arom) in the stromal cell catalyzes the conversion of androstenedione (A) to estrone (E_1), which is further reduced to E_2 by 17β-HSD type 1 in the endometriotic tissue. (At this time, the cell type that expresses 17β-HSD type 1 in endometriotic lesions is not known.) E_2 is normally inactivated by conversion to E_1 by 17β-HSD type 2 in epithelial cells of the eutopic endometrium during the secretory phase. In endometriotic tissue, however, E_2 is not metabolized owing to the lack of 17β-HSD type 2, giving rise to increased local concentration of this potent estrogen. Elevated E_2, in turn, will promote the growth of endometriotic tissue and, also, local PGE_2 formation in stromal cells.[24] Since PGE_2 is the most potent known inducer of aromatase in endometriosis, this will complete the positive feedback cycle that favors increased levels of E_2 in endometriosis through enhanced biosynthesis and deficient metabolism.

cells, as demonstrated in paired samples of eutopic endometrium and pelvic endometriosis obtained simultaneously during the luteal phase.[12] Consequently, this protective mechanism that lowers estradiol levels is lost in endometriotic tissue.[12] The aberrant expression of aromatase, the presence of 17β-HSD type 1, and the absence of 17β-HSD type 2 from endometriosis collectively give rise to elevated local levels of estradiol compared with eutopic endometrium. Additionally, 17β-HSD type 2 deficiency may also be viewed as a defective action of progesterone, which fails to induce this enzyme in endometriotic tissue (FIG. 4).

Rationale for Using Aromatase Inhibitors to Treat Endometriosis

Endometriosis is successfully suppressed by estrogen deprivation with GnRH analogs or the induction of surgical menopause. Control of pelvic pain with GnRH

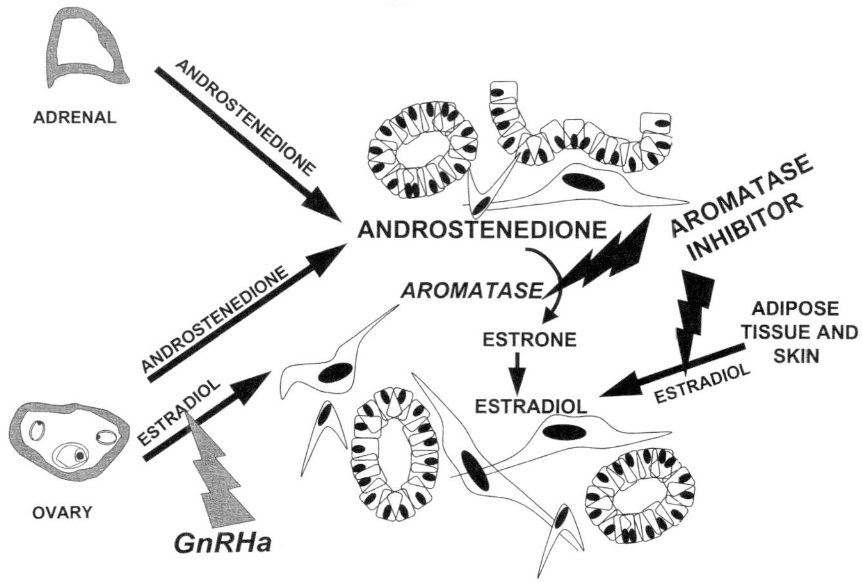

FIGURE 5. Site of action of GnRH agonists and aromatase inhibitors to treat endometriosis. This figure depicts the origin of estrogen in women with endometriosis: (*i*) delivery from the ovary and adipose tissue/skin via circulation and (*ii*) local biosynthesis in endometriosis. GnRH agonists will eliminate estradiol secreted by the ovary by downregulating the pituitary hypothalamic unit. In cases resistant to treatment with GnRH agonists or in postmenopausal endometriosis, the use of aromatase inhibitors to block estrogen formation in the skin and adipose tissue as well as in endometriotic stromal cells may be critical in controlling the growth of endometriotic tissue. Recurrent endometriosis, especially after surgical removal of the ovaries, may represent lesions that are sensitive to extremely low levels of estradiol and, thus, suppression of estradiol production in the periphery (adipose tissue/skin) and in endometriotic tissue may be mandatory for successful treatment of endometriosis.

agonists is usually successful during and immediately after the treatment, whereas pain associated with endometriosis returns in up to 75% of these women.[29,30] There may be multiple reasons for the failure of GnRH agonist treatment of endometriosis. One likely explanation is the presence of significant estradiol production that continues in the adipose tissue, skin, and endometriotic implant per se during the GnRH agonist treatment (FIG. 5). Therefore, blockage of aromatase activity in these extraovarian sites with an aromatase inhibitor may keep larger numbers of patients in remission for longer periods of time. The most striking evidence for the significance of extraovarian estrogen production is the recurrence of endometriosis after successfully completed hysterectomy and bilateral salpingo-oophorectomy in a number of women.[26,31] Endometriotic tissue in one such aggressive case was found to express much higher levels of aromatase mRNA compared with premenopausal endometriosis.[26] We recently reported the treatment of a 57-year-old overweight woman who had recurrence of severe endometriosis after hysterectomy and bilateral salpingo-oophorectomy. Two additional laparotomies were performed owing to persistent severe pelvic pain and bilateral ureteral obstruction, leading to left renal atrophy and right hydronephrosis. Treatment with megestrol acetate was ineffective. A large (3 cm) vaginal endometriotic lesion contained unusually high levels of aromatase mRNA. The patient was given anastrozole (an aromatase inhibitor) for 9 months. Despite the addition of calcium and alendronate (a nonsteroidal inhibitor of bone resorption), bone density in the lumbar spine decreased by 6.2%. The occurrence of significant bone loss in this particular case should be studied further. Dramatic relief of the pain and regression of the vaginal endometriotic lesion were observed within the first month of treatment. At the same time, circulating estradiol levels were reduced to 50% of the baseline value. Markedly high pretreatment levels of aromatase mRNA in the endometriotic tissue became undetectable in a repeat biopsy done 6 months later, and the lesion nearly disappeared after 9 months of therapy. Two potential mechanisms may have accounted for this strikingly successful result. First, there was evidence of suppression of peripheral (i.e., skin and adipose tissue) aromatase activity, giving rise to a significant decrease in serum estradiol level. Second, unusually high levels of aromatase expression in the endometriotic lesion disappeared after treatment with the aromatase inhibitor, anastrozole. Besides the expected direct inhibition of aromatase activity in endometriosis by anastrozole, the disappearance of aromatase mRNA expression in the lesion may be explicable by denial of estrogen that is known to stimulate local biosynthesis of PGE_2, which in turn stimulates aromatase expression (FIG. 2).

In summary, the recently developed potent aromatase inhibitors are candidate drugs in the treatment of endometriosis that is resistant to standard regimens. In fact, the use of aromatase inhibitors may be the only available treatment for aggressive postmenopausal endometriosis. It remains to be seen whether aromatase inhibitors alone or together with present lines of therapy in premenopausal women will increase the pain-free interval and time to recurrence after discontinuation (FIG. 5). Studies are under way to address these questions.

CONCLUSIONS

The development and growth of endometriotic lesions are estrogen-dependent. The mechanisms and effectiveness of hormonal treatments for endometriosis should be reevaluated in view of the new advances that increased our understanding of the body sites of estrogen production in a woman with endometriosis. In addition to ovarian secretion, estradiol is also produced in peripheral sites such as skin, adipose tissue, and endometriotic lesions per se. We suggest that the intracrine and paracrine effects of estradiol produced in the target tissue amplify the estrogenic action of steroid hormones delivered via the circulation. Additionally, defective inactivation of estradiol in endometriosis, in contrast to eutopic endometrium, may further enhance this local effect. Aberrant aromatase activity and defective estradiol metabolism in endometriosis are consequences of specific molecular aberrations such as inappropriate expression of a stimulatory transcription factor or progesterone resistance in this tissue. The clinical relevance of these findings was recently exemplified by the successful treatment of a severe case of recurrent postmenopausal endometriosis with an aromatase inhibitor. Future treatment strategies may be designed to target the signal transduction for aromatase expression in endometriosis or to enhance progesterone action in this tissue, and to eliminate bone loss that was an undesirable effect of aromatase inhibition in our otherwise successfully treated case of severe endometriosis.

ACKNOWLEDGMENTS

We thank Dee Alexander for providing expert editorial assistance. This research work was supported, in part, by NIH Grant No. HD38691 (to S. E. Bulun).

REFERENCES

1. VESSEY, M.P., L. VILLARD-MACKINTOSH & R. PAINTER. 1993. Epidemiology of endometriosis in women attending family planning clinics. Br. Med. J. **306:** 182–184.
2. KJERULFF, K.H., B.A. ERICKSON & P.W. LANGENBERG. 1996. Chronic gynecological conditions reported by U.S. women: findings from the National Health Information Survey, 1984 to 1992. Am. J. Public Health **86:** 195–199.
3. OLIVE, D.L. & L.B. SCHWARTZ. 1993. Endometriosis. N. Engl. J. Med. **328:** 1759–1769.
4. SAMPSON, J.A. 1927. Peritoneal endometriosis due to the menstrual dissemination of endometrial tissue into the peritoneal cavity. Am. J. Obstet. Gynecol. **14:** 422–425.
5. HALME, J. *et al.* 1988. Peritoneal macrophages from patients with endometriosis release growth factor activity *in vitro*. J. Clin. Endocrinol. Metab. **66:** 1044–1049.
6. NOBLE, L.S. *et al.* 1996. Aromatase expression in endometriosis. J. Clin. Endocrinol. Metab. **81:** 174–179.
7. ZEITOUN, K. *et al.* 1999. Stimulation of aromatase P450 promoter (II) activity in endometriosis and its inhibition in endometrium are regulated by competitive binding of SF-1 and COUP-TF to the same *cis*-acting element. Mol. Endocrinol. **13:** 239–253.
8. KHORRAM, O. *et al.* 1993. Peritoneal fluid concentrations of the cytokine RANTES correlate with the severity of endometriosis. Am. J. Obstet. Gynecol. **169:** 1545–1549.
9. SHARPE-TIMMS, K.L. *et al.* 1995. Partial purification and amino acid sequence analysis of endometriosis protein-II (ENDO-II) reveals homology with tissue inhibitor of metalloproteinases-1 (TIMP-1). J. Clin. Endocrinol. Metab. **80:** 3784–3787.
10. BRUNER, K.L. *et al.* 1997. Suppression of matrix metalloproteinases inhibits establishment of ectopic lesions by human endometrium in nude mice. J. Clin. Invest. **99:** 2851–2857.
11. OSTEEN, K.G. *et al.* 1996. Steroid and growth factor regulation of matrix metalloproteinase expression and endometriosis. Semin. Reprod. Endocrinol. **15:** 301–308.
12. ZEITOUN, K. *et al.* 1998. Deficient 17β-hydroxysteroid dehydrogenase type 2 expression in endometriosis: failure to metabolize estradiol-17β. J. Clin. Endocrinol. Metab. **83:** 4474–4480.
13. MICHAEL, M.D. *et al.* 1997. A CRE-like sequence that binds CREB and contributes to cAMP-dependent regulation of the proximal promoter of the human aromatase P450 (CYP19) gene. Mol. Cell. Endocrinol. **134:** 147–156.
14. MICHAEL, M.D. *et al.* 1995. Ad4BP/SF-1 regulates cyclic AMP–induced transcription from the proximal promoter (PII) of the human aromatase P450 (CYP19) gene in the ovary. J. Biol. Chem. **270:** 13561–13566.
15. SIMPSON, E.R. *et al.* 1994. Aromatase cytochrome P450, the enzyme responsible for estrogen biosynthesis. Endocr. Rev. **15:** 342–355.
16. ACKERMAN, G.E. *et al.* 1981. Aromatization of androstenedione by human adipose tissue stromal cells in monolayer culture. J. Clin. Endocrinol. Metab. **53:** 412–417.
17. MACDONALD, P.C. *et al.* 1967. Plasma precursors of estrogen. I. Extent of conversion of plasma Δ^4-androstenedione to estrone in normal males and non-pregnant normal, castrate, and adrenalectomized females. J. Clin. Endocrinol. Metab. **27:** 1103–1111.

18. MacDonald, P.C. *et al.* 1978. Effect of obesity on conversion of plasma androstenedione to estrone in postmenopausal women with and without endometrial cancer. Am. J. Obstet. Gynecol. **130:** 448–455.
19. Bulun, S.E. *et al.* 1993. A link between breast cancer and local estrogen biosynthesis suggested by quantification of breast adipose tissue aromatase cytochrome P450 transcripts using competitive polymerase chain reaction after reverse transcription. J. Clin. Endocrinol. Metab. **77:** 1622–1628.
20. Yue, W. *et al.* 1998. *In situ* aromatization enhances breast tumor estradiol levels and cellular proliferation. Cancer Res. **58:** 927–932.
21. Bulun, S.E. & E.R. Simpson. 1994. Expression of the CYP19 gene and its product aromatase cytochrome P450 in human leiomyoma tissues and cells in culture. J. Clin. Endocrinol. Metab. **78:** 736–743.
22. Noble, L.S. *et al.* 1997. Prostaglandin E_2 stimulates aromatase expression in endometriosis-derived stromal cells. J. Clin. Endocrinol. Metab. **82:** 600–606.
23. Bulun, S.E. *et al.* 1993. Polymerase chain reaction amplification fails to detect aromatase cytochrome P450 transcripts in normal human endometrium or decidua. J. Clin. Endocrinol. Metab. **76:** 1458–1463.
24. Huang, J.C. *et al.* 1996. Regulation of cyclooxygenase-2 gene in cultured endometrial stromal cells by sex steroids [abstract]. Proc. Am. Soc. Reprod. Med. Meeting S5.
25. Hill, J.A. 1992. Immunology and endometriosis. Fertil. Steril. **58:** 262–264.
26. Takayama, K. *et al.* 1998. Treatment of severe postmenopausal endometriosis with an aromatase inhibitor. Fertil. Steril. **69:** 709–713.
27. Andersson, S. & N. Moghrabi. 1997. Physiology and molecular genetics of 17β-hydroxysteroid dehydrogenases. Steroids **62:** 143–147.
28. Satyaswaroop, P.G. *et al.* 1982. Distribution of progesterone receptor, estradiol dehydrogenase, and 20α-dihydroprogesterone dehydrogenase activities in human endometrial glands and stroma: progestin induction of steroid dehydrogenase activities *in vitro* is restricted to the glandular epithelium. Endocrinology **111:** 743–749.
29. Henzl, M.R. *et al.* 1988. Administration of nasal nafarelin as compared with oral danazol for endometriosis. N. Engl. J. Med. **318:** 485–489.
30. Waller, K.G. & R.W. Shaw. 1993. Gonadotropin-releasing hormone analogues for the treatment of endometriosis: long-term follow-up. Fertil. Steril. **59:** 511–515.
31. Metzger, D.A. *et al.* 1991. Hormone-resistant endometriosis following total abdominal hysterectomy and bilateral salpingo-oophorectomy: correlation with histology and steroid receptor content. Obstet. Gynecol. **78:** 946–950.

Panel Discussion (Part II)

B.A. Lessey (*University of North Carolina, Chapel Hill, NC*): A question for Kevin Osteen. In many of the patients with endometriosis that I see and in the patients that other people see, they have a high frequency of endometrial spotting during the secretory phase, the mid-secretory phase, or mid-cycle, and you showed that MMPs are only partially suppressed at this time. Does this account for this and how does this relate to other molecules that have been described such as EBAF?

K.G. Osteen (*Vanderbilt University School of Medicine, Nashville, TN*): In the next lecture that I am going to deliver soon, I will talk a little bit more about the sort of local communication that is important for progesterone's ability to suppress MMPs. In the face of this increasing inflammatory environment that develops during the normal secretory phase, certainly any misexpression of a factor such as EBAF would block molecules that we know are stabilizing the endometrium and preventing MMP expression. In concert with Dr. Brenner's work, how far downstream the MMP misexpression is to other defects that occurred earlier also becomes a really important question. Are the MMPs among the first signs and do they get blocked; or if you block those by abnormal regulation, would that destabilize or did it take an earlier event for that to occur? Dr. Brenner may actually want to comment on that.

R.M. Brenner (*Oregon Regional Primate Research Center, Beaverton, OR*): The ability of progesterone to suppress endometrial MMPs may be limited by conditions that are not well understood during breakthrough bleeding. The recent literature, including work by Dr. Marbaix, suggests that there can be localized foci of endometrial bleeding and that only these foci may express MMPs. Hence, the mechanism controlling endometrial MMP expression probably involves local stimulatory factors that can override the suppressive effects of progesterone.

L.C. Giudice (*Stanford University, Stanford, CA*): I have a question for Dr. Bulun. Since our audience is very diverse and there is quite a bit of interest in the clinical use of aromatase inhibitors, I wonder if you could tell us in the context in which you and perhaps other investigators are administering this.

S.E. Bulun (*University of Illinois, Chicago, IL*): To my knowledge, we, at the University of Illinois at Chicago, are the only group conducting studies on the use of aromatase inhibitors to treat endometriosis. Two years ago, I remember seeing an Italian abstract in the ASRM meeting, but the investigators who sent the abstract did not show up; thus, I do not know if that study is still continuing. I suspect that there are other ongoing studies, but I am not aware of them. I am looking forward to studies on aromatase inhibitors and endometriosis to see if other investigators can also duplicate these data.

Giudice: With regard to that, do you recommend that these therapies be administered under approved protocols?

Bulun: That would be my recommendation. They are experimental at best. For example, I obtained permission from the FDA to perform these pilot studies, but none of them have been published. Neither have I completed them, so I would not recommend using them routinely at the moment unless the patient is postmenopausal.

I believe that if a postmenopausal patient is not responding to surgical treatment, an aromatase inhibitor is the treatment of choice.

R.N. TAYLOR (*University of California, San Francisco, CA*): I would like to make one comment. Even in the postmenopausal patient, I think it is very appropriate that you are treating for bone loss and watching bone loss carefully in your study. There is certainly some evidence that local aromatase activity within the bone itself might also be inhibited, so I think that it is still going to be an issue in these patients and should be a concern about this type of therapy.

K. CHWALISZ (*TAP Pharmaceutical Products, Lake Forest, IL*): I have a question for Dr. DeMayo. You mentioned in your talk that the coactivators might play a role here in endometriosis and in the regulation of steroid receptors. What about corepressors? Do you have any data suggesting that the differences in expression of corepressors could play a role?

F.J. DEMAYO (*Baylor College of Medicine, Houston, TX*): No, I don't have any data on corepressors. Most of the factors that we have been focusing on have been with regard to activation of gene expression and looking at the different coactivators. Right now, Dr. J. Xu (in collaboration with Drs. O'Malley and Chambon) is crossing all the different coactivator knockout mice to investigate potential reproductive and developmental defects in the multiple activator crosses. Thus, focusing on those and the multiple crosses will be pretty exciting.

V. MONTGOMERY RICE (*University of Kansas, Kansas City, KS*): Dr. Bulun, my question concerns the progesterone resistance. With the eutopic endometrium, you saw a cyclical fashion of the expression of progesterone receptor B and A. When you looked at the endometriotic tissue, you found no B. Did you look at that at different phases of the menstrual cycle? In other words, were those samples taken in different phases and were those women on any other medications, etc.?

BULUN: Yes. In fact, another group of investigators from Houston had looked at expression of PR-B and PR-A. I think it was Weigel and coworkers, and they found out that especially B is heavily regulated. For example, B levels are low during menstruation and then increase. They reach the highest levels right before the ovulation. They are decreased somewhat, but they are maintained during the luteal phase. We also biopsied eutopic endometria and endometriotic samples simultaneously from about, I believe, 12 patients from different phases of the menstrual cycle and these were all ovulatory patients. We were able to duplicate the work of Weigel and coworkers with respect to eutopic endometrium, but in endometriosis we could not demonstrate any PR-B.

K. YOSHINAGA (*National Institute of Child Health and Human Development, National Institutes of Health, Bethesda, MD*): If the aromatase inhibitor is effective in curing the endometriosis, is antiestrogen more effective?

BULUN: Possibly. I should not use the word "cure". Possibly, we are still far away from cure. I see aromatase inhibitors still as suppressors of endometriosis. It would be great if they did cure, but that is my bias. I really do not know much about the effects of new progestins on endometriosis. The available ones are not very effective; in fact, I choose all my patients deliberately from those who have not responded to Gn-rich agonists and/or progestins so that we could make a point.

N. BRACERO (*The Johns Hopkins Medical Center, Baltimore, MD*): In your studies, did you ever try or consider looking for the effect of blocking COX-2 and seeing what will happen in the development of the disease?

BULUN: That is an excellent suggestion. I think it should be done. It just makes sense to combine aromatase inhibitor treatment with a cyclic oxygenase inhibitor. Possibly, I would have chosen a general cyclic oxygenase inhibitor if the patient can tolerate it because this type is more effective than specific COX-2 inhibitors. To my knowledge, COX-2 inhibitors are used mostly for the lack of side effects, but that is an excellent suggestion.

S. PARTHASARATHY (*Emory University, Atlanta, GA*): In the patient whom you treated with the antiaromatase or the aromatase inhibitor, did you find any plasma lipid and lipoprotein changes that are proandrogenic?

BULUN: I really did not look at them at that moment. We were just doing this study with our own funds and we just did it in the most economic fashion. However, in the new studies that we are performing in premenopausal women, we are measuring their lipid profiles. Thus, we will have an answer.

Angiogenic Factors in Endometriosis

ROBERT N. TAYLOR, DAN I. LEBOVIC, AND MICHAEL D. MUELLER

Center for Reproductive Sciences, Department of Obstetrics, Gynecology, and Reproductive Sciences, University of California, San Francisco, San Francisco, California, USA

ABSTRACT: Similar to tumor metastases, endometriotic implants require neovascularization to establish, grow, and invade. The peritoneal environment is ideally suited to provide a proangiogenic milieu. Nevertheless, endometriotic lesions are found only in a minority of reproductive-age women (~10%) with retrograde menstruation. In this paper, we review the major cytokines, growth factors, steroid hormones, and eicosanoids responsible for angiogenesis in endometriosis. We postulate that interference with angiogenic principles expressed in the peritoneum may constitute novel therapeutic opportunities for the prevention, amelioration, or treatment of pelvic endometriosis.

KEYWORDS: neovascularization; vascular endothelial growth factor (VEGF); estrogen receptors; cytokines

INTRODUCTION

Endometriosis is a common gynecological disorder defined by the proliferation of endometrial tissue outside the uterine cavity. The disease affects about 10% of all reproductive-aged women and the prevalence rises to 20%–50% in infertile women. Genetic factors appear to influence susceptibility to endometriosis;[1] however, the mode of hereditary transmission is complex and likely multifactorial.[2] Recently, environmental factors, such as dioxin[3] and other presumed endocrine disrupters, have been implicated in its development.

The implantation hypothesis[4] is the most widely accepted etiology, supported by observations that retrograde menstruation[5] and intraperitoneal spillage of viable endometrial cells occur frequently in cycling women.[6] Some investigators proposed that microscopic peritoneal defects allow the cells to contact the submesothelial matrix[7] where they proliferate and invade the subperitoneal space. However, others demonstrated that endometrial fragments adhere directly to intact mesothelium.[8]

Using the analogy of tumor metastasis,[9] we postulated that the angiogenic potential of the derivative endometrium or the intraperitoneal environment might influence lesion establishment.[10] Indeed, endometriotic implants often are surrounded by vascularity (FIG. 1), and extrapelvic endometriosis, while rare, typically occurs in well-vascularized organs.[11] Microscopic studies have confirmed neovascularization around and within endometriosis implants.[12] The sprouting of capillaries from preexisting

Address for correspondence: Robert N. Taylor, Center for Reproductive Sciences, Department of Obstetrics, Gynecology, and Reproductive Sciences, University of California, San Francisco, San Francisco, CA 94143-0556. Fax: 415-753-3271.
rtaylor@socrates.ucsf.edu

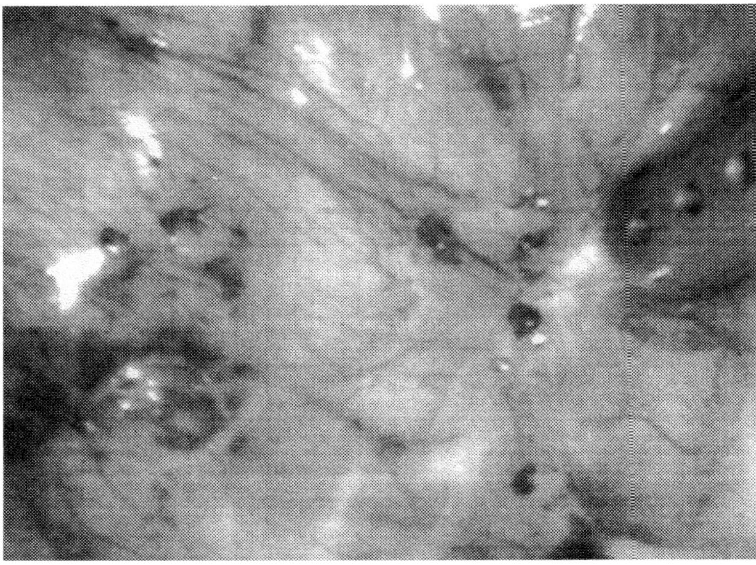

FIGURE 1. Laparoscopic photograph of endometriotic implants on peritoneal surface accompanied by neovascularization and subperitoneal hemorrhage. Tip of small probe is at the right of the field.

vessels requires proteolytic degradation of extracellular matrix, proliferation and migration of endothelial cells, and ultimately formation of a patent tubular network supplying the angiogenic stimulus (FIG. 2). Angiogenesis occurs when the balance of local factors favoring vascular growth exceeds those factors inhibiting angiogenesis.

PERITONEAL FLUID CYTOKINES: CLUES TO THE MICROENVIRONMENT OF ENDOMETRIOSIS

Although pelvic fluid is a complex medium containing and influenced by multiple cell types, we[13,14] and other investigators[15,16] have found this to be a useful biological fluid to define factors associated with endometriosis. Oosterlynck *et al.*,[15] using the chick chorioallantoic membrane bioassay, were the first to show that pelvic fluid from women with endometriosis had more angiogenic activity than pelvic fluid from normal controls. We confirmed this observation using an *in vitro* model of endothelial cell proliferation. [^{3}H]-Thymidine incorporation into nascent cellular

FIGURE 2. Cultured human endothelial cells recapitulate angiogenesis *in vitro* by formation of capillary-like tubular structures. **(A)** Endothelial cells grown on denatured collagen reveal a typical "cobblestone" morphology. **(B)** Exposure to a complex basement membrane (Matrigel®, Collaborative Research, Bedford, MA) for 8 hours begins to initiate 3-D reorganization. **(C)** After 48 hours on Matrigel®, mature tubular structures are manifested. Photomicrographs are reprinted with permission from the *American Journal of Physiology* and the American Physiological Society from the original studies of de Groot *et al.*[80]

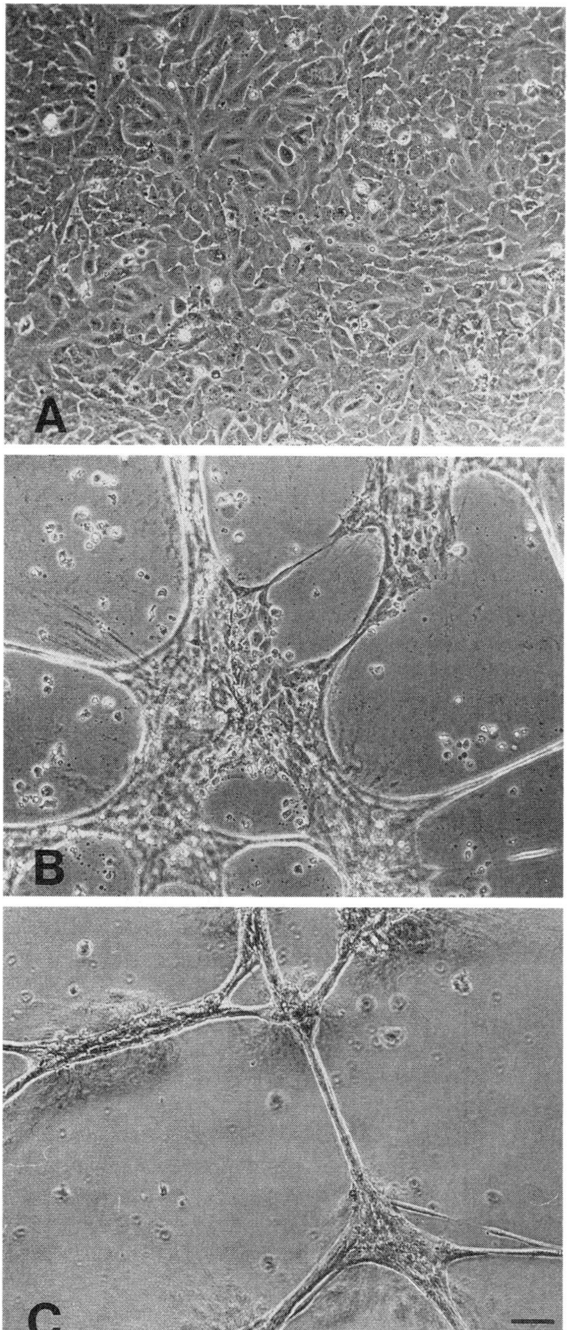

FIGURE 2. *See previous page for legend.*

DNA demonstrated that peritoneal fluid from women with endometriosis contained significantly more angiogenic activity than pelvic fluid from normal controls.[10]

ENDOCRINE COUPLING OF ENDOMETRIAL ANGIOGENESIS

Cyclical vascular changes within the primate endometrium have been recognized since the classical experiments of Markee,[17] who transplanted rhesus endometrium into the anterior chamber of the eye. These findings were supported by Noyes and colleagues,[18] who noted perivascular changes during the phases of the human endometrial cycle. Attempts to localize estrogen receptors (ER) or progesterone receptors (PR) in vascular endothelium have generally been negative.[10,19,20] These data will be reviewed later in the text. Most investigators suggest that steroid hormones indirectly promote angiogenesis via paracrine production of cytokines and growth factors.[10,21]

Interleukin-1

IL-1β is the dominant interleukin-1 secreted by activated peritoneal macrophages and its levels are elevated in endometriosis.[22] Studies report elevated levels in stage I and II endometriosis cases,[23,24] but this is not uniformly confirmed.[25] We showed that IL-1β produced by activated peritoneal macrophages plays an important role in the neovascularization that surrounds endometriotic lesions.[26] A 2.6-fold induction of vascular endothelial growth factor (VEGF) mRNA and a 6.3-fold increase in IL-6 mRNA transcripts in endometriotic stromal cells were noted after exposure to IL-1β. Normal endometrial stromal cells showed no induction. RT-PCR for the IL-1 receptor type I (IL-1RI) indicated that the differential effects of IL-1β were associated with more receptor mRNA in endometriosis-derived cells. Therefore, it appears that IL-1β activates an angiogenic phenotype in endometriosis stromal cells via IL-1RI.

Interleukin-6

Interleukin-6 (IL-6) is a multifunctional cytokine that is produced by endometrial epithelial and stromal cells.[27,28] IL-6 forms a complex with its receptor and associates with a transmembrane glycoprotein, gp130, that signals through the JAK-STAT cascade. IL-6 has immunomodulatory[28] and angiogenic[29] effects, some of which are mediated via the induction of VEGF expression.[30]

Stromal cells derived from ovarian endometriomas expressed higher basal and cytokine-induced IL-6 than stromal cells derived from normal endometrium,[28] whereas cells derived from eutopic endometrium of endometriosis patients had intermediate levels of IL-6. An attractive interpretation of this finding is that the endometrial lining of women destined to develop endometriosis manifests an "activated" angiogenic phenotype.

Interleukin-8

Interleukin-8 (IL-8) is an 8-kDa peptide of the α or C-X-C chemokine family produced in response to a variety of proinflammatory stimuli (e.g., IL-1 and TNF-α). IL-8 recruits and activates polymorphonuclear leukocytes and T lymphocytes and has angiogenic activity.[31] In the endometrium, IL-8 protein is localized predominantly in perivascular cells.[32] IL-8 gene expression and protein secretion were documented in cultured endometrial stromal cells stimulated with IL-1β, TNF-α, or serum.[33] Coincubation with progesterone increased IL-8 mRNA synthesis and stability.[34] Cultured epithelial cells also express IL-8 mRNA, although steady-state concentrations in stromal cells were higher. Therefore, both endometrial stromal and epithelial cells have the potential to recruit leukocytes[35] and especially neutrophils into the endometrium.

In endometriosis, correlations between IL-8 concentration and clinical disease stage were observed.[14,34] IL-8 derived from endometriotic lesions themselves or from pelvic macrophages[36] may promote the neovascularization of ectopic endometrial implants.

Epidermal Growth Factors

Epidermal growth factor (EGF) is a 6-kDa protein with homology to TGF-α, betacellulin, and amphiregulin proteins involved in embryonic development.[37] EGF[38] and TGF-α[39] have angiogenic activity. The human EGF receptor-1 (HER-1) is a 170-kDa transmembrane receptor tyrosine kinase. In the endometrium, EGF and HER-1 mediate estrogen-induced proliferative effects through coupled signaling pathways.[21,40,41] EGF and HER-1 are expressed in endometriosis implants.[42] In patients with endometriosis, treatment with a gonadotropin-releasing hormone analog caused a dramatic reduction of HER-1 expression in eutopic endometrium and in endometriotic implants.[43] Peritoneal fluid concentrations of EGF were highly variable and there was no significant difference in peritoneal fluids of women with or without endometriosis.[44]

Fibroblast Growth Factors

A family of more than nine related 17- to 38-kDa fibroblast growth factor (FGF) proteins play major roles in development, wound healing, and tumorigenesis. Four FGFs (1, 2, 4, and 7) have been identified in human endometrium.[45] FGF-1 (acidic FGF) and FGF-2 (basic FGF) are mitogenic for a variety of cell types, particularly capillary endothelial cells. However, FGF-2 does not induce proliferation in decidual endothelial cells.[46] FGF-2 is present in peritoneal fluid, but its concentration does not change during the menstrual cycle nor in the presence of endometriosis.[47]

Insulin-like Growth Factors

The insulin-like growth factors (IGFs), their receptors, and their binding proteins (IGFBPs) represent a complex system of growth-regulating factors in human endometrium. The IGFs are 7-kDa proteins related to insulin. The IGF type I receptor (IGF-I-R) is structurally similar to the classical insulin receptor. It forms a heterotetrameric transmembrane complex that binds IGF-I and -II ligands with high affinity (1–5 nM) and signals cellular mitogenesis via tyrosine kinase domains in its β-subunits.[48] Six human IGFBPs, ranging in size from 24 to 45 kDa, serve as IGF transporters and modulate local bioactive IGF concentrations. The bioactivity of the IGFBPs in turn may be modulated by endogenous serine proteases.[49] In human endometrium, IGF-I is expressed predominantly in the proliferative phase of the cycle, whereas IGF-II is abundant during the secretory phase. *In situ* hybridization analyses by Zhou *et al.*[50] suggest that IGF-1 and -II transcripts were predominantly stromal, whereas the two receptors were more abundant in the epithelium. Direct studies of the IGF system in endometriosis are very limited. IGF-I and -II and IGFBPs 2 and 3 are present in pelvic fluid from normal subjects,[49] but no differences are found in IGF-II or IGFBP 3 when compared to fluid from endometriosis patients.[51]

Platelet-Derived Growth Factor

Platelet-derived growth factor (PDGF) is a cationic protein of 32 kDa. Two related polypeptide chains, PDGF-A and PDGF-B, are linked by disulfide bonds. PDGF is chemotactic and mitogenic for cells of mesenchymal origin, including endothelial cells, although the latter effect may be indirect.[52] Normal human endometrium expresses PDGF ligand subunits and receptors.[53] Both endometrial epithelial[54] and stromal[55] cells proliferate *in vitro* in response to PDGF. Human peritoneal fluid and media conditioned by activated peritoneal macrophages[56] contain mitogenic activity with biochemical characteristics of PDGF. Pelvic fluid and purified PDGF stimulated [^{3}H]-thymidine incorporation into DNA of human endometrial stromal cell cultures.[55]

Platelet-Derived Endothelial Cell Growth Factor

Platelet-derived endothelial cell growth factor (PD-ECGF) is a cytoplasmic protein of 45 kDa that encodes the enzyme, thymidine phosphorylase.[57] PD-ECGF is chemotactic and mitogenic for vascular endothelial cells and is expressed strongly in endometrial glands during the luteal and menstrual phases of the cycle. PD-ECGF also has been localized to the epithelial cells lining ovarian endometriomas, near the subepithelial capillary plexus in these implants. Modulation of PD-ECGF during the menstrual cycle was not observed in endometriosis implants, suggesting that PD-ECGF may be a tonic angiogenic stimulator in these lesions.[58]

Vascular Endothelial Growth Factor

Vascular endothelial growth factor (VEGF) is the prototypic and most potent angiogenic factor. The biochemistry and molecular biology of VEGF are well described.[59] VEGF binds to a family of tyrosine kinase receptors, particularly Flt-1 and KDR, leading to dimer formation, autophosphorylation, and activation of mitogen-activated protein kinases.[60] In human endometrium, VEGF mRNA reaches a maximum in late proliferative and secretory endometrium.[61] We and others demonstrated that VEGF is an estrogen- and progestin-responsive angiogenic factor.[61,62] Ovarian steroids appear to increase VEGF mRNA transcriptional activity and stability. Putative estrogen-responsive elements have been identified in the VEGF gene promoter.[63,64] VEGF protein is secreted apically by polarized human endometrial epithelial cells *in vitro*.[65] Hypoxia,[66] IL-1β,[26] PDGF,[67] EGF,[68] and PGE_2[69] also upregulate VEGF expression.

Peritoneal fluid concentrations of soluble VEGF from patients with endometriosis[61,70] correlate significantly with the stage of disease. Endometriotic lesions themselves[61] produce VEGF, predominantly in the epithelial cell layer (FIG. 3). Moreover, activated peritoneal macrophages[70] and neutrophils[71] also have the capacity to synthesize and secrete VEGF. Donnez *et al.*[72] demonstrated that

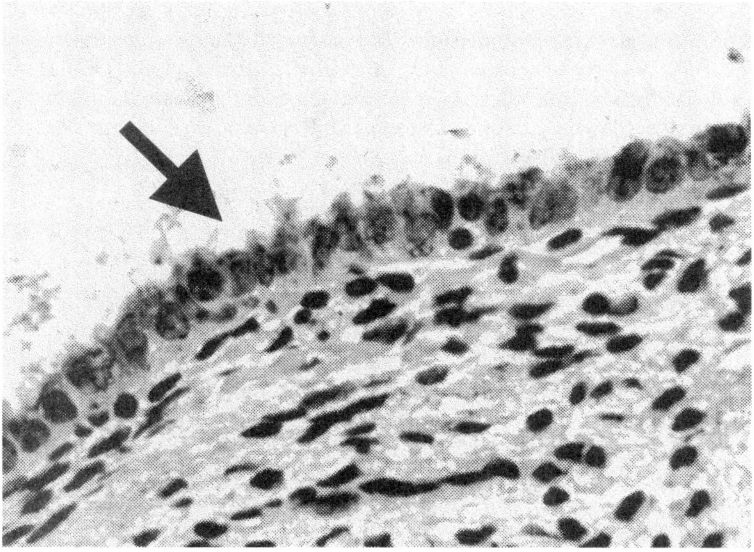

FIGURE 3. Endometriotic lesions express VEGF. Intense immunohistochemical staining for VEGF is observed in the cytoplasm of the epithelial layer of an endometriotic implant (*arrow*). Note that the underlying stromal cells contain lighter immunopositive reaction products. The cell nuclei were counterstained with hematoxylin.

eutopic glandular epithelium of endometriosis patients had significantly higher VEGF content during the late secretory phase compared to the endometrium of patients without endometriosis.

Endometriosis Protein-I

Endometriosis protein-I (ENDO-I) is preferentially synthesized and secreted by ectopic endometrial tissues.[73] Sequence analysis identified ENDO-I as a haptoglobin-like protein.[74] ENDO-I transcript levels are significantly higher in ectopic pelvic endometrium than in eutopic endometrium of the same individuals, independent of the stage of the reproductive cycle.[74] Local peritoneal production of ENDO-I may be associated with angiogenesis and altered immune phenomena related to endometriosis.

Ovarian Steroids

It is unlikely that ovarian steroids are direct mediators of endometrial or endometriosis angiogenesis. Most investigators have failed to identify detectable levels of classical estrogen (α) or progesterone (A and B) receptors in endometrial vascular endothelial cells.[19,75] However, recent reports demonstrated PR and ER-β expression in human endometrial endothelial cells by RT-PCR and immunohistochemistry, respectively.[76,77] In the former study, PR complexes appeared to inhibit endothelial mitotic activity.[76]

Indirect angiogenic effects of estrogen and progesterone were shown in the rat uterus[62,63] and human endometrium.[61,78] Estrogens and progestins upregulate VEGF mRNA and protein production in uterine tissues and cells. These studies support the obligatory role of ovarian steroids on endometriosis implants[79] and the observation that downregulating doses of GnRH analogs decrease the size and vascularity of endometriosis lesions.[11]

SUMMARY

Endometriosis is a fascinating and complex disease resulting from a dysregulation between exfoliated menstrual endometrium and the intra-abdominal environment. Increased concentrations of activated pelvic macrophages and lymphocytes and elevated levels of specific cytokines and growth factors reviewed above support this hypothesis. The precise roles of these soluble factors are currently unknown, but we propose that a complex network of locally produced cytokines, growth factors, steroids, and eicosanoids modulate the growth and inflammatory behavior of ectopic endometrial implants via neovascularization. The enhanced secretion of local pro-angiogenic proteins by endometriosis lesions and associated immune cells (and the concomitant reduction of antiangiogenic principles) promotes the recruitment of capillaries toward the growing lesions. Ultimately, a cascade of effects on the peritoneal microenvironment results in implant proliferation and invasion. Future therapeutic strategies to target these angiogenic stimuli have the potential to block the vascular pathogenesis of endometriosis. However, we must not ignore the likely physiological actions of these same antiangiogenic molecules in eutopic endometrial function. Indeed, unless these agents are selectively or preferentially reversible in the eutopic endometrium, angiosuppressive therapy may be more amenable for the treatment of endometriosis-associated pain than for infertility.

ACKNOWLEDGMENTS

Our original studies summarized in this review were supported by NIH Grant Nos. HD33238, HD08517, and HD37321, through the Specialized Cooperative Centers Program in Reproductive Research, and by a grant from the Swiss National Science Foundation (to M. D. Mueller).

REFERENCES

1. Treloar, S., D. O'Connor, V. O'Connor & N. Martin. 1999. Genetic influences on endometriosis in an Australian twin sample. Fertil. Steril. **71:** 701–710.
2. Malinak, L.R., V.C. Buttram, Jr., S. Elias & J.L. Simpson. 1980. Heritage aspects of endometriosis. II. Clinical characteristics of familial endometriosis. Am. J. Obstet. Gynecol. **137:** 332–337.
3. Rier, S.E., D.C. Martin, R.E. Bowman *et al.* 1993. Endometriosis in rhesus monkeys (*Macaca mulatta*) following chronic exposure to 2,3,7,8-tetrachlorodibenzo-*p*-dioxin. Fundam. Appl. Toxicol. **21:** 433–441.
4. Sampson, J. 1927. Peritoneal endometriosis due to the menstrual dissemination of endometrial tissue into the peritoneal cavity. Am. J. Obstet. Gynecol. **14:** 422–469.

5. HALME, J., M. HAMMOND, J. HULKA *et al.* 1984. Retrograde menstruation in healthy women and in patients with endometriosis. Obstet. Gynecol. **64:** 151–154.
6. KRUITWAGEN, R., L. POELS, W. WILLEMSEN *et al.* 1991. Endometrial epithelial cells in peritoneal fluid during the early follicular phase. Fertil. Steril. **55:** 297–303.
7. GROOTHUIS, P., C. KOKS, A. DE GOEIJ *et al.* 1999. Adhesion of human endometrial fragments to peritoneum *in vitro*. Fertil. Steril. **71:** 1119–1124.
8. WITZ, C.A., M.R. THOMAS, I.A. MONTOYA-RODRIGUEZ *et al.* 2001. Short-term culture of peritoneum explants confirms attachment of endometrium to intact peritoneal mesothelium. Fertil. Steril. **75:** 385–390.
9. HANAHAN, D. & J. FOLKMAN. 1996. Patterns and emerging mechanisms of the angiogenic switch during tumorigenesis. Cell **86:** 353–364.
10. TAYLOR, R., I. RYAN, E. MOORE *et al.* 1997. Angiogenesis and macrophage activation in endometriosis. Ann. N.Y. Acad. Sci. **828:** 194–207.
11. RYAN, I. & R. TAYLOR. 1997. Endometriosis and infertility: new concepts. Obstet. Gynecol. Surv. **52:** 365–371.
12. NISOLLE, M., B. CASANAS ROUX, V. ANAF *et al.* 1993. Morphometric study of the stromal vascularization in peritoneal endometriosis. Fertil. Steril. **59:** 681–684.
13. KHORRAM, O., R. TAYLOR, I. RYAN *et al.* 1993. Peritoneal fluid concentrations of the cytokine RANTES correlate with the severity of endometriosis. Am. J. Obstet. Gynecol. **169:** 1545–1549.
14. RYAN, I., J. TSENG, E. SCHRIOCK *et al.* 1995. Interleukin-8 concentrations are elevated in peritoneal fluid of women with endometriosis. Fertil. Steril. **63:** 929–932.
15. OOSTERLYNCK, D.J., C. MEULEMAN, H. SOBIS *et al.* 1993. Angiogenic activity of peritoneal fluid from women with endometriosis. Fertil. Steril. **59:** 778–782.
16. RAMEY, J.W. & D.F. ARCHER. 1993. Peritoneal fluid: its relevance to the development of endometriosis. Fertil. Steril. **60:** 1–14.
17. MARKEE, J. 1940. Menstruation in intraocular endometrial transplants in the rhesus monkey. Contrib. Embryol. **177:** 220–230.
18. NOYES, R.W., A.T. HERTIG & J. ROCK. 1950. Dating the endometrial biopsy. Fertil. Steril. **1:** 3–25.
19. PERROT-APPLANAT, M., M. DENG, H. FERNANDEZ *et al.* 1994. Immunohistochemical localization of estradiol and progesterone receptors in human uterus throughout pregnancy: expression in endometrial blood vessels. J. Clin. Endocrinol. Metab. **78:** 216–224.
20. BAKER, V.L., V.A. CHAO, J.T. MURAI *et al.* 1997. Human umbilical vessels and cultured umbilical vein endothelial and smooth muscle cells lack detectable protein and mRNA encoding estrogen receptors. J. Soc. Gynecol. Invest. **4:** 316–324.
21. NELSON, K., T. TAKAHASHI, N. BOSSERT *et al.* 1991. Epidermal growth factor replaces estrogen in the stimulation of female genital-tract growth and differentiation. Proc. Natl. Acad. Sci. U.S.A. **88:** 21–25.
22. MORI, H., M. SAWAIRI, M. NAKAGAWA *et al.* 1992. Expression of interleukin-1 (IL-1) beta messenger ribonucleic acid (mRNA) and IL-1 receptor antagonist mRNA in peritoneal macrophages from patients with endometriosis. Fertil. Steril. **57:** 535–542.
23. FAKIH, H., B. BAGGETT, G. HOLTZ *et al.* 1987. Interleukin-1: a possible role in the infertility associated with endometriosis. Fertil. Steril. **47:** 213–217.
24. TAKETANI, Y., T.M. KUO & M. MIZUNO. 1992. Comparison of cytokine levels and embryo toxicity in peritoneal fluid in infertile women with untreated or treated endometriosis. Am. J. Obstet. Gynecol. **167:** 265–270.
25. KEENAN, J.A., T.T. CHEN, N.L. CHADWELL *et al.* 1995. IL-1 beta, TNF-alpha, and IL-2 in peritoneal fluid and macrophage-conditioned media of women with endometriosis. Am. J. Reprod. Immunol. **34:** 381–385.
26. LEBOVIC, D., F. BENTZIEN, V. CHAO *et al.* 2000. Induction of an angiogenic phenotype in endometriosis stromal cell cultures by interleukin-1β. Mol. Hum. Reprod. **6:** 269–275.
27. TABIBZADEH, S., Q.F. KONG, A. BABAKNIA & L.T. MAY. 1995. Progressive rise in the expression of interleukin-6 in human endometrium during menstrual cycle is initiated during the implantation window. Hum. Reprod. **10:** 2793–2799.
28. TSENG, J., I. RYAN, T. MILAM *et al.* 1996. Interleukin-6 secretion *in vitro* is up-regulated in ectopic and eutopic endometrial stromal cells from women with endometriosis. J. Clin. Endocrinol. Metab. **81:** 1118–1122.

29. MOTRO, B., A. ITIN, L. SACHS & E. KESHET. 1990. Pattern of interleukin 6 gene expression *in vivo* suggests a role for this cytokine in angiogenesis. Proc. Natl. Acad. Sci. U.S.A. **87:** 3092–3096.
30. COHEN, T., D. NAHARI, L.W. CEREM *et al.* 1996. Interleukin 6 induces the expression of vascular endothelial growth factor. J. Biol. Chem. **271:** 736–741.
31. KOCH, A., P. POLVERINI, S. KUNKEL *et al.* 1992. Interleukin-8 as a macrophage-derived mediator of angiogenesis. Science **258:** 1798–1801.
32. MILNE, S., H. CRITCHLEY, T. DRUDY *et al.* 1999. Perivascular interleukin-8 messenger ribonucleic acid expression in human endometrium varies across the menstrual cycle and in early pregnancy decidua. J. Clin. Endocrinol. Metab. **84:** 2563–2567.
33. ARICI, A., J. HEAD, P. MACDONALD & M. CASEY. 1993. Regulation of interleukin-8 gene expression in human endometrial cells in culture. Mol. Cell. Endocrinol. **94:** 195–204.
34. ARICI, A., P. MACDONALD & M. CASEY. 1996. Progestin regulation of interleukin-8 mRNA levels and protein synthesis in human endometrial stromal cells. J. Steroid Biochem. Mol. Biol. **58:** 71–76.
35. BULMER, J., M. LONGFELLOW & A. RITSON. 1991. Leukocytes and resident blood cells in endometrium. Ann. N.Y. Acad. Sci. **622:** 57–68.
36. RANA, N., D.P. BRAUN, R. HOUSE *et al.* 1996. Basal and stimulated secretion of cytokines by peritoneal macrophages in women with endometriosis. Fertil. Steril. **65:** 925–930.
37. MIYAUCHI, A., M. MOMOEDA, M. NAKABAYASHI *et al.* 1995. Regulation of the plasminogen activator/plasmin system by epidermal growth factor in cultured human endometrial cells. Hum. Reprod. **10:** 3284–3288.
38. GOSPODAROWICZ, D., K. BROWN, C. BIRDWELL & B. ZETTER. 1978. Control of proliferation of human vascular endothelial cells: characterization of the response of human umbilical vein endothelial cells to fibroblast growth factor, epidermal growth factor, and thrombin. J. Cell Biol. **77:** 774–788.
39. FOLKMAN, J. 1995. Clinical applications of research on angiogenesis. N. Engl. J. Med. **333:** 1757–1764.
40. IMAI, T., H. KURACHI, K. ADACHI *et al.* 1995. Changes in epidermal growth factor receptor and the levels of its ligands during menstrual cycle in human endometrium. Biol. Reprod. **52:** 928–938.
41. CURTIS, S., T. WASHBURN, C. SEWALL *et al.* 1996. Physiological coupling of growth factor and steroid receptor signaling pathways: estrogen receptor knockout mice lack estrogen-like response to epidermal growth factor. Proc. Natl. Acad. Sci. U.S.A. **93:** 12626–12630.
42. HUANG, J. & J. YEH. 1994. Quantitative analysis of epidermal growth factor receptor gene expression in endometriosis. J. Clin. Endocrinol. Metab. **79:** 1097–1101.
43. DI LIETO, A., G. DE ROSA, G. ALBANO *et al.* 1997. Influence of goserelin depot therapy on epidermal growth factor receptor expression in pelvic endometriosis. Gynecol. Endocrinol. **11:** 17–20.
44. HUANG, J.C., C. PAPASAKELARIOU & M.Y. DAWOOD. 1996. Epidermal growth factor and basic fibroblast growth factor in peritoneal fluid of women with endometriosis. Fertil. Steril. **65:** 931–934.
45. FERRIANI, R.A., D.S. CHARNOCK-JONES, A. PRENTICE *et al.* 1993. Immunohistochemical localization of acidic and basic fibroblast growth factors in normal human endometrium and endometriosis and the detection of their mRNA by polymerase chain reaction. Hum. Reprod. **8:** 11–16.
46. GRIMWOOD, J., R. BICKNELL & M. REES. 1995. The isolation, characterization, and culture of human decidual endothelium. Hum. Reprod. **10:** 2142–2148.
47. SELI, E., H.B. ZEYNELOGLU, L.M. SENTURK *et al.* 1998. Basic fibroblast growth factor: peritoneal and follicular fluid level and its effect on early embryonic development. Fertil. Steril. **69:** 1145–1148.
48. LE ROITH, D. 1996. Insulin-like growth factor receptors and binding proteins. Bailliere's Clin. Endocrinol. Metab. **10:** 49–73.
49. GIUDICE, L., B. DSUPIN, S. GARGOSKY *et al.* 1994. The insulin-like growth factor system in human peritoneal fluid: its effects on endometrial stromal cells and its potential relevance to endometriosis. J. Clin. Endocrinol. Metab. **79:** 1284–1293.

50. ZHOU, J., B. DSUPIN, L. GIUDICE & C. BONDY. 1994. Insulin-like growth factor system gene expression in human endometrium during the menstrual cycle. J. Clin. Endocrinol. Metab. **79:** 1723–1734.
51. GURGAN, T., O. BUKULMEZ, H. YARALI *et al.* 1999. Serum and peritoneal fluid levels of IGF I and II and insulin-like growth binding protein-3 in endometriosis. J. Reprod. Med. **44:** 450–454.
52. NICOSIA, R., S. NICOSIA & M. SMITH. 1994. Vascular endothelial growth factor, platelet-derived growth factor, and insulin-like growth factor-1 promote rat aortic angiogenesis *in vitro*. Am. J. Pathol. **145:** 1023–1029.
53. CHEGINI, N., M. ROSSI & B. MASTERSON. 1992. Platelet-derived growth factor (PDGF), epidermal growth factor (EGF), and EGF and PDGF beta-receptors in human endometrial tissue: localization and *in vitro* action. Endocrinology **130:** 2373–2385.
54. MUNSON, L., N. UPADHYAYA & S. VAN METER. 1995. Platelet-derived growth factor promotes endometrial epithelial cell proliferation. Am. J. Obstet. Gynecol. **173:** 1820–1825.
55. SURREY, E. & J. HALME. 1991. Effect of platelet-derived growth factor on endometrial stromal cell proliferation *in vitro*: a model for endometriosis? Fertil. Steril. **56:** 672–679.
56. OLIVE, D., I. MONTOYA, R. RIEHL & R. SCHENKEN. 1991. Macrophage-conditioned media enhance endometrial stromal cell proliferation *in vitro.* Am. J. Obstet. Gynecol. **164:** 953–958.
57. MOGHADDAM, A., H.T. ZHANG, T.P. FAN *et al.* 1995. Thymidine phosphorylase is angiogenic and promotes tumor growth. Proc. Natl. Acad. Sci. U.S.A. **92:** 998–1002.
58. FUJIMOTO, J., H. SAKAGUCHI, R. HIROSE & T. TAMAYA. 1999. Expression of platelet-derived endothelial cell growth factor (PD-ECGF) related to angiogenesis in ovarian endometriosis. J. Clin. Endocrinol. Metab. **84:** 359–362.
59. FERRARA, N. 1999. Vascular endothelial growth factor: molecular and biological aspects. Curr. Top. Microbiol. Immunol. **237:** 1–30.
60. D'ANGELO, G., I. STRUMAN, J. MARTIAL & R. WEINER. 1995. Activation of mitogen-activated protein kinases by vascular endothelial growth factor and basic fibroblast growth factor in capillary endothelial cells is inhibited by the antiangiogenic factor 16-kDa-terminal fragment of prolactin. Proc. Natl. Acad. Sci. U.S.A. **92:** 6374–6378.
61. SHIFREN, J., J. TSENG, C. ZALOUDEK *et al.* 1996. Ovarian steroid regulation of vascular endothelial growth factor in the human endometrium: implications for angiogenesis during the menstrual cycle and in the pathogenesis of endometriosis. J. Clin. Endocrinol. Metab. **81:** 3112–3118.
62. CULLINAN-BOVE, K. & R. KOOS. 1993. Vascular endothelial growth factor/vascular permeability factor expression in the rat uterus: rapid stimulation by estrogen correlates with estrogen-induced increases in uterine capillary permeability and growth. Endocrinology **133:** 829–837.
63. HYDER, S.M., Z. NAWAZ, C. CHIAPPETTA & G.M. STANCEL. 2000. Identification of functional estrogen response elements in the gene coding for the potent angiogenic factor vascular endothelial growth factor. Cancer Res. **60:** 3183–3190.
64. MUELLER, M.D., J-L. VIGNE, A. MINCHENKO *et al.* 2000. Regulation of vascular endothelial growth factor (VEGF) gene transcription by estrogen receptors alpha and beta. Proc. Natl. Acad. Sci. U.S.A. **97:** 10972–10977.
65. HORNUNG, D., D. LEBOVIC, J. SHIFREN *et al.* 1998. Vectorial secretion of vascular endothelial growth factor by polarized human endometrial epithelial cells. Fertil. Steril. **69:** 909–915.
66. LIU, Y., S. COX, T. MORITA & S. KOUREMBANAS. 1995. Hypoxia regulates vascular endothelial growth factor gene expression in endothelial cells: identification of a 5′ enhancer. Circ. Res. **77:** 638–643.
67. BROGI, E., T. WU, A. NAMIKI & J. ISNER. 1994. Indirect angiogenic cytokines upregulate VEGF and bFGF gene expression in vascular smooth muscle cells, whereas hypoxia upregulates VEGF expression only. Circulation **90:** 649–652.
68. GOLDMAN, C., J. KIM, W. WONG *et al.* 1993. Epidermal growth factor stimulates vascular endothelial growth factor production by human malignant glioma cells: a model of glioblastoma multiform pathophysiology. Mol. Biol. Cell **4:** 121–133.

69. BEN-AV, P., L. CROFFORD, R. WILDER & T. HLA. 1995. Induction of vascular endothelial growth factor expression in synovial fibroblasts by prostaglandin E and interleukin-1: a potential mechanism for inflammatory angiogenesis. FEBS Lett. **372:** 83–87.
70. MCLAREN, J., A. PRENTICE, D. CHARNOCK-JONES *et al.* 1996. Vascular endothelial growth factor is produced by peritoneal fluid macrophages in endometriosis and is regulated by ovarian steroids. J. Clin. Invest. **98:** 482–489.
71. MUELLER, M.D., D.I. LEBOVIC, E. GARRETT & R.N. TAYLOR. 2000. Neutrophils infiltrating the endometrium express vascular endothelial growth factor (VEGF): potential role in endometrial angiogenesis. Fertil. Steril. **74:** 107–112.
72. DONNEZ, J., P. SMOES, S. GILLEROT *et al.* 1998. Vascular endothelial growth factor (VEGF) in endometriosis. Hum. Reprod. **13:** 1686–1690.
73. SHARPE, K., R. ZIMMER, W. GRIFFIN & L. PENNEY. 1993. Polypeptides synthesized and released by human endometriosis differ from those of the uterine endometrium in cell and tissue explant culture. Fertil. Steril. **60:** 839–851.
74. PIVA, M. & K. SHARPE-TIMMS. 1999. Peritoneal endometriotic lesions differentially express a haptoglobin-like gene. Mol. Hum. Reprod. **5:** 71–78.
75. TAYLOR, R., I. RYAN, J. TSENG *et al.* 1999. Ovarian steroids and angiogenesis. *In* Understanding Endometriosis: Advances in Research and Practice, pp. 131–137. Parthenon. Carnforth.
76. IRUELA-ARISPE, M.L., J. RODRIGUEZ-MANZANEQUE & G. ABU-JAWDEH. 1999. Endometrial endothelial cells express estrogen and progesterone receptors and exhibit a tissue specific response to angiogenic growth factors. Microcirculation **6:** 127–140.
77. LECCE, G., G. MEDURI, M. ANCELIN *et al.* 2001. Presence of estrogen receptor beta in the human endometrium through the cycle: expression in glandular, stromal, and vascular cells. J. Clin. Endocrinol. Metab. **86:** 1379–1386.
78. CHARNOCK-JONES, D., A. SHARKEY, J. RAJPUT-WILLIAMS *et al.* 1993. Identification and localization of alternately spliced mRNAs for vascular endothelial growth factor in human uterus and estrogen regulation in endometrial carcinoma cell lines. Biol. Reprod. **48:** 1120–1128.
79. DIZEREGA, G., D. BARBER & G. HODGEN. 1980. Endometriosis: role of ovarian steroids in initiation, maintenance, and suppression. Fertil. Steril. **33:** 649–653.
80. DE GROOT, C.J.M., V.A. CHAO, J.M. ROBERTS & R.N. TAYLOR. 1995. Human endothelial cell morphology and autacoid expression. Am. J. Physiol. **268**(Heart Circ. Physiol. 37)**:** H1613–H1620.

Local Cytokines in Endometrial Tissue: The Role of Interleukin-8 in the Pathogenesis of Endometriosis

AYDIN ARICI

Division of Reproductive Endocrinology, Department of Obstetrics and Gynecology, Yale University School of Medicine, New Haven, Connecticut, USA

ABSTRACT: Endometriosis, defined by the presence of viable endometrial tissue outside the uterine cavity, is among the most common gynecologic disorders affecting women of reproductive age. Endometriosis is associated with an inflammatory peritoneal environment, where multiple cytokines and growth factors are found at elevated levels. Interleukin-8 (IL-8) is a cytokine that induces chemotaxis of neutrophils and is a potent angiogenic agent. In addition, IL-8 was recently found to stimulate proliferation of various cells. We have observed that IL-8 is elevated in the peritoneal fluid of women with endometriosis and the levels correlate with the severity of the disease. We hypothesized that IL-8 may play a role in the growth and maintenance of ectopic endometrial tissue not only by chemoattracting and stimulating leukocytes to secrete growth factors and cytokines, but also by directly affecting endometrial cell proliferation. We found that IL-8 mRNA and protein levels in the endometrium were significantly higher during early proliferative and late secretory phases than during the mid-cycle. IL-8 receptors A and B are also expressed in the endometrium mostly localized in the stroma. Interestingly, IL-8 receptor expression is higher in the eutopic endometrium of women with endometriosis compared to the endometrium of women without endometriosis. Endometrial cells in culture proliferate significantly when treated with IL-8, which is inhibited by anti-IL-8 neutralizing antibody. More convincingly, IL-8 antisense oligonucleotide treatment decreases IL-8 production by endometrial cells as well as cell proliferation when compared to non-sense oligonucleotide treatment. The addition of IL-8 reverses the inhibitory effect of IL-8 antisense oligonucleotides on cell proliferation. These findings suggest that IL-8 may act as an autocrine growth factor in the endometrium. We have also studied the effect of endometrial cell adhesion on IL-8 expression and observed that IL-8 stimulates the adhesion of endometrial cells to fibronectin. Treatment of the cells with anti-IL-8 neutralizing antibody inhibited partially the cell adhesion. Thus, IL-8 may also be relevant for stimulating the attachment of endometrial implants in the pathogenesis of endometriosis. In addition, adherence of endometrial cells induced further IL-8 expression by an integrin-dependent mechanism. In summary, IL-8 may act as an autocrine growth factor in the endometrium and may also play a role in the pathogenesis of endometriosis by promoting the vicious circle of endometrial cell attachment, cell growth, and further secretion of this cytokine.

KEYWORDS: endometriosis; endometrium; interleukin-8; cytokines; chemokines

Address for correspondence: Aydin Arici, M.D., Division of Reproductive Endocrinology and Infertility, Department of Obstetrics and Gynecology, Yale University School of Medicine, 333 Cedar Street, New Haven, CT 06520-8063.Voice: 203-785-4005; fax: 203-785-7134.
aydin.arici@yale.edu

INTRODUCTION

Endometriosis, defined by the presence of viable endometrial tissue outside the uterine cavity, is among the most common gynecologic disorders affecting women of reproductive age.[1] The pathogenesis of endometriosis involves retrograde dissemination of endometrium and/or development *in situ* by metaplasia and there is evidence suggesting that genetic and hormonal factors may play a role.[2] There is also substantial evidence that immunologic factors, namely, peritoneal macrophages, T cells, natural killer cells, and soluble products secreted by these cells, are involved in the pathogenesis of endometriosis. The immunologic profile of endometriosis is typical of an inflammatory disease.[3] What role these secretory products may play in the pathogenesis of endometriosis is not yet known. They have been indirectly implicated as adversely affecting fertility and/or stimulating the implantation and proliferation of endometrial cells. One such factor is interleukin-8 (IL-8), a cytokine that induces chemotaxis of neutrophils and a potent angiogenic agent. In addition to its chemotactic and angiogenic properties, IL-8 was recently found to stimulate proliferation of various other cells such as epidermal cells,[4] melanoma cells,[5] and smooth muscle cells.[6] We and others have previously shown that IL-8 is elevated in the peritoneal fluid of women with endometriosis.[7–10] We also observed that IL-8 levels correlated with the severity of the disease.[8] Besides mesothelial cells that form the majority of the peritoneal cells, macrophages and endometrial cells themselves are potential sources of this chemokine.[8,11] We hypothesized that IL-8 may play a role in the growth and maintenance of ectopic endometrial tissue not only by stimulating leukocytes to secrete growth factors and cytokines, but also by directly affecting endometrial cell attachment and proliferation.

IL-8 IN THE HUMAN ENDOMETRIUM

We initially studied the regulation of IL-8 production by human endometrial stromal and epithelial cells in culture.[11] We then investigated menstrual cycle–dependent expression of IL-8 mRNA and protein in the endometrium.[12] Endometrial tissue (n = 52) was obtained from human uteri after hysterectomy conducted for reasons other than endometrial disease or from endometrial biopsies. The day of the menstrual cycle was established from women's menstrual history and confirmed by histology. Half of the tissues (n = 26) were snap-frozen in liquid nitrogen, cellular RNA extracted, and Northern blots hybridized with a riboprobe complementary to a specific sequence of IL-8 mRNA. Remaining tissues (n = 26) were processed for frozen sections and immunohistochemistry was performed using mouse antihuman IL-8 antibody. Comparison of IL-8 mRNA levels throughout the menstrual cycle revealed that late secretory and early-to-mid proliferative phase IL-8 expression was significantly greater than mid-cycle expression (see FIG. 1; $p < 0.02$). Analysis of the IL-8 immunohistochemistry revealed that IL-8 protein is found in the surface epithelium and glands throughout the menstrual cycle. There was no detectable immunoreactive IL-8 in the stromal cells. In summary, IL-8 is produced in the human endometrium *in vivo* and the variations of IL-8 mRNA throughout the menstrual cycle suggest that sex hormones may regulate its gene expression.

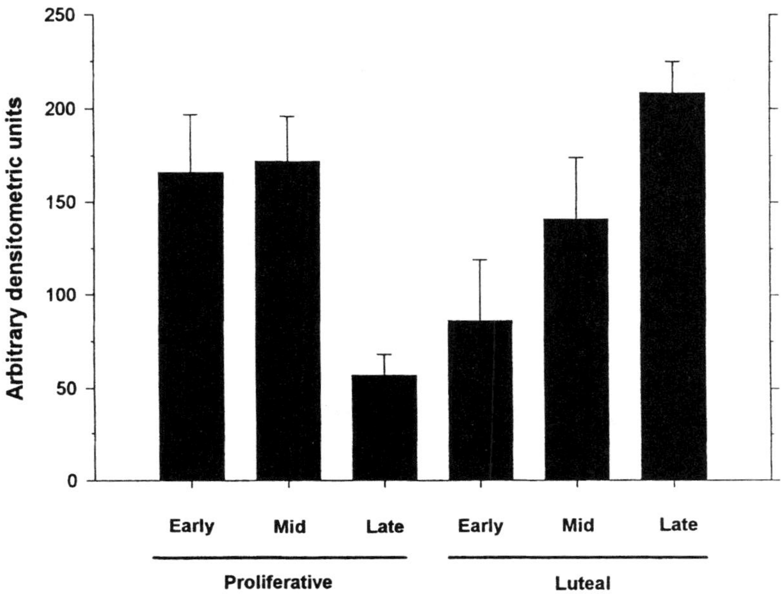

FIGURE 1. Northern analysis of IL-8 mRNA in human endometrial tissue. Total RNA (20 μg per lane) isolated from endometrial tissues was evaluated. Samples are arranged according to menstrual cycle phase. *Graphic bars* represent the mean value of densitometric units for each group normalized to G3PDH; $p < 0.02$ for late secretory and early-to-mid proliferative vs. mid-cycle.

IL-8 STIMULATES ADHESION OF ENDOMETRIAL CELLS

To implant and grow, endometrial cells need to establish cell-cell or cell–extracellular matrix interactions with the peritoneum. Recent evidence suggests that, after the initial cell attachment, early endometriosis lesions invade the extracellular matrix of the peritoneum.[13] Most of these interactions between endometrial cells and extracellular matrix are mediated by the integrin family of cell surface receptors,[14] which are capable of transducing intracellular signals.

The most effective tissue samples for the transplantation of endometrium in the primate endometriosis model are the late secretory menstrual/early proliferative endometrial samples[15] and these are the phases when the highest levels of endometrial IL-8 are observed.[12] We thus studied the effect of IL-8 and mouse antihuman IL-8 monoclonal antibody on endometrial stromal cell adhesion to fibronectin.[16] To determine the effect of IL-8 in regulating endometrial cell adhesion, stromal cell cultures were incubated in serum-free medium for 24 h and then were treated with various concentrations of IL-8 (0.001–10 ng/mL) or with PBS (control) for 24 h. The adhesion of the cells to fibronectin matrix was evaluated by labeling the cells with calcein. There was a dose-dependent increase of cell adhesion with IL-8 treatment (2-fold at 10 ng/mL; $p < 0.05$) (FIG. 2). Because endometrial stromal cells in culture produce IL-8 constitutively (in the range of 0.1–1 ng/mL), we also investigated

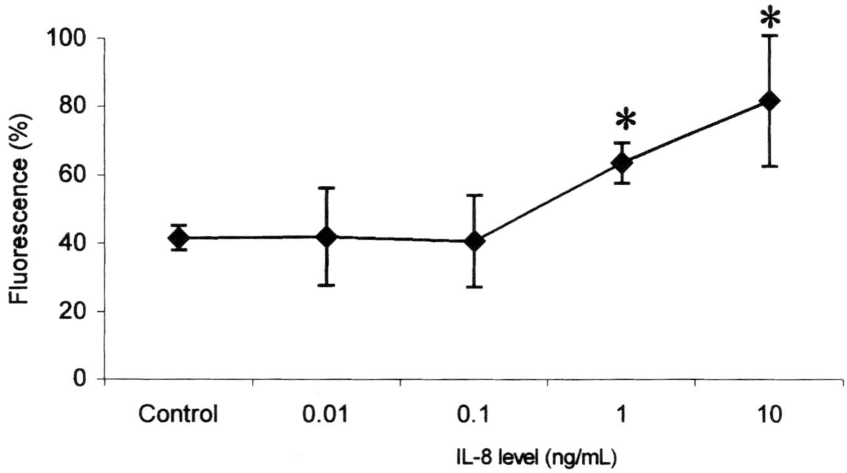

FIGURE 2. IL-8 induces a dose-dependent increase in endometrial cell adhesion to fibronectin (2-fold at 10 ng/mL); $*p = 0.006$ compared to control. Bars represent means ± SD.

whether the neutralization of IL-8 produced by these cells would affect their adhesion. Endometrial stromal cells in serum-free medium for 24 h were treated with various concentrations of mouse antihuman IL-8 neutralizing antibody (0.01–1 μg/mL) or with nonspecific mouse IgG (control) for 24 h, and adhesion was evaluated by calcein prelabeling. We observed a significant trend towards concentration-dependent inhibition of cell adhesion with anti-IL-8 neutralizing antibody compared to control ($p = 0.014$). We thus conclude that IL-8 stimulates the adhesion of endometrial stromal cells to fibronectin in a concentration-dependent manner. IL-8 may therefore be relevant for the attachment of endometrial implants in the pathogenesis of endometriosis.

ADHESION OF ENDOMETRIAL CELLS STIMULATES IL-8 EXPRESSION

Adhesion of endometrial cells to the peritoneal extracellular matrix may result in the transmission of the necessary signals for cell migration and invasion. Additionally, it has been shown that the mesothelial cells of the peritoneum express integrins *in vitro* as well as *in vivo*.[17] Several integrins are expressed by the mesothelium of the peritoneum, with different expression observed *in vivo* and *in vitro* in monolayer and explant cultures. This recent identification of integrins along the surface of the mesothelium suggests that these mesothelial integrins may have a role in the initial attachment of ectopic endometrium to the peritoneal lining. We hypothesized that cell adhesion itself may enhance the expression of IL-8, thus contributing to the inflammation in the peritoneal cavity, and as a consequence may play a role in the pathogenesis of endometriosis. We therefore have investigated the role that the inter-

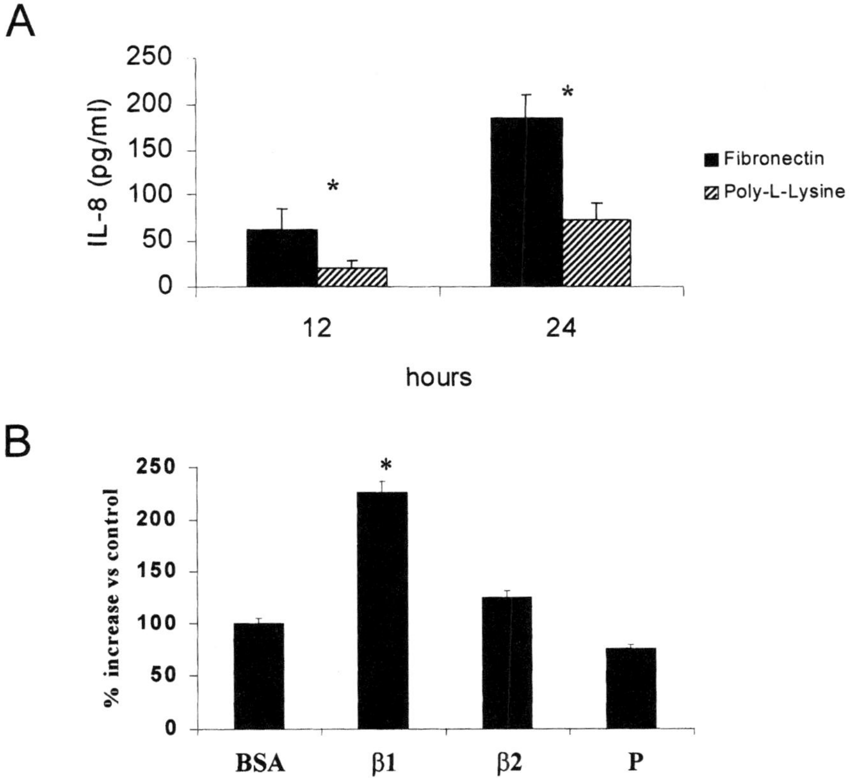

FIGURE 3. **(A)** IL-8 protein secretion by endometrial stromal cells is upregulated by adhesion in a time-dependent manner. Twenty-four hours after the adhesion process starts, fibronectin induces a significantly higher IL-8 secretion compared to a nonintegrin-dependent substrate (poly-L-lysine). $*p < 0.05$ at 12 h; $p < 0.01$ at 24 h fibronectin vs. poly-L-lysine. **(B)** Engagement with the β_1 (but not the β_2) integrin subunit upregulates IL-8 protein secretion in endometrial stromal cells. BSA: bovine serum albumin; β_1: mouse antihuman integrin β_1 monoclonal antibody; β_2: mouse antihuman integrin β_2 monoclonal antibody; P: poly-L-lysine. $*p < 0.01$ β_1 vs. other groups.

action between endometrial stromal cells and extracellular matrix components may have in the regulation of IL-8 gene expression and secretion.[18]

Endometrial stromal cells were plated on culture dishes coated with fibronectin (20 μg/mL), laminin (20 μg/mL), collagen IV (20 μg/mL), poly-L-lysine (0.1 mg/mL), or mouse antihuman integrin β_1 and β_2 monoclonal antibodies. Adherence of endometrial stromal cells to various extracellular matrix substrates induced the expression of both IL-8 mRNA and protein, except for poly-L-lysine, a nonintegrin-dependent adhesion matrix. Engagement of β_1-containing integrins was associated with cell adhesion and resulted in upregulation of IL-8 gene expression and protein secretion (FIG. 3). Disruption of the actin cytoskeleton by treating cells with cytochalasin D (5 μg/mL) completely blocked the increase of IL-8 that was induced in response to integrin activation. These findings indicate a novel mechanism of IL-8 regulation. Cell adhesion to extracellular matrix is an important event that leads to stimulation of IL-8 expression, and this process is mediated by integrins. Our findings that IL-8 stimulates the adhesion of endometrial cells and, in turn, cell attachment leads to further stimulation of IL-8 expression suggest a positive feedback mechanism, which may play a role in the progression of endometriosis.

IL-8 STIMULATES INVASIVENESS OF ENDOMETRIAL CELLS

The pathogenesis of endometriosis involves local invasion of peritoneal surfaces by endometrial implants. Recent evidence suggests that, after the initial cell attachment, endometrial cells invade the extracellular matrix of the peritoneum by way of increased metalloproteinase activity. We thus evaluated the effect of IL-8 and different extracellular matrix proteins on the protease activity of endometrial stromal cells in culture.[19] Cells were cultured on plates coated with poly-L-lysine (0.1 mg/mL), fibronectin (1 μg/cm^2), or vitronectin (0.1 μg/cm^2). Uncoated and poly-L-lysine-coated wells were compared to fibronectin- and vitronectin-coated wells. In addition, some uncoated, poly-L-lysine-, fibronectin-, or vitronectin-coated wells were treated with IL-8 (1 ng/mL) or vehicle for 24 h. Metalloproteinase activity in endometrial stromal cell conditioned media was measured using the thiopeptolide substrate in a spectrophotometric assay. Samples were also analyzed with substrate gel zymography.

Endometrial stromal cells that were grown in fibronectin- and vitronectin-coated dishes demonstrated 1.4- and 1.8-fold increases, respectively, in metalloproteinase activity as compared to cells grown in uncoated or poly-L-lysine-coated dishes. IL-8 increased the protease activity in uncoated dishes by 1.7-fold. In fibronectin- and vitronectin-coated dishes, protease activity was increased by 2-fold and 2.4-fold, respectively, with IL-8 treatment. Results obtained in spectrophotometry were confirmed in zymograms: 72-kDa bands in zymograms showed that MMP-2 is the major metalloproteinase regulated by IL-8. We thus conclude that IL-8 may also play a role in the pathogenesis of endometriosis by increasing metalloproteinase activity in endometrial cells and by potentiating the integrin-dependent protease activity of these cells.

IL-8 INDUCES PROLIFERATION OF ENDOMETRIAL CELLS

Comparison of IL-8 mRNA levels throughout the menstrual cycle revealed that early-to-mid proliferative and late secretory phase IL-8 expression was significantly higher than mid-cycle expression.[12] The cyclicity of IL-8 expression is similar to the one that is observed for the number of mitoses in the endometrial stroma throughout the menstrual phases. Although endometrial proliferation is dependent on sex steroid hormones, specific growth factors are likely to play an important role in regulating this process. We thus hypothesized that IL-8, which has been shown to stimulate growth in other cell types, may directly stimulate proliferation of endometrial cells. We first investigated the effect of IL-8 and mouse antihuman IL-8 neutralizing antibody on endometrial stromal cell proliferation using both a colorimetric assay and thymidine uptake. We then investigated the modulation of endometrial stromal cell

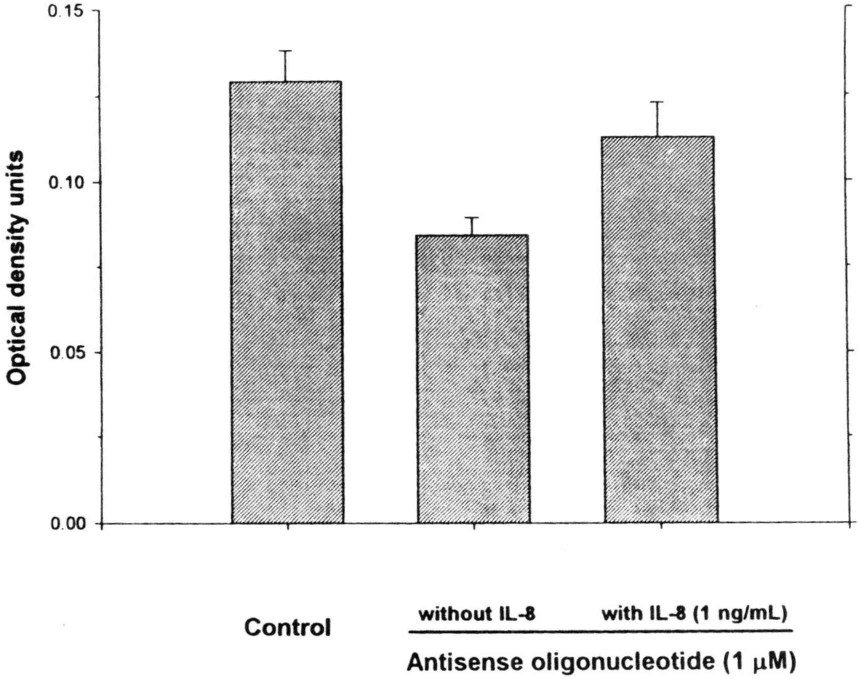

FIGURE 4. The effect of recombinant IL-8 on the IL-8 antisense oligonucleotide-induced inhibition of proliferation of endometrial stromal cells in culture. Confluent cells were placed in serum-free medium for 24 h and were incubated for 2 h with culture medium containing IL-8 antisense oligonucleotide (1 μM) in the presence or absence of IL-8 (1 ng/mL). After that, 1% FBS was added. Cell proliferation was assessed by MTT colorimetric method. Data are means ± SEM. IL-8 antisense oligonucleotide induced a decrease in the proliferation of endometrial stromal cells in culture ($p < 0.01$). The addition of IL-8 reversed the proliferation inhibitory effect of the IL-8 antisense oligonucleotide.

IL-8 production and proliferation by antisense oligonucleotides specific for IL-8.[20] There was a concentration-dependent increase of cell proliferation with IL-8 (2-fold at 1 ng/mL; $p < 0.01$ between control and concentrations above 0.01 ng/mL) and a concentration-dependent inhibition of cell proliferation with anti-IL-8 antibody (to 30% of the control at 1 μg/mL; $p < 0.01$ between control and concentrations above 0.1 μg/mL). IL-8 antisense oligonucleotide treatment decreased IL-8 production by endometrial stromal cells in culture as well as cell proliferation when compared to scrambled (non-sense) oligonucleotide treatment ($p < 0.01$). Addition of IL-8 (1 ng/mL) reversed the proliferation inhibitory effect of IL-8 antisense oligonucleotides (see FIG. 4). We thus propose that IL-8 may act as an autocrine growth factor in the endometrium and suggest that it may also play a role in the pathogenesis of endometriosis.

CONCLUSIONS

Despite intense interest in the endometriosis, there are many gaps in our understanding of its pathogenesis. Nevertheless, there is substantial evidence that immunologic factors play a role in the pathogenesis of endometriosis and endometriosis-associated reproductive failure. It has been established that the overwhelming majority of women regurgitate menstrual debris into the peritoneal cavity, but only few develop endometriosis. The initiation of endometriosis may be a function of the quantity of refluxed endometrium that is viable. Furthermore, the environment of the peritoneal cavity may play a decisive role in the development of endometriosis. An altered response, characterized by an increased inflammatory environment, will allow endometrial cells to implant and grow more easily in ectopic sites. Activated peritoneal leukocytes and their secreted growth factors and cytokines will also induce proliferation of the endometrial implants, while they may be inhibiting early reproductive events.

We have obtained and presented *in vivo* evidence for a potential relationship between IL-8 and endometriosis: levels of IL-8 are significantly higher in the peritoneal fluid from women who have endometriosis than in the peritoneal fluid from women who do not have endometriosis. We have also observed the highest expression of IL-8 in late secretory and early proliferative phase endometrium (which is also the most effective endometrial sample for inducing endometriosis via transplantation in the primate model). We have obtained evidence that IL-8 stimulates endometrial cell proliferation and attachment to extracellular matrix. Endometrial cell adhesion to extracellular matrix stimulates further IL-8 production by these

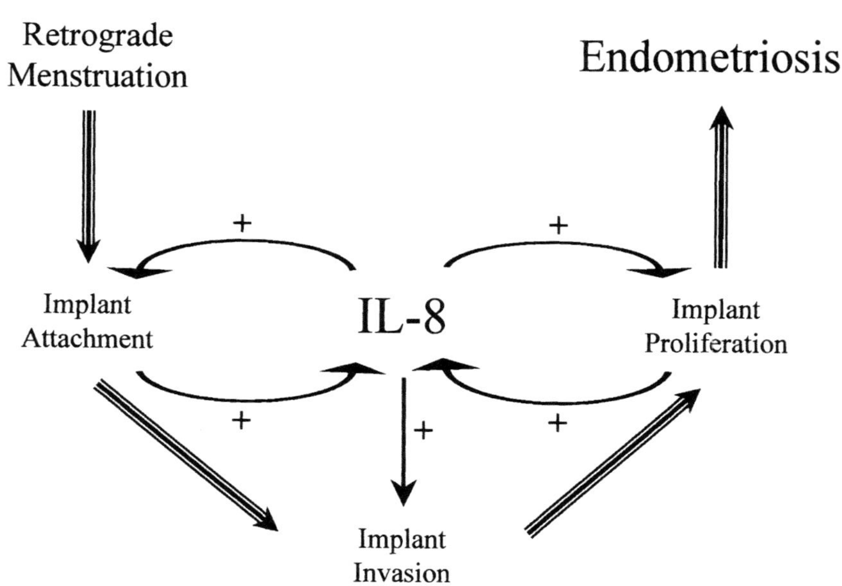

FIGURE 5. The role of IL-8 in the pathogenesis of endometriosis.

cells, thus creating a vicious cycle (FIG. 5). Since the development of endometriosis requires cell attachment and growth, our findings strongly suggest that IL-8 may play a role in the pathogenesis of endometriosis. Although these findings do not prove a cause-and-effect relationship, they suggest an association that needs to be further investigated.

REFERENCES

1. DUIGNAN, N., J. JORDAN, B. COUGHLAN & R. LOGAN-EDWARDS. 1972. One thousand consecutive cases of diagnostic laparoscopy. J. Obstet. Gynaecol. Br. Commonw. **79:** 1016–1024.
2. ORAL, E. & A. ARICI. 1997. Pathogenesis of endometriosis. Obstet. Gynecol. Clin. North Am. **24:** 219–233.
3. SENTURK, L.M. & A. ARICI. 1999. Immunology of endometriosis. J. Reprod. Immunol. **43:** 67–83.
4. TUSCHIL, A., C. LAM, A. HASLBERGER & I. LINDLEY. 1992. Interleukin-8 stimulates calcium transients and promotes epidermal cell proliferation. J. Invest. Dermatol. **99:** 294–298.
5. SCHADENDORF, D., A. MOLLER, B. ALGERMISSEN *et al.* 1993. IL-8 produced by human malignant melanoma cells *in vitro* is an essential autocrine growth factor. J. Immunol. **151:** 2667–2675.
6. YUE, T-L., X. WANG, C-P. SUNG *et al.* 1994. Interleukin-8: a mitogen and chemoattractant for vascular smooth muscle cells. Circ. Res. **75:** 1–7.
7. RYAN, I.P., J.F. TSENG, E.D. SCHRIOCK *et al.* 1995. Interleukin-8 concentrations are elevated in peritoneal fluid of women with endometriosis. Fertil. Steril. **63:** 929–932.
8. ARICI, A., S.I. TAZUKE, E. ATTAR *et al.* 1996. Interleukin-8 concentration in peritoneal fluid of patients with endometriosis and modulation of interleukin-8 expression in human mesothelial cells. Mol. Hum. Reprod. **2:** 40–45.
9. GAZVANI, M.R., S. CHRISTMAS, S. QUENBY *et al.* 1998. Peritoneal fluid concentrations of interleukin-8 in women with endometriosis: relationship to stage of disease. Hum. Reprod. **13:** 1957–1961.
10. IWABE, T., T. HARADA, T. TSUDO *et al.* 1998. Pathogenetic significance of increased levels of interleukin-8 in the peritoneal fluid of patients with endometriosis. Fertil. Steril. **69:** 924–930.
11. ARICI, A., J. HEAD, P.C. MACDONALD & M.L. CASEY. 1993. Regulation of interleukin-8 gene expression in human endometrial cells in culture. Mol. Cell. Endocrinol. **94:** 195–204.
12. ARICI, A., E. SELI, L.M. SENTURK *et al.* 1998. Interleukin-8 in the human endometrium. J. Clin. Endocrinol. Metab. **83:** 1783–1787.
13. SPUIJBROEK, M.D.E.H., G.A.J. DUNSELMAN, P.P.J.A. MENHEERE & J.L.H. EVERS. 1992. Early endometriosis invades the extracellular matrix. Fertil. Steril. **58:** 929–933.
14. JULIANO, R.L. & S. HASKILL. 1993. Signal transduction from the extracellular matrix. J. Cell Biol. **120:** 577–585.
15. D'HOOGHE, T.M., C.S. BAMBRA, B.M. RAEYMAEKERS *et al.* 1995. Intrapelvic injection of menstrual endometrium causes endometriosis in baboons (*Papio cynocephalus* and *Papio anubis*). Am. J. Obstet. Gynecol. **173:** 125–134.
16. GARCIA-VELASCO, J.A. & A. ARICI. 1999. Interleukin-8 stimulates the adhesion of endometrial stromal cells to fibronectin. Fertil. Steril. **72:** 336–340.
17. WITZ, C.A., I.A. MONTOYA-RODRIGUEZ, D.M. MILLER *et al.* 1998. Mesothelium expression of integrins *in vivo* and *in vitro*. J. Soc. Gynecol. Invest. **5:** 87–93.
18. GARCIA-VELASCO, J.A. & A. ARICI. 1999. Interleukin-8 expression in endometrial stromal cells is regulated by integrin-dependent cell adhesion. Mol. Hum. Reprod. **5:** 1135–1140.
19. MULAYIM, N., A. SAVLU & A. ARICI. 2000. Interleukin-8 increases endometrial stromal cell metalloproteinase activity: possible role in endometriosis. Fertil. Steril. **74:** S22.
20. ARICI, A., E. SELI, H.B. ZEYNELOGLU *et al.* 1998. Interleukin-8 induces proliferation of endometrial stromal cells: a potential autocrine growth factor. J. Clin. Endocrinol. Metab. **83:** 1201–1205.

Control of Growth and Differentiation of the Endometrium: The Role of Tissue Interactions

ROBERT M. BIGSBY

Indiana University School of Medicine, Indianapolis, Indiana 46202, USA

ABSTRACT: Early work with neonatal mice showed that estrogen receptor–negative uterine epithelium responded to estrogen treatment. Since the underlying mesenchymal cells were estrogen receptor–positive, it was suggested that these cells mediated the hormonal response through elaboration of a paracrine factor. Cell culture work showed that mesenchymal cells produced soluble factors that stimulate uterine epithelium, but hormonal regulation was absent or minimal. The paracrine hypothesis of estrogen action has been proved by the use of tissue recombinant studies in which epithelium from estrogen receptor–alpha knockout mice was combined with wild-type mesenchyme; estrogen stimulated the ERα-negative epithelium if the underlying stromal cells were receptor-positive. Also, it is hypothesized that there is a reciprocal paracrine interaction during stimulation with progesterone and estrogen. Accordingly, under progesterone dominance, the epithelium elaborates factors that direct the underlying stroma to proliferate when estrogen is administered. Although this hypothesis needs further testing, it has been shown that the uterine epithelium is required for stromal responsiveness to hormones. The question arises: What are the factors that mediate the effects of the steroid hormones in the uterus? Several peptide growth factors are regulated by estrogen and/or progesterone. Use of knockout animals will allow a determination of the role that these factors play in the uterus. However, ablation of many of these growth factor genes has proved lethal to the newborn animals, making it impossible to study hormonal effects using standard techniques. Tissue xenograft and tissue recombination studies offer a means of defining the role of specific growth factors in uterine physiology.

KEYWORDS: tissue interactions; paracrine factors; cell proliferation; estrogen; progesterone; tissue recombinations; xenograft; gene knockout

One of the hallmarks of endometriosis is the inclusion of endometrial stroma in the ectopic tissue implant. Is this merely a diagnostic tool for pathologists or does it point to a biologically important aspect of the disease process? Endometriomas are responsive to hormonal changes, but the hormonal effects are not always identical to those occurring in the normal endometrium. Do the hormonal responses of endometrioma tissues derive from an interaction of the stromal and epithelial tissues and

Address for correspondence: Robert M. Bigsby, Ph.D., Department of Obstetrics and Gynecology, Indiana University School of Medicine, 975 West Walnut Street (IB360), Indianapolis, IN 46202-5121. Voice: 317-274-8970; fax: 317-278-2884.
rbigsby@iupui.edu

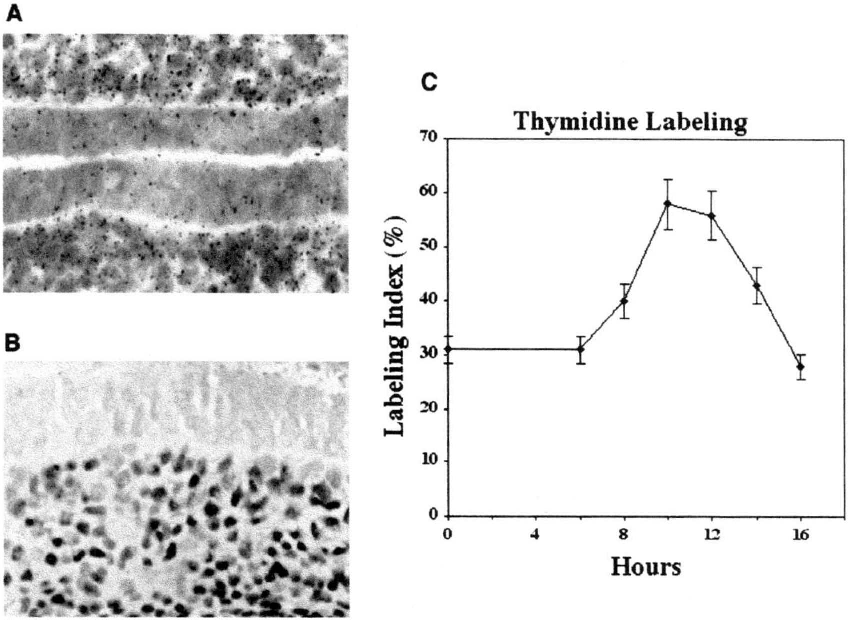

FIGURE 1. Estrogen-induced DNA synthesis in ER-negative epithelium of the neonatal mouse uterus. **(A)** Estradiol autoradiography shows that the epithelial cells of the 4-day-old Balb/C mouse do not concentrate the steroid in their nuclei as do the underlying mesenchymal cells. **(B)** Immunohistochemistry of ERα likewise shows that there is a lack of this receptor in the epithelium, while it is abundantly expressed in the mesenchyme. **(C)** Thymidine labeling index of the uterine epithelium of 4-day-old mice following estradiol treatment indicates that the ER-negative epithelium has responded with a transient increase in proliferative activity. (Modified from references 1 and 2.)

are the altered responses due to disrupted tissue interactions? This review will emphasize the role of tissue interactions in the estrogen and progesterone regulation of cellular proliferation and gene expression.

It is now well established that uterine mesenchymal cells, that is, the stroma, direct certain epithelial responses to estrogen. Using the mouse as an experimental model, it was shown that the uterine epithelium of the neonatal animal is devoid of estrogen-binding activity and yet it responds to estradiol stimulation with an increased rate of cell proliferation; the fact that the underlying mesenchymal cells do express estrogen receptor (ERα) suggests that the stroma mediates the effect of the hormone (FIG. 1).[1,2] Although useful in demonstrating the elaboration of stromal factors that stimulate epithelial proliferation, coculture experiments were unsuccessful in demonstrating estrogen enhancement of this tissue interaction (FIG. 2).[3] However, in a more recent report, it was shown that estradiol stimulated DNA synthesis in human endometrial epithelial cells grown with stromal cells in a transfilter system.[4] Using tissue recombinant experiments in which tissues from ER knockout (ERαKO) and wild-type mice were recombined in heterologous fashion, Cooke, Cunha, and colleagues confirmed the paracrine mode of estrogen action.[5] As part of

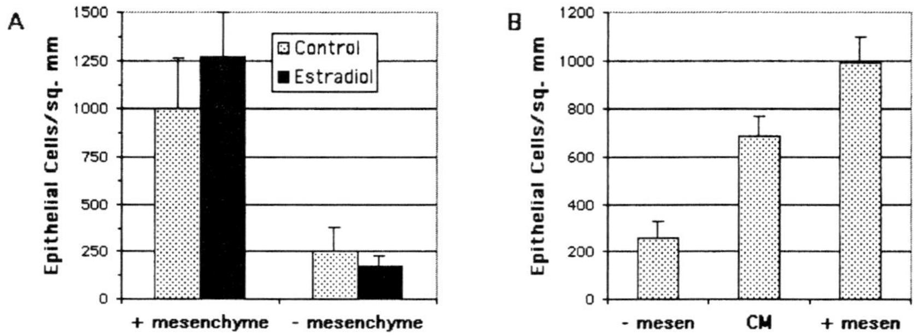

FIGURE 2. Transfilter cocultures of uterine epithelium and mesenchyme. Uteri derived from 2- to 4-day-old Balb/C mice were enzymatically separated into the epithelial and mesenchymal components and these were further digested into single cell suspensions. The mesenchymal cells were seeded onto the underside of a nitrocellulose (Millipore) filter and the epithelial cells were seeded onto the top of the filter. The epithelial cell density was assessed after 5 days in culture (mean ± SD, $n = 3$). Epithelial cells grew at a rate approximately 4-fold higher when mesenchymal cells were present (**A**). Although there was a tendency for increased epithelial growth in response to estradiol when mesenchyme was present, this was not statistically different. Inclusion of conditioned medium (CM) from cultures of mesenchymal cells increased epithelial cell growth to an intermediate level compared to that achieved when the mesenchymal cells were present (+ mesen) (**B**), indicating that the growth factors elaborated by the mesenchyme are soluble factors. (Reproduced with permission from reference 3.)

our own investigation of tissue interactions in the uterus, we have repeated the study presented by Cooke *et al.* and the results are depicted in FIGURE 3. In these experiments, epithelium and mesenchyme are separated, recombined in hetero- or homotypic fashion, and grown as xenograft in athymic host mice. When ER-negative epithelium derived from ERαKO uterus was recombined with wild-type, ER-positive mesenchyme, the resulting mature epithelium was responsive to estrogen; however, wild-type epithelium recombined with ERαKO mesenchyme was not responsive. Thus, the ER-positive stroma behaves as the interpreter of the estrogen signal, translating it into a growth-stimulating message that is sent to the epithelium. In contrast, progesterone will block estrogen-induced epithelial proliferation. Tissue recombination experiments using wild-type and progesterone receptor knockout (PRKO) tissues have shown that this inhibitory effect is mediated by the stromal PR,[6] implying that progesterone is blocking stromal expression of the epithelial growth-stimulating factor or that it is inducing the production of a growth-inhibitory factor.

For the most part, hormonal regulation of gene expression in the epithelium appears to be a direct action through the cognate receptor within the responding cell rather than through a paracrine mechanism. Estrogen-induced c-fos expression in the uterine epithelium is rapid, occurring within minutes of steroid administration;[7] this time course suggests that this response is a direct effect of the hormone within the responding cells. In the neonatal CD-1 mouse, ER expression is restricted to about 40% of the epithelial cells; the estrogen-induced gene, lactoferrin, is expressed only

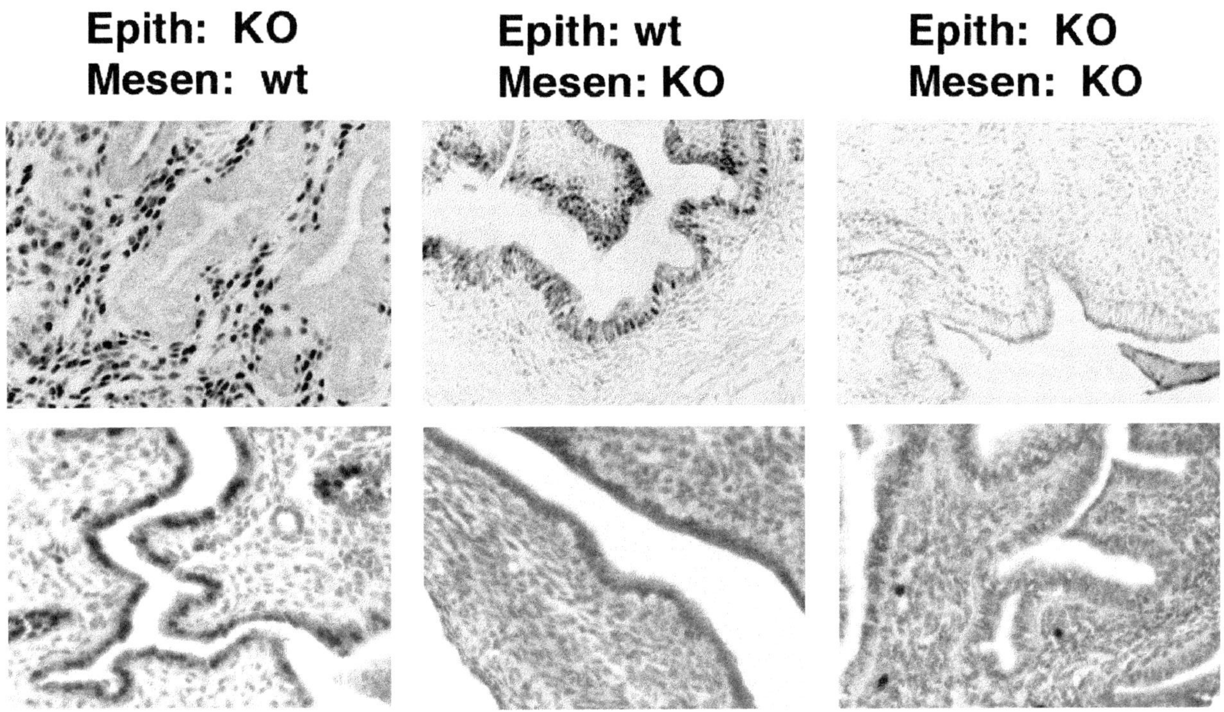

FIGURE 3. Tissue recombinants made of ERαKO and wild-type tissues demonstrate the paracrine mode of estrogen action. Uterine tissues taken from neonatal wild-type or ERαKO mice were recombined in hetero- or homotypic fashion so that the resultant uterine recombinant was composed of ER-positive (wt) or ER-negative (KO) epithelium (Epith) growing on ER-positive or ER-negative stroma (Mesen). The recombinants were grown in intact athymic female mice for 5 weeks, at which time the hosts were ovariectomized, and then left untreated for 3 additional weeks. Hosts were then treated with estradiol and then [^{3}H]-thymidine 20 hours later. Immunostaining of tissue recombinants confirms the ER status of the tissues (upper row). Thymidine autoradiography (lower row) indicates that the ER-negative epithelium responded to estrogen stimulation (dark grains over nuclei) if it was grown in apposition to ER-positive stroma, but the ER-positive epithelium was unresponsive when the stroma was ER-negative. These figures are representative of 4–6 replicates each.

in those cells coexpressing ER.[8] Estrogen-induced expression of epithelial secretory products, lactoferrin and complement C3, require both epithelial and stromal ER.[9] Progesterone inhibits estrogen-induced lactoferrin in the epithelium; full inhibition requires both stromal and epithelial PR.[10] On the other hand, estrogen down-regulates epithelial PR in the uterus of ovariectomized mice; this effect depends on stromal ER.[11] Thus, there is a clear difference in the way that cellular proliferation and gene expression are regulated by steroids in the uterus.

Tissue-tissue interactions are likely to occur in the reciprocal direction as well; that is, uterine epithelium sends regulatory signals to the underlying stroma. This was first illustrated by experiments investigating the role of the epithelium in establishing the decidual cell reaction (DCR) in the stroma. During early pregnancy, embryo attachment induces cell proliferation and differentiation of the stromal cells immediately adjacent to the site of attachment; this stromal response is referred to as decidualization. Deciduoma formation is an artificial decidualization; it is a hyperproliferative response that occurs in the stroma following experimentally inflicted trauma to the uterus in ovariectomized animals (rats or mice) that have been primed with progesterone and estrogen. DCR does not occur if the epithelium has been ablated, suggesting that an epithelially derived signal is required.[12] Even in the absence of trauma, estrogen induces cell proliferation in the stroma of ovariectomized rodents that have been suitably primed with progesterone. Tissue recombinant studies utilizing developmentally committed epithelia, that is, epithelium that is morphologically and functionally determined as either uterine or vaginal, showed that this stromal response requires uterine epithelium (FIG. 4).[13] Thus, an epithelial signal directs or permits hormonal stimulation of the stroma. Further studies are under way to determine the requirement for tissue-specific expression of estrogen or progesterone receptors in this stromal response.

The question arises: What are the hormonally regulated growth factors that mediate these tissue interactions? Several peptide growth factors whose expression is

TABLE 1. Uterine growth factor expression and regulation

Growth factor	Tissue expression[a]	Hormonal regulation[b]	Reference
IGF-I	Epithelium Stroma	E2 + (epithelium) PE2 + (stroma)	14
EGF	Epithelium	E2 +	15
TGF-α	Epithelium	P +	16
HB-EGF	Epithelium, (stroma)	E2 + (PE2 +)	17
Amphiregulin	Epithelium	P +	18
Betacellulin & epiregulin	Epithelium Subepithelial stroma	PE2 & blastocyst +	19
TGF-$\beta_{1,2,3}$	Epithelium	E2 +	20
Prostaglandin/COX-2	Epithelium Subepithelial stroma	PE2 & blastocyst +	21

[a]Predominant site of expression.

[b]Hormonal regulation: E2 or PE2 +, expression increased by estradiol or progesterone plus estradiol treatment in ovariectomized animals (increase occurs in specific tissue); PE2 & blastocyst +, expression increased by hormones when blastocyst is present.

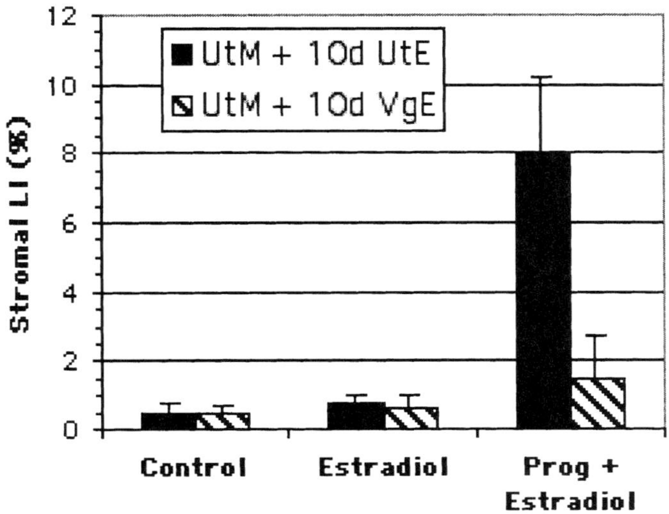

FIGURE 4. Hormone-induced stromal cell proliferation requires uterine epithelial factors. Uterine or vaginal epithelium was harvested from Balb/C mice at 10–15 days of age (10d UtE or 10d VgE) and these were combined with mesenchyme derived from 2-day-old uterus (UtM). Use of epithelia from 10- to 15-day-old mice insures that this epithelium is already developmentally determined; thus, the VgE retains its squamous phenotype in the presence of uterine mesenchyme. These tissue recombinants were grown in female athymic mice for 5 weeks and then the host animals were ovariectomized. At 2 weeks post-ovariectomy, the hosts were treated with vehicle (control) or estradiol for 1 day, or with progesterone for 2 days followed by progesterone plus estradiol. At 20 hours after the last hormone injection, each host received an injection of [^{3}H]-thymidine and the grafted tissues were harvested 1 hour later. The percentage of stromal cells labeled with [^{3}H]-thymidine was determined in microautoradiographs. The stroma responded to the combined progesterone plus estrogen treatment only when uterine epithelium was present. (Modified from reference 13.)

hormonally responsive have been identified in the uterus, for example, EGF, IGF-I, TGF-α, TGF-β, amphiregulin, and HB-EGF (TABLE 1). In addition, COX-2, an enzyme involved in the production of prostaglandins, has been shown to be hormonally responsive in the uterus.[22] Are these the mediators of stromal-epithelial interaction in the uterus?

Although descriptive studies have implicated several potential mediators of tissue interactions, it is difficult to make further progress in determining the exact growth factor requirements for hormone action in the uterus using standard techniques. The importance of IGF-I for estradiol-induced mitosis in the uterus was demonstrated using IGF-I knockout animals; however, this is an extremely difficult model to use because only a small percentage of IGF-I null mice survive to maturity.[23] Similarly, EGF receptor (EGF-R) null animals die soon after birth, making this knockout model unworkable for studies on estradiol action in adult animals. However, by grafting the uterus of neonatal EGF-R knockout animals to athymic mice, Hom *et al.*[24] were able to grow the tissue to maturity and perform a hormone replacement experiment in ovariectomized hosts. They found that EGF-R was required for the stromal response to estrogen, while not for the epithelial response. Experiments using knockout tissues in xenograft, either whole tissues or tissue recombinants, are well suited to approach the question of how single growth factors are involved in mediating hormone action. Tissues derived from gene-ablated, knockout animals can be taken at term or immediately after birth and they can be grown in xenograft, either intact or recombined, to ascertain the specific role of the ablated gene. Utilizing tissue recombinants derived from growth factor null animals, we can determine the importance of that growth factor in hormonally regulated tissue interactions.

It appears likely that stromal-epithelial interactions are key to hormonal regulation of growth in endometrial tissues. Over the past three decades, we have learned a great deal about steroid receptors and their molecular mechanisms of action in the uterus and other target tissues. Knowledge of hormonally enhanced expression of growth-related immediate-early genes and peptide growth factors supplies us with the materials for building a concept of direct and paracrine control of tissue growth. The task at hand is first to construct the framework of this concept in a way that explains normal endometrial physiology and then to determine how that framework may have come undone in the pathophysiology of endometriosis.

REFERENCES

1. BIGSBY, R.M. & G.R. CUNHA. 1986. Estrogen stimulation of deoxyribonucleic acid synthesis in uterine epithelial cells which lack estrogen receptors. Endocrinology **119:** 390–396.
2. BIGSBY, R.M., L. AIXIN, K. LUO & G.R. CUNHA. 1990. Strain differences in the ontogeny of estrogen receptors in murine uterine epithelium. Endocrinology **126:** 2592–2596.
3. EVERETT, L.M., A. CAPERELL-GRANT & R.M. BIGSBY. 1997. Mesenchymal-epithelial interactions in an *in vitro* model of neonatal mouse uterus. Proc. Soc. Exp. Biol. Med. **214:** 49–53.
4. PIERRO, E., F. MINICI, O. ALESIANI *et al.* 2001. Stromal-epithelial interactions modulate estrogen responsiveness in normal human endometrium. Biol. Reprod. **64:** 831–838.
5. COOKE, P.S., D.L. BUCHANAN, P. YOUNG *et al.* 1997. Stromal estrogen receptors mediate mitogenic effects of estradiol on uterine epithelium. Proc. Natl. Acad. Sci. U.S.A. **94:** 6535–6540.
6. KURITA, T., P. YOUNG, J.R. BRODY *et al.* 1998. Stromal progesterone receptors mediate the inhibitory effects of progesterone on estrogen-induced uterine epithelial cell deoxyribonucleic acid synthesis. Endocrinology **139:** 4708–4713.
7. BIGSBY, R.M. & A. LI. 1994. Differentially regulated immediate early genes in the rat uterus. Endocrinology **134:** 1820–1826.
8. YAMASHITA, S., R.R. NEWBOLD, J.A. MCLACHLAN & K.S. KORACH. 1990. The role of the estrogen receptor in uterine epithelial proliferation and cytodifferentiation in neonatal mice. Endocrinology **127:** 2456–2463.
9. BUCHANAN, D.L., T. SETIAWAN, D.B. LUBAHN *et al.* 1999. Tissue compartment–specific estrogen receptor–alpha participation in the mouse uterine epithelial secretory response. Endocrinology **140:** 484–491.
10. KURITA, T., K.J. LEE, P.S. COOKE *et al.* 2000. Paracrine regulation of epithelial progesterone receptor and lactoferrin by progesterone in the mouse uterus. Biol. Reprod. **62:** 831–838.
11. KURITA, T., K.J. LEE, P.S. COOKE *et al.* 2000. Paracrine regulation of epithelial progesterone receptor by estradiol in the mouse female reproductive tract. Biol. Reprod. **62:** 821–830.

12. LEJEUNE, B. & F. LEROY. 1980. Role of the uterine epithelium in inducing the decidual cell reaction. Prog. Reprod. Biol. **7:** 92–101.
13. BIGSBY, R.M., L. AIXIN & L. EVERETT. 1993. Stromal-epithelial interactions regulating cell proliferation in the uterus. *In* Local Systems in Reproduction, pp. 171–188. Raven Press. New York.
14. KAPUR, S., H. TAMADA, S.K. DEY & G.K. ANDREWS. 1992. Expression of insulin-like growth factor-I (IGF-I) and its receptor in the peri-implantation mouse uterus, and cell-specific regulation of IGF-I gene expression by estradiol and progesterone. Biol. Reprod. **46:** 208–219.
15. HUET-HUDSON, Y.M., I. CHAKRABORTY, S.K. DAS *et al.* 1990. Estrogen regulates the synthesis of epidermal growth factor in mouse uterine epithelial cells. Mol. Endocrinol. **4:** 510–523.
16. PARIA, B.C., S.K. DAS, Y.M. HUET-HUDSON & S.K. DEY. 1994. Distribution of transforming growth factor alpha precursors in the mouse uterus during the peri-implantation period and after steroid hormone treatments. Biol. Reprod. **50:** 481–491.
17. WANG, X.N., S.K. DAS, D. DAMM *et al.* 1994. Differential regulation of heparin-binding epidermal growth factor–like growth factor in the adult ovariectomized mouse uterus by progesterone and estrogen. Endocrinology **135:** 1264–1271.
18. DAS, S.K., I. CHAKRABORTY, B.C. PARIA *et al.* 1995. Amphiregulin is an implantation-specific and progesterone-regulated gene in the mouse uterus. Mol. Endocrinol. **9:** 691–705.
19. DAS, S.K., N. DAS, J. WANG *et al.* 1997. Expression of betacellulin and epiregulin genes in the mouse uterus temporally by the blastocyst solely at the site of its apposition is coincident with the "window" of implantation. Dev. Biol. **190:** 178–190.
20. TAKAHASHI, T., B. EITZMAN, N.L. BOSSERT *et al.* 1994. Transforming growth factors β1, β2, and β3 messenger RNA and protein expression in mouse uterus and vagina during estrogen-induced growth: a comparison to other estrogen-regulated genes. Cell Growth Differ. **5:** 919–935.
21. SCHERLE, P.A., M. WEGLE, H. LIM *et al.* 2000. Regulation of cyclooxygenase-2 induction in the mouse uterus during decidualization: an event of early pregnancy. J. Biol. Chem. **275:** 37086–37092.
22. CHAKRABORTY, I., S.K. DAS, J. WANG & S.K. DEY. 1996. Developmental expression of the cyclo-oxygenase-1 and cyclo-oxygenase-2 genes in the peri-implantation mouse uterus and their differential regulation by the blastocyst and ovarian steroids. J. Mol. Endocrinol. **16:** 107–122.
23. ADESANYA, O.O., J. ZHOU, C. SAMATHANAM *et al.* 1999. Insulin-like growth factor 1 is required for G2 progression in the estradiol-induced mitotic cycle. Proc. Natl. Acad. Sci. U.S.A. **96:** 3287–3291.
24. HOM, Y.K., P. YOUNG, J.F. WIESEN *et al.* 1998. Uterine and vaginal organ growth requires epidermal growth factor receptor signaling from stroma. Endocrinology **139:** 913–921.

Panel Discussion (Part III)

B.A. LESSEY (*University of North Carolina, Chapel Hill, NC*): A quick comment for Bob Bigsby. Your point is well taken about the difficulty in showing stromal effects on proliferation in culture. We reported in *Human Reproduction* (2001. **16:** 836) that the stromal cells placed in contact with basement membrane showed an exaggerated response in that setting. Since basement membrane has two sides, and one side contacts stroma, this may be a signal for stromal cells to become more paracrine in their nature.

R.M. BIGSBY (*Indiana University School of Medicine, Indianapolis, IN*): May I ask what was the basement membrane?

LESSEY: Matrigel.

BIGSBY: Which is full of growth factors.

R.N. TAYLOR (*University of California, San Francisco, CA*): Just a comment to that. Your conditioned media experiments did not seem to quite reach the stimulation that you saw when the two cocultures were in direct contact with each other.

BIGSBY: No. I just consider that a dilution factor. I am not sure if that is true, but it is a simple explanation.

B. ATTARDI (*Bioqual, Rockville, MD*): I have a question for Dr. Taylor. Does the estrogen receptor bind directly to this variant ERE and the VEGF promoter?

TAYLOR: Yes. In our *PNAS* paper (2000. **9:** 10972–10977), we proved that by gel-shift experiments and we mutagenized that site to show that it is a direct ERE.

ATTARDI: Can you block the induction by antiestrogens?

TAYLOR: Yes, to some extent, but it depends on whether you are using ERα or ERβ.

C.R. LYTTLE (*Wyeth Ayerst Research, Radnor, PA*): Can I ask Bob Bigsby a question? You showed a slide looking at the responses in the human cells when you had the combination cultures. The concentration of estradiol seemed to go from 10^{-8} to 10^{-6} molar. Is that correct and isn't that rather nonphysiologic?

BIGSBY: That is correct. It is not my study, so I do not have to defend it, but that is the way they reported it.

S. PARTHASARATHY (*Emory University, Atlanta, GA*): In the interest of the VEGF, we have a paper demonstrating that VEGF gene expression is potentially angiogenic. Considering that glycodelin levels are increased in endometriosis, this would be a significant addition to the contribution of VEGF in stimulating neovascularization. What we described is glycodelin inducing VEGF gene expression.

Circulating Ovarian Steroids and Endometrial Matrix Metalloproteinases (MMPs)

PATRICK HENRIET,[a] PATRICIA B. CORNET,[a] PASCALE LEMOINE,[a] CHRISTINE GALANT,[a,b] CHRISTIAN F. SINGER,[a,c] PIERRE J. COURTOY,[a] YVES EECKHOUT,[a] AND ETIENNE MARBAIX[a,b]

[a]*Cell Biology Unit, Christian de Duve Institute of Cellular Pathology, Université Catholique de Louvain, Brussels, Belgium*

[b]*Department of Pathology, Saint Luc University Clinics, Université Catholique de Louvain, Brussels, Belgium*

ABSTRACT: Recent studies strongly suggest that matrix metalloproteinases (MMPs) play a key role in the initiation of menstrual bleeding in the human endometrium upon the fall of ovarian steroid serum concentrations by inducing the degradation of the extracellular matrix of this mucosa. MMPs are also involved in abnormal endometrial bleeding and have been identified in endometriotic foci. In all cases, they are associated with areas of extracellular matrix breakdown. This paper reviews the literature on the regulation by estradiol and progesterone of the expression and activation of MMPs, and of the expression of their tissue inhibitors (TIMPs), (i) in the endometrium *in situ* during normal cycle, (ii) during artificial cycles in spayed monkeys, and (iii) in cultures of endometrial explants or purified cells. Whereas progesterone consistently decreases the activity of endometrial MMPs, its effects vary in intensity, duration, and pattern between MMPs as well as among experimental systems. The contribution and limitations of the various investigations are therefore discussed. The focal heterogeneity points to additional local controls of the expression and activation of MMPs in human endometrium, acting beyond the general inhibitory role of progesterone, for example, by cytokines. Focal changes in type or abundance of sex steroid receptors also could be responsible for spatial variation in the expression of MMPs in the endometrium and endometriotic lesions.

KEYWORDS: endometrium; estradiol; progesterone; matrix metalloproteinases; tissue inhibitors

INTRODUCTION

Topic of the Review

Throughout reproductive years, the human endometrium undergoes cyclic degradation and renewal in response to ovarian steroids. Estrogens induce tissue

Address for correspondence: Etienne Marbaix, Department of Pathology, Saint Luc University Clinics, Université Catholique de Louvain, Avenue Hippocrate, 10, B-1200 Brussels, Belgium. Voice: +32 2 764 1784; fax: +32 2 764 8924.

marbaix@cell.ucl.ac.be

[c]Present address: Christian F. Singer, Division of Special Gynecology, Department of Obstetrics and Gynecology, University of Vienna, Vienna, Austria.

TABLE 1. Expression, localization, and regulation of MMPs and TIMPs in fresh cycling endometrium and in cultured endometrial explants and purified endometrial cells

MMP #	Noncultured tissue		Explant culture			Cell culture		
	Cellular origin	Expression during the menstrual cycle	- H	+E+P Expression	+E+P Activation	- H	+E+P	P withdrawal
MMP-1	• stroma ; focal, periglandular or (peri)vascular (mRNA and protein)	restricted to M	↗	↘ except if sampled in M	↘	stromal cells	↘ in most experiments	↗ sustained
MMP-2	• stroma ; focal, periglandular or (peri)vascular (mRNA and protein) • in epithelium	strongly enhanced around M ; mRNA residual throughout the cycle	↗	↘ except if sampled in M	↘	stromal cells	=	↗ transient
MMP-3	• stroma ; focal, periglandular or (peri)vascular (mRNA and protein)	restricted to M	↗	↘ except if sampled in M	↘	stromal cells	↘ in most experiments	↗ sustained
MMP-7	• epithelium	strongly enhanced around M residual mRNA in MP+LP	↗	↘		epithelial cells	↘ requires a stromal cell-derived factor	
MMP-9	• stroma (inflammatory cells) • epithelium • vessels	• restricted to around M ¥ • secretory phase • MP and LS	↗	↘	↘	stromal cells		↗
MMP-10	• stroma (mRNA)	restricted to M						
MMP-11	• stroma (mRNA)	strongly enhanced around M, residual in MP+LP				stromal cells	↘	
MMP-14	• stroma (mRNA) (inflammatory cells) • epithelium (protein)	strongly enhanced ¥ around M, residual throughout the cycle				stromal cells		
MMP-15	• widespread • epithelium (abundant)	no clear-cut variation						
TIMP-1	• stroma (mRNA) • stroma, epithelium and arteries (protein)	strongly enhanced ¥ around M, residual throughout the cycle	↘ with time of culture	= or slow ↘	N/A	stromal cells	↗	=
TIMP-2	• stroma (mRNA) • stroma, epithelium and arteries (protein)	enhanced around M ¥ residual throughout the cycle	=	=	N/A	stromal cells	↗	=
TIMP-3	• stroma (mRNA) • epithelium (mRNA) • stroma, epithelium and arteries (protein)	• ES, MS and LS ¥ • along the cycle except in LS			N/A	stromal cells	↗ ¥	=

NOTE: M, menstruation; MP+LP, proliferative; MP, mid-proliferative; LP, late proliferative; ES, early secretory; MS, mid-secretory; LS, late secretory; +E+P, in presence of 1 nM estradiol and 100 nM progesterone; ↗, increase; ↘, decrease; =, unchanged; ¥, conflicting results (see text). This table summarizes our current interpretation of published studies at the risk of oversimplification.

proliferation during the proliferative phase, whereas progesterone acts on estradiol-primed endometrium to induce glandular secretion and stromal decidualization. In the absence of pregnancy, the fall of both ovarian steroids in late secretory phase triggers a cascade of events leading to proteolytic breakdown and shedding of the functional layer, associated with bleeding. This review summarizes studies published in the last decade on the control by ovarian steroids of the expression, activation, and inhibition of matrix metalloproteinases (MMPs) in the endometrium. These enzymes are thought to play a critical role in the degradation of the extracellular matrix (ECM) of eutopic endometrium at menstruation, as well as of "active" and bleeding endometriotic lesions. MMPs also play important roles in other processes controlled by ovarian steroids, such as implantation, trophoblast invasion, labor, and postpartum involution. These roles have been thoroughly surveyed by Hulboy, Rudolph, and Matrisian[1] and are beyond the scope of this review.

Matrix Metalloproteinases (MMPs)

MMPs are a family of enzymes able to degrade *in vitro* all ECM constituents of the endometrium at neutral pH.[2] MMPs are classified into five groups according to structural homologies and substrate specificities. Members of all groups have been detected in the human endometrium:

(i) Interstitial collagenase (MMP-1) belongs to the group of collagenases, the only mammalian enzymes (with neutrophil elastase and cathepsin K) able to cleave the triple-helical structure of native fibrillar collagen such as type I and type III collagens, major components of endometrial ECM.
(ii) Gelatinase A (MMP-2) and gelatinase B (MMP-9) form the group of gelatinases that bind to and further degrade collagen denatured after initial cleavage by collagenase.
(iii) Stromelysin-1 (MMP-3), stromelysin-2 (MMP-10), and matrilysin-1 (MMP-7) belong to the group of stromelysins that degrade many components of the basement membranes and the protein core of proteoglycans.
(iv) Membrane type-1 MMP (MT-1-MMP or MMP-14) and membrane type-2 MMP (MT-2-MMP or MMP-15) are members of the membrane-associated MMPs. MMP-14 has been shown *in vitro* to play a crucial role in the activation of proMMP-2 in the vicinity of the plasma membrane. In addition, MMP-2 and MMP-14 are capable of collagenolytic triple-helicase activity, although more slowly than the so-called "true" collagenases.
(v) Stromelysin-3 (MMP-11), which degrades the decidualization-associated insulin-like growth factor–binding protein-1 (IGFBP-1),[3] and matrilysin-2 (or endometase, MMP-26), recently identified in endometrial carcinoma cell lines,[4] belong to the last group of enzymes whose substrates are diverse or unknown.

Tissue Inhibitors of Metalloproteinases (TIMPs)

MMPs are potent enzymes that need to be controlled by specific physiological inhibitors, referred to as tissue inhibitors of metalloproteinases (TIMPs).[5] Expression of MMPs often correlates in time and space with that of TIMPs. TIMP-1, -2, and -4 are secreted as soluble molecules, whereas TIMP-3 is associated with the ECM. These four TIMPs are able to inhibit the proteolytic activity of all mature MMPs, albeit with unequal potency. Notably, TIMP-1 is a poor inhibitor of MMP-14.[6] In addition, combinations between TIMPs and latent MMP zymogens can occur, thereby regulating MMP activation. TIMP-1, -2, and -3 have been identified in the human endometrium.

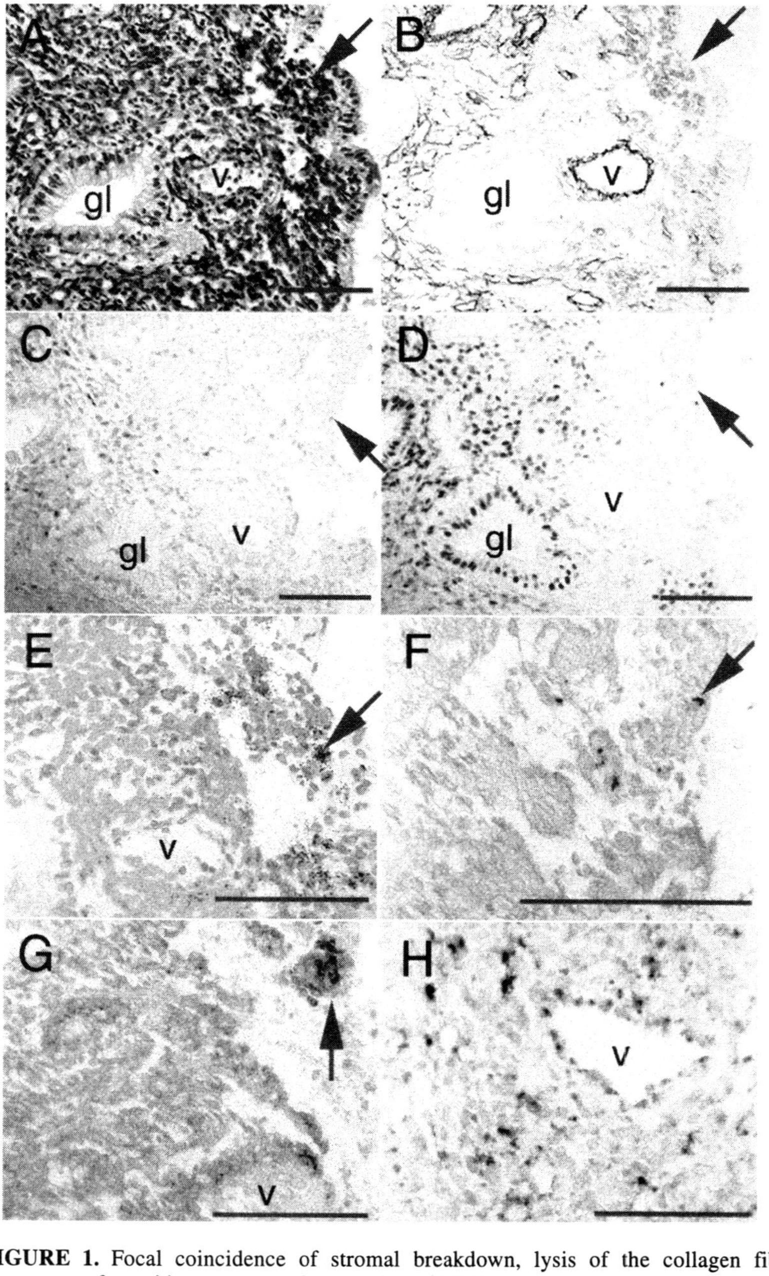

FIGURE 1. Focal coincidence of stromal breakdown, lysis of the collagen fibers, disappearance of steroid receptors, and expression of MMPs in menstrual endometrium. Serial histological sections of a menstrual endometrium were stained with hematoxylin and eosin (**A**), impregnated with silver (**B**), immunolabeled with antiprogesterone receptors (**C**) or anti-estrogen receptor-α monoclonal antibodies (**D**), hybridized with an MMP-1 mRNA antisense riboprobe (**E**), or immunostained with anti-MMP-3 (**F**) or anti-MMP-2 (**G**) monoclonal anti-

SPONTANEOUS MMP AND TIMP EXPRESSION IN THE CYCLING HUMAN ENDOMETRIUM

Several MMPs and TIMPs Are Predominantly, if Not Exclusively, Expressed around Menses

The expression profile of most endometrial MMPs and TIMPs, as measured at mRNA and protein level in tissue homogenates, shows consistent variations during the menstrual cycle, strongly suggesting a tight control of their expression by ovarian steroids (TABLE 1). As a logical consequence of our first studies on endometrial explants (see below), Hampton and Salamonsen[7] clearly showed that the expression of MMP-1 and MMP-3 mRNAs is restricted to the menstrual phase of the cycle. This was confirmed in our laboratory[8] [C. F. Singer *et al.*, unpublished data] and we further observed that only perimenstrual endometria secrete MMP-1 protein during the first day of explant culture, that is, in conditions that presumably reflect the *in vivo* status of the tissue.[8,9]

The fall of serum concentration of ovarian steroids around menstruation is also associated with a strikingly increased expression of MMP-2, MMP-11, MMP-14, and TIMP-1 mRNAs, as well as (although less convincingly) of TIMP-2 mRNA[7,10] [C. F. Singer *et al.*, unpublished data]. These MMP and TIMP mRNAs are expressed at residual levels throughout the menstrual cycle, except MMP-11 mRNA, which is observed essentially during the proliferative phase. In contrast, TIMP-3 mRNA showed no evident pattern of regulation throughout the cycle using RNase protection assays [C. F. Singer *et al.*, unpublished data], although it was found in mid-secretory (but not proliferative) endometria in a Northern blotting study that did not explore the other phases of the cycle.[11]

In their comprehensive study by *in situ* hybridization, Rodgers and coworkers also observed that expression of these and other MMPs was restricted to or enhanced at the menstrual phase.[12] These results were subsequently confirmed by several other morphological studies, including immunohistochemistry (FIG. 1). Thus, the expression of MMP-1, -3, and -10 mRNAs is largely restricted to the perimenstrual phase, at which time expression of MMP-2 mRNA and protein increases.[12–14] Furthermore, a prominent expression of MMP-7 and MMP-11 is observed at menstruation, which persists and declines during the proliferative phase.[12,15] Stromal cells express all endometrial MMPs, except MMP-7, which is exclusively expressed by epithelial cells.[12,15,16] Increased expression of TIMP-1 and -2 mRNAs and proteins is also observed in the endometrial stroma at menstruation.[13,17]

---

bodies. The same area is shown in a further nonserial histological section immunolabeled with anti-MMP-1 monoclonal antibody (**H**). Uterine lumen is at right. Note higher enlargements in panels E–H (bars correspond to 100 μm). *Arrows* point to the same focus combining stromal breakdown, lysis of argyrophilic collagen fibers, disappearance of steroid receptors, and expression of MMP-1 mRNA, as well as immunolabeling of MMP-2 and -3. Note also the immunolabeling of MMP-2 in the wall of vessels (G). Terms: gl, gland; v, vessel.

Discrepancies in Reported Studies

However, several discrepancies appeared between quantitative and morphological analyses and, among the latter studies, regarding the expression pattern of MMPs and TIMPs. First, conflicting results exist for MMP-9 expression along the menstrual cycle. Indeed, the protein could be extracted from endometrial tissue collected throughout the cycle, albeit only in latent form during the nonmenstrual phases and in larger amounts and partially in an active form at menstruation.[18,19] Although (pro)MMP-9 could originate from circulating leukocytes at some phases of the cycle, the protein has also been immunolocalized in epithelial glandular cells during the secretory phase and in a few stromal cells at menstruation, in addition to the neutrophils, eosinophils, and macrophages.[13,16,19,20] In contrast, MMP-9 mRNA appeared restricted to foci of stromal cells at the perimenstrual phase in one study[12] and was not detected in another study that only explored the nonmenstrual phases of the cycle.[21]

The second discrepancies are related to MT-MMPs. Whereas an *in situ* hybridization study disclosed MMP-14 mRNA only in stromal cells of late secretory endometria,[17] an immunohistochemical study reported a patchy MMP-14 localization to epithelial cells and to subsets of macrophages, neutrophils, and large granular lymphocytes at the mid-proliferative, mid-secretory, and menstrual phases of the cycle.[22] The apparent lack of variation in MMP-14 immunolabeling throughout the cycle does not fit very well with its presumed role in proMMP-2 activation, which increases at menstruation.[18] MMP-15 was reported to be more widely and abundantly expressed throughout the cycle in glandular epithelium.[22]

The third discrepancies are related to TIMPs. TIMP-1 and -2 mRNAs were detected only in stromal cells of late secretory endometria in one study,[17] in agreement with an immunohistochemical study.[13] However, another *in situ* hybridization study showed TIMP-1 mRNA in stromal cells throughout the cycle and, additionally, in epithelial cells at menstruation.[12] Immunohistochemical studies found TIMP-1, -2, and -3 in all tissue compartments, including glandular and luminal epithelium, stroma, and vasculature, throughout the cycle.[13,23] TIMP-3 mRNA was weakly detected in epithelial cells of proliferative endometria, in both epithelial and stromal cells of early secretory endometria, and was abundant in (but restricted to) stromal cells in late secretory endometria.[17] Thus, it seems difficult to derive from morphological studies alone a coherent picture for TIMPs that is consistent with biochemical data.

FOCAL EXPRESSION OF MMPs AND TIMPs

Despite these conflicting results in relative intensity of expression throughout the cycle, morphological studies showed that MMP and TIMP expression is heterogeneous within a section, pointing to additional local factors modulating the overall regulation by circulating ovarian steroids. MMP-1 expression is exclusively localized to the functional layer at menstruation; when the menstrual process starts, expression of MMP-1 is limited to foci of stromal cells in the superficial zone. As menstruation proceeds, expression of MMP-1 increases and extends towards the entire functionalis; it is maximal at the periphery of shed fragments.[9,12–14] MMP-2 and -3 expression is also focal, but more extended than that of MMP-1, and limited to stromal cells in the functionalis.[12,13,16,20,21] However, in one report, immunoreactive MMP-2 was detected in some glandular epithelial cells throughout the cycle.[22]

MMP-1-expressing stromal cells show a remarkable colocalization with areas of reduced stromal and epithelial expression of receptors for estrogen and progesterone[14] (FIG. 1). This points to local heterogeneity of tissue hormonal impregnation and suggests that MMP-1 becomes only expressed when this impregnation falls below a critical threshold for hormone suppression. Foci of MMP-1 expression coincide with foci of disruption of the argyrophilic fibrillar network, consistent with a role of MMP-1 in ECM breakdown.[9,14] Preferential expression of MMP-1, -2, and -3 in stromal cells surrounding receptor-negative glands points to pericellular communication between epithelial cells and MMP-producing stromal cells.[12,14]

Menses are characterized by bleeding. At menstruation, several MMPs, including MMP-1, -2, -3, and -9, are preferentially localized around and even in arteriolar walls.[9,13,14,22] In one of these studies, MMP-1 and -2 were observed in vessel walls throughout the cycle, but MMP-9 was restricted to the mid-proliferative, secretory, and menstrual phases.[13] TIMP-1 and -2 have also been preferentially immunolocalized in vessel walls throughout the menstrual cycle.[13,23] Provided their activity can override the inhibitory potential of TIMPs, the preferential localization of MMP expression along some arterioles supports the hypothesis that bleeding is a consequence of the ECM degradation in the vessel wall.

A general conclusion emerges from all these studies. Transcription of most endometrial MMPs seems to be turned on just before the onset of menstruation and suppressed, or at least inhibited, from the beginning of the proliferative phase to the late secretory phase. Around menstruation, activity of the expressed MMPs is probably no longer balanced by TIMPs, whose expression appears either unchanged or increased to a lesser extent. These observations thus suggest that activity of members from all MMP groups is boosted upon ovarian steroid withdrawal at the end of the secretory cycle, resulting in multiple and major proteolytic activities that are able in concert to quickly degrade the various endometrial ECM components.[24] However, local substantial overexpression of the TIMPs may occur to inhibit the proteolytic activity released from shed fragments and prevent unregulated degradation of the endometrial basal layer or of the wall of some vessels.

REGULATION OF MMP AND TIMP EXPRESSION BY OVARIAN STEROIDS IN THE MONKEY

In their elegant study, Brenner and colleagues addressed the hormonal regulation of MMPs *in vivo* in ovariectomized rhesus macaques.[25] Estrogen- and progesterone-secreting devices were implanted subcutaneously to mimic proliferative and secretory phases. Upon progesterone removal, MMP-1, -2, -3, -7, -10, -11, and -14 were quickly upregulated, peaking at the second or third day after progesterone withdrawal, except for MMP-7, which was maximally expressed after 5 days. Interestingly, expression of all these MMPs declined spontaneously after menstruation in the absence of progesterone. Two patterns of expression upon progesterone removal were observed. Expression of MMP-1, -3, and -10 was brief, being strongly induced for only 3 days and then almost abolished after 5 days. On the other hand, expression of MMP-2, -7, -11, and -14 was more sustained, remaining detectable after 3 weeks of artificially extended proliferative phase, except for MMP-7, which decreased after 10 days. Only MMP-7 and -11 were further suppressed when resuming progesterone treatment at the end of a 2-week pseudo-proliferative phase. Moreover, removal of the estradiol-releasing implant in addition to progesterone withdrawal increased and prolonged expression levels of MMP-2, -11, and -14 for up to 2 weeks, but not those of MMP-1, -3, and -10.

These investigations clearly demonstrate, at least in monkeys, that progesterone and (to a lesser extent) estradiol tightly control the expression of these MMPs and that the fall of progesterone serum concentration at the end of the menstrual cycle is the main factor triggering the expression of MMPs in the functionalis of the endometrium, as was suspected for humans.

LESSONS FROM *IN VITRO* STUDIES

Complementarity of In Vitro *Systems*

Two experimental *in vitro* models are widely used to test the role of MMPs in endometrial ECM breakdown and their regulation upon ovarian steroid withdrawal: *ex vivo* endometrial explants and purified cells alone or in coculture. Both allow for strict control of the environment and analysis of secretory products by collecting the conditioned medium. The culture of endometrial explants offers the advantage of maintaining the tissue in a similar environment as *in situ*. Stromal and epithelial cells are indeed surrounded by their native ECM so that the natural cell-cell and cell-ECM contacts are maintained.[26] This system is probably the best suited for identifying the key relevant interactions for human tissue studies. These can then be defined using purified stromal or epithelial cells alone or in physical or chemical contact through a porous membrane. In general, epithelial cells are isolated from aggregates of glandular or superficial epithelium, whereas stromal cells are collected as individual cells after proteolytic digestion of the tissue. Several studies based on the culture of explants or isolated endometrial cells have greatly enriched our knowledge on the effect of ovarian steroids on endometrial MMP and TIMP production (see TABLE 1).

When endometrial explants are cultured in the presence of ovarian steroids, the ECM fibrillar structure is well preserved, except when tissue is sampled around menstruation.[24] Conversely, when ovarian steroids are omitted from the culture, collagen-rich argyrophilic fibers are degraded and explants shrink, as in the endometrium *in situ*. Consistently, ECM degradation is preceded by the release in the conditioned medium of various MMPs, at least partially in active form. These observations are entirely consistent with the *in vivo* experiments with monkeys and demonstrate that ECM breakdown is controlled by ovarian steroids, except at menses, presumably because of the drop of ovarian steroid receptors.

Central Role of MMPs in Endometrial ECM Breakdown

Endometrial explants cultured without ovarian steroids express the same MMPs and TIMPs as found in noncultured perimenstrual endometrium. Expression of MMP-1, -2, and -3 is focal in stromal cells surrounding glands devoid of ovarian steroid receptors. Degradation of ECM that can be monitored by the disappearance of argyrophilic fibers at the end of the culture and by measurements of hydroxyproline release in the culture medium is severely decreased by inhibitors of metalloproteinases, but not by inhibitors of serine, cysteine, or aspartate proteinases.[24] These observations demonstrate that MMPs are responsible for initiating the breakdown of the network of collagen-rich fibers in endometrial explants and strongly support their involvement in menstruating tissue *in situ* as well. Whether other classes of proteinases act downstream in some degradative processes is of course not excluded by these experiments.

Abundant Secretion of Activated MMPs in the Absence of Ovarian Steroids ex Vivo

Secretion of latent and active forms of MMPs is considerable. When cultured for >2 days without ovarian steroids, endometrial explants produce from 10 to 200 mU of (pro)collagenase per day and per mg tissue.[8,9,27] Most of it is readily released in the culture medium (FIG. 2A). Procollagenase secretion during the first day of culture is influenced by the phase of the menstrual cycle at sampling: the highest levels of enzyme are measured in medium conditioned by explants from perimenstrual or menstrual endometria. Spontaneous activation of collagenase occurs in variable proportions in media conditioned by menstrual explants, but not in media conditioned by nonmenstrual explants.[9] From the second day of culture, enzyme release is abundant in all media, with an up to 10-fold enhancement between the first and the fourth day of culture for nonperimenstrual samples. Activation of collagenase then also occurs in media conditioned by nonmenstrual explants (FIG. 2B). Collagenase activity is unlikely to result from the release or production of MMP-8, but is rather provided by *de novo* synthesis of MMP-1 since it is inhibited by cycloheximide, but not by *N*-ethylmaleimide. This conclusion is also supported by the enhanced MMP-1 mRNA expression in nonperimenstrual endometria when cultured in the absence of ovarian steroids.[8]

A concomitant production of gelatinolytic activity is measured in conditioned media and is associated with a significant increase in the release of both latent and active forms of MMP-2 and MMP-9 (FIG. 2C).[27] In nonperimenstrual explant cultures, an up to 50-fold upregulation of gelatinase activity is measured between the first and the fourth day of culture. Osteen and coworkers reported that immunoreactive proMMP-3 and proMMP-7 are released during the second day of culture only by explants from proliferative endometrium, and not by explants from secretory endometrium.[28] In our hands, endometrial explants from the secretory phase also produced MMP-3 in both latent and active forms, detectable by both casein zymography (FIG. 2B) and Western blotting.[18] TIMP-1 and -2 are released by endometrial explants. Secretion of TIMP-1 decreases with time in culture, whereas that of TIMP-2 is more sustained (FIG. 2D).

Overall Control by Ovarian Steroids of MMP Expression, Activation, and Inhibition by TIMPs ex Vivo

In nonmenstrual explants, progesterone almost abolishes the expression of MMP-1,[8] largely suppresses that of MMP-3 and -7,[28] and moderately decreases the amount of MMP-2 and -9 released in the medium[27] (FIGS. 2A–2C). Estradiol by itself

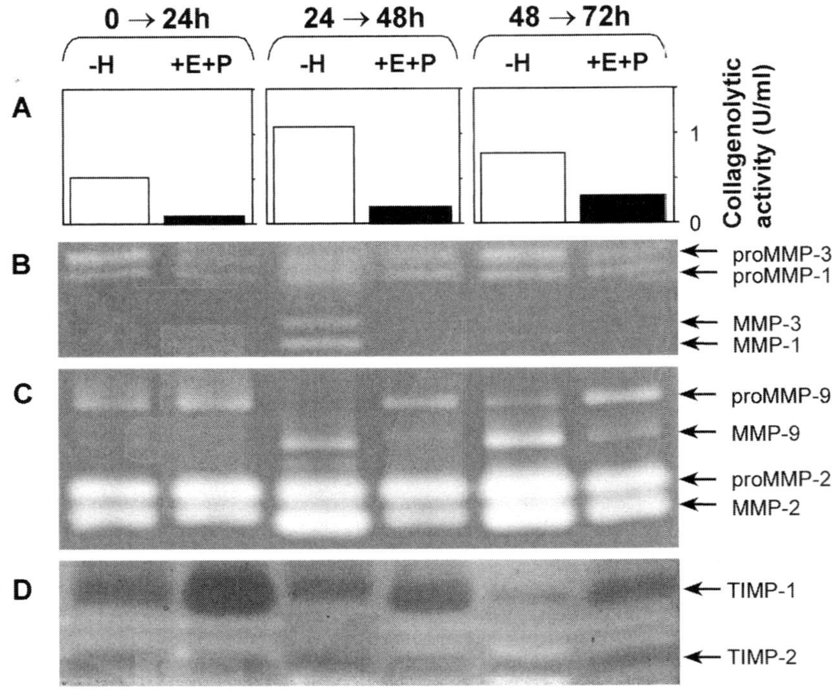

FIGURE 2. Characterization of endometrial MMPs and TIMPs in explant culture. Explants were prepared from a mid-to-late secretory endometrium as described[24] and cultured for 3 days in the absence or presence of 1 nM estradiol and 100 nM progesterone, with daily medium change. Medium collected after 1, 2, or 3 days of culture was submitted to total collagenase assay (after APMA activation) (**A**), casein zymography (**B**), gelatin zymography (**C**), and reverse gelatin zymography (**D**), as previously described.[27] In part A, values above 0.35 U/mL (maximal level of trypsin blank) can be formally attributed to authentic collagenase.

moderately decreases collagenase and gelatinase production[9] and fails to inhibit the expression of MMP-3 and -7.[28] However, when combined at physiologically relevant concentrations, estradiol potentiates the inhibition by progesterone of the production of MMP-1, -3, and -7.[8,9,29] As observed in noncultured cycling endometrium, the expression of progesterone and estradiol receptors in cultured explants is decreased in focal areas of MMP-1 production. Progesterone receptors are even absent in epithelial cells in such foci.[14] On the other hand, MMP-1 expression in explants is focally repressed where ovarian steroid receptors are detected.[14]

Ovarian steroids further inhibit MMP activation. In the absence of added hormones, conditioned media usually contain the active forms of MMP-1, -2, -3, and -9, with variable proportions between individuals. Addition of progesterone with or without estradiol during culture severely inhibits the activation of MMP-1, -3, and -9 and decreases that of MMP-2 (FIG. 2).[9,27] Since MMP-3 appears to be a key activator of endometrial proMMP-9, inhibition by progesterone of its expression and activation may account for the strong decrease of MMP-9 activation by this hormone.[18] Combination of estradiol and progesterone slows down the decline of TIMP-1 release in the medium, but does not seem to affect TIMP-2 production (FIG. 2D).

Progesterone Inhibits MMP Production by Purified Endometrial Cells

Purified endometrial stromal cells express and secrete variable amounts of several MMPs and TIMPs in the absence of added ovarian steroids. The mRNAs encoding MMP-1, -2, -3, -9, -11, and -14 as well as most corresponding immunoreactive proteins (predominantly in latent forms) are generally,[28,30–32] but not always, observed.[33] Conversely, progesterone and its derivatives inhibit the expression of MMP-1, -3, and -11 mRNA and the secretion of MMP-1 and -3 proteins by stromal cells.[28,31,32,34–36] Progesterone does not affect MMP-2 mRNA level[33,34] nor proMMP-2 release,[22] but decreases its secreted active form.[22] Although progesterone does not inhibit the expression of MMP-14,[22,33] which is thought to activate proMMP-2 *in vivo*, it increases the release of TIMP-2 (see below),[35] which could be responsible for the decreased activation of proMMP-2. As for explants, estradiol has no effect on its own on MMP-3 production by purified stromal cells, but potentiates the inhibition by progesterone.[32,36] Epithelial cells purified from proliferative endometria produce only MMP-7.[28] This is not affected by progesterone or estradiol, but MMP-7 production by epithelial cells is inhibited by a soluble factor produced by stromal cells in response to progesterone, as was nicely shown by Osteen and colleagues in cocultures of purified cells.[28]

Stromal cells express TIMP-1 and -2 mRNAs when cultured without hormone,[33,34] and TIMP-3 mRNA was also detected by RNase protection assay,[33] but not by Northern blotting.[11] Addition of estradiol to the culture medium did not affect the level of expression of TIMP-1 and TIMP-3 mRNAs as analyzed by Northern blotting,[11,34] and secretion of TIMP-1 protein (but not of TIMP-2 and -3) was disclosed by reverse zymography.[35] Progesterone alone or combined with estradiol had no effect on the expression of TIMP-1 and -2 mRNAs,[33,34] but increased the secretion of TIMP-1 and induced that of TIMP-2 and -3.[35] High concentrations of progesterone were necessary to induce the expression of TIMP-3 mRNA as assessed by Northern blotting,[11] although another study showed no effect of combined estradiol and progesterone by RNase protection assay.[33] When cultured in the presence of progesterone and estradiol, stromal cells secrete large amounts of TIMP-1 and significant amounts of TIMP-2 and -3, and the rate of secretion seems to increase steadily with the time of culture.[23,35,37]

Progesterone Withdrawal Induces MMP Production by Purified Endometrial Cells

The release of the progesterone block increases the production of MMP-1, -2, -3, and -9, but does not change TIMP production by cultured stromal cells.[10,32,34,37] Secretion of MMP-2 upon progesterone withdrawal is abundant, but transient,[10] whereas that of MMP-1 and -3 is more sustained:[32,34] after 8 days without added hormone, higher concentrations were still detected for MMP-1 and -3, but not for MMP-2 mRNAs.[34] Interestingly, enhanced MMP-3 secretion upon progesterone withdrawal follows the increase in corresponding mRNA level after a delay of several days, suggesting an additional posttranscriptional control.[32] However, MMP-1 and -3 mRNA expression and protein secretion are quickly upregulated by the progesterone receptor antagonist, mifepristone (RU486), alone or in combination with a progestin.[34,36]

Factors Contributing to the Variability of MMP and TIMP Expression in Cell Culture

As mentioned above, important variations, if not discrepancies, occur in cultures of endometrial cells. Moreover, the response of MMP production to ovarian steroids in cell culture only partially mimics the observations with explants. While variability among patients certainly comes into play, there are also differences in cell environment and/or methodological aspects that need to be carefully evaluated.

Sampling of the Endometrial Cell Source

The phase of the cycle at which endometrial samples are collected should be systematically assessed (and reported), at least histologically, since Osteen and coworkers reported the production of MMPs by explants from proliferative (but not secretory) endometria.[28] In addition to morphological analysis, decidualization of stromal cells can be monitored by measuring the expression level of prolactin or of other markers such as IGFBP-1.[38]

General Culture Conditions

When cultured in plain plastic wells, cells are devoid of their original physiological environment. Cell-matrix and cell-cell interactions are modified and responses to treatment can, accordingly, diverge from the *in vivo* situation. To improve culture conditions, cells can be plated on, or within, a reconstituted ECM. Moreover, different cell types can be cocultured either with physical contact or with only chemical communication through a porous membrane.[28,39] The composition of the culture medium can also significantly affect cell behavior and gene expression. Expression of endometrial MMPs is influenced by the presence of insulin[8,27] and other culture medium components.[34] Serum should be deprived in estrogen and progesterone by charcoal treatment. In addition, parameters related to the history of cultured cells should not be neglected. In particular, initial cell number, cell passage, and addition of hormones should be carefully monitored. MMP-1 response to ovarian steroid is already significantly modified in stromal cells after one passage, compared to cells in primary culture.[34]

Effective Hormone Concentration in Culture

The actual concentration of hormones in the culture medium can significantly diverge from the concentration initially supplied because of direct adsorption to the culture support or steroid metabolism by the cultured cells. To evaluate adsorption on the plastic wells, culture medium supplemented with estradiol or progesterone was first incubated for 24 h in the absence of cells. We noted that $91\pm6\%$ of the initial concentration of estradiol remained at the end of the incubation, but that progesterone dropped to $66\pm1\%$. Thus, decrease in progesterone can be due, at least in part, to plastic adsorption. We next checked the variation of steroid concentrations

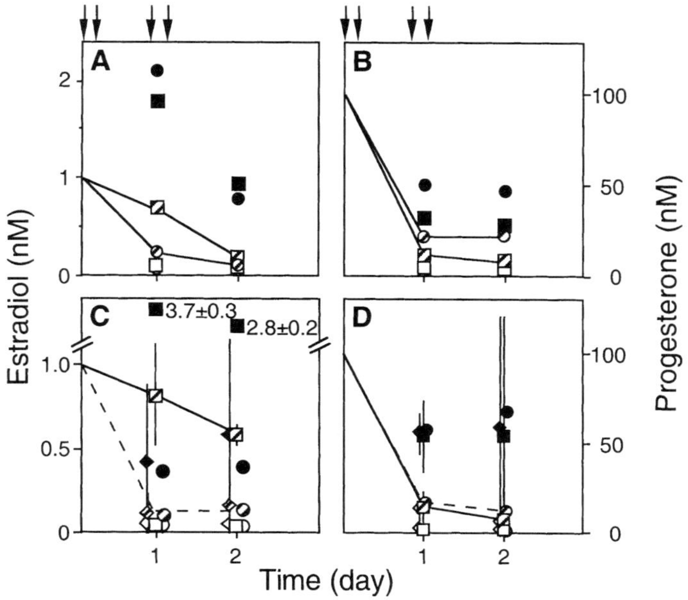

FIGURE 3. Decrease of estradiol and progesterone concentrations in culture. Estradiol (A, C) and progesterone (B, D) concentrations were measured by radioimmunoassay in culture media of endometrial explants (A, B) or of purified endometrial cells (C, D). Concentrations were assayed at the end of the first and second days of culture, without change of the culture media. Media received (i) no hormone addition (open symbols), (ii) 1 nM estradiol together with 100 nM progesterone (nominal) once at the start of the culture (hatched symbols), or (iii) the same addition at four consecutive times throughout culture (arrows; closed symbols). Water-soluble complexes of steroids and 2-hydroxypropyl-β-cyclodextrin were used. Cultured explants (A, B) were from a mid-secretory endometrium (circles) and from a late secretory endometrium (squares); the symbols correspond to assays performed in pools of 4–6 conditioned media. Purified endometrial cells (C, D) were isolated from the same endometria and from another late secretory endometrium. The experiments were performed on primary cultures started on the day of endometrial sampling in two cases and after 4 days of culture in the presence of 10% fetal calf serum in the third culture. Culture media were devoid of serum during the experiment. Squares: purified stromal cells (n = 3, mean ± SD); circles: purified epithelial cells (mean of two cultures); diamonds: cocultures of stromal and epithelial cells (n = 3, mean ± SD). The lines indicate the fall of estradiol and progesterone concentrations after a single addition of the steroids at the start of the culture in each culture of explants in panels A and B and for the purified stromal cells (solid lines) and epithelial cells (dashed lines) in panels C and D.

in the medium during cultures of explants and of purified epithelial and stromal cells (FIG. 3). After 1 day of culture, the concentration of progesterone dramatically dropped from an initial nominal concentration of 100 nM to below 20 nM in all types of cultures tested: explants, purified stromal cells, purified epithelial cells, as well as in cocultures of stromal and epithelial cells. Repeated additions of 100 nM progesterone to the culture medium maintained a mean concentration around 50 nM. These results are compatible with a fall of progesterone concentration secondary to adsorption to the plastic surfaces of the culture devices since it occurred at similar levels in all types of cultures. In contrast, the decline of estradiol concentration varied between explant cultures and its extent also largely differed between stromal and epithelial cells. The drop was particularly rapid with epithelial cells, pointing to a faster metabolism of estradiol by these cells. This could be attributed to 17β-hydroxysteroid dehydrogenase, which catabolizes estradiol into estrone. This enzyme is present in the glandular epithelium and its expression is induced by progesterone.[40]

Despite the large drop in ovarian steroid concentrations that occurs after 1 day of culture, the production of many MMPs can still be controlled by progesterone, in particular in cultures of explants, indicating either that low concentrations remain sufficient to block the expression of these MMPs or that the higher concentrations present during the first hours of culture induce a remanent inhibitory effect that could be mediated by long-acting intracellular or extracellular secondary mediators, such as cytokines.

GENERAL AND LOCAL REGULATION BY PROGESTERONE RECEPTORS AND CYTOKINES

DNA and Protein Targets of Progesterone Receptors

The mechanisms by which estrogen and progesterone regulate the expression of MMPs and TIMPs are still unclear, but both likely involve progesterone receptors. As mentioned above, MMP-1-expressing foci correspond to areas of reduced receptors for estrogen and progesterone, in the endometrium *in situ* as well as in cultured explants. The potentiating effect of estradiol on progesterone-induced inhibition of MMP production may be attributed to an enhanced expression of progesterone receptors.[41] Conversely, the decreased expression of progesterone receptors at menstruation likely accounts for the failure of menstrual explants to respond to hormonal treatment.[42]

Together with the receptors for estrogen (hER) and glucocorticoids (hGR), human receptors for progesterone (hPR) belong to the family of the nuclear steroid hormone receptors. Two distinct isoforms of the progesterone receptor (hPR-A and hPR-B) are encoded from a single gene by alternative promoter usage. Both hPR-A and hPR-B isoforms contain the same ligand-binding domain (and therefore display undistinguishable hormone interactions), as well as identical DNA-binding domains and transcriptional activation domains AF-1 and AF-2. However, an additional activation domain AF-3 occurs only in the N-terminal segment of hPR-B, leading to distinct transcriptional activity.[43] In addition, the two isoforms interact: an inhibitory receptor domain, located at the N-terminus of hPR-A, mediates hPR-A *trans*-repression of hPR-B-induced gene transcription.[44] Although also present in hPR-B, this domain shows no intramolecular inhibitory activity due to constraints imparted by AF-3.[44,45]

Steroid hormone receptors modulate gene expression by a variety of inducing or repressing mechanisms, with most protranscriptional effects resulting from the docking of the occupied receptor to specific hormone-responsive elements. According to the classical concept of action, progesterone binding induces a conformational change in the receptor molecule that leads to dissociation from a complex of heat-shock proteins, phosphorylation of the receptor, dimerization, and binding to specific DNA sequences termed progesterone-responsive elements (PRE).[46] Homo- and possibly heterodimerization can occur and are likely to induce different responses. Focal variations in the type of progesterone receptor expressed, or in the relative amount of each type, could thus be responsible for a specific spatial pattern of expression of some MMPs in human endometrium throughout the menstrual cycle.

Although PRE may occur in MMP and TIMP promoters (e.g., MMP-1 and -9), the control of MMP and TIMP gene expression apparently does not involve direct binding of the dimerized progesterone receptors with the DNA of their promoters. One possible relay is interaction with components of the AP-1 complex. Another mechanism could be the control of inducing or repressing cytokines. This will be addressed in a subsequent section.

AP-1 is controlled by phorbol esters. Tetradecanoyl phorbol acetate (TPA)–responsive elements (TRE) occur in the promoters of several MMP and TIMP genes (e.g., MMP-1, -3, and -9, as well as TIMP-1) and mediate transcriptional upregulation by TPA *in vitro*.[2,3] Progesterone receptor could therefore block AP-1 activation of MMP gene by directly preventing AP-1 binding to TREs or by inhibiting its transactivation function.[47] It is still unknown whether such interaction requires dimerization of hPR. Recent observations based on a promoter derived from the collagenase gene show that both hPR-A and hPR-B interact with hER at the AP-1 site and suggest that opposing steroid influences are integrated at this TRE.[48] Moreover, unlike hER and hGR, hPR is able to influence AP-1-mediated transcription even in the absence of ligand and could itself exert opposite effects, depending on progesterone binding. For example, transfection of hPR-B in hPR-negative human endometrial adenocarcinoma cells (HEC-1B) induces AP-1-controlled expression in the absence of ligand, and addition of progesterone reverses this effect.[49]

Whether hPR directly interacts with AP-1 is still unclear. Coactivators of the AP-1 complex such as Jun-activation domain-binding protein-1 (JAB-1) can also interact with both hPR and the steroid receptor coactivator-1 (SRC-1), a member of the large family of nuclear receptor coactivators. However, JAB-1 is not likely to play a major role in the hPR inhibitory effect on AP-1 transcription.[50]

Interplay between Cytokines and Ovarian Steroids

Although progesterone is a key regulator of endometrial MMP expression, the focal response upon ovarian steroid withdrawal argues against a direct effect and implies heterogeneity in hormone responsiveness by the unequal occurrence of hormone receptors or in the intracellular relay as discussed above and/or additional local (e.g., paracrine) controls. Recent lines of evidence have demonstrated that cytokines control endometrial MMP expression in response to progesterone and estradiol, in particular interleukin-1α (IL-1α) and transforming growth factors β (TGF-β). They can either mediate or potentiate the progesterone block, or instead trigger MMP production despite progesterone impregnation.

The induction of stromal MMP-1 and -3, as well as of epithelial MMP-7 expression, appears to be mediated by IL-1α, likely released from the epithelial cells and acting through autocrine/paracrine effects.[30,39,51,52] Similarly, IL-1β induces MMP-3 production by stromal cells.[36] Interestingly, Osteen and coworkers have recently demonstrated that the ability of progesterone to inhibit MMP expression depends on the extent and/or duration of steroid exposure, suggesting local balances between agonist and antagonist cytokines. The working hypothesis is therefore that IL-1α is abundantly expressed in the endometrium during the secretory phase to prepare induction of MMPs for rapid matrix turnover at the end of the cycle and that its prodegradative function is fully silenced until menstruation by progesterone impregnation.[51,53]

Cytokines of the TGF-β family seem to cooperate with progesterone to limit MMP expression. Recombinant TGF-β1 inhibits MMP-3 and -7 production in endometrial organ culture.[29] TGF-β1 and -β2 inhibit MMP-7 production by isolated epithelial cells.[54] In coculture, TGF-β1 potentiates the inhibition mediated by stromal cells of MMP-7 expression in epithelial cells, in response to combined estradiol and progesterone.[54] Conversely, anti-TGF-β antibody fully prevents the progesterone block on both MMP-3 and -7 in cell coculture as well as in organ cultures. Since TGF-β2 expression is enhanced during the secretory phase, these observations suggest that TGF-β2 may be a major mediator of progesterone-induced suppression of MMP-3 and -7.[54]

Although progesterone analogues reproduce the inhibition of progesterone on MMP-1 and -3 expression in isolated stromal cells,[32,35,37] the endometrium of patients under long-term progestin-only contraception focally escapes the tight hormonal control of the expression of MMP-1 and -3, as well as of the activation of MMP-2 and -9, despite persistent levels of progestin concentration in the serum,[55,56] Interestingly, the serum concentration of estradiol is slightly, but significantly, decreased at the start of bleeding episodes, and progesterone receptors are generally not detectable in the foci of stromal breakdown, suggesting that a local decrease of the expression of progesterone receptors induced by a fall of estradiol level is responsible for the loss of control of MMP activity at the sites of bleeding. Bleeding episodes are generally associated with a strong increase of IL-1α release,[55] suggesting that this cytokine plays a similar prodegradative function in normal and abnormal endometrial ECM turnover and bleeding.

GENERAL CONCLUSION AND PERSPECTIVES

It is now clear that MMPs play a major role in the endometrial ECM breakdown *ex vivo* upon ovarian steroid withdrawal, thereby strongly suggesting that they trigger physiological menstruation as well as abnormal uterine bleeding *in vivo*. Bleeding is also thought to be a critical event in the clinical expression of endometriotic lesions.[57] Despite considerable advances contributed by several active laboratories, there are still some significant discrepancies that must be clarified and important questions that remain to be answered in order to integrate the already known molecular players. Since several MMPs from at least three different groups are turned on upon progesterone withdrawal (i.e., collagenase, gelatinases, and stromelysins), further experiments are required to investigate their respective contribution to ECM breakdown. Moreover, assuming that proMMP activation and degradative action result from a cascade of events, their sequence needs to be clarified. From a medical perspective, the most important issue is to clarify the mechanisms of the local control of MMP (in)activation, in particular the temporal and spatial modulation of cytokine expression, their involvement as progesterone mediators, and their mutual interactions. For example, although endometriotic foci are still overall responsive to ovarian steroids, they appear to escape the control of estrogen and progesterone at some point, so as to unpredictably express MMP-1 and engage in stromal breakdown even between menses,[58] by a mechanism comparable to that found in the eutopic endometrium at menstruation. An interplay between ovarian steroids and local cytokines is thus likely to control the local expression of MMPs in endometriotic foci as in the eutopic endometrium. Finally, it is surprising to realize how little we understand about the control of MMP and TIMP gene expression by ovarian steroids. These numerous questions will certainly keep the growing number of involved laboratories busy for many years to come.

ACKNOWLEDGMENTS

We are grateful to R. de Hertogh and staff members of the Laboratory of Gynecological Endocrinology, Medical School of the Université Catholique de Louvain, for assaying steroid concentrations in culture media and to J. Donnez and the whole staff of the Gynecology Department at Saint Luc University Clinics, Medical School of the Université Catholique de Louvain, for providing human tissues. Our investigations have been supported by grants from the FSR (Université Catholique de Louvain), the Belgian Fonds National de la Recherche Scientifique (FNRS), Concerted Research Action (French Speaking Belgian Community), and Interuniversity Attraction Poles (Belgian State), as well as scientific grants from Ipsen-Biotech (Paris, France), Novo-Nordisk (Bagsvaerd, Denmark), and WHO (Geneva, Switzerland). P. B. Cornet is a Research Fellow of the FNRS.

REFERENCES

1. Hulboy, D.L., L.A. Rudolph & L.M. Matrisian. 1997. Matrix metalloproteinases as mediators of reproductive function. Mol. Hum. Reprod. **3:** 27–45.
2. Eeckhout, Y. & P. Henriet. 2002. Matrix metalloproteinases. *In* The Encyclopedia of Molecular Medicine. Wiley. New York. In press.
3. Manes, S., E. Mira, M.M. Barbacid *et al.* 1997. Identification of insulin-like growth factor–binding protein-1 as a potential physiological substrate for human stromelysin-3. J. Biol. Chem. **272:** 25706–25712.
4. Park, H.I., J. Ni, F.E. Gerkema *et al.* 2000. Identification and characterization of human endometase (matrix metalloproteinase-26) from endometrial tumor. J. Biol. Chem. **275:** 20540–20544.
5. Henriet, P. & Y. Eeckhout. 2002. Tissue inhibitors of matrix metalloproteinases. *In* The Encyclopedia of Molecular Medicine. Wiley. New York. In press.
6. Will, H., S.J. Atkinson *et al.* 1996. The soluble catalytic domain of membrane type 1 matrix metalloproteinase cleaves the propeptide of progelatinase A and initiates autoproteolytic activation: regulation by TIMP-2 and TIMP-3. J. Biol. Chem. **271:** 17119–17123.
7. Hampton, A.L. & L.A. Salamonsen. 1994. Expression of messenger ribonucleic acid encoding matrix metalloproteinases and their tissue inhibitors is related to menstruation. J. Endocrinol. **141:** R1–R3.
8. Marbaix, E., I. Kokorine, P. Henriet *et al.* 1995. The expression of interstitial collagenase in human endometrium is controlled by progesterone and by oestradiol and is related to menstruation. Biochem. J. **305:** 1027–1030.

9. MARBAIX, E., I. KOKORINE, J. DONNEZ *et al.* 1996. Regulation and restricted expression of interstitial collagenase suggest a pivotal role in the initiation of menstruation. Hum. Reprod. **11**(suppl. 2): 134–143.
10. IRWIN, J.C., D. KIRK, R.B.L. GWATKIN *et al.* 1996. Human endometrial matrix metalloproteinase-2, a putative menstrual proteinase: hormonal regulation in cultured stromal cells and messenger RNA expression during the menstrual cycle. J. Clin. Invest. **97:** 438–447.
11. HIGUCHI, T., H. KANZAKI, H. NAKAYAMA *et al.* 1995. Induction of tissue inhibitor of metalloproteinase 3 gene expression during *in vitro* decidualization of human endometrial stromal cells. Endocrinology **136:** 4973–4981.
12. RODGERS, W.H., L.M. MATRISIAN, L.C. GIUDICE *et al.* 1994. Patterns of matrix metalloproteinase expression in cycling endometrium imply differential functions and regulation by steroid hormones. J. Clin. Invest. **94:** 946–953.
13. FREITAS, S., G. MEDURI *et al.* 1999. Expression of metalloproteinases and their inhibitors in blood vessels in human endometrium. Biol. Reprod. **61:** 1070–1082.
14. KOKORINE, I., E. MARBAIX, P. HENRIET *et al.* 1996. Focal cellular origin and regulation of interstitial collagenase (matrix metalloproteinase-1) are related to menstrual breakdown in the human endometrium. J. Cell Sci. **109:** 2151–2160.
15. RODGERS, W.H., K.G. OSTEEN, L.M. MATRISIAN *et al.* 1993. Expression and localization of matrilysin, a matrix metalloproteinase, in human endometrium during the reproductive cycle. Am. J. Obstet. Gynecol. **168:** 253–260.
16. KOKS, C.A., P.G. GROOTHUIS, P. SLAATS *et al.* 2000. Matrix metalloproteinases and their tissue inhibitors in antegradely shed menstruum and peritoneal fluid. Fertil. Steril. **73:** 604–612.
17. MAATTA, M., Y. SOINI, A. LIAKKA *et al.* 2000. Localization of MT1-MMP, TIMP-1, TIMP-2, and TIMP-3 messenger RNA in normal, hyperplastic, and neoplastic endometrium: enhanced expression by endometrial adenocarcinomas is associated with low differentiation. Am. J. Clin. Pathol. **114:** 402–411.
18. RIGOT, V., E. MARBAIX, P. LEMOINE *et al.* 2001. *In vivo* perimenstrual activation of progelatinase B (proMMP-9) in the human endometrium and its dependence on stromelysin 1 (MMP-3) *ex vivo.* Biochem. J. **358:** 275–280.
19. SKINNER, J.L., S.C. RILEY, A.E. GEBBIE *et al.* 1999. Regulation of matrix metalloproteinase-9 in endometrium during the menstrual cycle and following administration of intrauterine levonorgestrel. Hum. Reprod. **14:** 793–799.
20. JEZIORSKA, M., H. NAGASE, L.A. SALAMONSEN *et al.* 1996. Immunolocalization of the matrix metalloproteinases gelatinase B and stromelysin 1 in human endometrium throughout the menstrual cycle. J. Reprod. Fertil. **107:** 43–51.
21. SOINI, Y., E. ALARAKKOLA & H. AUTIO-HARMAINEN. 1997. Expression of messenger RNAs for metalloproteinases 2 and 9, type IV collagen, and laminin in nonneoplastic and neoplastic endometrium. Hum. Pathol. **28:** 220–226.
22. ZHANG, J., A.L. HAMPTON, G. NIE *et al.* 2000. Progesterone inhibits activation of latent matrix metalloproteinase (MMP)–2 by membrane-type 1 MMP: enzymes coordinately expressed in human endometrium. Biol. Reprod. **62:** 85–94.
23. ZHANG, J. & L.A. SALAMONSEN. 1997. Tissue inhibitor of metalloproteinases (TIMP)–1, –2, and –3 in human endometrium during the menstrual cycle. Mol. Hum. Reprod. **3:** 735–741.
24. MARBAIX, E., I. KOKORINE, P. MOULIN *et al.* 1996. Menstrual breakdown of human endometrium can be mimicked *in vitro* and is selectively and reversibly blocked by inhibitors of matrix metalloproteinases. Proc. Natl. Acad. Sci. U.S.A. **93:** 9120–9125.
25. RUDOLPH-OWEN, L.A., O.D. SLAYDEN, L.M. MATRISIAN *et al.* 1998. Matrix metalloproteinase expression in *Macaca mulatta* endometrium: evidence for zone-specific regulatory tissue gradients. Biol. Reprod. **59:** 1349–1359.
26. CORNILLIE, F., I. BROSENS, E.M. BELSEY *et al.* 1991. Lysosomal enzymes in the human endometrium: a biochemical study in untreated and levonorgestrel-treated women. Contraception **43:** 387–400.
27. MARBAIX, E., J. DONNEZ, P.J. COURTOY *et al.* 1992. Progesterone regulates the activity of collagenase and related gelatinases A and B in human endometrial explants. Proc. Natl. Acad. Sci. U.S.A. **89:** 11789–11793.

28. OSTEEN, K.G., W.H. RODGERS, M. GAIRE *et al.* 1994. Stromal-epithelial interaction mediates steroidal regulation of metalloproteinase expression in human endometrium. Proc. Natl. Acad. Sci. U.S.A. **91:** 10129–10133.
29. BRUNER, K.L., E. EISENBERG, F. GORSTEIN *et al.* 1999. Progesterone and transforming growth factor–β coordinately regulate suppression of endometrial matrix metalloproteinases in a model of experimental endometriosis. Steroids **64:** 648–653.
30. RAWDANOWICZ, T.J., A.L. HAMPTON, H. NAGASE *et al.* 1994. Matrix metalloproteinase production by cultured human endometrial stromal cells: identification of interstitial collagenase, gelatinase-A, gelatinase-B, and stromelysin-1 and their differential regulation by interleukin-1α and tumor necrosis factor-α. J. Clin. Endocrinol. Metab. **79:** 530–536.
31. SCHATZ, F., C. PAPP, E. TOTH-PAL *et al.* 1994. *In vitro* regulation of stromelysin-1 in human endometrial stromal cells. Ann. N.Y. Acad. Sci. **732:** 479–481.
32. SCHATZ, F., C. PAPP, E. TOTH-PAL *et al.* 1994. Ovarian steroid–modulated stromelysin-1 expression in human endometrial stromal and decidual cells. J. Clin. Endocrinol. Metab. **78:** 1467–1472.
33. SINGER, C.F., E. MARBAIX, P. LEMOINE *et al.* 1999. Local cytokines induce differential expression of matrix metalloproteinases but not their tissue inhibitors in human endometrial fibroblasts. Eur. J. Biochem. **259:** 40–45.
34. LOCKWOOD, C.J., G. KRIKUN, V.A. HAUSKNECHT *et al.* 1998. Matrix metalloproteinase and matrix metalloproteinase inhibitor expression in endometrial stromal cells during progestin-initiated decidualization and menstruation-related progestin withdrawal. Endocrinology **139:** 4607–4613.
35. HAMPTON, A.L., G. NIE & L.A. SALAMONSEN. 1999. Progesterone analogues similarly modulate endometrial matrix metalloproteinase-1 and matrix metalloproteinase-3 and their inhibitor in a model for long-term contraceptive effects. Mol. Hum. Reprod. **5:** 365–371.
36. SCHATZ, F., C. PAPP, S. AIGNER *et al.* 1997. Biological mechanisms underlying the clinical effects of RU 486: modulation of cultured endometrial stromal cell stromelysin-1 and prolactin expression. J. Clin. Endocrinol. Metab. **82:** 188–193.
37. SALAMONSEN, L.A., A.R. BUTT, F.R. HAMMOND *et al.* 1997. Production of endometrial matrix metalloproteinases, but not their tissue inhibitors, is modulated by progesterone withdrawal in an *in vitro* model for menstruation. J. Clin. Endocrinol. Metab. **82:** 1409–1415.
38. BRYANT-GREENWOOD, G.D., E-M. RUTANEN, S. PARTANEN *et al.* 1993. Sequential appearance of relaxin, prolactin, and IGFBP-1 during growth and differentiation of the human endometrium. Mol. Cell. Endocrinol. **95:** 23–29.
39. SINGER, C.F., E. MARBAIX, I. KOKORINE *et al.* 1997. Paracrine stimulation of interstitial collagenase (MMP-1) in the human endometrium by interleukin 1α and its dual block by ovarian steroids. Proc. Natl. Acad. Sci. U.S.A. **94:** 10341–10345.
40. TSENG, L. 1979. Physiologic changes in binding and metabolism of estradiol and progesterone in human endometrium during the menstrual cycle. Obstet. Gynecol. Annu. **8:** 1–17.
41. ARONICA, S.M. & B.S. KATZENELLENBOGEN. 1991. Progesterone receptor regulation in uterine cells: stimulation by estrogen, cyclic adenosine 3′,5′-monophosphate, and insulin-like growth factor I and suppression by antiestrogens and protein kinase inhibitors. Endocrinology **128:** 2045–2052.
42. TAMAYA, T., T. MURAKAMI & H. OKADA. 1986. Concentrations of steroid receptors in normal human endometrium in relation to the day of the menstrual cycle. Acta Obstet. Gynecol. Scand. **65:** 195–198.
43. SARTORIUS, C.A., M.Y. MELVILLE, A.R. HOVLAND *et al.* 1994. A third transactivation function (AF3) of human progesterone receptors located in the unique N-terminal segment of the B-isoform. Mol. Endocrinol. **8:** 1347–1360.
44. GIANGRANDE, P.H., G. POLLIO & D.P. MCDONNELL. 1997. Mapping and characterization of the functional domains responsible for the differential activity of the A and B isoforms of the human progesterone receptor. J. Biol. Chem. **272:** 32889–32900.
45. HOVLAND, A.R., R.L. POWELL, G.S. TAKIMOTO *et al.* 1998. An N-terminal inhibitory function, IF, suppresses transcription by the A-isoform, but not the B-isoform of human progesterone receptors. J. Biol. Chem. **273:** 5455–5460.

46. CONNEELY, O.M. & J.P. LYDON. 2000. Progesterone receptors in reproduction: functional impact of the A and B isoforms. Steroids **65:** 571–577.
47. BEATO, M. 1991. Transcriptional control by nuclear receptors. FASEB J. **5:** 2044–2051.
48. UHT, R.M., C.M. ANDERSON, P. WEBB *et al.* 1997. Transcriptional activities of estrogen and glucocorticoid receptors are functionally integrated at the AP-1 response element. Endocrinology **138:** 2900–2908.
49. BAMBERGER, A.M., C.M. BAMBERGER, B. GELLERSEN *et al.* 1996. Modulation of AP-1 activity by the human progesterone receptor in endometrial adenocarcinoma cells. Proc. Natl. Acad. Sci. U.S.A. **93:** 6169–6174.
50. CHAUCHEREAU, A., M. GEORGIAKAKI, M. PERRIN-WOLFF *et al.* 2000. JAB1 interacts with both the progesterone receptor and SRC-1. J. Biol. Chem. **275:** 8540–8548.
51. KELLER, N.R., E. SIERRA-RIVERA, E. EISENBERG *et al.* 2000. Progesterone exposure prevents matrix metalloproteinase-3 (MMP-3) stimulation by interleukin-1α in human endometrial stromal cells. J. Clin. Endocrinol. Metab. **85:** 1611–1619.
52. OSTEEN, K.G., E. SIERRA-RIVERA, N.R. KELLER *et al.* 1997. Interleukin-1α opposes progesterone-mediated suppression of MMP-7: a possible role of this cytokine during human implantation. Ann. N.Y. Acad. Sci. **828:** 137–145.
53. OSTEEN, K.G., N.R. KELLER, F.A. FELTUS *et al.* 1999. Paracrine regulation of matrix metalloproteinase expression in the normal human endometrium. Gynecol. Obstet. Invest. **48**(suppl. 1)**:** 2–13.
54. BRUNER, K.L., W.H. RODGERS, L.I. GOLD *et al.* 1995. Transforming growth factor β mediates the progesterone suppression of an epithelial metalloproteinase by adjacent stroma in the human endometrium. Proc. Natl. Acad. Sci. U.S.A. **92:** 7362–7366.
55. GALANT, C., M. VEKEMANS, P. LEMOINE *et al.* 2000. Temporal and spatial association of matrix metalloproteinases with focal endometrial breakdown and bleeding upon progestin-only contraception. J. Clin. Endocrinol. Metab. **85:** 4827–4834.
56. MARBAIX, E., M. VEKEMANS, C. GALANT *et al.* 2000. Circulating sex hormones and endometrial stromelysin-1 (matrix metalloproteinase-3) at the start of bleeding episodes in levonorgestrel-implant users. Hum. Reprod. **15**(suppl. 3)**:** 120–134.
57. BROSENS, I.A. 1997. Endometriosis: a disease because it is characterized by bleeding. Am. J. Obstet. Gynecol. **176:** 263–267.
58. KOKORINE, I., M. NISOLLE, J. DONNEZ *et al.* 1997. Expression of interstitial collagenase (matrix metalloproteinase-1) is related to the activity of human endometriotic lesions. Fertil. Steril. **68:** 246–251.

Paracrine Mediators of Endometrial Matrix Metalloproteinase Expression

Potential Targets for Progestin-Based Treatment of Endometriosis

KEVIN G. OSTEEN, KAYLON L. BRUNER-TRAN, DAVID ONG, AND ESTHER EISENBERG

Women's Reproductive Health Research Center, Department of Obstetrics and Gynecology, and Department of Biochemistry, Vanderbilt University of Medicine, Nashville, Tennessee, USA

ABSTRACT: The endometrial lining of the human uterus is a highly specialized, steroid-sensitive tissue. Throughout the reproductive years, the endometrium undergoes dramatic cycles of growth, differentiation, and breakdown under the influence of ovarian steroids. In response to changes in steroid exposure throughout the menstrual cycle, the endometrium produces an array of bioactive growth factors and other cytokines that are critical components of paracrine communication. For example, cell-cell communication via paracrine factors directs the expression of matrix metalloproteinases (MMPs), enzymes that mediate tissue remodeling during the menstrual cycle. The disease endometriosis is thought to occur as a consequence of retrograde menstruation, and MMPs appear to contribute to the establishment and progression of ectopic endometrial growth in the peritoneal cavity. Although the risk for developing endometriosis is linked to a woman's steroid exposure, locally produced paracrine factors can modify steroid action on multiple gene targets, including the MMPs. Estrogen-associated growth factors as well as inflammatory cytokines are potent stimulators of MMP expression and may contribute to the ability of endometrial fragments to invade the peritoneal surface and establish ectopic sites of growth. In contrast, paracrine factors associated with progesterone action during early pregnancy inhibit MMP expression and prevent ectopic endometrial growth in an experimental model. For example, locally produced retinoic acid and transforming growth factor-β (TGF-β) act in concert with progesterone to suppress MMPs, while enhancing expression of MMP inhibitors (TIMPs) during endometrial differentiation. Targeting pregnancy-associated factors that inhibit endometrial-specific MMP expression and action may enhance the effectiveness of progestin-related treatments for endometriosis.

KEYWORDS: MMPs; retinoic acid; transforming growth factor-β; endometriosis

Address for correspondence: Kevin G. Osteen, Ph.D., Director, Women's Reproductive Health Research Center, B-1100 Medical Center North, Department of Obstetrics and Gynecology, Vanderbilt University School of Medicine, Nashville, TN 37232. Voice: 615-322-4196; fax: 615-343-7913.

kevin.osteen@mcmail.vanderbilt.edu

INTRODUCTION

Endometriosis is a complex disease, defined rather simply by pathologists as the growth of glandular and stromal elements of endometrial tissue at an extrauterine site, which is often accompanied by hemosiderin. Although the etiology of this disease remains poorly understood, certain biological factors can be linked to the development of endometriosis. For example, the disease occurs naturally only in menstruating species, and the process of tissue loss at menstruation is clearly related to a woman's risk of developing endometriosis. In 1927, Sampson theorized that the development of endometriosis occurs as a consequence of the mechanical transfer of endometrial tissue to the peritoneum via retrograde menstruation.[1] In an attempt to address Sampson's theory of retrograde menstruation, a human study induced endometriosis in 2 of 15 women who voluntarily allowed peritoneal injection of their own menstrual tissue several months prior to scheduled surgery.[2] Although Ridley and Edward's study would be highly inappropriate by today's standards, their findings suggest that endometrial tissue transport into the peritoneal cavity provides the necessary biological opportunity for the establishment of endometriosis as proposed by Sampson.[1] In further support of the retrograde menstruation theory, endometriosis is more common among women whose menstrual flow is excessive or of long duration,[3] and reproductive surgeons have obtained viable endometrial tissue fragments from the peritoneal cavity following normal menstruation.[4]

The mechanical distribution of endometrial tissue appears to be required for initiation of endometriosis; however, the progression of the disease process clearly depends on continued steroid support. Endometriosis is generally observed only during the reproductive years of a woman's life,[5] and the risk of developing the disease reflects a woman's endogenous and exogenous steroid exposure. Exposure to estrogen represents the principal endocrine risk factor for developing endometriosis,[6] and a lower incidence of the disease is noted in women with decreased estrogen production subsequent to extensive exercise or smoking.[3] Medical therapy for endometriosis frequently includes the reduction of endogenous estrogen production,[7] and the disease usually regresses in concert with the demise of ovarian estrogen synthesis following menopause.[8] In contrast to the role of estrogen as a positive risk factor for endometriosis, progesterone exposure during pregnancy is recognized as a negative risk factor[6] and progestin-based therapies often lead to a regression of this disease.[9,10] Although retrograde menstruation and steroid exposure each represent relatively clear biological risk factors for developing endometriosis, cellular mechanisms linking specific elements of endometrial biology to these risk factors remain elusive. In an attempt to connect the pathophysiology of this disease to more clearly defined elements of endometrial biology, our research group has focused on the interactive roles of steroids and local tissue factors in the cyclic expression of multiple matrix metalloproteinases (MMPs).

MMPs AND ENDOMETRIAL BIOLOGY

The extensive degree of cellular growth and turnover associated with the menstrual cycle in humans and nonhuman primates is rare among other mammalian species. This constant remodeling of the endometrial extracellular matrix in response to changing patterns of ovarian steroids potentially explains the occurrence of endometriosis only in menstruating species. Although steroids are critical mediators of endometrial biology, our studies have shown that steroids act in concert with locally produced growth factors and cytokines to direct a unique, cell-type specific pattern of MMP expression during each phase of the menstrual cycle.[11] The highest expression of numerous endometrial MMPs occurs in response to the loss of progesterone support at menstruation;[12,13] however, these enzymes are focally expressed during tissue repair processes[14] as well as during early endometrial growth.[12,13] Viable fragments of endometrium have been identified in the peritoneum as a component of retrograde menses[4] and the expression of MMPs by these fragments could promote the establishment of sites of ectopic peritoneal growth. Our research group has developed an experimental model of endometriosis in athymic, nude mice to determine the role of MMPs in the establishment of ectopic lesions. Since human menses contains a complex mixture of blood and cellular debris, a more homogenous endometrial tissue source for experimentation can be obtained by biopsy during the proliferative phase of the menstrual cycle. Using proliferative human endometrium, we have demonstrated that the expression and enzymatic action of MMPs are required for the establishment of ectopic sites of endometrial growth within the peritoneum of mice.[15] Among the most interesting early findings obtained using this experimental model has been the ability to distinguish the actions of estradiol versus progesterone on human endometrium relative to the establishment of tissue growth in mice. Specifically, short-term treatments of human endometrium with estradiol maintain expression of endometrial MMPs and subsequently promote the establishment of experimental endometriosis, while progesterone treatments inhibit MMP expression and prevent the experimental disease.

Our experimental model of endometriosis suggests that progesterone-mediated inhibition of endometrial MMPs can prevent ectopic growth of human tissue in nude mice, although steroidal regulation of MMP expression associated with endometriosis appears more complicated. For example, stromal cells isolated from the endometrium of women with this disease exhibit an increased sensitivity to inflammatory cytokines,[16] and an altered pattern of endometrial MMP expression in response to progesterone is apparent *in vivo* and *in vitro*.[17] Although the etiology of endometriosis clearly involves numerous risk factors, differences in the action of local endometrial factors,[14] in combination with a reduced steroid responsiveness,[18] could contribute to the development of endometriosis in some women. In support of this possibility, we have shown that cotreatments of normal human endometrium with the inflammatory cytokine IL-1α interfere with the ability of progesterone to suppress MMP expression *in vitro* and subsequently promote the *in vivo* development of ectopic lesions in mice.[19] It remains to be established whether defects in progesterone-mediated MMP expression represent a complication in predicting the success or failure of progestin-based therapy for women with endometriosis.

RETINOIC ACID AND ENDOMETRIAL BIOLOGY

Progesterone action has been linked by numerous laboratories to the suppression of MMPs during the normal menstrual cycle.[11] Additionally, progesterone acts to block the stimulatory impact of inflammatory cytokines on these enzymes, preventing endometrial breakdown in response to these factors at the maternal-fetal interface.[20,21] Taken together with the ability of progesterone to prevent the establishment of experimental endometriosis,[15] these studies suggest that a failure of normal progestin-mediated MMP regulation may be associated with the pathophysiology of endometriosis. By developing a better understanding of how locally produced paracrine factors mediate endometrial responses to progesterone, we may be able to strengthen the success of progestin-based treatments for this disease. In a search for such factors, our research group has identified the local synthesis of retinoic acid from retinol precursor as a progesterone-dependent component of stromal cell differentiation into their specialized decidual phenotype.[14,22] Retinoic acid, the most active form of vitamin A, has been recognized for more than 75 years as being necessary for normal endometrial function.[23] The retinoids bind to specific receptors, RAR and RXR, which are members of the steroid receptor superfamily and have been localized within the human endometrium.[24] The action of retinoids is additionally controlled by the local expression of carrier proteins, including cellular retinoid binding proteins (CRBP I and CRBP II) and the retinoic acid binding proteins (CRABP I and CRABP II), each found within the endometrium.[22,25] During the human menstrual cycle, expression of CRABP II and the cell-specific synthesis of retinoic acid appear to be regulated by the changing pattern of steroid exposure.[14,25,26] Although local retinoic acid synthesis likely regulates numerous facets of endometrial behavior, decidual cell synthesis of retinoic acid during progesterone-induced differentiation may contribute to MMP regulation during early pregnancy. For example, retinoic acid has been shown to repress MMP-3 gene transcription[27] and treatments of isolated human endometrial stromal cells with retinoic acid inhibit secretion of MMP-3 protein in the absence of progesterone.[14] Additionally, the ability of both progesterone and retinoic acid to regulate endometrial MMP expression is intriguing since combinations of steroids and cytokines are known to provide a balanced environment during different stages of inflammation in many tissues. In the endometrium, early pregnancy represents an inflammatory-like environment and *in vitro* treatments of isolated human stromal/decidual cells with either progesterone or retinoic acid inhibit MMP-3 protein secretion and block the expression of this enzyme in response to IL-1α.[20,21] Although these results suggest that the local synthesis of endometrial retinoic acid may enhance or even duplicate the regulatory action of progesterone on MMP-3 expression, other local factors are equally necessary for normal endometrial function.

TGF-β AND ENDOMETRIAL BIOLOGY

The invasive events required for the establishment of ectopic endometrial growth involve the breakdown of extracellular matrix within the peritoneal cavity,[28] and the expression of numerous MMPs within menstrual tissue may provide a sufficient quantity of bioactive agents for this process. However, the extracellular matrix is not simply a structural element of tissue architecture, but an active component of local cellular communication as well. Altered cell-cell relationships are a common feature of ectopic lesions of endometriosis and may, to some degree, provide an architectural limit to steroid-sensitive MMP regulation in ectopic tissues.[29,30] Although our initial findings indicate that the local synthesis of retinoic acid may enhance progesterone-

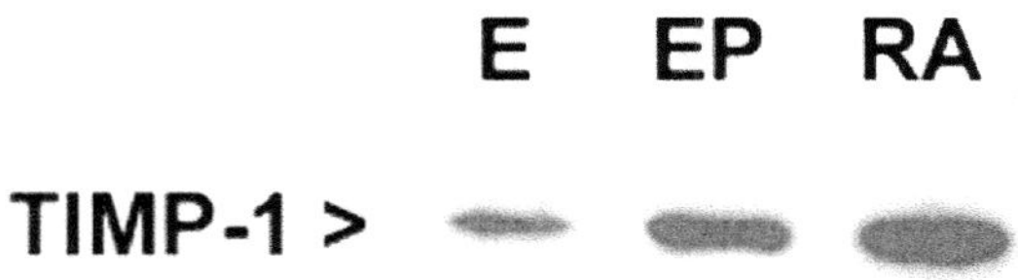

FIGURE 1. Western analysis of expression and regulation of TIMP-1 in proliferative-phase endometrial organ cultures. Tissues were maintained for 48 h in estradiol (E, 1 nM), estradiol plus progesterone (EP; E = 1 nM, P = 500 nM), or estradiol plus retinoic acid (RA; E = 1 nM, RA = 10 nM).

mediated inhibition of endometrial MMPs, *in vitro* studies demonstrate that members of the transforming growth factor-β (TGF-β) family are required for MMP regulation by retinoic acid or progesterone.[14,31] At present, the role of specific isotypes of TGF-β in the pathophysiology of endometriosis remains unclear; however, changes in TGF-β isotype expression are associated with alterations in cell-cell communication, resulting in a loss of growth control in endometrial cancers.[32] In our studies with this growth factor family, we find that *in vitro* exposure to progesterone increases the specific expression of TGF-β2 by human endometrium[31] and that retinoic acid can also specifically induce TGF-β2 under similar experimental conditions.[14] These results suggest that progesterone may act through the local synthesis of retinoic acid to regulate the expression of specific TGF-β isotypes during normal endometrial differentiation in preparation for pregnancy. Interestingly, vitamin A deficiency and loss of TGF-β2 expression have each been independently associated with early pregnancy loss.[33,34] While the relationship of these findings to endometriosis is not yet established, both retinoic acid and TGF-β appear to be required in our experimental model of the disease for the prevention of establishment of human lesions in nude mice.[17]

The regulation of MMP gene and protein expression by progesterone in conjunction with locally produced growth factors and cytokines appears to represent a unique control system related to the complex biology of endometrial function in humans and primates. Furthermore, in all tissues, the activity of MMP proteins is potentially destructive and these enzymes are often inhibited locally by tissue inhibitors of MMPs (TIMPs).[11] The expression of TIMPs is frequently regulated by paracrine factors, such as the TGF-β's, which also mediate MMP expression,[35] ensuring a tissue balance between matrix degradation and matrix stability.[36] Not unexpectedly, in short-term organ cultures, either progesterone or retinoic acid may contribute to endometrial tissue stability by inhibiting MMP expression,[14] as well as by increasing TIMP-1 expression (FIG. 1).

As indicated by each of the many studies discussed in this review, steroid control over endometrial biology involves the cooperative actions of numerous, locally produced cytokines and growth factors that are critical for normal tissue behavior. FIGURE 2 summarizes our emerging understanding of the interrelationships among progesterone, retinoic acid, and TGF-β2 in the regulation of members of the MMP and TIMP family in the normal endometrium. Defining the individual and interactive roles of these paracrine factors in the regulation of endometrial MMPs should allow

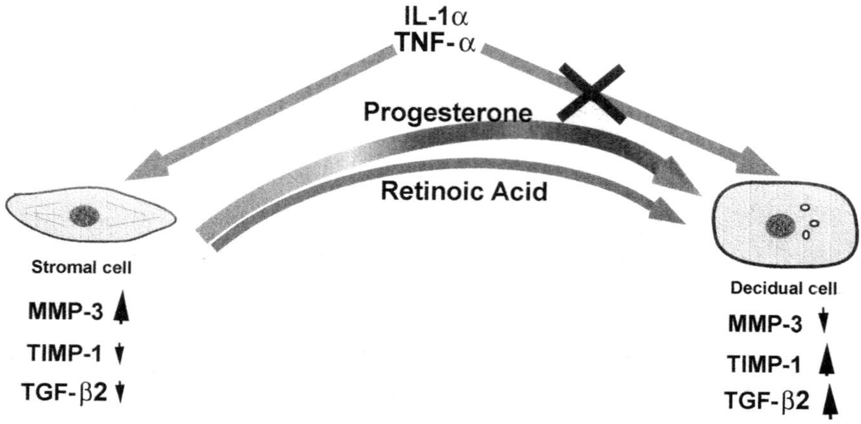

FIGURE 2. Illustration of our current understanding of progesterone and retinoic acid regulation of endometrial sensitivity to IL-1α and TNF-α.

the development of novel therapeutic approaches for the treatment of endometriosis based on a more complete understanding of progesterone action.

SUMMARY

Although mechanical tissue displacement may explain the development of endometriosis only in menstruating species, the epidemiology and natural history of this disease are complex. The discriminating factor(s) in determining who may develop endometriosis may involve a complex array of potentially interactive influences, including endogenous and exogenous steroid exposure, environmental toxin exposure, immunological disturbances, and genetic predisposition. Nevertheless, steroid support is central to the development and progression of this disease and stromal-epithelial communication is critical to the endometrium's normal response to steroids. In the endometrium, the stroma appears to be the cell type most closely aligned with steroid sensitivity, often directing the behavior of adjacent cells during the cycle and in the complex cellular environment of pregnancy. Normal cell-cell communication in the endometrium requires the specific production of locally active factors that act to modulate steroid-directed tissue behavior. The control of MMP expression provides a mechanism for steroid-directed endometrial restructuring during the reproductive cycle, but may also provide a mechanism for ectopic endometrial invasion and growth. By targeting endometrial MMP expression therapeutically, it may be possible to regulate critical molecules that are necessary for the establishment and progression of endometriosis, perhaps resulting in more successful medical treatments for this disease.

ACKNOWLEDGMENTS

We gratefully acknowledge the donors who provided endometrial samples and the physicians of our department who performed these critical biopsies. This work was supported in part through cooperative agreement (No. U54-HD-37321) as part of the Specialized Cooperative Centers Program in Reproduction Research. Additional support was provided by grants from the United States Environmental Protection Agency (No. R826300) and The Endometriosis Association Research Program at Vanderbilt.

REFERENCES

1. SAMPSON, J.A. 1927. Peritoneal endometriosis due to menstrual dissemination of endometrial tissue into the peritoneal cavity. Am. J. Obstet. Gynecol. **14:** 422–469.
2. RIDLEY, J.H. & I.K. EDWARDS. 1958. Experimental endometriosis in the human. Am. J. Obstet. Gynecol. **76:** 783–790.
3. CRAMER, D.W., E. WILSON, R.J. STILLMAN *et al.* 1986. The relation of endometriosis to menstrual characteristics, smoking, and exercise. J. Am. Med. Assoc. **255:** 1904–1908.
4. LUI, D.T.Y. 1986. Endometriosis: its association with retrograde menstruation, dysmenorrhea, and tubal pathology. Br. J. Obstet. Gynaecol. **93:** 859–864.
5. HOUSTON, D.E. 1984. Evidence for the risk of pelvic endometriosis by age, race, and socioeconomic status. Epidemiol. Rev. **6:** 167–180.
6. HALME, J. & D. STOVALL. 1995. Endometriosis and its medical management. *In* Reproductive Medicine and Surgery, pp. 695–710. Mosby. St. Louis.
7. SPEROFF, L., R.H. GLASS & N.G. KASE. 1998. Clinical Gynecologic Endocrinology and Infertility. Fifth edition, pp. 1063–1067. Williams & Wilkins. Baltimore.
8. PUNNONEN, R., P.J. KLEMI & V. NIKKANEN. 1980. Postmenopausal endometriosis. Eur. J. Obstet. Gynecol. Reprod. Biol. **11:** 195–200.
9. OLIVE, D.L. 1989. Medical treatment: alternatives to danazol. *In* Endometriosis: Contemporary Concepts and Clinical Management, p. 60. Lippincott. Philadelphia.
10. KAUNITZ, A.M. 1998. Injectable depot medroxyprogesterone acetate contraception: an update for U.S. clinicians. Int. J. Fertil. Women's Med. **43:** 73–83.
11. CURRY, T.E. & K.G. OSTEEN. 2001. Cyclic changes in the matrix metalloproteinase system in the ovary and uterus. Biol. Reprod. **64:** 1285–1296.
12. RODGERS, W.H., L.M. MATRISIAN, L.C. GIUDICE *et al.* 1994. Patterns of matrix metalloproteinase expression in cycling endometrium imply differential functions and regulation by steroids. J. Clin. Invest. **94:** 946–953.
13. RODGERS, W.H., K.G. OSTEEN, L.M. MATRISIAN *et al.* 1993. Expression and localization of matrilysin (Pump-1, MMP-7), a matrix metalloproteinase in the human endometrium. Am. J. Obstet. Gynecol. **168:** 253–260.
14. OSTEEN, K.G., N.R. KELLER, F.A. FELTUS & M.H. MELNER. 1999. Paracrine regulation of matrix metalloproteinase expression in the normal human endometrium. Gynecol. Obstet. Invest. **48**(1)**:** 2–13.
15. BRUNER, K.L., L.M. MATRISIAN, W.H. RODGERS *et al.* 1997. Suppression of matrix metalloproteinases inhibits establishment of ectopic lesions by human tissue in nude mice. J. Clin. Invest. **99:** 2851–2857.
16. TSENG, J.F., I.P. RYAN, T.D. MILAM *et al.* 1996. Interleukin-6 secretion *in vitro* is up-regulated in ectopic and eutopic endometrial stromal cells from women with endometriosis. J. Clin. Endocrinol. Metab. **81:** 1118–1122.
17. BRUNER-TRAN, K.L., E. EISENBERG & K.G. OSTEEN. 2000 (October). Establishment of experimental endometriosis by eutopic or ectopic endometrial tissue acquired from women with endometriosis cannot be prevented by progesterone treatments [abstract]. Presented at the Fifty-sixth Annual Meeting of the American Society for Reproductive Medicine, San Diego.

18. SEGARS, J.H. 1997. Endometriosis and nuclear hormone receptors. *In* Endometrium and Endometriosis, pp. 321–332. Blackwell Science. Malden, MA.
19. BRUNER, K.L., N.R. KELLER & K.G. OSTEEN. 1999. Interleukin-1α opposes suppression of human endometrial matrix metalloproteinases by progesterone in a model of experimental endometriosis. *In* Understanding and Managing Endometriosis: Advances in Research and Practice, pp. 123–130. Parthenon. Pearl River, NY.
20. KELLER, N.R., E. SIERRA-RIVERA, E. EISENBERG & K.G. OSTEEN. 2000. Progesterone exposure prevents matrix metalloproteinase-3 (MMP-3) stimulation by interleukin-1α in human endometrial stromal cells. J. Clin. Endocrinol. Metab. **85:** 1611–1619.
21. OSTEEN, K.G., K.L. BRUNER-TRAN, D.E. ONG & E. EISENBERG. 2000. Progesterone or retinoic acid treatment of human endometrial tissue reduces basal and cytokine-stimulated MMP expression and increases TIMP-1 secretion. Biol. Reprod. **62**(1)**:** 230.
22. ZHENG, W.L., E. SIERRA-RIVERA, J. LUAN *et al.* 2000. Retinoic acid synthesis and expression of cellular retinol-binding protein and cellular retinoic acid–binding protein type II are concurrent with decidualization of rat uterine stromal cells. Endocrinology **141:** 802–808.
23. WOLBACH, S.B. & P.R. HOWE. 1925. Tissue changes following deprivation of fat soluble vitamin A. J. Exp. Med. **43:** 753–777.
24. GIGUERE, V. 1994. Retinoic acid receptors and cellular retinoid binding proteins: complex interplay in retinoid signaling. Endocr. Rev. **15:** 61–79.
25. SIDDIQUI, N.A., A. LOUGHNEY, E.J. THOMAS *et al.* 1994. Cellular retinoid binding proteins and nuclear retinoic acid receptors in endometrial epithelial cells. Hum. Reprod. **9:** 1410–1416.
26. LOUGHNEY, A.D., M.K. KUMARENDRAN, E.J. THOMAS & C.P. REDFERN. 1995. Variation in the expression of cellular retinoid binding proteins in human endometrium throughout the menstrual cycle. Hum. Reprod. **10:** 1297–1304.
27. BENBOW, U. & C.E. BRINCKERHOFF. 1997. The AP-1 site and MMP gene regulation: what is all the fuss about? Matrix Biol. **15:** 519–526.
28. SPUIJBROEK, M.D.E.H., G.A.J. DUNSELMAN, P.P.C.A. MENHEERE & J.L.H. EVERS. 1992. Early endometriosis invades the extracellular matrix. Fertil. Steril. **58:** 929–933.
29. OSTEEN, K.G., K.L. BRUNER & K.L. SHARPE-TIMMS. 1996. Steroid and growth factor regulation of matrix metalloproteinase expression and endometriosis. Semin. Reprod. **14:** 247–255.
30. OSTEEN, K.G., K.L. BRUNER, E. SIERRA-RIVERA & L.I. GOLD. 1997. Progesterone and transforming growth factor-β co-mediate matrix metalloproteinase expression in a model of endometriosis. *In* International Congress, Symposium, and Seminar Series, Vol. 13, Endometriosis Today, pp. 200–209. Parthenon. Lancaster.
31. BRUNER, K.L., W.H. RODGERS, M. KORC *et al.* 1995. Transforming growth factor-β mediates the progesterone suppression of an epithelial metalloproteinase by adjacent stroma. Proc. Natl. Acad. Sci. U.S.A. **92:** 7362–7366.
32. GOLD, L.I. 1999. The role for transforming growth factor-β (TGF-β) in human cancer. Crit. Rev. Oncog. **10:** 303–360.
33. SIMSEK, M., M. NAZIROGLU, H. SIMSEK *et al.* 1998. Blood plasma levels of lipoperoxides, glutathione peroxidase, beta carotene, vitamin A and E in women with habitual abortion. Cell. Biochem. Funct. **16:** 227–231.
34. LEA, R.G., J. UNDERWOOD, K.C. FLANDERS *et al.* 1995. A subset of patients with recurrent spontaneous abortion is deficient in transforming growth factor beta-2–producing "suppressor cells" in uterine tissue near the placental attachment site. Am. J. Reprod. Immunol. **34:** 52–64.
35. MAUVIEL, A. 1993. Cytokine regulation of metalloproteinase gene expression. J. Cell. Biochem. **53:** 288–295.
36. VINCENTI, M. 2001. The matrix metalloproteinase (MMP) and tissue inhibitor of metalloproteinase (TIMP) genes: transcriptional and posttranscriptional regulation, signal transduction, and cell-type-specific expression. Methods Mol. Biol. **151:** 121–148.

Paracrine Regulation of Matrix Metalloproteinase Expression in Endometriosis

KATHY L. SHARPE-TIMMS AND KATHRYN E. COX

Department of Obstetrics and Gynecology, University of Missouri-Columbia, Columbia, Missouri 65212, USA

ABSTRACT: Following retrograde menstruation, shed endometrial tissue fragments attach to and invade the peritoneal surface to form established endometriotic lesions. With disease progression, the biochemically active lesions undergo remodeling and become fibrotic. Matrix metalloproteinase enzymes (MMPs) and the tissue inhibitors of metalloproteinases (TIMPs) play a significant role in normal endometrial remodeling during menses. Anomalous expression of MMPs and TIMPs has been identified in endometriotic lesions as compared to their highly regulated expression in eutopic endometrium. The paracrine mechanisms regulating misexpression of MMPs and TIMPs by endometriotic lesions are, however, not well defined. Misexpression of the MMPs and TIMPs may be due to innate anomalies in the eutopic endometrium from women with endometriosis, in the resident immune cells and peritoneal cells that juxtapose the ectopic endometrium, and/or numerous substances present in peritoneal fluid of women with endometriosis. The majority of MMPs are under strict transcriptional regulation. Steroid hormones and cytokines appear to act on the MMP promoter, either independently or in consort, to provide both positive and negative regulation of these genes. Misregulated expression of MMPs and TIMPs is associated with a more aggressive phenotype and a cascade of events facilitating peritoneal extracellular matrix degradation and establishment or remodeling of endometriotic lesions. The mechanisms by which MMP and TIMP expression are misregulated warrant further investigation as such information may provide insight into novel therapeutic modalities for endometriosis.

KEYWORDS: matrix metalloproteinases; tissue inhibitors of metalloproteinases; MMP; TIMP; regulation; steroids; cytokines

CURRENT STATE OF KNOWLEDGE

The pathogenic mechanisms of endometriosis are incompletely understood. The prevailing hypothesis involves that, following retrograde menstruation, shed endometrial tissues attach, invade the peritoneal surface, become vascularized, and form established endometriotic lesions.[1–3] The most biochemically active lesions are the red or proposed early lesions and, with disease progression, the endometriotic lesions

Address for correspondence: K. L. Sharpe-Timms, Department of Obstetrics and Gynecology, University of Missouri-Columbia, 1 Hospital Drive, Columbia, MO 65212. Voice: 573-882-7937; fax: 573-882-9010.
timmsk@health.missouri.edu

undergo remodeling and eventually become more fibrotic and less biochemically active.[4,5]

Matrix metalloproteinase enzymes (MMPs) and their inhibitors, the tissue inhibitors of matrix metalloproteinases (TIMPs), play a significant role in normal endometrial remodeling that accompanies menses.[6–8] The MMP family consists of several structurally related, Zn^{2+}-dependent secreted endopeptidases, which collectively are responsible for degrading a variety of extracellular matrix components, including several types of collagen, gelatins, proteoglycans, laminin, fibronectin, and elastin.[6–12] The TIMPs are the natural inhibitors of MMPs; in combination, they inhibit all members of the MMP family.[6,10–12] The expression of MMPs and TIMPs is tightly regulated in the uterine endometrium.[7,9] A significant upregulation of MMP expression is coincident with tissue breakdown and remodeling occurring at menses and during the early proliferative stage of the menstrual cycle.[7,9]

Anomalous expression of specific members of the MMP and TIMP families has been identified in endometriotic lesions as compared to their highly regulated expression in eutopic endometrium.[13–18] For example, studies of human tissues and studies using animal models have shown that MMP-1, MMP-3, and MMP-7 are constitutively expressed by endometriotic lesions, but are highly regulated in the eutopic endometrium during the menstrual cycle.[9,13,18] Also, while endometriotic lesions *de novo* synthesize and secrete TIMP-1 protein *in vitro*,[19] *in vivo* TIMP-1 protein concentrations are lower in the peritoneal fluid of women with endometriosis.[20] A possible explanation for these differences is that, *in vivo*, TIMP-1 may be selectively localized within the endometriotic lesions or other peritoneal tissues and cells. We have previously shown that TIMP-1 protein can be immunohistochemically identified in endometriotic lesions throughout the menstrual cycle.[4] Interestingly, addition of TIMP protein to the peritoneal cavity of nude mice prevented the establishment of endometriosis.[21]

As the expression of MMPs and TIMPs is highly regulated by steroids in the eutopic endometrium, altered biochemical characteristics in the ectopic endometrial tissue may affect production of these enzymes and their inhibitors. Endometriotic lesions are biochemically different from normal uterine endometrium in several ways, including steroid production, responsiveness, and receptor content; growth factor responsiveness and receptor content; and synthesis and secretion of several proteins such as haptoglobin, monocyte chemotactic protein-1, and complement component 3.[22–25] During the past decade, a variety of studies, using various techniques, have shown that steroid receptor content in endometriotic lesions is more heterogeneous than in eutopic endometrium.[22] More recently, work from Bulun and colleagues[24,25] has shown that endometriotic lesions produce aromatase, which endows them with the capability to produce estrogen, and express the progesterone isoform A, but not the isoform B. Evidence is now emerging that shows the eutopic endometrial tissue of women with endometriosis may innately display some of these differences.[26]

In addition to the biochemical differences, endometriotic lesions also differ structurally and spatially from eutopic endometrium. They are located distally to the uterine-ovarian vasculature and are not likely receiving the same level of steroid stimulation as the eutopic endometrium. Further, the epithelial cell to stromal cell ratio is often disturbed in endometriotic lesions. As specific endometrial epithelial cell and stromal cell interactions have been shown to affect MMP production, it is possible that this altered ratio may change the response of the ectopic tissues to particular stimuli as compared to the response of the uterine endometrium. For example, progesterone acts on endometrial stromal cells to increase production of TGF-β. In turn, the TGF-β acts on the endometrial epithelial cells to decrease MMP-7 production.[4] If the stromal component of the endometriotic lesion is reduced, progesterone-induced TGF-β stimulus may be lessened and may subsequently alter MMP-7 expression by the ectopic lesion.

Endometriotic lesions also differ in the number and activity of their resident immune cells and are juxtaposed among peritoneal mesothelial and subserosal cells. Both resident endometrial and endometriotic immune cells and peritoneal immune cells produce growth factors and cytokines that alter MMP and TIMP expression.[2,22,27–29] Further, the immune cells also produce certain MMPs.[30–32] Human mesothelial cells synthesize and secrete MMPs and TIMP-1 too.[33] The state of the mesothelial cell differentiation has a striking influence on the expression of these enzymes and their inhibitors. Characteristic of the normal early response to serosal injury, reactive cuboidal mesothelium may manifest a matrix-degrading phenotype favoring normal repair as opposed to fibrosis. It is not known how the combination of MMPs and TIMPs produced by endometrial tissue fragments, immune cells, and peritoneal cells might alter the balance of these substances in the peritoneal cavity and subsequently contribute to the development of endometriosis.

Endometriotic lesions are also bathed in peritoneal fluid. Numerous substances are present in peritoneal fluid of women with endometriosis and may originate from a variety of sources.[3,22] These substances might originate from the ovary, peritoneal mesothelial or subserosal cells, or peritoneal immune cells, or from the shed endometrial tissue fragments or endometriotic epithelial and stromal cells. They include gonadal hormones, prostaglandins, enzymes and inhibitors, growth factors, inflammatory mediators, and various other proteins. Many of these factors are known regulators of MMP and TIMP production. Both epidermal growth factor (EGF) and transforming growth factor-α (TGF-α), known upregulators of MMPs, have been found in endometriotic lesions of rats with surgically induced disease.[34] Rat lesions also express TGF-β, a downregulator of MMP expression.[35] Women with endometriosis have elevated levels of interleukin-1α (IL-1α), another well-recognized upregulator of MMP, in their peritoneal fluid.[36–38] This IL-1α is believed to originate from activated peritoneal immune cells, macrophages, and T cells, which are responding to the inflammation of the peritoneal cavity.[39] We recently found that IL-1α mRNA and protein are expressed in increasing amounts over time when rat uterine tissues are placed into tissue explant culture. The increased IL-α specifically coincides with an increase in MMP-3 mRNA levels and protein synthesis, but not MMP-2 nor TIMP-1 mRNA or protein (FIG. 1).

The majority of MMPs are under strict transcriptional regulation by certain growth factors, tumor promoters, hormones, and oncogenes.[40] Transcriptional activation can result in up to 50-fold changes in MMP mRNA expression. There are both positive and negative transcriptional regulators upstream from the transcription site and include AP-1, PEA, TIE, and TATA box consensus sequences for transcription factor binding. There are differences in promoter regions between members of the MMP family.[41–45] Factors, including IL-1α, IL-1β, tumor necrosis factor-α (TNF-α), platelet-derived growth factor (PDGF), TGF-α, EGF, basic fibroblast growth factor

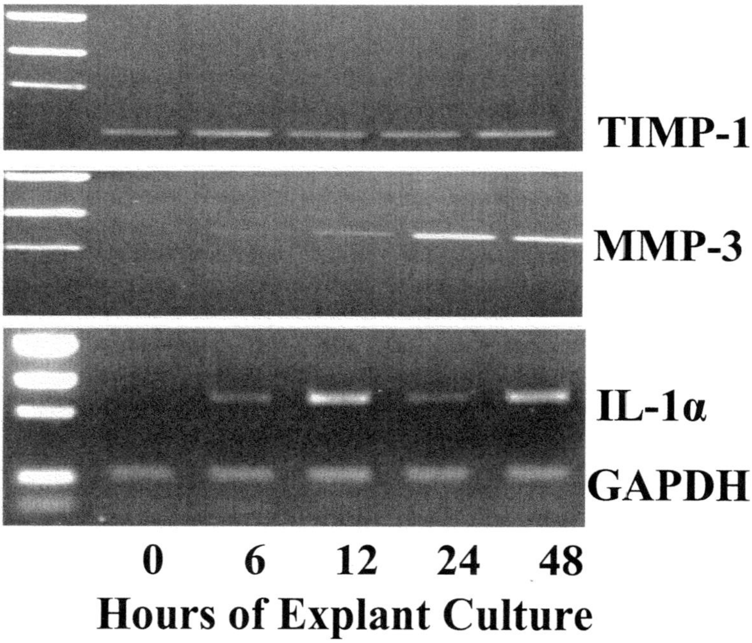

FIGURE 1. Increased endometrial MMP-3 mRNA levels coincide with increased endometrial IL-1α mRNA levels *in vitro*. To study the effects of an ectopic location free from confounding peritoneal influences, rat uterine tissues were placed into tissue explant culture for 48 hours. Tissues were harvested and snap-frozen. The mRNA was isolated and reverse-transcribed. RT-PCR was performed with gene-specific primers. GAPDH levels were evaluated as load controls. IL-1α mRNA was expressed in increasing amounts over time when rat uterine tissues were placed into tissue explant culture. The increased IL-1α specifically coincided with an increase in MMP-3 mRNA levels, but not MMP-2 nor TIMP-1 mRNA levels.

(bFGF), and phorbol esters, induce MMP gene by increasing the levels of c-fos and c-jun, two transcription factors.[10,40,46] With the exception of MMP-2, MMP genes contain an AP-1-binding site, 5′ to the translation start site.[42,44] It is at this AP-1 consensus sequence where c-fos and c-jun heterodimers bind.[47–51] This site is also where most growth factor and cytokine regulatory pathways converge for both positive and negative regulation.[40,52] The AP-1 site is a necessary, but not sufficient, element for transcriptional activation and basal MMP expression.[53–55] The MMP-3 promoter also contains a binding site where Ets family transcription factors bind. This Ets (or PEA3) site acts synergistically with the AP-1 site to result in maximal positive transcriptional induction.[50,56–58]

There are also negative regulatory elements in the MMP promoter.[10,51,59] Whereas IL-1α-induced c-fos binding at the AP-1 site results in positive MMP transcription, c-fos also plays a role in the AP-1-independent downregulation of MMPs by TGF-β at the TGF-β inhibitory element (TIE) site of the promoter.[10,60,61] While

TGF-β downregulation of MMPs is independent of AP-1, the downregulation of MMPs by glucocorticoids and retinoic acid occurs through the AP-1 site and binding of the Jun/Fos complex.[62–68] It has also recently been shown that MMP-1 and MMP-3 mRNAs can be inhibited by urinary trypsin inhibitor (UTI), a member of the Kunitz-type proteinase inhibitors, although the method of action has not yet been elucidated.[69] The novel discovery of a cytokine-induced repressor of IL-1-stimulated expression of MMP-3 in that promoter suggests that activation and repression are tightly controlled and in some cases intertwined.[59]

As previously noted, progesterone is a potent inhibitor of MMP-3 expression in endometrial stromal cells and MMP-7 in endometrial epithelial cells both *in vivo* and *in vitro*.[70,71] Curiously, IL-1α is a potent stimulator of MMP-3 in proliferative-phase endometrium in organ culture, yet progesterone exposure *in vivo* reduces the IL-1α stimulation of MMP-3 in secretory-phase tissue.[70] This loss of sensitivity to IL-1α was duplicated in isolated stromal cells treated with progesterone *in vitro*, and IL-1α stimulation of MMP-3 was restored in a dose-dependent manner with progesterone withdrawal. It has been proposed that inflammatory cytokines, such as IL-1α, may block or interfere with steroid-mediated MMP regulation at ectopic sites.[72]

We repeated these experiments with cells from a rat model for endometriosis. Purified rat uterine and endometriotic stromal cells were cultured with 0, 0.1, 1.0, and 10×10^{-8} M concentrations of medroxyprogesterone for 48 hours. Compared to the cultured endometriotic cells, MMP-3 mRNA levels were lower in the cultured endometrial stromal cells (FIG. 2). The elevated and persistent MMP-3 expression by endometriotic stromal cells cultured in the presence of progesterone was correlated with elevated levels of IL-1α mRNA detected in the endometriotic cells (FIG. 2) and IL-1α protein in their culture media. Little or no IL-1α expression was found in the uterine stromal cells, except for the highest dose of progesterone tested (10×10^{-8} M, FIG. 2). Thus, we hypothesize that production of IL-1α by the endometriotic lesions was able to overcome the progesterone-induced suppression of MMP-3 in these cells, a phenomenon that was not observed in the cultured uterine stromal cells. Preliminary studies from our laboratory suggest that IL-1α and progesterone act in consort to change binding at the AP-1 site on the MMP-3 promoter, the site required for upregulation of MMP expression, and that this phenomenon is different comparing uterine and endometriotic MMP-3. While further work is mandated, these preliminary data offer a plausible IL-1α-related mechanism for the perpetuation of MMP-3 production by endometriotic cells in the presence of progesterone.

Overall, these studies support the hypothesis that misregulated expression of MMPs and TIMPs in women with endometriosis is associated with a more aggressive phenotype and a cascade of events facilitating degradation and remodeling of the peritoneal extracellular matrix and establishment or remodeling of endometriotic lesions in the peritoneal cavity. The mechanisms by which MMP and TIMP expression are misregulated in endometriosis are, however, not well understood.

EMERGING ISSUES AND CONTINUING GAPS IN KNOWLEDGE

It has been established that ectopic endometrial tissue fragments possess the mechanisms by which they can attach to and invade an intact peritoneal surface.[73–75]

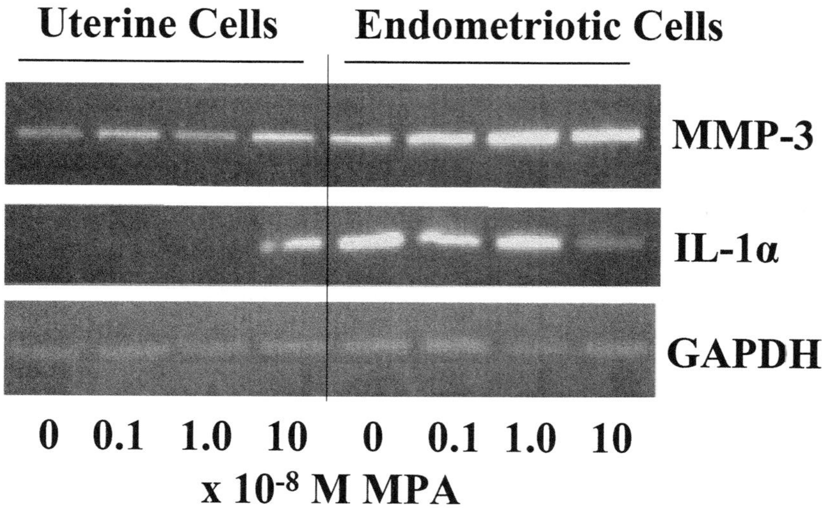

FIGURE 2. An IL-1α-induced mechanism for the perpetuation of MMP-3 production by endometriotic cells in the presence of progesterone. Purified rat uterine stromal cells and rat endometriotic stromal cells were cultured with 0, 0.1, 1.0, and 10×10^{-8} M concentrations of medroxyprogesterone (MPA) for 48 hours. Compared to the cultured endometriotic cells, MMP-3 mRNA levels were lower in the cultured endometrial stromal cells. The elevated and persistent MMP-3 expression by endometriotic stromal cells cultured in the presence of progesterone was correlated with elevated levels of IL-1α mRNA detected in the endometriotic cells. Little or no IL-1α mRNA was found in the uterine stromal cells, except at the highest dose of progesterone tested (10×10^{-8} M). The production of IL-1α by the endometriotic lesions offers a plausible mechanism by which MMP-3 mRNA levels remain elevated in endometriotic lesions in the presence of progesterone, a phenomenon that is not observed in cultured uterine stromal cells.

It is evident that products of endometrial and endometriotic tissues, including MMPs and TIMPs as well as cytokines that regulate production of these enzymes and inhibitors, may actively participate in establishment and remodeling of endometriotic lesions.[4] Also, while studies have recognized that eutopic endometrium from women with endometriosis is innately aberrant compared to women without endometriosis,[26] it is unclear if this is true for the expression of MMPs and/or TIMPs. It would also be of interest to know if immune cells or peritoneal cells from women with endometriosis have defects in MMP and TIMP expression and if these cells alter such expression by ectopic endometrial cells. Either of these mechanisms could contribute to the establishment of the disease or remodeling of the lesions during disease progression.

There are still many questions to be answered. Is misexpression of MMPs and TIMPs caused by an innate anomaly in endometrial, immune, or peritoneal components in women with endometriosis or a consequence of tangential and highly interrelated factors that elicit this aberrant expression in the peritoneal cavity? Why, when MMP and TIMP expression is altered to a more invasive phenotype, are endometriotic lesions not more like cancer and more aggressive in their invasion? As endometriotic lesions undergo remodeling much like the eutopic endometrium, why do the lesions progress through a series of phenotypes and become fibrotic and scar-like? As it is plausible that MMPs and TIMPs participate in these events, what mechanisms control their expression? Are defects in the peritoneal surface architecture important for MMP activity to be effective in extracellular matrix breakdown? Further research is required to answer these questions.

REFERENCES

1. SAMPSON, J.A. 1927. Peritoneal endometriosis due to menstrual dissemination of endometrial tissue into the peritoneal cavity. Am. J. Obstet. Gynecol. **14:** 422–469.
2. SAMPSON, J.A. 1940. The development of the implantation theory for the origin of peritoneal endometriosis. Am. J. Obstet. Gynecol. **40:** 549–557.
3. GIUDICE, L.C., S.I. TAZUKE & L. SWIERSZ. 1998. Status of current research on endometriosis. J. Reprod. Med. **43**(suppl. 3)**:** 252–262.
4. OSTEEN, K.G., K.L. BRUNER & K.L. SHARPE-TIMMS. 1996. Steroid and growth factor regulation of matrix metalloproteinase expression and endometriosis. Semin. Reprod. Endocrinol. **14:** 247–255.
5. D'HOOGHE, T.M., C.S. BAMBRA, B.M. RAEYMAEKERS & P.R. KONINCKX. 1996. Serial laparoscopies over 30 months show that endometriosis in captive baboons (*Papio anubis, Papio cynocephalus*) is a progressive disease. Fertil. Steril. **65**(3)**:** 645–649.
6. WOESSNER, J.F. 1991. Matrix metalloproteinases and their inhibitors in connective tissue remodeling. FASEB J. **5:** 2145–2154.
7. SALAMONSEN, L.A. & D.E. WOOLLEY. 1996. Matrix metalloproteinases in normal menstruation. Hum. Reprod. **11**(suppl. 2)**:** 124–133.
8. HULBOY, D.L., L.A. RUDOLPH & L.M. MATRISIAN. 1997. Matrix metalloproteinases as mediators of reproductive function. Mol. Hum. Reprod. **3**(1)**:** 27–45.
9. RODGERS, W.H., K.G. OSTEEN, L.M. MATRISIAN *et al.* 1993. Expression and localization of matrilysin, a matrix metalloproteinase, in human endometrium during the reproductive cycle. Am. J. Obstet. Gynecol. **168:** 253–260.
10. MATRISIAN, L.M. 1990. Metalloproteinases and their inhibitors in matrix remodeling. Trends Genet. **6**(4)**:** 121–125.
11. BIRKEDAL-HANSEN, H., W.G.I. MOORE, M.K. BODDEN *et al.* 1993. Matrix metalloproteinases: a review. Crit. Rev. Oral Biol. Med. **4**(2)**:** 197–250.
12. MATRISIAN, L. 1992. The matrix-degrading metalloproteinases. Bioessays **14**(7)**:** 455–463.
13. KOKORINE, I., M. NISOLLE, J. DONNEZ *et al.* 1997. Expression of interstitial collagenase (matrix metalloproteinase-1) is related to the activity of human endometriotic lesions. Fertil. Steril. **68:** 246–251.
14. SPUIJBROEK, M.D.E.H., G.J. DUNSELMAN, P.P.C.A. MENHEERE & J.L.H. EVERS. 1992. Early endometriosis invades the extracellular matrix. Fertil. Steril. **58:** 929–933.
15. SAITO, T., H. MIZUMOTO *et al.* 1995. Expression of MMP-3 and TIMP-1 in the endometriosis and the influence of danazol. Acta Obstet. Gynecol. Jpn. **47:** 495–496.
16. KOKS, C.A., P.G. GROOTHUIS *et al.* 2000. Matrix metalloproteinases and their tissue inhibitors in antegradely shed menstruum and peritoneal fluid. Fertil. Steril. **73**(3)**:** 604–612.
17. MARBAIX, E., J. DONNEZ, P.J. COURTOY & Y. EECKHOUT. 1992. Progesterone regulates the activity of collagenase and related gelatinases A and B in human endometrial explants. Proc. Natl. Acad. Sci. U.S.A. **89:** 11789–11793.
18. COX, K.E., M. PIVA & K.L. SHARPE-TIMMS. 2001. Differential regulation of matrix metalloproteinase-3 (MMP-3) gene expression in endometriotic lesions as compared to endometrium. Biol. Reprod. In press.
19. SHARPE-TIMMS, K.L., L.L. PENNEY, R.L. ZIMMER *et al.* 1995. Partial purification and amino acid sequence analysis of endometriosis protein-II (ENDO-II) reveal homology with tissue inhibitor of metalloproteinases-1 (TIMP-1). J. Clin. Endocrinol. Metab. **80**(12)**:** 3784–3787.

20. SHARPE-TIMMS, K.L., L. KEISLER, E. MCINTUSH & D. KEISLER. 1998. Tissue inhibitor of metalloproteinase-1 concentrations are attenuated in peritoneal fluid and sera of women with endometriosis and restored in sera by gonadotropin-releasing hormone agonist therapy. Fertil. Steril. **69:** 1128–1134.
21. BRUNER, K.L., L.M. MATRISIAN, W.H. RODGERS *et al.* 1997. Suppression of matrix metalloproteinases inhibits establishment of ectopic lesions by human endometrium in nude mice. J. Clin. Invest. **99:** 2851–2857.
22. SHARPE-TIMMS, K.L. 1997. Basic research in endometriosis. Obstet. Gynecol. Clin. North Am. **24:** 269–290.
23. SHARPE-TIMMS, K.L., E.A. RICKE, M. PIVA & G.M. HOROWITZ. 2000. Differential *in vivo* expression and localization of endometriosis protein-I (ENDO-I), a haptoglobin homologue, in endometrium and endometriotic lesions. Hum. Reprod. **15**(10)**:** 101–105.
24. BULUN, S.E., K. ZEITOUN, K. TAKAYAMA *et al.* 1999. Estrogen production in endometriosis and use of aromatase inhibitors to treat endometriosis. Endocr. Relat. Cancer **6**(2)**:** 293–301.
25. ATTIA, G.R., K. ZEITOUN, D. EDWARDS *et al.* 2000. Progesterone receptor isoform A, but not B is expressed in endometriosis. J. Clin. Endocrinol. Metab. **85**(8)**:** 2897–2902.
26. SHARPE-TIMMS, K.L. 2001. Endometrial anomalies in women with endometriosis. Proc. Natl. Acad. Sci. U.S.A. In press.
27. HILL, J.A. 1997. Immunology and endometriosis: fact, artifact, or epiphenomenon? Obstet. Gynecol. Clin. North Am. **24**(2)**:** 291–306.
28. NOTHNICK, W.B. & P.D. SOLOWAY. 1998. Novel implications in the development of endometriosis: biphasic effect of macrophage activation on peritoneal tissue expression of tissue inhibitor of metalloproteinase-1. Am. J. Reprod. Immunol. **40**(5)**:** 364–369.
29. JEZIORSKA, M., H. NAGASE, L.A. SALAMONSEN & D.E. WOOLLEY. 1996. Immunolocalization of the matrix metalloproteinases gelatinase B and stromelysin 1 in human endometrium throughout the menstrual cycle. J. Reprod. Fertil. **107**(1)**:** 43–51.
30. JONES, R.K., J.N. BULMER & R.F. SEARLE. 1998. Phenotypic and functional studies of leukocytes in human endometrium and endometriosis. Hum. Reprod. Update **4**(5)**:** 702–709.
31. VINCENT, A.J., N. MALAKOOTI, J. ZHANG *et al.* 1999. Endometrial breakdown in women using Norplant is associated with migratory cells expressing matrix metalloproteinase-9 (gelatinase B). Hum. Reprod. **14**(3)**:** 807–815.
32. KIM, M.H., R.P. KITSON, P. ALBERTSSON *et al.* 2000. Secreted and membrane-associated matrix metalloproteinases of IL-2-activated NK cells and their inhibitors. J. Immunol. **164**(11)**:** 5883–5889.
33. MA, C., R.W. TARNUZZER & N. CHEGINI. 1999. Expression of matrix metalloproteinases and tissue inhibitor of matrix metalloproteinases in mesothelial cells and their regulation by transforming growth factor-β1. Wound Repair Regeneration **7**(6)**:** 477–485.
34. SIMMS, J.S., N. CHEGINI, R.S. WILLIAMS *et al.* 1991. Identification of epidermal growth factor, transforming growth factor-alpha, and epidermal growth factor receptor in surgically induced endometriosis in rats. Obstet. Gynecol. **78:** 850–857.
35. CHEGINI, N., L.I. GOLD, R.S. WILLIAMS & B.J. MASTERSON. 1994. Localization of transforming growth factor beta isoforms TGF-beta 1, TGF-beta 2, and TGF-beta 3 in surgically induced pelvic adhesions in the rat. Obstet. Gynecol. **83:** 449–454.
36. FAKIH, H., B. BAGGETT, G. HOLTZ *et al.* 1987. Interleukin-1: a possible role in the infertility associated with endometriosis. Fertil. Steril. **47**(2)**:** 213–217.
37. HILL, J.A. & D.J. ANDERSON. 1989. Lymphocyte activity in the presence of peritoneal fluid from fertile women and infertile women with and without endometriosis. Am. J. Obstet. Gynecol. **161:** 861–864.
38. TAKETANI, Y., T.M. KUO & M. MIZUNO. 1992. Comparison of cytokine levels and embryo toxicity in peritoneal fluid in infertile women with untreated or treated endometriosis. Am. J. Obstet. Gynecol. **167:** 265–270.
39. CHRISTMAN, G. & J. HALME. 1992. Pathophysiology of Endometriosis-Associated Symptoms. Saunders. Philadelphia.
40. CORCORAN, M.L., D.E. KLEINER & W.G. STETLER-STEVENSON. 1995. Regulation of matrix metalloproteinases during extracellular matrix turnover. Adv. Exp. Med. Biol. **385:** 151–159.

41. Brinckerhoff, C.E., K.L. Sirum-Connolly, M.J. Karmilowicz & D.T. Auble. 1992. Expression of stromelysin and stromelysin-2 in rabbit and human fibroblasts. Matrix Suppl. **1:** 165–175.
42. Huhtala, P., L.T. Chow & K. Tryggvason. 1990. Structure of the human type IV collagenase gene. J. Biol. Chem. **265**(19)**:** 11077–11082.
43. Sato, H., M. Kita & M. Seiki. 1993. v-Src activates the expression of 92-kDa type IV collagenase gene through the AP-1 site and the GT box homologous to retinoblastoma control elements: a mechanism regulating gene expression independent of that by inflammatory cytokines. J. Biol. Chem. **268**(31)**:** 23460–23468.
44. Templeton, N.S. & W.G. Stetler-Stevenson. 1991. Identification of a basal promoter for the human Mr 72,000 type IV collagenase gene and enhanced expression in a highly metastatic cell line. Cancer Res. **51**(22)**:** 6190–6193.
45. Twining, S.S. 1994. Regulation of proteolytic activity in tissues. Crit. Rev. Biochem. Mol. Biol. **29**(5)**:** 315–383.
46. Frisch, S.M. & H.E. Ruley. 1987. Transcription from the stromelysin promoter is induced by interleukin-1 and repressed by dexamethasone. J. Biol. Chem. **262**(34)**:** 16300–16304.
47. Angel, P., I. Baumann, B. Stein *et al.* 1987. 12-*O*-Tetradecanoyl-phorbol-13-acetate induction of the human collagenase gene is mediated by an inducible enhancer element located in the 5′-flanking region. Mol. Cell. Biol. **7:** 2256–2266.
48. Angel, P., M. Imagawa, R. Chiu *et al.* 1987. Phorbol ester–inducible genes contain a common *cis* element recognized by a TPA-modulated *trans*-acting factor. Cell **49:** 729–739.
49. Buttice, G. & M. Kurkinen. 1994. Oncogenes control stromelysin and collagenase gene expression. Contrib. Nephrol. **107:** 101–107.
50. Gutman, A. & B. Wasylyk. 1990. The collagenase promoter contains a TPA and oncogene-responsive unit encompassing the PEA3 and AP-1 binding sites. EMBO J. **9**(7)**:** 2241–2246.
51. Quinones, S., J. Saus, Y. Otani *et al.* 1989. Transcriptional regulation of human stromelysin. J. Biol. Chem. **264**(14)**:** 8339–8344.
52. Sassone-Corsi, P., L.J. Ransone & I.M. Verma. 1990. Cross-talk in signal transduction: TPA-inducible factor jun/AP-1 activates cAMP-responsive enhancer elements. Oncogene **5**(3)**:** 427–431.
53. Fini, M.E., J.R. Cook, R. Mohan & C.E. Brinckerhoff. 1998. Regulation of matrix metalloproteinase gene expression. *In* Matrix Metalloproteinases, pp. 300–339. Academic Press. San Diego.
54. Lafyatis, R., S.J. Kim, P. Angel *et al.* 1990. Interleukin-1 stimulates and all-*trans*-retinoic acid inhibits collagenase gene expression through its 5′ activator protein-1 binding site. Mol. Endocrinol. **4**(7)**:** 973–980.
55. White, L.A. & C.E. Brinckerhoff. 1995. Two activator protein-1 elements in the matrix metalloproteinase-1 promoter have different effects on transcription and bind Jun D, c-Fos, and Fra-2. Matrix Biol. **14**(9)**:** 715–725.
56. Logan, S.K., M.J. Garabedian, C.E. Campbell & Z. Werb. 1996. Synergistic transcriptional activation of the tissue inhibitor of metalloproteinases-1 promoter via function interaction of AP-1 and Ets-1 transcription factors. J. Biol. Chem. **271**(2)**:** 774–782.
57. Wasylyk, C., A. Gutman, R. Nicholson & B. Wasylyk. 1991. The c-Ets oncoprotein activates the stromelysin promoter through the same elements as several non-nuclear oncoproteins. EMBO J. **10**(5)**:** 1127–1134.
58. Wasylyk, C. & B. Wasylyk. 1992. Oncogenic conversion alters the transcriptional properties of Ets. Cell Growth Differ. **3**(9)**:** 617–625.
59. Borghaei, R.C., C. Sullivan & E. Mochan. 1999. Identification of a cytokine-induced repressor of interleukin-1 stimulated expression of stromelysin 1 (MMP-3). J. Biol. Chem. **274:** 2126–2131.
60. Kerr, L.D., N.E. Olashaw & L.M. Matrisian. 1988. Transforming growth factor beta 1 and cAMP inhibit transcription of epidermal growth factor– and oncogene-induced transin RNA. J. Biol. Chem. **263**(32)**:** 16999–17005.
61. Kerr, L.D., D.B. Miller & L.M. Matrisian. 1990. TGF-β inhibition of transin/stromelysin gene expression is mediated through a Fos binding sequence. Cell **61**(2)**:** 267–278.

62. PAN, L., S.H. CHAMBERLAIN, D.T. AUBLE & C.E. BRINCKERHOFF. 1992. Differential regulation of collagenase gene expression by retinoic acid receptors–alpha, beta, and gamma. Nucleic Acids Res. **20**(12)**:** 3105–3111.
63. PFAHL, M. 1993. Nuclear receptor/AP-1 interaction. Endocr. Rev. **14**(5)**:** 651–658.
64. SALBERT, G., A. FANJUL, F.J. PIEDRAFITA *et al.* 1993. Retinoic acid receptors and retinoid X receptor-alpha down-regulate the transforming growth factor-beta 1 promoter by antagonizing AP-1 activity. Mol. Endocrinol. **7**(10)**:** 1347–1356.
65. SCHROEN, D.J. & C.E. BRINCKERHOFF. 1996. Inhibition of rabbit collagenase (matrix metalloproteinase-1; MMP-1) transcription by retinoid receptors: evidence for binding of RARs/RXRs to the –77 AP-1 site through interaction with c-Jun. J. Cell. Physiol. **169**(2)**:** 320–332.
66. SCHULE, R., P. RANGARAJAN, N. YANG *et al.* 1991. Retinoic acid is a negative regulator of AP-1 responsive genes. Proc. Natl. Acad. Sci. U.S.A. **88**(14)**:** 6092–6096.
67. TRUSS, M. & M. BEATO. 1993. Steroid hormone receptors: interactions with deoxyribonucleic acid and transcription factors. Endocr. Rev. **14**(4)**:** 459–479.
68. YANG-YEN, H.F., J.C. CHAMBARD, Y.L. SUN *et al.* 1990. Transcriptional interference between c-Jun and the glucocorticoid receptor: mutual inhibition of DNA binding due to direct protein-protein interaction. Cell **62**(6)**:** 1205–1215.
69. IMADA, K., A. ITO, N. KANAYAMA *et al.* 1997. Urinary trypsin inhibitor suppresses the production of interstitial procollagenase/proMMP-1 and pro-stromelysin 1/proMMP-3 in human uterine cervical fibroblasts and chorionic cells. FEBS Lett. **417**(3)**:** 337–340.
70. KELLER, N.R., E. SIERRA-RIVERA, E. EISENBERG & K.G. OSTEEN. 2000. Progesterone exposure prevents matrix metalloproteinase-3 (MMP-3) stimulation by interleukin-1α in endometrial stromal cells. J. Clin. Endocrinol. Metab. **85**(4)**:** 1611–1619.
71. OSTEEN, K.G., E. SIERRA-RIVERA, N.R. KELLER & D.B. FOX. 1997. Interleukin-1α opposes progesterone-mediated suppression of MMP-7. Ann. N.Y. Acad. Sci. **828:** 137–145.
72. OSTEEN, K.G., N.R. KELLER, F.A. FELTUS & M.H. MELNER. 1999. Paracrine regulation of matrix metalloproteinase expression in the normal endometrium. Gynecol. Obstet. Invest. **48**(suppl. 1)**:** 2–13.
73. WITZ, C.A., A. TAKAHASHI, I.A. MONTOYA-RODRIGUEZ *et al.* 2000. Expression of the $\alpha2\beta1$ and $\alpha3\beta1$ integrins at the surface of mesothelial cells: a potential attachment site of endometrial cells. Fertil. Steril. **74**(3)**:** 579–584.
74. WITZ, C.A., I.A. MONTOYA-RODRIGUEZ & R.S. SCHENKEN. 1999. Whole explants of peritoneum and endometrium: a novel model of the early endometriosis lesion. Fertil. Steril. **71**(1)**:** 56–60.
75. WITZ, C.A. 1999. Current concepts in the pathogenesis of endometriosis. Clin. Obstet. Gynecol. **42**(3)**:** 566–585.

Panel Discussion (Part IV)

S. PARTHASARATHY (*Emory University, Atlanta, GA*): With the MMP being a zinc-dependent enzyme and also zinc being a metal that can turn Th1 helper cells into Th2 cell types that will completely shift the balance of cytokines, is there any evidence in the literature that zinc might play a role in endometriosis or in the development of the MMP problem?

K.G. OSTEEN (*Vanderbilt University School of Medicine, Nashville, TN*): It is certainly possible. There are effects of certain types of zinc in terms of activation of the MMPs and other reproductive function. It is possible, but I am not aware of specific evidence of that.

E. MARBAIX (*Université Catholique de Louvain, Brussels, Belgium*): I have no knowledge of it.

C.R. LYTTLE (*Wyeth Ayerst Research Institute, Radnor, PA*): This is a question for Dr. Sharpe-Timms. I am not sure if I understood your gel-shift experiment. You had an AP-1 consensus region that you were shifting and you shifted that with a nuclear extract from cells treated with IL-1α and/or progesterone. Is that correct?

K.L. SHARPE-TIMMS (*University of Missouri, Columbia, MO*): The purpose of our gel-shift experiments was to determine the possible binding sites for IL-1α and progesterone-dependent transcription factors on the MMP-3 promoter. Nuclear extracts were prepared from treated uterine and endometriotic cells and subjected to electrophoretic mobility shift assays with double-stranded oligonucleotides constructed from sequences of the AP-1, Ets, and TGF-β promoter of the MMP-3 promoter. We actually did not see any shift in electrophoretic mobility. If you noticed, all of the bands were still at the same level. For the AP-1 site, we observed a single band in the nontreated cells. This same primary band plus a smaller band, indicating the formation of two transcription factor complexes, were seen when the cells were treated with IL-1α, progesterone, or both. Densitometric analysis of the primary band showed more binding at the primary site in the treated cells. It was thus a change in binding.

LYTTLE: I still do not understand. How did you measure the change in binding?

SHARPE-TIMMS: What I showed was a representative gel of five different replicates that were then evaluated by densitometric analysis. The mean was then calculated and statistically compared with both background binding and binding in the nontreated cells. All of the binding was specific as evaluated by competition with both a nonspecific competitor and an unlabeled AP-1 consensus site. I should have shown the negative controls in my presentation; my slide was remiss.

LYTTLE: Okay. Thank you.

P. GROOTHUIS (*University of Maastricht, Maastricht, the Netherlands*): This is a question for Dr. Osteen. It is very interesting to see that a role is emerging for retinoids in this whole mechanism of cell control and differentiation control. You probably know that retinoic acid needs to be produced inside the cell and you need a substrate for it. In the swine uterus just prior to implantation, retinol levels increase dramatically, as do the retinol binding proteins. Do you have any information as to what the concentrations of retinoids are in the uterine fluid in women?

OSTEEN: No, we do not. This is sort of a recent finding. We are looking at a lot of different carrier proteins and binding proteins that might be involved in regulating a synthetic capacity versus a reaction of each of these cell types. We have got some data in that regard, but nothing about the levels just because of the way that we measure retinoids with HPLC. It is not completely quantitative.

QUESTION: Is there any evidence that the myometrium can control endometrial growth? We tend to forget that the eutopic endometrium is located within the uterus and is surrounded by the myometrial cells. Thus, we are all missing this aspect. Years ago, I did an experiment in rabbits. Rabbits are difficult for dissection of the endometrium from the myometrium and we just transplanted a part of the uterus. After a couple of weeks, the myometrium surrounded the endometrium because there was an intensive proliferation of myometrial cells and then the endometrial lesion disappeared. Hence, there might be an additional mechanism that could be important for controlling the endometrial growth and this factor might also rise from the myometrium.

SHARPE-TIMMS: I can address that comment. I have looked in the literature for studies of MMP and TIMP production in the myometrium. I found two papers, but I am remiss as I cannot cite the authors' names at this time. There is some evidence in the literature that the myometrium produces MMPs and TIMPs, which may have paracrine interaction with the endometrium. Certainly, there are a myriad of other factors that might be produced by the myometrium that also affect the endometrium as well.

QUESTION: Thank you again. When we talk about endometrial stromal cells, we talk about a very dynamic cell that can turn into a decidual cell. Has the process of decidualization been looked at? Specifically, what happens in terms of the control of these MMPs when the cells become decidual cells?

OSTEEN: In other words, do they become decidual cells in ectopic endometrium? It is highly variable. The most endometrial-like tissue is probably in the endometriomas. The peritoneal lesions are often very fibroblastic. Thus, part of the failure of stromal cells to actually produce many of the factors that they would normally produce is part of what is probably not happening in ectopic growth of endometrium. Maybe this occurs in eutopic women with endometriosis. We just do not know yet.

Regulation and Modulation of Abnormal Immune Responses in Endometriosis

NEIL SIDELL, SHOU WEI HAN, AND SAMPATH PARTHASARATHY

Department of Gynecology and Obstetrics, Emory Center for Advanced Research on Women's Health, Emory University, Atlanta, Georgia 30322, USA

ABSTRACT: There is ample evidence demonstrating that endometriosis is accompanied by inflammatory reactions in the peritoneum, resulting in abnormal levels of a variety of cytokines and chemokines in the peritoneal fluid. Among the immunological parameters that have been shown to be altered in the peritoneal cavity of women with endometriosis, an increase in the number of activated nonadherent macrophages that show reduced surface expression of scavenger receptors has been observed. The cause-and-effect relationship between aberrant peritoneal macrophage activity and endometriosis is still unknown. We have demonstrated that steroid hormone receptor agonists and antagonists [e.g., retinoids, antiglucocorticoids, ligands to peroxisome proliferator activated receptors (PPARs)] can regulate macrophage functions in ways that could either suppress or stimulate the growth of ectopic endometrial lesions. Our studies include a number of relevant findings: (1) RU486, acting as an antioxidant, can suppress activation of NFκB, a nuclear transcription factor that affects the expression of several inflammatory genes such as those for MCP-1, GM-CSF, CSF-1, and various adhesion molecules; (2) IL-6 secretion from a variety of cell types including endometrial cells is inhibited by retinoic acid; and (3) retinoids and PPARγ ligands can upregulate the expression of scavenger receptors in cells of the monocyte/macrophage lineage. These observations, combined with the possibility that macrophage activity may play a fundamental role in endometriosis, suggest that pharmacologic manipulation of macrophage function may provide a novel mechanism for treating this disease.

KEYWORDS: endometriosis; PPARγ; RU486; IL-6; CD36; scavenger receptor; monocytes

ENDOMETRIOSIS: AN IMMUNE-MEDIATED SYNDROME?

Despite the abundance of evidence that endometriosis is associated with a variety of abnormal immunological changes, a causative role for aberrant immune responses in the etiology and/or progression of endometriosis remains speculative. A primary role for abnormal macrophage activity in endometriosis is supported by numerous studies showing altered macrophage-dependent cytokine levels and functional activity that can affect the survival and growth of ectopic endometrial cells.[1] To this end, a number of growth-promoting factors have been demonstrated to be elevated

Address for correspondence: Neil Sidell, Ph.D., Department of Gynecology and Obstetrics, 4303 Woodruff Memorial Research Building, 1639 Pierce Drive, Emory University School of Medicine, Atlanta, GA 30322. Voice: 404-727-9155; fax: 404-727-8615.
nsidell@emory.edu

in the peritoneal fluid (PF) of women with endometriosis. These include platelet-derived growth factor (PDGF), endothelial cell growth factor (EGF), vascular endothelial cell–derived growth factor (VEGF), basic fibroblast growth factor (bFGF), interleukin-6 (IL-6), and colony-stimulating factor-1 (CSF-1).[1–3] Although the contribution of some of these to the growth of ectopic endometrium has been questioned, there is nonetheless ample evidence that both monocytes and macrophages can stimulate the growth of endometrial cells.[4,5]

Another mechanism by which abnormally functioning macrophages could contribute to the growth of ectopic endometrial cells is through defective scavenging activity. One of the vital functions of macrophages in the face of an invading "foreign" material or when encountering cellular debris and apoptotic cells is the scavenger function.[6,7] A variety of surface structures such as the Fc receptor, the acetyl LDL receptor (scavenger receptor type A), macrosialin, and CD36 (scavenger receptor type B) are involved in this activity.[6–9] This fact gives rise to a fundamental question in endometriosis research: although endometrial cells at various stages of apoptosis are present in menstrual blood of women with endometriosis, why are they not cleared from ectopic sites by macrophages? Is it possible that peritoneal macrophages from women with endometriosis do not express fully functional scavenger receptors (SCR)? These receptors are highly regulated by a number of factors, including cytokines, glucocorticoids, lipopolysaccharides, interferons, M-CSF, and retinoids.[10–12] Since these cytokines and hormones are present in abnormal levels in the PF of women with endometriosis, it is tempting to speculate that the altered levels may then give rise to defective scavenger receptor function that might exacerbate the disease.

Yet another suggestion for the potentially altered scavenger function in PF macrophages associated with endometriosis comes from the studies of Gordon and coworkers.[13–15] They demonstrated that scavenger receptors can play a role in cellular adhesion processes and showed that an antibody to SCR can block the adhesion of cells to culture dishes. Accordingly, macrophages that are not adherent and are not attached to extracellular matrix in tissues do not express scavenger receptors of the A-type (SRA).[16] Thus, in contrast to tissue macrophages, the PF macrophages that are not attached to extracellular matrix components, despite their differentiated status, may not be competent scavengers. A decreased expression of several integrins, the alpha-v beta-3 vitronectin receptor integrin in particular, has been noted in the endometrium of women with endometriosis.[17] Moreover, these women show an increased number of nonadherent macrophages in their peritoneal cavity (PC).[18] Whether this property is an inherent defect in women with endometriosis, and thus may play a causal role in the etiology of this disease through decreased macrophage scavenger activity, is an important question that we are presently addressing. Correspondingly, the ability to regulate the expression of scavenger receptors on PF macrophages may be another method for using immune modulation as a tool for treating endometriosis. In recent studies described below, we have demonstrated that expression of CD36, a member of the scavenger receptor type B (SRB) family implicated in the uptake and degradation of apoptotic cells and other debris,[19] can be upregulated in human monocytes and nonadherent macrophages by a novel mechanism of action that does not require cell adherence. Pharmacologic modulation of this function, as well as other immune functions associated with the inflammatory activity of endometriosis, may provide a novel mechanism for treating this disease.

REGULATION OF CD36 EXPRESSION ON NONADHERENT MONOCYTES/MACROPHAGES BY RETINOIDS

Regulation of CD36 expression is a complex process resulting from the coordinated interplay between multiple soluble factors and cell surface adhesion molecules.[20–22] In cells of the monocyte/macrophage lineage, expression of CD36 has been shown to be regulated through the peroxisome-proliferator-activated-receptor gamma (PPARγ) pathway and to be directly correlated with the maturational stage of the cells. CD36 expression is dramatically increased on monocytes upon their interaction with activated endothelium and by treatment of monocytes with macrophage colony-stimulating factor or IL-4. Furthermore, it has been shown that a variety of specific PPARγ ligands can, by themselves, upregulate CD36, indicating that activation of PPARγ is sufficient for inducing the expression of this scavenger receptor.[23,24] A common feature that appears to accompany CD36 upregulation on macrophages induced by different methodologies (e.g., interaction with activated endothelium or treatment with M-CSF) is the differentiation of the cells as reflected by increased adherence and a variety of morphologic criteria.[22] The fact that monocytes/macrophages from the PF of women with endometriosis seem to have reduced adherent properties[18] may therefore be inconsistent with their ability to express high levels of CD36 and their resultant scavenging activity. We now demonstrate a heretofore undescribed mechanism of CD36 induction that involves neither PPARγ nor an association with monocyte adherence. This mechanism is represented by the ability of the naturally occurring morphogen, retinoic acid (RA), to enhance CD36 mRNA levels and surface protein expression on human monocytic cells. A thorough understanding of this novel mechanism of action may lead to the discovery of a new class of drugs that can be utilized for clinical applications of selective CD36 modulation and increased scavenger activity in nonadherence macrophages.

In our initial experiments to investigate regulation of CD36 expression on cells of the monocyte/macrophage lineage, we have utilized the well-characterized human monocyte cell line THP-1, which can be induced to differentiate into macrophages by a variety of stimuli including PMA, GM-CSF, and IL-4.[21,25,26] To assess surface protein levels of CD36, cells were stained with *R*-phycoerythrin (*R*-PE)–conjugated mouse antihuman CD36 monoclonal antibody (PharMingen) and analyzed by flow cytometry. FIGURE 1 shows that untreated THP-1 cells show little, if any, surface expression of CD36. As reported, when these cells are cultured in the presence of PMA (100 nM), they undergo major differentiation changes beginning at 12 h of treatment, which corresponds to the cells taking on the characteristics of mature macrophages as assessed by their morphologic, antigenic, and adherence properties.[27] FIGURE 1 demonstrates that these cells also show a dramatic increase in surface CD36 expression that correlates with this differentiation process. Thus, THP-1 cells appear to possess the same characteristics as normal human monocytes of increased CD36 expression as they differentiate into macrophages.[26,28]

Studies from a number of laboratories have indicated that CD36 expression is regulated through the PPARγ pathway and that its expression can be induced by ligands to this nuclear receptor.[23,24] Both normal monocytes and THP-1 cells have been shown to express PPARγ. As expected, FIGURE 1 demonstrates that the natural PPARγ ligand, 15-deoxy-δ prostaglandin J_2 (15dd-PGJ2), can significantly induce surface expression of CD36 in THP-1 cells. Since retinoids have been extensively

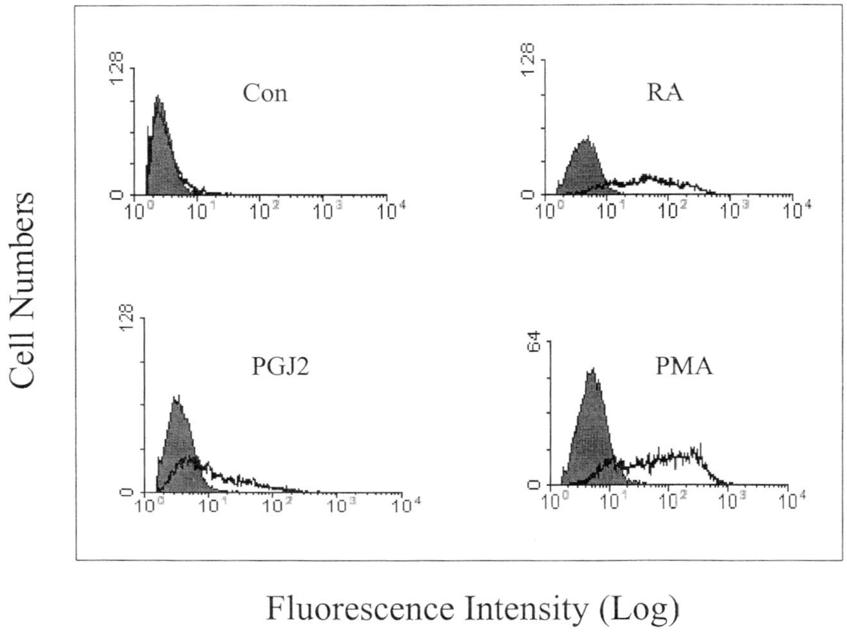

FIGURE 1. Flow cytometry analysis of surface CD36 protein on THP-1 cells. Cells were treated for 48 h with 5 µM RA, 10 µM 15dd-PGJ2, 100 nM PMA, or solvent control (Con) as indicated and analyzed using a PE-conjugated anti-CD36 monoclonal antibody (open histograms). The solid histograms represent cells incubated with PE-conjugated isotype control Ab.

studied as differentiation inducers in a variety of cell systems, we were also interested to evaluate the effects of these compounds on CD36 expression in THP-1 cells. In these experiments, we cultured the cells with RA (5 µM), 15dd-PGJ2 (10 µM), and/or PMA (100 nM) for up to 48 h. As shown in FIGURE 1, RA, like PPARγ ligands and PMA, markedly upregulated CD36 expression in a time- and dose-dependent manner. Unlike cultures with PMA where the cells became substrate-adherent and took on the morphologic features of macrophages (flattened morphology with multiple pseudopodia formation), treatment with RA produced no apparent differentiation changes and the cells remained nonadherent. These results support those of Zhu *et al.*, who observed that 9-*cis*-RA also did not induce differentiation of THP-1 cells.[29]

EFFECTS OF RA ON CD36 mRNA LEVELS

To determine whether the observed RA-induced increase in CD36 surface protein on THP-1 reflects regulation at the transcriptional level, mRNA levels were assessed by semiquantitative RT-PCR.[30,31] Positive controls for these experiments included cells treated with PMA and 15dd-PGJ2. As exemplified in FIGURE 2, 1-day treat-

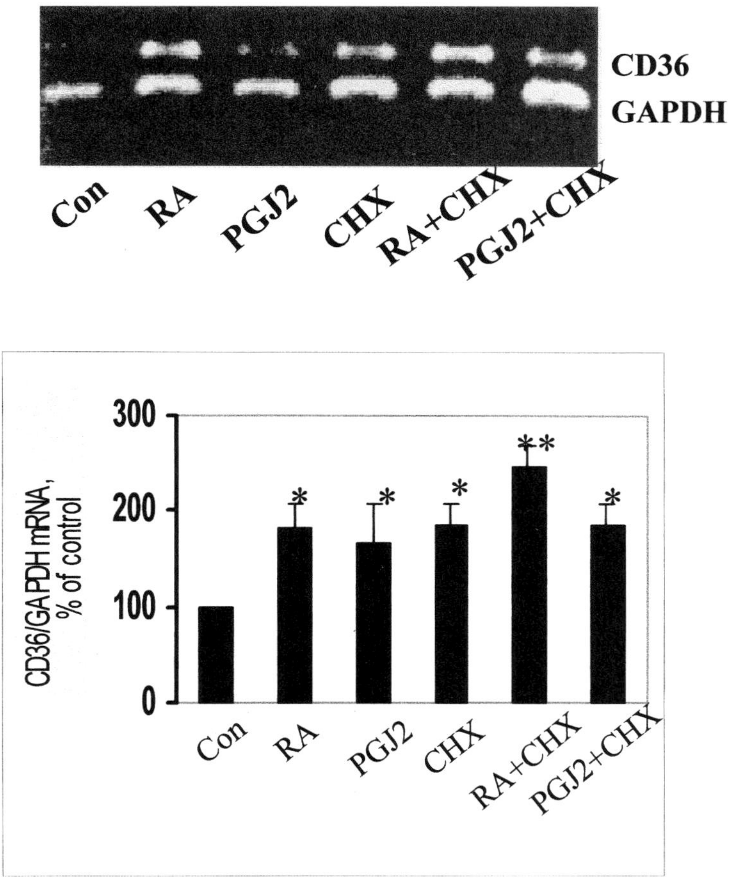

FIGURE 2. Upregulation of CD36 mRNA levels. THP-1 cells were cultured for 24 h with RA (5 μM), 15dd-PGJ2 (10 μM), cycloheximide (CHX; 10 μM), RA (5 μM) + CHX (10 μg/mL), or 15dd-PGJ2 (10 μM) + CHX (10 μg/mL) as indicated and analyzed by semi-quantitative RT-PCR for steady-state levels of CD36 mRNA. GAPDH mRNA was used as an internal control for normalization purposes. Graphic bars (below) represent the CD36/GAPDH ratio (±SD) for each treatment. *Significant difference between single treatments and control. **Significance between cells treated with more than one agent and singly treated values ($p < 0.05$).

ment with 5 μM RA, as well as that with 100 nM PMA and 10 μM 15dd-PGJ2, caused a marked increase in steady-state levels of CD36 mRNA. Changes induced by RA were found to be rapid; THP-1 cells exposed to RA for less than 24 h showed a significant increase in the levels of CD36 mRNA, while maximal stimulation occurred after 2 days of treatment (data not shown). To ascertain whether the increase of CD36 mRNA by RA required concurrent protein synthesis, we tested the effect of cycloheximide (CHX) on this induction. In these experiments, THP-1 cells were cultured with 5 μM RA for 24 h in the absence or presence of 10 μg/mL CHX, which inhibited protein synthesis by >90% (data not shown). As shown in FIGURE 2, CHX alone resulted in a 2-fold increase in CD36 transcripts over this 24-h period, suggesting that a specific labile protein may affect steady-state CD36 mRNA levels. As expected, RA alone caused a 2-fold induction of mRNA levels, while exposure to RA in the presence of CHX resulted in a further increase in receptor expression. These results indicate that CD36 is subject to CHX superinduction in human monocytes and that protein synthesis is not required for increased expression by RA.

RA INDUCTION OF CD36 IS NOT MEDIATED THROUGH THE PPARγ SIGNALING PATHWAY

Our results have shown that RA induces CD36 expression in THP-1 cells. Previous studies by Zhu *et al.* have shown that the 9-*cis*-RA isomer can upregulate PPARγ in these cells.[29] Since CD36 is known to be regulated through PPARγ activation,[32] this finding supports the contention that upregulation of CD36 by RA is caused by upregulation of PPARγ. However, we now have evidence that this is, in fact, not the case. The culture medium of normally passaged THP-1 cells and in the experiments described above included RPMI 1640 plus 10% fetal bovine serum (FBS). Both FBS and RPMI 1640 contain ligands for PPARγ, for example, modified (e.g., oxidized) LDL, HDL, VLDL, and fatty acids in the former and *p*-aminobenzoic acid in the latter. Since it has been shown that PPARγ-mediated gene activation requires liganded receptor,[23,32] we determined whether upregulation of CD36 by RA could be accomplished in Hanks balanced salt solution (i.e., whether RA induction could be accomplished in the complete absence of any possible PPARγ ligands). FIGURES 3 and 4 demonstrate that RA increased CD36 surface protein (mean fluorescence intensity) and CD36 mRNA levels as compared to the control under these conditions.

SOME CONCLUSIONS REGARDING RA INDUCTION OF CD36 AS REPRESENTING A NOVEL MECHANISM OF CD36 GENE REGULATION

The *in vitro* studies described on the preceding pages demonstrate that RA can upregulate the expression of CD36 surface expression and mRNA levels in the human monocyte cell line THP-1. This effect occurs in the absence of cellular differentiation. CD36 induction by RA is protein synthesis–independent, suggesting a mechanism directly mediated by retinoid nuclear receptors on the transcriptional machinery of CD36 rather than through intermediary proteins. A link between RA-induced upregulation of PPARγ and the activation of CD36 has been discounted by the finding that RA remained a potent inducer of CD36 surface protein and mRNA expression in the complete absence of any possible ligands for PPARγ. Taken together, it is our hypothesis that RA induction of CD36 represents a new mechanism of regulation of this gene that is, at least partly, independent of the PPARγ pathway and can occur in the absence of cellular adhesion and differentiation. The ability to selectively up-

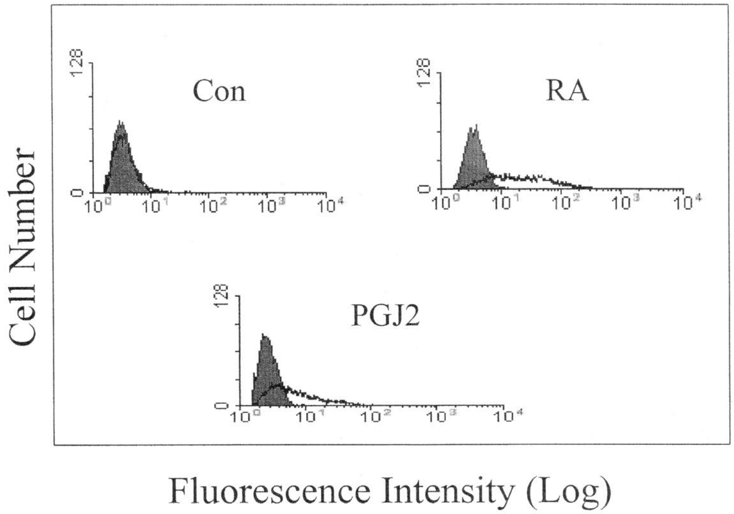

FIGURE 3. RA induction of CD36 protein in the absence of PPARγ ligands. Flow cytometry analysis of surface CD36 expression of cells cultured in Hanks balanced salt solution. THP-1 cells were treated for 24 h with RA (5 μM), 15dd-PGJ2 (10 μM), or solvent control (Con) as indicated and analyzed using a PE-conjugated anti-CD36 monoclonal antibody (open histograms). The solid histograms represent cells incubated with PE-conjugated isotype control Ab.

regulate CD36 expression in nonadherent cells of the monocyte/macrophage lineage suggests the possibility of increasing the scavenging function of PF macrophages of women with endometriosis as a means of altering the course of their disease.

EFFECTS OF RU486 ON MACROPHAGE DIFFERENTIATION AND FUNCTION

The hypotheses of how inflammatory cytokines and macrophage function may play a role in supporting the growth of ectopic endometrial cells are thoroughly discussed in other chapters of this volume. Therefore, any discussion of how steroid family members may impact on endometriosis should address the question of how such compounds affect immune function such as presented above for the case of RA on macrophage scavenger receptor expression. One steroid derivative that has already been utilized in women with endometriosis is the antiprogesterone/antiglucocorticoid compound, RU486. This agent appears to have significant clinical potential in the medical management of endometriosis. Although RU486 has been shown to alleviate the pain associated with endometriosis[33] and to inhibit endometrial cell growth,[34] direct evidence that RU486 may affect macrophage function is lacking. Studies by us and others have shown that RU486 has a variety of effects on macrophage function, including growth inhibition, alteration of production of a variety of cytokines, and upregulation of scavenger receptor activity.[35,36] Although

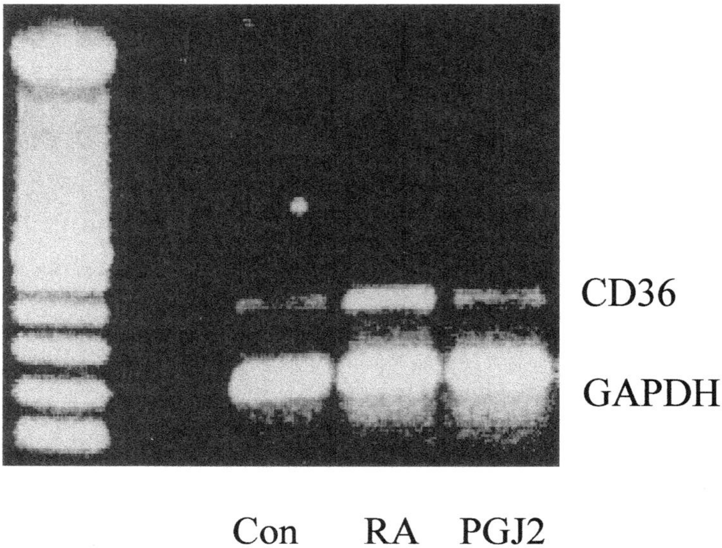

FIGURE 4. RA induction of CD36 mRNA in the absence of PPARγ ligands. THP-1 cells were cultured for 24 h with RA (5 μM), 15dd-PGJ2 (10 μM), or solvent control (Con) as indicated and then analyzed by semiquantitative RT-PCR for steady-state levels of CD36 mRNA. GAPDH mRNA analysis was performed on the same samples as an internal control.

RU486 is known to act by binding to progesterone and glucocorticoid receptors, studies from our group have demonstrated that RU486 can function as a potent antioxidant by a mechanism distinguished from its activity as an antiprogesterin and antiglucocorticoid.[37] The following data indicate that this compound, acting as an antioxidant, can suppress activation of NFκB, a nuclear transcription factor that affects the expression of several inflammatory genes such as those for IL-6, MCP-1, GM-CSF, CSF-1, and various adhesion molecules.[38] For this work, we utilized the mouse macrophage cell line RAW and activated it with the linoleate oxidative product HPODE. In these experiments, HPODE was prepared by oxidizing 1 mM linoleic acid using 100 U/mL of soybean lipoxygenase in a total volume of 1 mL of PBS.[39] The oxidation product (13-HPODE) was followed by the formation of conjugated diene at OD 234 nm in a spectrophotometer.[40]

RAW macrophages were placed in 60-mm dishes and were grown to confluence in RPMI medium containing 10% FCS. After washing, the cells were treated as indicated in FIGURE 5 with RU486 (antiglucocorticoid with antioxidant function) or probucol (antioxidant without antiglucocorticoid activity) in the absence and presence of HPODE for 24 h. Compounds were added at 10 μM levels. Cells were washed and nuclear extracts were prepared by detergent treatment. Equal amounts of nuclear proteins (which will contain NFκB) were incubated with ^{32}P-labeled NFκB-binding motifs as described by the manufacturer of the kit (GIBCO). Gel-shift assays were performed on 1% agarose and the gel was subjected to autoradiography.

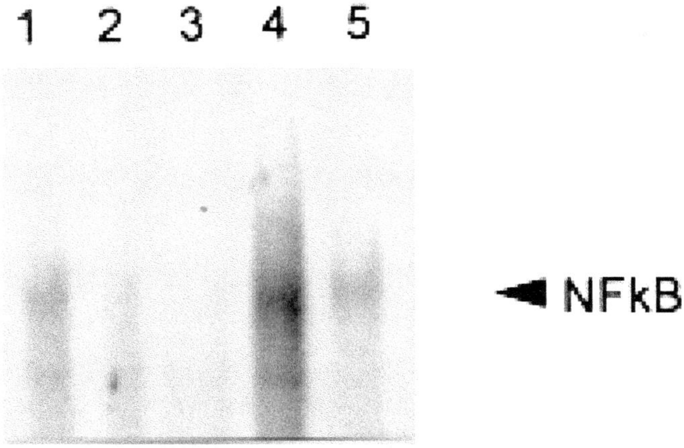

FIGURE 5. Suppression of NFκB binding in RAW macrophages. Cells were treated for 24 h with solvent control (lane 1), 10 μM RU486 (lane 2), 10 μM probucol (lane 3), 50 μM 13-HPODE (lane 4), and 10 μM RU486 + 50 μM 13-HPODE (lane 5).

Results presented in FIGURE 5 show that control cells expressed low levels of available NFκB in the nucleus, while cells incubated with RU486 as well as with probucol (antioxidant without antisteroid activity) demonstrated a marked decrease in the presence of this transcription factor. Treatment of these cells with 13-HPODE dramatically increased NFκB availability as compared to control cells. Finally, the addition of RU486 to the HPODE-treated cultures again induced a marked reduction in NFκB binding. These results suggest that, in a biologically active system, RU486 can retard oxidation-induced increases in the nuclear availability of NFκB. Since RU486 can gain access to the nucleus by its ability to bind to a variety of steroid hormone receptors including the progesterone, glucocorticoid, and androgen receptors,[41] it is tempting to speculate whether its nuclear presence is responsible for its action on NFκB as opposed to general antioxidant activity in the cell or in the extracellular milieu. This contention is supported by our observation that vitamin E had no effect on NFκB binding (unpublished data). If this is the case, RU486 should have superior or unique cell-type-specific antioxidant functions that would depend on hormone receptor phenotype or expression. As such, the ability of hormone-receptor-binding antioxidants such as RU486 could define these compounds as members of a new group of antioxidants that might be known as "target-specific nuclear antioxidants".

DIRECT EFFECTS ON HUMAN ENDOMETRIAL CELLS

Along with their ability to alter the functional activity of cells of the monocyte/macrophage lineage, there is ample evidence showing that compounds of the steroid hormone family can affect the progression of endometriosis through direct action on

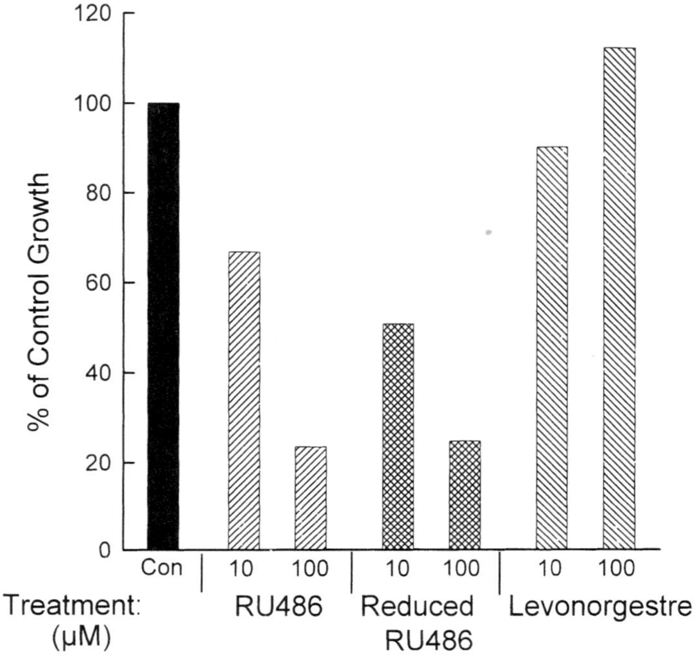

FIGURE 6. Inhibition by RU486 of endometrial cell proliferation. The human endometrial carcinoma cell line RL-95-2 was plated in triplicate in 24-well dishes (10^4 cells/well) and treated for 24 h with solvent control (Con), RU486, reduced RU486, or levonorgestrel at the concentrations indicated. During the last 6 h of culture, the cells were pulsed with 1 μCi ^{3}H-thymidine/well and incorporation was assessed by standard procedures. Results are expressed as percent of control growth and represent average values of three independent experiments.

endometrial cells. Thus, although the clinical effectiveness of RU486 in the treatment of endometriosis may be partly (or largely) mediated by its potent activity on immunological components of the disease (e.g., PF macrophages), we have hypothesized that direct inhibition of endometrial cell proliferation may also come into play.[34] Moreover, a complete understanding of the clinical potential of retinoids, antioxidants, or similar compounds in endometriosis will require a thorough knowledge of their direct effects on the growth and function of relevant endometrial cell types. To this end, we present data here suggesting that both RU486 and RA can alter the biology of endometriosis through direct actions on endometrial cells.

EFFECTS OF RU486 ON HUMAN ENDOMETRIAL CELL PROLIFERATION

To test the hypothesis that part of the clinical efficacy of RU486 in endometriosis is through direct inhibition of cell growth, we assessed its effects on the growth of endometrial cell lines and primary tissue.[34] An example of our results is shown in

FIGURE 6. These data demonstrate the ability of RU486 to modulate the growth of the human endometrial carcinoma cell line RL-95-2 and we compare the results with those obtained with reduced RU486 and levonorgestrel, another potent antiglucocorticoid compound, but which does not, like RU486, possess antioxidant properties.[37] Reduced RU486 has been shown to retain potent antioxidant properties; however, with the reduction of the progesterone ring, it loses antiprogesterone and antiglucocorticoid activity.[34,37] As shown in FIGURE 6, RU486 decreased endometrial cell proliferation in a dose-dependent fashion: 10 μM and 100 μM of RU486 reduced cell proliferation to 65% and 25% of controls, respectively. Levonorgestrel did not consistently modify cell proliferation. A similar lack of activity has also been demonstrated with the "pure" antiprogesterone, ZK112,993, which is structurally similar to RU486, but lacks the dimethylaminophenyl group and is therefore devoid of antioxidant properties.[37] In contrast, reduced RU486 significantly decreased endometrial cell proliferation to 50% and 25% of control growth using 10 μM and 100 μM, respectively. These results demonstrate the direct growth-inhibitory effects of RU486 on endometrial cells and suggest that this activity, similar to its inhibition of NFκB activity in macrophages described above, may be mediated at least partly through its antioxidant properties. These results have now been confirmed using primary human endometrial cells as well as other cell lines.[34]

RETINOIDS SUPPRESS IL-6 PRODUCTION IN HUMAN ENDOMETRIAL CELLS

The multifunctional cytokine, IL-6, has been implicated in the autocrine growth of myeloma and other neoplasms, and may be involved in the ectopic growth of endometrial cells in endometriosis.[42] This effect may be mediated directly through its action as a growth factor on endometrial cell proliferation or through its ability to act as a coactivator of macrophages and lymphocytes, resulting in the sustained production of cytokines involved in chemotaxis and cellular growth. Women with endometriosis have markedly elevated levels of IL-6 in their PF. Increased levels of IL-6 have also been observed in Paget's disease (characterized by increased osteoclastogenesis), rheumatoid arthritis, Castleman's disease, and POEMS syndrome, and may play an important role in the aging process.[42] Findings by Shanti *et al.* that certain autoantibodies are increased in endometriosis suggest an additional systemic implication of increased IL-6 levels in humans.[43] It is clear that IL-6 may play a significant role in the overall clinical features of endometriosis. We have recently shown that retinoids can induce a marked decrease in IL-6 secretion from endometrial cells.[44] The data demonstrated that RA inhibition of IL-6 expression in endometrial cell lines and primary cultures occurred in a time- and dose-dependent fashion, showing maximal effects at pharmacologically achievable blood serum concentrations (μM range) (FIG. 7). Mutational analysis of reporter gene constructs indicated that RA suppression of IL-6 expression was mediated, at least in part, through functional antagonism with the nuclear factor IL-6 (NF-IL-6) binding site located in the IL-6 promoter.[42] The ability of retinoids to affect IL-6 production by infiltrating hematopoietic cells associated with endometriosis has not yet been determined. Nonetheless, the demonstrated ability of these compounds to inhibit IL-6 in a variety of cell types, including peripheral T and B lymphocytes, Kaposi's sarcoma

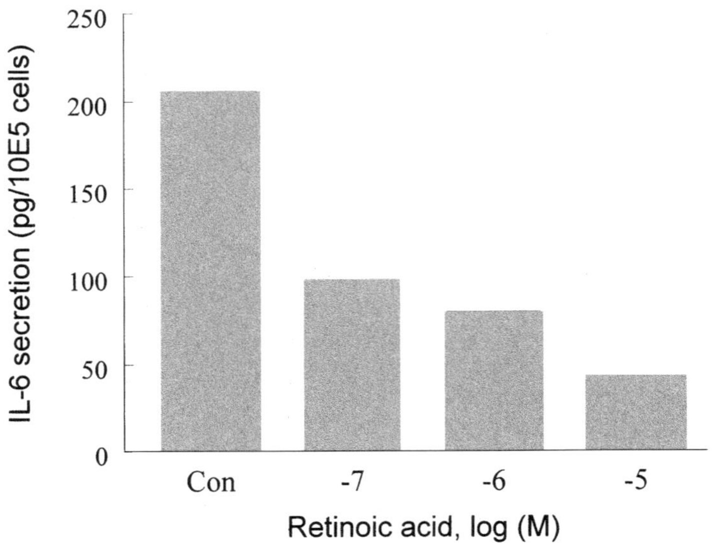

FIGURE 7. Suppression of IL-6 secretion from the endometrial cell line EM42 by RA. Cells were treated for 3 days with the indicated concentration of RA, at which time the medium was changed and the cultures were treated for an additional 24 h. The IL-6 in this 3- to 4-day culture supernatant was assessed by ELISA.

cells, myeloma cells, fibroblasts, and osteogenic cells, suggests the general nature of this retinoid activity.[45–47] Thus, although the contribution of IL-6 secretion from ectopic endometrial cells to the high levels noted in the PF of women with endometriosis is not yet known, a reduction of these levels by RA would appear likely. Whether a reduction in IL-6 will help ameliorate the disease process is unknown. However, at the very least, reduction of IL-6 levels should help to normalize the abnormal immunologic milieu that can play a direct role in the aberrant growth of endometriotic lesions.

SOME CONCLUSIONS REGARDING THE ABILITY OF STEROID COMPOUNDS TO ALTER THE BIOLOGY OF ENDOMETRIOSIS

In endometriosis, it is generally assumed that the endometriotic implants are steroid hormone–dependent (estrogen and progesterone) and, in the absence of these steroids, endometriosis undergoes regression.[48] In this light, the demonstrated antiprogesterone and antiestrogenic activity of RU486 led to the hypothesis that this compound may be potentially beneficial in modulating the growth of ectopic endometrial cells. Subsequent clinical trials supported this contention and pointed to a potentially promising new use for antiprogesterones/antiglucocorticoids, of which more than 400 different analogues have been synthesized by different pharmaceutical companies worldwide. Recent evidence from our laboratory suggests that increased therapeutic benefits in endometriosis can be obtained by targeting the abnormal immune responses associated with this disease. Reduced PF macrophage scavenger receptor activity and markedly elevated levels of IL-6 in the PF are two examples of an aberrant immunologically mediated phenomenon that, if corrected, might beneficially alter the course of the disease. What is desperately needed is a precise knowledge of the mechanism(s) of action of biologically active steroids on endometrial cells and on the inflammatory reactions associated with endometriosis. Gaining such knowledge is essential for understanding how these compounds may be clinically utilized and for designing future pharmacologic agents.

[NOTE ADDED IN PROOF: Since submission of this report, a new study by Wuttge *et al.* (2001. *FASEB J.* **15:** 1221–1223) also showed that RA upregulates CD36 expression in human monocytes.]

REFERENCES

1. LEBOVIC, D.I., M.D. MUELLER & R.N. TAYLOR. 2001. Immunobiology of endometriosis. Fertil. Steril. **75:** 1–10.
2. ORAL, E. & A. ARICI. 1996. Peritoneal growth factors and endometriosis. Semin. Reprod. Endocrinol. **14:** 257–267.
3. MCLAREN, J., A. PRENTICE, D.S. CHARNOCK-JONES *et al.* 1996. Vascular endothelia growth factor (VEGF) concentrations are elevated in peritoneal fluid of women with endometriosis. Hum. Reprod. **11:** 220–223.
4. OLIVE, D.L., I. MONTOYA, R.M. RIEHL *et al.* 1991. Macrophage-conditioned media enhance endometrial stromal cell proliferation *in vitro*. Am. J. Obstet. Gynecol. **164:** 953–958.
5. BRAUN, D.P., A. MURIANA, H. GEBEL *et al.* 1994. Monocyte-mediated enhancement of endometrial cell proliferation in women with endometriosis. Fertil. Steril. **61:** 78–84.
6. RAMPRASAD, M.P., W. FISHER, J.L. WITZTUM *et al.* 1995. The 94- to 97-kDa mouse macrophage membrane protein that recognizes oxidized low density lipoprotein and phosphatidylserine-rich liposomes is identical to macrosialin, the mouse homologue of human CD68. Proc. Natl. Acad. Sci. U.S.A. **92:** 9580–9584.
7. OTTNAD, E., S. PARTHASARATHY, G.R. SAMBRANO *et al.* 1995. A macrophage receptor for oxidized low density lipoprotein distinct from the receptor for acetyl low density lipoprotein: partial purification and role in recognition of oxidatively damaged cells. Proc. Natl. Acad. Sci. U.S.A. **92:** 1391–1395.
8. STANTON, L.W., R.T. WHITE, C.M. BRYANT *et al.* 1992. A macrophage Fc receptor for IgG is also a receptor for oxidized low density lipoprotein. J. Biol. Chem. **267:** 22446–22451.
9. ENDEMANN, G., L.W. STANTON, K.S. MADDEN *et al.* 1993. CD36 is a receptor for oxidized low density lipoprotein. J. Biol. Chem. **268:** 11811–11816.
10. MOULTON, K.S., H. WU, J. BARNETT *et al.* 1992. Regulated expression of the human acetylated low density lipoprotein receptor gene and isolation of promoter sequences. Proc. Natl. Acad. Sci. U.S.A. **89:** 8102–8106.
11. WU, H., K. MOULTON, A. HORVAI *et al.* 1994. Combinatorial interactions between AP-1 and Ets domain proteins contribute to the developmental regulation of the macrophage scavenger receptor gene. Mol. Cell. Biol. **14:** 2129–2139.
12. DE VILLIERS, W.J., I.P. FRASER & S. GORDON. 1994. Cytokine and growth factor regulation of macrophage scavenger receptor expression and function. Immunol. Lett. **43:** 73–79.
13. HUGHES, D.A., I.P. FRASER & S. GORDON. 1995. Murine macrophage scavenger receptor: *in vivo* expression and function as receptor for macrophage adhesion in lymphoid and non-lymphoid organs. Eur. J. Immunol. **25:** 466–473.
14. DE VILLIERS, W.J., I.P. FRASER, D.A. HUGHES *et al.* 1994. Macrophage-colony-stimulating factor selectively enhances macrophage scavenger receptor expression and function. J. Exp. Med. **180:** 705–709.

15. Fraser, I., D. Hughes & S. Gordon. 1993. Divalent cation–independent macrophage adhesion inhibited by monoclonal antibody to murine scavenger receptor. Nature **364:** 343–346.
16. Kim, J.G., C. Keshava, A.A. Murphy *et al.* 1997. Fresh mouse peritoneal macrophages have low scavenger receptor activity. J. Lipid Res. **38:** 2207–2215.
17. Lessey, B.A., J.J. Casterbaum, S.W. Sawin *et al.* 1994. Aberrant integrin expression in the endometrium of women with endometriosis. J. Clin. Endocrinol. Metab. **79:** 643–649.
18. Olive, D.L., J.B. Weinberg & A.F. Haney. 1985. Peritoneal macrophages and infertility: the association between cell number and pelvic pathology. Fertil. Steril. **44:** 772–777.
19. Fadok, V.A., M.L. Warner, D.L. Bratton *et al.* 1998. CD36 is required for phagocytosis of apoptotic cells by human macrophages that use either a phosphatidylserine receptor or the vitronectin receptor (alpha v beta 3). J. Immunol. **161:** 6250–6257.
20. Tontonoz, P., L. Nagy, J.G. Alvarez *et al.* 1998. PPAR-gamma promotes monocyte/macrophage differentiation and uptake of oxidized LDL. Cell **93:** 241–252.
21. Feng, J., J. Han, S.F. Pearce *et al.* 2000. Induction of CD36 expression by oxidized LDL and IL-4 by a common signaling pathway dependent on protein kinase C and PPAR-gamma. J. Lipid. Res. **41:** 688–696.
22. Huh, H.Y., S.K. Lo, L.M. Yesner *et al.* 1995. CD36 induction on human monocytes upon adhesion to tumor necrosis factor–activated endothelial cells. J. Biol. Chem. **270:** 6267–6271.
23. Han, J., D.P. Ajar, J.M. Tauras *et al.* 2000. Transforming growth factor-β1 (TGF-β1) and TGF-β2 decrease expression of CD36, the type B scavenger receptor, through mitogen-activated protein kinase phosphorylation of peroxisome proliferator-activated receptor-γ. J. Biol. Chem. **275:** 1241–1246.
24. Huang, J.T., J.S. Welch, M. Ricote *et al.* 1999. Interleukin-4-dependent production of PPAR-gamma ligands in macrophages by 12/15-lipoxygenase. Nature **400:** 378–382.
25. Keisari, Y., G. Robin *et al.* 2000. Role of cytokines in the maturation and function of macrophages: effect of GM-CSF and IL-4. Adv. Exp. Med. Biol. **476:** 73–89.
26. Scaccabarozzi, A., P. Arosio, G. Weiss *et al.* 2000. Relationship between TNF-alpha and iron metabolism in differentiating human monocytic THP-1 cells. Br. J. Haematol. **110:** 978–984.
27. Tsuchiya, S., Y. Kobayashi, Y. Goto *et al.* 1982. Induction of maturation in cultured human monocytic leukemia cells by a phorbol diester. Cancer Res. **42:** 1530–1536.
28. Auwerx, J. 1991. The human leukemia cell line, THP-1: a multifaceted model for the study of monocyte-macrophage differentiation. Experientia **47:** 22–31.
29. Zhu, L., B. Gong, C. Bisgaier *et al.* 1998. Induction of PPARγ1 expression in human THP-1 monocytic leukemia cells by 9-*cis*-retinoic acid is associated with cellular growth suppression. Biochem. Biophys. Res. Commun. **251:** 842–848.
30. Ricciarelli, R., J.M. Aingg & A. Azzi. 2000. Vitamin E reduces the uptake of oxidized LDL by inhibiting CD36 scavenger receptor expression in cultured aortic smooth muscle cells. Circulation **102:** 82–87.
31. Goswami, P.C., L.D. Albee, D.R. Spitz *et al.* 1997. A polymerase chain reaction assay for simultaneous detection and quantitation of proto-oncogene and GAPD mRNAs in different cell growth rates. Cell Proliferation **30:** 271–282.
32. Tontonoz, P. & L. Nagy. 1999. Regulation of macrophage gene expression by peroxisome proliferator-activated receptor gamma: implications for cardiovascular disease. Curr. Opin. Lipidol. **10:** 485–490.
33. Kettel, L.M., A.A. Murphy, A. Morales *et al.* 1998. Preliminary report on the treatment of endometriosis with low-dose mifepristone (RU 486). Am. J. Obstet. Gynecol. **178:** 1151–1156.
34. Murphy, A.A., M.H. Zhou, S. Malkapuram *et al.* 2000. RU486-induced growth inhibition of human endometrial cells. Fertil. Steril. **74:** 1014–1019.
35. Roberts, C.P., S. Parthasarathy, R. Hulati *et al.* 1995. Effect of RU-486 and related compounds on the proliferation of cultured macrophages. Am. J. Reprod. Immunol. **34:** 248–256.
36. Roberts, C.P., A. Murphy, N. Santanam *et al.* 1996. The effect of RU 486 and related compounds on cultured macrophage differentiation and function. Am J. Obstet. Gynecol. **175:** 248–259.

37. PARTHASARATHY, S., A.J. MORALES & A.A. MURPHY. 1994. Antioxidant: a new role for RU486 and related compounds. J. Clin. Invest. **94:** 1990–1995.
38. BARNES, P.J. & M. KARIN. 1997. Nuclear factor-kappaB: a pivotal transcription factor in chronic inflammatory diseases. N. Engl. J. Med. **336:** 1066–1071.
39. FRUEBIS, J., S. PARTHASARATHY & D. STEINBERG. 1992. Evidence for a concerted reaction between lipid hydroperoxides and polypeptides. Proc. Natl. Acad. Sci. U.S.A. **89:** 10588–10592.
40. SANTANAM, N. & S. PARTHASARATHY. 1995. Paradoxical actions of antioxidants in the oxidation of low density lipoprotein by peroxidases. J. Clin. Invest. **95:** 2594–2600.
41. KIM, R.S., C.L. ZABORNIAK, A. BEGLEITER *et al.* 1992. Antiproliferative properties of aminosteroid antioxidants on cultured cancer cells. Cancer Lett. **64:** 61–66.
42. KELLER, E.T., J. WANAGAT & W.B. ERSHLER. 1996. Molecular and cellular biology of interleukin-6 and its receptor. Front. Biosci. **1:** 340–357.
43. SHANTI, A., N. SANTANAM, A.J. MORALES *et al.* 1999. Autoantibodies to markers of oxidative stress are elevated in women with endometriosis. Fertil. Steril. **71:** 1115–1118.
44. SAWATSRI, S., N. DESAI, J.A. ROCK *et al.* 2000. Retinoic acid suppresses interleukin-6 production in human endometrial cells. Fertil. Steril. **73:** 1012–1019.
45. OGATA, A., N. NISHIMOTO, Y. SHIMA *et al.* 1994. Inhibitory effect of all-*trans* retinoic acid on the growth of freshly isolated myeloma cells via interference with interleukin-6 signal transduction. Blood **84:** 3040–3046.
46. ZITNIK, R.J., R.M. KOTLOFF, J. LATIFPOUR *et al.* 1994. Retinoic acid inhibition of IL-1-induced IL-6 production by human lung fibroblasts. J. Immunol. **152:** 1419–1427.
47. BLOMHOFF, H.K., E.B. SMELAND, B. ERIKSTEIN *et al.* 1992. Vitamin A is a key regulator for cell growth, cytokine production, and differentiation in normal B cells. J. Biol. Chem. **267:** 23988–23992.
48. DIZEREGA, G.S., D.L. BARBER & G.D. HODGEN. 1980. Endometriosis: role of ovarian steroids in initiation, maintenance, and suppression. Fertil. Steril. **33:** 649–653.

Autoantibody Responses to Carbohydrate Epitopes in Endometriosis

GRANT R. YEAMAN, JANE E. COLLINS, AND GILLIAN A. LANG

Department of Microbiology and Immunology, Dartmouth Medical School, Lebanon, New Hampshire 03756, USA

ABSTRACT: Autoantibody responses to endometrial and serum antigens are a common feature of endometriosis. We have shown that the serum autoantibody response in endometriosis to a number of previously identified antigens, including α_2-Heremans Schmidt glycoprotein and carbonic anhydrase, is specific for a carbohydrate epitope common to these proteins. Removal of carbohydrate moieties from these antigens resulted in a loss of antibody binding. Antibody reactivity was abolished following adsorption with the lectin jacalin, which specifically binds the Thomsen-Friedenreich (T) antigen (Galβ1-3GalNAc). Demonstration that the autoantibodies also reacted with other Thomsen-Friedenreich antigen–bearing proteins, such as serum IgA1, hemopexin, and MMP-9, confirmed that this glycotope is involved in the autoantibody response. However, the autoantibody binding requires the presence of at least one sialic acid residue. Thus, the glycotope involved may be a sialylated T antigen. These findings allow us to hypothesize a number of mechanisms whereby the autoimmune response plays a direct role in several aspects of the disease process. The proposed mechanisms take into account the salient endocrine dependency of endometriotic lesions and other aspects of the disease process such as aberrant matrix metalloproteinase function and the ability of endometrial cells to implant at ectopic sites. The anti-T-like response may also be indicative of an underlying genetic defect in glycosylation or in the control of glycosylation by steroid sex hormones. Further characterization of this autoimmune response may prove useful in the development of serum-based diagnostic tests for endometriosis and may lead to the development of therapeutic strategies.

KEYWORDS: endometriosis; autoantibodies; Thomsen-Friedenreich antigen; carbohydrate antigen; glycosylation

INTRODUCTION

Although the etiology of endometriosis remains enigmatic, altered cellular and humoral immune function is clearly a feature of established disease.[1–3] Autoantibodies to endometrial antigens and deposition of complement components have been described in a number of studies, and a number of serum, peritoneal fluid, and endometrial antigens have been described.[1] Recognized tissue antigens include the

Address for correspondence: Grant R. Yeaman, Ph.D., Department of Microbiology, Dartmouth Medical School, 1 Medical Center Drive, Lebanon, NH 03756. Voice: 603-650-6329, ext. 6329; fax: 603-650-6223.

grant.yeaman@dartmouth.edu

human chorionic gonadotropin receptor, isoforms I and II of the enzyme carbonic anhydrase, and CA125.[4–12] Antibodies to serum transferrin and α_2-Heremans Schmidt glycoprotein (α_2-HSG) have also been described and proposed as diagnostic markers.[13,14]

The nature of the epitopes on these diverse proteins had not been previously studied. In particular, the possibility that carbohydrate epitopes (glycotopes) were involved in the autoantibody response had not been evaluated. We have recently shown that a common carbohydrate epitope is recognized on α_2-HSG, carbonic anhydrase, hemopexin, and the α-chain of IgA1.[15] This conclusion was based on the finding that removal of the carbohydrate moieties from the antigens abolished the ability of endometriosis sera to bind these antigens. All of the identified antigens are known to bind the lectin jacalin. Adsorption of purified serum antigens and peritoneal fluid antigen preparations with solid-phase jacalin removed antibody-binding activity. Carbonic anhydrase was not tested by deglycosylation or jacalin binding; however, purified α_2-HSG and fetuin competed with the binding of autoantibodies to this protein.

The carbohydrate structure recognized by jacalin is very specific and binding is dependent on the presence of T antigen. Jacalin recognizes the disaccharide Galβ1-3GalNAc, which is the type 1 core of *O*-linked oligosaccharides. Galβ1-3GalNAc is expressed by a limited number of plasma proteins, including IgA1, IgD, C1-inhibitor, hemopexin, plasminogen, α1-antitrypsin, α2-macroglobulin, 8S-α3 glycoprotein, chorionic gonadotropin (hCG), and α_2-HSG.[16]

Structures expressing this epitope in the uterus are less well defined. Both T and sialosyl-T epitopes are expressed on epithelial cells of the uterus.[17,18] The sialylated form of T is referred to as cryptic since most lectins (jacalin being an exception) and monoclonal antibodies are unable to bind to this form of the antigen without prior removal of the sialic acid.[18] Our results indicate that, in contrast to T antigen–specific monoclonal antibodies, the autoantibodies in endometriosis require some level of sialylation for this binding since extensive neuraminidase treatment abolished autoantibody binding. This is in contrast to the binding of jacalin, which generally increases following the removal of terminal sialic acid residues.[19] Our data suggest that autoantibody binding to the epitope(s) is dependent on D-galactose and, in this respect, is similar to jacalin binding.[16] The precise structures recognized by the endometrial autoantibodies remain to be determined and oligosaccharide inhibition studies are in progress.

IgM antibodies specific for the T antigen are designated natural antibodies since they are found in the sera of most healthy individuals.[20] The anti-T-like antibodies found in the sera of endometriosis patients differ from those of normal sera in that significant titers of IgG antibodies are present. Preliminary subclass analysis indicates that these IgG antibodies are not only of the IgG2 and IgG4 subclasses, typical of an anticarbohydrate response, but also of the IgG1 subclass. The utility of the anti-T autoantibody response for the diagnosis and monitoring of disease activity in endometriosis is also currently under evaluation.

Whether or not the expression of this epitope and the attendant autoantibody response play a role in the pathogenesis of endometriosis is not known. Here, we will review what is known about the T epitope and its recognition by mammalian lectins. We will summarize the role of T antigens and anti-T antibodies in cancers. Finally, we will present potential mechanisms whereby an increase in the expression of

T antigen and subsequent anti-T antibody responses could account for some of the known immunological and endocrine features of endometriosis.

ANTI-T ANTIBODIES IN CANCER

In addition to characteristics common to autoimmune diseases, the development of endometriotic lesions shows certain similarities to tumor development. Similar to metastatic tumor development, in endometriosis, cells must be capable of migration, of implantation, and of promoting angiogenesis. Thus, in this respect, endometriosis can be thought of as metastasis of untransformed endometrial cells. The observation that high levels of T antigen expression are seen in several types of cancer and that T antigen expression levels correlate with increased metastasis and a poor prognosis may indicate that T or T-like antigen is of relevance to the pathogenesis of endometriosis in the context of establishment of ectopic lesions.[21] Furthermore, using mouse tumor models, it has been shown that anti-T antibodies are effective in preventing metastasis, and a number of studies have evaluated the use of T antigen as a cancer vaccine.[21]

MAMMALIAN LECTINS WITH SPECIFICITY FOR T ANTIGEN

A number of mammalian lectins expressed in the human uterus recognize T antigen. The most prominent of these are members of the human galectin family, of which galectins-1 and -3 are the best characterized.[22] Galectins bind a number of glycotopes bearing terminal β-galactosyl residues, and galectin-3 binds T antigen with high affinity.[23] They mediate diverse functions, including immune modulation, extracellular matrix interactions, and angiogenesis.[22,24,25] These are some of the very processes implicated in the pathogenesis of endometriosis.

Immunomodulatory activities of galectins include roles in leukocyte trafficking: for example, galectin-3 is a chemotactic factor for monocytes and macrophages and mediates interaction of T cells with the dendritic cells following L-selectin interaction.[26,27] Galectins play antagonistic roles in both promoting (galectin-1) and inhibiting (galectin-3) the apoptosis of activated memory T cells.[26,28] As a consequence of CD45 binding, galectin-1 can also modulate B cell function[29] and potentiate inflammatory cytokine synthesis following interaction with CD4 on T cells and macrophages.[30–32] Binding of galectin-3 to CD66b primes neutrophils for increased oxidative burst activity.[33,34]

CD23, the low-affinity IgE receptor (FcεRII), in addition to its immunoglobulin domains, contains an N-terminal lectin domain. The lectin domain, which is credited with much of the receptor's biologic activity, binds β-Gal glycotopes and preferentially T antigen. Therefore, CD23 shows a similar specificity to both jacalin and galectin-3, which both bind cell surface and soluble IgE.[35,36] B cell–expressed CD23 is shed in soluble form following cleavage by an as yet unidentified transmembrane MMP upon B cell activation.[37–39] Thus, it is perhaps of significance that levels of soluble CD23 are elevated in both the serum and peritoneal fluid of patients with endometriosis, indicating ongoing B cell activation.[40–42] This is consistent with our finding of significant numbers of CD23-negative B cells of an activated phenotype in the eutopic and ectopic endometrium of endometriosis patients, in contrast to the largely unactivated phenotype of B cells observed in the endometrium of control subjects (unpublished observations).

Thus, it is possible that anti-T antibody responses could block or mimic some of the biological functions of galectins and CD23. Binding of anti-T-like antibodies to T-bearing ligands on leukocytes may have different biological effects from those observed upon binding of galectins since the Fc portion of the anti-T-like antibodies may also trigger FcR signaling. Whether or not galectins are abnormally expressed in eutopic endometrium from endometriosis patients, or in ectopic lesions, is unknown. However, expression of uterine galectins is under either direct or indirect steroid sex hormone control.[43–46]

IMMUNE-ENDOCRINE INTERACTIONS

In recent studies, it has become apparent that ectopic lesions can be self-sustaining with respect to estradiol production.[47–49] Ectopic lesions synthesize estrogens through the conversion of androstenedione (produced in the adrenal gland) by the enzyme aromatase (P450 CYP19) to the weak estrogen, estrone. Estrone is then further converted to 17β-estradiol by a second enzyme, 17β-hydroxysteroid dehydrogenase (type I). In support of this mechanism, aromatase is expressed in stromal cells of both eutopic and ectopic endometrium from endometriosis patients, but expression is low or absent in control uterine endometrium.[50,51] 17β-Hydroxysteroid dehydrogenase (type I) expression is also evident in epithelial cells in endometriotic lesions. In contrast, expression of 17β-hydroxysteroid dehydrogenase (type II), which catalyzes the conversion of estradiol to the less biologically active estrone, is deficient in ectopic lesions.[52]

We hypothesize that, in endometriosis, the persistent expression of aromatase and 17β-hydroxysteroid dehydrogenase is driven by the T-like autoantibody response. Control of expression of these two enzymes by cytokines and immunological mediators, such as prostaglandin E_2 (PGE_2), is well established.[47] Cytokines that induce aromatase (through the aromatase type I promoter) and 17β-hydroxysteroid dehydrogenase expression include IL-1, TNF-α, and IL-6.[47–49] In some tissues, these cytokines can directly upregulate aromatase expression; however, in ectopic endometrium, it is likely these cytokines act indirectly by inducing prostaglandin synthase-2 (COX-II) expression.[53] This enzyme, which catalyzes the production of PGE_2 from its arachidonic acid precursor, upregulates aromatase gene expression through its type II promoter. Production of these same proinflammatory cytokines is increased in endometriosis.[54–68] Furthermore, autoantibodies recognizing the T-like antigen could directly trigger the synthesis of these cytokines. When peripheral blood mononuclear cells are cultured in the presence of the T antigen–specific lectin jacalin, monocytes secrete high levels of IL-6, IL-1, and IFN-γ.[69–71] Taken together with our studies, the potential for T-like interactions indicates that β-Gal-bearing epitopes may play a role in the pathogenesis of endometriosis. Higher levels of expression of T or sT antigen may arise from aberrant galactosylation or sialylation of carbohydrates in endometriosis patients.

A number of published studies indicate that the degrees of sialylation and galactosylation in both rats and humans are under strict sex steroid hormone control.[18,72–75] Indeed, the presence of sT antigen varies during the menstrual cycle in the human uterus: it is absent throughout the menstrual cycle in normal endometrium, except in the early to mid-secretory phase.[18] It remains to be determined whether such epitopes are expressed in an abnormal manner in the eutopic endometrium of endometriosis patients. We find that serum autoantibodies from patients with endometriosis bind to antigens in normal endometrium from the secretory phase. These antigens are not expressed in endometrium from the proliferative phase. A similar profile is present when endometria from endometriosis patients are analyzed, except that the secretory phase binding is greater than that with the normal endometria (unpublished observations). It is intriguing that one genetic lesion that has been inconsistently associated with endometriosis is the increased occurrence of a mutant allele of galactose-1-phosphate uridyl transferase, indicating that galactose metabolism may play a role in disease pathogenesis.[76]

IMPLANTATION AND ANGIOGENESIS—POTENTIAL ROLES OF ANTI-T-LIKE ANTIBODIES IN MMP FUNCTION

The development of ectopic lesions requires that endometrial cells are able to implant at nonuterine sites. Subsequent growth of the lesion is dependent on the ability of the ectopic tissue to promote vascularization. Thus, the mechanisms of implantation and angiogenesis are of importance in the pathogenesis of endometriosis. Matrix metalloproteinase (MMP) activity is an integral part of these processes and has been shown to be disrupted in endometriosis.[77–80]

Our finding that hemopexin is an autoantigen recognized by the T-like autoantibodies found in endometriosis has led us to consider other proteins that contain conserved hemopexin domains as additional potential autoantigens. All members of the MMP family (with the exception of MMP-7) contain a hemopexin domain. The *O*-linked oligosaccharides of MMP-9 have been sequenced and multiple T epitopes are present.[81] Western blotting analysis of natively glycosylated pro-MMP-9 dimer revealed reactivity with both jacalin and IgG antibodies present in serum from endometriosis patients (unpublished observations). Given the conservation of potential *O*-glycosylation sites on the hemopexin domains of MMPs, we predict that many members of this family of enzymes will be recognized by the T-like autoantibodies. Such a contention is supported by reports that galectins bind to, and that their lectin-binding function is modulated by, both MMP-2 and MMP-3.[82,83] Hemopexin domains (termed PEX) are released from MMPs by proteolysis in tissues and have been shown to play a role in the regulation of angiogenesis.[84]

In summary, expression of MMP and tissue inhibitors of matrix proteinases is dysregulated in ectopic lesions, and both galectins and the PEX domain play a role in angiogenesis. Thus, the possibility exists that autoantibody binding to MMPs could interfere with normal activation or inhibition of MMP function.

SUMMARY AND CONCLUSIONS

The identification of an autoimmune response against a T antigen–containing epitope in endometriosis may lead to the development of serum-based tests useful for both the diagnosis and monitoring of disease activity. Whether this response is merely an epiphenomenon or is an integral part of the disease pathogenesis remains to be determined. We have outlined possible immunological interactions and how these may impact the local endocrine conditions that may be involved in the pathogenesis of endometriosis. Clearly, mechanistic studies need to be undertaken to determine whether any of these hypotheses will hold true. It is possible that the autoantibody response is a consequence of aberrant glycosylation in susceptible women. This may arise as a consequence of genetic abnormalities in the glycosylation pathways or in the hormonal control of these pathways. Studies to evaluate whether biochemical and/or genetic differences in glycosylation pathways are present in endometriosis patients versus controls would begin to address this issue. Given the recognized features of endometriosis, we are of the opinion that endometriosis is both an endocrine- and autoimmune-based disease such that endocrine conditions contribute to the establishment of the autoimmune response, which in turn promotes the local endocrine conditions evident in ectopic lesions. Thus, future therapeutic approaches may have to combine both endocrine- and immune-based approaches.

ACKNOWLEDGMENTS

This work was supported by a research grant from the Endometriosis Association and by the National Institutes of Health (Grant No. AI34478).

REFERENCES

1. BURNS, W.N. & R.S. SCHENKEN. 1999. Pathophysiology of endometriosis-associated infertility. Clin. Obstet. Gynecol. **42:** 586–610.
2. RIER, S.E. & G.R. YEAMAN. 1997. Immune aspects of endometriosis: relevance of the uterine mucosal immune system. Semin. Reprod. Endocrinol. **15:** 209–220.
3. WITZ, C.A. 1999. Current concepts in the pathogenesis of endometriosis. Clin. Obstet. Gynecol. **42:** 566–585.
4. MONCAYO, H. *et al.* 1989. Ovarian failure and autoimmunity: detection of autoantibodies directed against both the unoccupied luteinizing hormone/human chorionic gonadotropin receptor and the hormone-receptor complex of bovine corpus luteum. J. Clin. Invest. **84:** 1857–1865.
5. BRINTON, D.A., T.M. QUATTROCIOCCHI-LONGE & F.L. KIECHLE. 1996. Endometriosis: identification by carbonic anhydrase autoantibodies and clinical features. Ann. Clin. Lab. Sci. **26:** 409–420.
6. D'CRUZ, O.J. *et al.* 1996. Antibodies to carbonic anhydrase in endometriosis: prevalence, specificity, and relationship to clinical and laboratory parameters. Fertil. Steril. **66:** 547–556.
7. KIECHLE, F.L., T.M. QUATTROCIOCCHI-LONGE & D.A. BRINTON. 1994. Carbonic anhydrase antibody in sera from patients with endometriosis. Am. J. Clin. Pathol. **101:** 611–615.
8. BARBIERI, R.L. 1986. CA-125 in patients with endometriosis. Fertil. Steril. **45:** 767–769.
9. BARBIERI, R.L. *et al.* 1986. Elevated serum concentrations of CA-125 in patients with advanced endometriosis. Fertil. Steril. **45:** 630–634.
10. GIUDICE, L.C. *et al.* 1986. Serum levels of CA-125 in patients with endometriosis. Gynecol. Oncol. **25:** 256–258.
11. PATTON, P.E. *et al.* 1986. CA-125 levels in endometriosis. Fertil. Steril. **45:** 770–773.
12. KONINCKX, P.R., S.H. KENNEDY & D.H. BARLOW. 1998. Endometriotic disease: the role of peritoneal fluid. Hum. Reprod. Update **4:** 741–751.

13. MATHUR, S.P. *et al.* 1998. Levels of antibodies to transferrin and α2-HS glycoprotein in women with and without endometriosis. Am. J. Reprod. Immunol. **40:** 69–73.
14. PILLAI, S. *et al.* 1996. Antibodies to endometrial transferrin and α2-Heremans Schmidt (HS) glycoprotein in patients with endometriosis. Am. J. Reprod. Immunol. **35:** 483–494. [1997. Erratum. Am. J . Reprod. Immunol. **37**(3): 277.]
15. LANG, G.A. & G.R. YEAMAN. 2001. Autoantibodies in endometriosis sera recognize a Thomsen-Friedenreich-like carbohydrate antigen. J. Autoimmun. **16:** 151–161.
16. KABIR, S. 1998. Jacalin: a jackfruit (*Artocarpus heterophyllus*) seed–derived lectin of versatile applications in immunobiological research. J. Immunol. Methods **212:** 193–211.
17. CAO, Y. *et al.* 1996. Thomsen-Friedenreich-related carbohydrate antigens in normal adult human tissues: a systematic and comparative study. Histochem. Cell Biol. **106:** 197–207.
18. RAVN, V. & H. JENSEN. 1988. Thomsen-Friedenreich-related antigen in human endometrium: an immunohistochemical study employing the monoclonal antibody 49H.8—a preliminary report. Acta Pathol. Microbiol. Immunol. Scand. **C96:** 552–558.
19. HORTIN, G.L. & B.L. TRIMPE. 1990. Lectin affinity chromatography of proteins bearing *O*-linked oligosaccharides: application of jacalin-agarose. Anal. Biochem. **188:** 271–277.
20. ZANETTI, M., G. LENERT & G.F. SPRINGER. 1993. Idiotypes of pre-existing human anti-carcinoma anti-T and anti-Tn antibodies. Int. Immunol. **5:** 113–119.
21. SPRINGER, G.F. 1997. Immunoreactive T and Tn epitopes in cancer diagnosis, prognosis, and immunotherapy. J. Mol. Med. **75:** 594–602.
22. BARONDES, S.H. *et al.* 1994. Galectins: structure and function of a large family of animal lectins. J. Biol. Chem. **269:** 20807–20810.
23. LEFFLER, H. & S.H. BARONDES. 1986. Specificity of binding of three soluble rat lung lectins to substituted and unsubstituted mammalian beta-galactosides. J. Biol. Chem. **261:** 10119–10126.
24. RABINOVICH, G.A. *et al.* 1999. Galectins: a key intersection between glycobiology and immunology. Braz. J. Med. Biol. Res. **32:** 383–393.
25. NANGIA-MAKKER, P. *et al.* 2000. Galectin-3 induces endothelial cell morphogenesis and angiogenesis. Am. J. Pathol. **156:** 899–909.
26. SANO, H. *et al.* 2000. Human galectin-3 is a novel chemoattractant for monocytes and macrophages. J. Immunol. **165:** 2156–2164.
27. SWARTE, V.V. *et al.* 1998. Lymphocyte triggering via L-selectin leads to enhanced galectin-3-mediated binding to dendritic cells. Eur. J. Immunol. **28:** 2864–2871.
28. PERILLO, N.L., M.E. MARCUS & L.G. BAUM. 1998. Galectins: versatile modulators of cell adhesion, cell proliferation, and cell death. J. Mol. Med. **76:** 402–412.
29. FOUILLIT, M. *et al.* 2000. Regulation of CD45-induced signaling by galectin-1 in Burkitt lymphoma B cells. Glycobiology **10:** 413–419.
30. RABINOVICH, G.A. *et al.* 1999. Specific inhibition of T-cell adhesion to extracellular matrix and proinflammatory cytokine secretion by human recombinant galectin-1. Immunology **97:** 100–106.
31. CORTEGANO, I. *et al.* 2000. Interaction between galectin-3 and FcγRII induces down-regulation of IL-5 gene: implication of the promoter sequence IL-5REIII. Glycobiology **10:** 237–242.
32. JENG, K.C., L.G. FRIGERI & F.T. LIU. 1994. An endogenous lectin, galectin-3 (epsilon BP/Mac-2), potentiates IL-1 production by human monocytes. Immunol. Lett. **42:** 113–116.
33. KARLSSON, A. *et al.* 1998. Galectin-3 activates the NADPH-oxidase in exudated, but not peripheral blood neutrophils. Blood **91:** 3430–3438.
34. YAMAOKA, A. *et al.* 1995. A human lectin, galectin-3 (epsilon bp/Mac-2), stimulates superoxide production by neutrophils. J. Immunol. **154:** 3479–3487.
35. KIJIMOTO-OCHIAI, S. & T. UEDE. 1995. CD23 molecule acts as a galactose-binding lectin in the cell aggregation of EBV-transformed human B-cell lines. Glycobiology **5:** 443–448.
36. KIJIMOTO-OCHIAI, S., E. HORIMOTO & T. UEDE. 1994. Demonstration of the interaction between the CD23 molecule and the galactose residue of glycoproteins. Immunol. Lett. **40:** 49–53.

37. Bailey, S. *et al.* 1998. Selective inhibition of low affinity IgE receptor (CD23) processing. Bioorg. Med. Chem. Lett. **8:** 29–34.
38. Guedez, L., L. Courtemanch & M. Stetler-Stevenson. 1998. Tissue inhibitor of metalloproteinase (TIMP)–1 induces differentiation and an antiapoptotic phenotype in germinal center B cells. Blood **92:** 1342–1349.
39. Wheeler, D.J. *et al.* 1998. Inhibition of sCD23 and immunoglobulin E release from human B cells by a metalloproteinase inhibitor, GI 129471. Immunology **95:** 105–110.
40. Odukoya, O.A. *et al.* 1996. Soluble CD23 protein in the peritoneal fluid of patients with endometriosis. Hum. Reprod. **11:** 2018–2021.
41. Odukoya, O., A. Bansal & I. Cooke. 1996. Serum endometrial IgG antibodies and soluble CD23 concentrations in patients with endometriosis. Acta Obstet. Gynecol. Scand. **75:** 927–931.
42. Odukoya, O.A. *et al.* 1995. Serum-soluble CD23 in patients with endometriosis and the effect of treatment with danazol and leuprolide acetate depot injection. Hum. Reprod. **10:** 942–946.
43. Lee, V.H. *et al.* 1998. Spatio-temporal pattern for expression of galectin-3 in the murine utero-placental complex: evidence for differential regulation. Biol. Reprod. **58:** 1277–1282.
44. Choe, Y.S. *et al.* 1997. Expression of galectin-1 mRNA in the mouse uterus is under the control of ovarian steroids during blastocyst implantation. Mol. Reprod. Dev. **48:** 261–266.
45. Maquoi, E. *et al.* 1997. Changes in the distribution pattern of galectin-1 and galectin-3 in human placenta correlate with the differentiation pathways of trophoblasts. Placenta **18:** 433–439.
46. Phillips, B. *et al.* 1996. Differential expression of two beta-galactoside-binding lectins in the reproductive tracts of pregnant mice. Biol. Reprod. **55:** 548–558.
47. Zeitoun, K.M. & S.E. Bulun. 1999. Aromatase: a key molecule in the pathophysiology of endometriosis and a therapeutic target. Fertil. Steril. **72:** 961–969.
48. Bulun, S.E. *et al.* 1999. Estrogen production in endometriosis and use of aromatase inhibitors to treat endometriosis. Endocr. Relat. Cancer **6:** 293–301.
49. Bulun, S.E. *et al.* 2000. Estrogen biosynthesis in endometriosis: molecular basis and clinical relevance. J. Mol. Endocrinol. **25:** 35–42.
50. Kitawaki, J. *et al.* 1999. Expression of aromatase cytochrome P450 in eutopic endometrium and its application as a diagnostic test for endometriosis. Gynecol. Obstet. Invest. **48:** 21–28.
51. Noble, L.S. *et al.* 1996. Aromatase expression in endometriosis. J. Clin. Endocrinol. Metab. **81:** 174–179.
52. Zeitoun, K. *et al.* 1998. Deficient 17β-hydroxysteroid dehydrogenase type 2 expression in endometriosis: failure to metabolize 17β-estradiol. J. Clin. Endocrinol. Metab. **83:** 4474–4480.
53. Noble, L.S. *et al.* 1997. Prostaglandin E2 stimulates aromatase expression in endometriosis-derived stromal cells. J. Clin. Endocrinol. Metab. **82:** 600–606.
54. Keenan, J.A. *et al.* 1995. IL-1β, TNF-α, and IL-2 in peritoneal fluid and macrophage-conditioned media of women with endometriosis. Am. J. Reprod. Immunol. **34:** 381–385.
55. Awadalla, S.G. *et al.* 1987. Local peritoneal factors: their role in infertility associated with endometriosis. Am. J. Obstet. Gynecol. **157:** 1207–1214.
56. Mori, H. *et al.* 1992. Expression of interleukin-1 (IL-1) beta messenger ribonucleic acid (mRNA) and IL-1 receptor antagonist mRNA in peritoneal macrophages from patients with endometriosis. Fertil. Steril. **57:** 535–542.
57. Taketani, Y., T.M. Kuo & M. Mizuno. 1992. Comparison of cytokine levels and embryo toxicity in peritoneal fluid in infertile women with untreated or treated endometriosis. Am. J. Obstet. Gynecol. **167:** 265–270.
58. Fakih, H. *et al.* 1987. Interleukin-1: a possible role in the infertility associated with endometriosis. Fertil. Steril. **47:** 213–217.
59. Hill, J.A. & D.J. Anderson. 1989. Lymphocyte activity in the presence of peritoneal fluid from fertile women and infertile women with and without endometriosis. Am. J. Obstet. Gynecol. **161:** 861–864.

60. KOYAMA, N., K. MATSUURA & H. OKAMURA. 1993. Cytokines in the peritoneal fluid of patients with endometriosis. Int. J. Gynaecol. Obstet. **43:** 45–50.
61. OVERTON, C. *et al.* 1996. Peritoneal fluid cytokines and the relationship with endometriosis and pain. Hum. Reprod. **11:** 380–386.
62. HARADA, T. *et al.* 1997. Increased interleukin-6 levels in peritoneal fluid of infertile patients with active endometriosis. Am. J. Obstet. Gynecol. **176:** 593–597.
63. RIER, S.E., A.K. PARSONS & J.L. BECKER. 1994. Altered interleukin-6 production by peritoneal leukocytes from patients with endometriosis. Fertil. Steril. **61:** 294–299.
64. RIER, S.E. *et al.* 1995. Dysregulation of interleukin-6 responses in ectopic endometrial stromal cells: correlation with decreased soluble receptor levels in peritoneal fluid of women with endometriosis. J. Clin. Endocrinol. Metab. **80:** 1431–1437.
65. BUYALOS, R.P. *et al.* 1992. Elevated interleukin-6 levels in peritoneal fluid of patients with pelvic pathology. Fertil. Steril. **58:** 302–306.
66. RANA, N. *et al.* 1996. Basal and stimulated secretion of cytokines by peritoneal macrophages in women with endometriosis. Fertil. Steril. **65:** 925–930.
67. EISERMANN, J. *et al.* 1988. Tumor necrosis factor in peritoneal fluid of women undergoing laparoscopic surgery. Fertil. Steril. **50:** 573–579.
68. HALME, J. 1989. Release of tumor necrosis factor-alpha by human peritoneal macrophages *in vivo* and *in vitro*. Am. J. Obstet. Gynecol. **161:** 1718–1725.
69. CRANE, I. *et al.* 1984. The preparation of interferon gamma–producing T-cell hybridomas from jacalin-stimulated T lymphocytes and the SH9 T-cell line. Immunology **53:** 855–859.
70. BLASCO, E. *et al.* 1995. Proliferative response of human CD4+ T lymphocytes stimulated by the lectin jacalin. Eur. J. Immunol. **25:** 2010–2018.
71. TAIMI, M. *et al.* 1994. Involvement of CD4 in interleukin-6 secretion by U937 monocytic cells stimulated with the lectin jacalin. J. Leukocyte Biol. **55:** 214–220.
72. GANGULY, S., D. SARKAR & J.J. GHOSH. 1976. Sialic acid and sialidase activity in human endometrial tissue, uterine fluid, and plasma under different conditions of uterine dysfunction. Acta Endocrinol. **81:** 574–579.
73. NELSON, J.D. *et al.* 1977. Glycosyltransferase and UDP-galactose pyrophosphatase activities in the endometrium during oestrous cycle of the rat. J. Endocrinol. **73:** 53–58.
74. ZHU, Z. *et al.* 1990. Glycosphingolipids of human myometrium and endometrium and their changes during the menstrual cycle, pregnancy, and ageing. J. Reprod. Fertil. **88:** 71–79.
75. RAVN, V. *et al.* 1992. The distribution of type-2 chain histo-blood group antigens in normal cycling human endometrium. Cell Tissue Res. **270:** 425–433.
76. CRAMER, D.W. *et al.* 1996. Endometriosis associated with the N314D mutation of galactose-1-phosphate uridyl transferase (GALT). Mol. Hum. Reprod. **2:** 149–152.
77. SHARPE-TIMMS, K.L. *et al.* 1998. Gonadotropin-releasing hormone agonist (GnRH-a) therapy alters activity of plasminogen activators, matrix metalloproteinases, and their inhibitors in rat models for adhesion formation and endometriosis: potential GnRH-a-regulated mechanisms reducing adhesion formation. Fertil. Steril. **69:** 916–923.
78. OSTEEN, K.G. *et al.* 1999. Paracrine regulation of matrix metalloproteinase expression in the normal human endometrium. Gynecol. Obstet. Invest. **48:** 2–13.
79. BRUNER, K.L. *et al.* 1995. Transforming growth factor beta mediates the progesterone suppression of an epithelial metalloproteinase by adjacent stroma in the human endometrium. Proc. Natl. Acad. Sci. U.S.A. **92:** 7362–7366.
80. BRUNER, K.L. *et al.* 1999. Progesterone and transforming growth factor-beta coordinately regulate suppression of endometrial matrix metalloproteinases in a model of experimental endometriosis. Steroids **64:** 648–653.
81. VAN DEN STEEN, P. *et al.* 1998. Oligosaccharides of recombinant mouse gelatinase B variants. Biochim. Biophys. Acta **1425:** 587–598.
82. OCHIENG, J. *et al.* 1994. Galectin-3 is a novel substrate for human matrix metalloproteinases-2 and -9. Biochemistry (Mosc.) **33:** 14109–14114.
83. OCHIENG, J. *et al.* 1998. Modulation of the biological functions of galectin-3 by matrix metalloproteinases. Biochim. Biophys. Acta **1379:** 97–106.
84. BROOKS, P.C. *et al.* 1998. Disruption of angiogenesis by PEX, a noncatalytic metalloproteinase fragment with integrin binding activity. Cell **92:** 391–400.

Macrophages, Oxidation, and Endometriosis

NALINI SANTANAM, ANA A. MURPHY, AND SAMPATH PARTHASARATHY

Department of Gynecology and Obstetrics, Emory University, Atlanta, Georgia, USA

ABSTRACT: Retrograde menstruation has been suggested to be the cause for the presence of endometrial cells in the peritoneal cavity. However, little is known about the events that lead to the adhesion and growth of these cells that ultimately result in endometriosis, considering the fact that the disease occurs only in certain women despite the common occurrence of retrograde menstruation in most women. We postulate that, in normal women, the endometrial cells and tissue that arrive in the peritoneal cavity during menstruation are effectively removed by macrophages that are chemoattracted and become resident tissue macrophages in the peritoneal cavity. In contrast, the peritoneal macrophages in women with endometriosis are nonadherent and ineffectively scavenged, resulting in the sustained presence and growth of the endometrial cells. We also postulate that the peritoneal fluid is not a passive reservoir of the factors secreted by cells of the peritoneum, but actively promotes endometriosis. The peritoneal fluid is rich in lipoproteins, particularly low-density lipoprotein, which generates oxidized lipid components in a macrophage-rich inflammatory milieu. The oxidants exacerbate the growth of endometriosis by inducing chemoattractants such as MCP-1 and endometrial cell growth-promoting activity. We provide evidence for the presence of oxidative milieu in the peritoneal cavity of women with endometriosis, the nonscavenging properties of macrophages that are nonadherent, and the synergistic interaction between macrophages, oxidative stress, and the endometrial cells. For example, the peritoneal fluid lipoproteins of subjects with endometriosis have increased the propensity to undergo oxidation as compared with plasma lipoproteins, and the subjects also have increased titer of autoantibodies to oxidatively modified proteins. If the oxidative proinflammatory nature of the peritoneal fluid is an important mediator of endometriosis growth, anti-inflammatory agents and antioxidants might afford protection against endometriosis.

KEYWORDS: macrophages; oxidation; endometriosis; endometrial cells; growth factors; lipoproteins; peritoneal fluid; cytokines

Endometriosis is a disease that afflicts women of reproductive age. It is defined as the presence of endometrial glands and stroma outside the endometrial cavity. Endometriosis has been noted in 10% to 50% of patients undergoing gynecologic laparotomies. The pathophysiology of this disease still remains elusive. The three common theories of its causes are (a) retrograde menstruation with subsequent implantation, (b) coelomic metaplasia, and (c) hematogenous or lymphatic transport of endometrial tissue.

Address for correspondence: Sampath Parthasarathy, Ph.D., Department of Gynecology and Obstetrics, Emory University School of Medicine, Atlanta, GA 30322. Voice: 404-727-8604; fax: 404-727-8615.

spartha@emory.edu

CELLULAR COMPONENTS ATTRIBUTED TO ENDOMETRIOSIS

Human endometrium is composed of glandular and surface epithelia that are invested by endometrial stroma. Lymphoid cells are scattered as single cells in endometrial stroma or within endometrial glands in the basalis T lymphocytes, while monocytes/macrophages constitute the major portion and the B cells, dendritic cells, and NK cells form a smaller population of the lymphoid cells. Both the lymphoid cells and the endometrial stromal and epithelial cells have proliferative activity.

ORIGIN OF ENDOMETRIAL CELLS IN THE PERITONEAL CAVITY

The presence of menstrual blood in the peritoneal cavity (PC) is a common occurrence and retrograde menstruation has been suggested to be the source of endometrial tissue in the PC.[1–5] Epithelial cells of menstrual origin have been noted in the PC[6–8] and endometrial cells have been cultured from the peritoneal fluid (PF).[9] A number of studies have shown that menstrual flow correlates with endometriosis.[1–5] The presence of menstrual blood in the PC is not restricted to women with endometriosis. Thus, it is unlikely that the mere presence of menstrual blood or endometrial cells will contribute to an antigenic response or to endometriosis. It would therefore seem that, if menstrual blood is an etiologic factor in endometriosis, the menstrual blood in the subjects with endometriosis is likely to have components that are unique and pathogenic.

To our knowledge, no one has ever speculated the basis for altered immunogenicity or the need for removal of the endometrial cells in the PC. A number of possibilities exist for endometrial cells in the PC to represent a foreign entity resulting in the recruitment of monocytes into the PC of endometriosis subjects. These include (a) the very presence of the endometrial tissue outside of the uterine endometrium, (b) changes in the cellularity (undigested tissue pieces as opposed to individual cells), and (c) alterations in cell phenotype (apoptotic endometrial cells and "damaged" red blood cells), which may represent a foreign presence and account for their chemotactic recruitment. Yet another possibility—that these cells are normal when they arrived at the PC, but are somehow altered in the PC to elicit a chemotactic response—should also be considered. The possibility that acellular components in the menstrual blood, for example, the menstrual blood plasma, may contain increased amounts of chemokines or might be capable of generating chemotactic activity for monocytes also cannot be ignored.

ARE THERE CHANGES IN THE ENDOMETRIAL CELLS THAT ARE DRAINED INTO THE PC?

Substantial quantities of endometrial cells are shed with blood during menstruation. Very little is known regarding the nature of these cells in menstrual blood or in the peritoneal milieu. The uterine endometrium undergoes considerable cyclic variations during the monthly cycle and the endometrial cells are destined for a programmed death at the end of the cycle. During the late proliferative and menstrual phase of the cycle, TNF-α and its receptor activity go up and the expression of Bcl-

2, a marker gene for protection against apoptosis, is reduced. More apoptotic endometrial cells appear at this phase.[10–14] Digestion of the extracellular matrix and disruption of blood supply to the endometrium would isolate the tissue from the uterus, thus depriving the cells of nutrients. Whether the apoptosis is augmented as a result of this nutritional deprivation process and whether the endometrial cells that are drained into the PC include a substantial proportion of apoptotic cells are not known.

Regardless of the proximal cause for apoptosis in the endometrium during late secretory menstrual phase, a growing body of evidence now suggests that apoptosis may involve oxidation mechanisms.[15–20] A number of oxidants induce apoptosis in cultured cells and antioxidants appear to protect against apoptotic cell death.[21] High levels of expression of Bcl-2 (Bcl-2 has now been recognized to act via antioxidant mechanisms) protect cells against apoptosis.[22] Lack of blood supply, hormonal factors, and the presence of heme and its products, including free iron, may contribute to oxidative stress and promote apoptotic cell death. It is thus likely that the endometrial cells that are shed during menstruation are apoptotic and are "programmed" to die. Yet, since the growth of the ectopic endometrium is the basis of endometriosis, it is possible that their new environment in the PC is conducive to their revival and growth.

MACROPHAGES RECRUITED IN THE PC

The presence of macrophages in the PC of rodents is well known. Their presence is assumed to be a normal physiological occurrence. Usually about 7% of monocytes in circulation are constantly drained, although not exclusively into the PC. The introduction of irritants such as thioglycollate, talc, bacteria, and others results in a greater recruitment of these cells into the PC. The presence of macrophages in human PC, however, is commonly associated with an inflammatory process. For example, the presence of pathogens or the growth of tumors in the PC is often accompanied by an increase in the presence of macrophages in the ascites fluid.[23–26] The well-documented increased presence of macrophages in women suffering from endometriosis[2,27–33] is unexpected as no pathogens have been implicated in the disease. Obviously, the ectopic endometrium itself represents an alien presence that results in the influx of monocytes into the PC. Macrophages in the PC can serve a variety of functions. The immunological association of macrophages and T lymphocytes may demand that macrophages process the foreign invading endometrial cells and present suitable antigenic targets for the generation of antibodies. A corollary to the immune theory of endometriosis is the obligatory recognition, uptake, and processing of endometrial cells by macrophages. In other words, the scavenger function of macrophages may be synonymous with their immunological role. However, the a priori assumption that "normal" endometrial cells may be recognized by macrophages in the PC as an alien entity is not supported by the observation that macrophages are normal constituents of the endometrium.[34–36] Macrophages and endometrial cells coexist in the endometrium and there are cyclic variations in the presence and number of macrophages in the normal uterus.

The increased number of PC macrophages in women with endometriosis[2,27–33] may indicate that, for some reason, the presence of endometrial tissue in the PC represents a foreign entity and needs to be removed. A number of studies have documented that normal women have fewer mononuclear cells in the PF[2,27–33] and most of these cells may represent a less-differentiated monocytic phenotype. In contrast, cells in the PF of endometriosis subjects are more differentiated macrophages. The PC macrophages are nonadherent and can be easily lavaged. The increased number of mononuclear cells in the PF of endometriosis subjects may be due to increased chemotactic activity of the PF.[37–39] A number of studies have documented an increase in specific chemotactic agents such as monocyte chemotactic protein-1 (MCP-1),[38,40] RANTES,[39,41] and lyso-phosphatidylcholine (lyso-PC) in the PF of endometriosis subjects.[42] Conversely, the decreased lavageable mononuclear cells in the PC of normal women could be due to their increased efflux from the PC or increased presence of adherent cells.

OXIDIZED RED BLOOD CELLS (RBC) IN THE MENSTRUUM?

There is a considerable loss of blood during menstruation. The hemoglobin content of RBC and their ability to carry oxygen make these cells particularly vulnerable to oxidation. The peroxidase activity of heme to catalyze oxidation reactions is well founded.[43,44] If the digestion of extracellular matrix and disruption of blood supply result in nutritional deprivation and promote apoptosis in endometrial cells, similar changes may occur in RBC. In normal RBC, phosphatidylserine (PS) is asymmetrically exposed facing the inside of the bilayer membrane and is maintained by the enzyme translocase.[45,46] This is an ATP-requiring enzyme and its inactivation results in the exposure of PS on the outside. In senescent RBC, high levels of PS are exposed at the surface, presumably as a result of inactivation of this enzyme. Oxidation of RBC mimics *in vivo* aging and exposes PS at the surface. However, in the menstrual blood, outside the arterioles and venules, the RBC are nutritionally deprived and are also subjected to the actions of digestive enzymes released by the degrading endometrium. Thus, it is likely that the damaged RBC would provide an ideal target for the recruitment of monocytes; however, the very definition of chemotaxis (directional movement across a soluble chemical gradient) precludes intact "damaged RBC" or "apoptotic" endometrial cells themselves to act as chemotactic stimuli. The chemotactic agent must be secreted by the endometrial cells or by the RBC. In the latter case, the shedding of a membrane protein, peroxidized lipid components, or lyso-PC may represent it.

MACROPHAGES AS SCAVENGERS OF ENDOMETRIAL COMPONENTS IN THE PC

One of the vital functions of the mononuclear phagocytes in the face of an invading "foreign" material is the scavenger function. A variety of receptors such as the Fc receptor, the acetyl LDL receptor, macrosialin, SR-B1, and CD36 may be involved in this function (unpublished observation).[47–52] The Fc receptor–mediated clearance would require antigen-antibody complexes and the role of CD36 is yet poorly defined. The acetyl LDL receptor has been cloned, sequenced, and expressed in cells and can perform as a true endocytotic receptor.[50,53–55] This receptor has been suggested to be involved in the recognition and uptake of a variety of polyanionic molecules.[50] Our recent studies have revealed yet another scavenger receptor on macrophages that recognizes, among other ligands, oxidatively modified lipoproteins, PS, oxidatively damaged RBC, and apoptotic cells.[47,51]

Even if abnormal RBC and apoptotic endometrial cells are present in menstrual blood of women with endometriosis, why are they not cleared by the macrophage scavenger receptor(s)? Is it possible that the peritoneal macrophages from women with endometriosis do not express fully functional scavenger receptors? The scavenger receptor of macrophages is highly regulated by a number of factors, including cytokines, glucocorticoids, LPS, TNF-α, γ-interferon (IFN-γ), M-CSF, and retinoids.[56–66] These cytokines and hormones are present in altered levels in the PF of endometriosis and may play a role in the expression of SCR.

Yet another suggestion for the potential altered scavenger function in the macrophages of the PF may come from the studies of Gordon and coworkers.[66–69] They demonstrated that scavenger receptor may also play a role in the cellular adhesion process, and an antibody to the scavenger receptor also blocked the adhesion of cells to culture dishes. Accordingly, macrophages that are not adherent and are not attached to extracellular matrix in tissues do not express scavenger receptors.[70] Studies from Krieger and coworkers have shown that the scavenger receptor is expressed at the surface as a trimeric protein.[53,71] The binding of ligands to monomers has not been demonstrated. It is likely that adherence of the cell may be due to both new synthesis of the protein as well as the export of the monomers to the cell surface or their trimerization. Thus, in contrast to tissue macrophages, the PF macrophages that are not attached to extracellular matrix components, despite their differentiated status, may not be competent scavengers. A decreased expression of several integrins, $\alpha_V\beta_3$ in particular, has been noted in the endometrium of women with endometriosis.[72,73] Whether such low expression is an inherent defect in women with endometriosis is an important question that has to be addressed.

DO MACROPHAGES PLAY A ROLE IN THE ECTOPIC GROWTH OF ENDOMETRIAL CELLS?

A number of growth-promoting activities have been noted in the PF. These include platelet-derived growth factor (PDGF), endothelial cell growth factor (EGF), vascular endothelial cell–derived growth factor (VEGF), and basic fibroblast growth factor (bFGF).[74–78] The contribution of some of these to the growth of the ectopic endometrium has been questioned recently. In addition, both monocytes and macrophages stimulate the growth of endometrial cells[79,80] by mechanisms not known. However, it does not appear to be an intrinsic nature of monocytes/macrophages to secrete growth-promoting activity for endometrial cells. It has been noted that peripheral blood monocytes from women with endometriosis may support growth of endometrial cells, whereas cells from control subjects failed to support endometrial growth.[80] This finding would suggest that there might be factors in the peripheral blood of endometriosis subjects that activate the synthesis of growth factors. In other words, the monocytes from these subjects are already primed to generate growth-promoting activity. The identity of such activity or the factors that control the expression of such activity are not known at present. The preliminary results presented here would suggest that macrophages from the same subjects also promote the growth of endometrial cells.

PF OF ENDOMETRIOSIS SUBJECTS

The PF of endometriosis subjects has been studied with great interest for a long time. As a result, a plethora of information is available on the presence and levels of hormones, prostanoids, cytokines, growth factors, chemokines, and various biochemical parameters. There is a long list of components that are present at higher or lower levels in the PF of endometriosis subjects and, as a result, some type of association is suggested between their presence and the disease process itself. These components include prostaglandin products, IL-1, IL-6, glycodelin, MCP-1, RANTES, TNF-α, IFN-γ, M-CSF, various growth-promoting activities, iron, enzymes, hormones, and others.[31,39,74,75,79,81–99] The reason that these components are elevated or decreased in the PF is not understood—for example, the reason why MCP-1 or M-CSF genes are induced has not been studied.

IS THERE A CONNECTION BETWEEN ENDOMETRIOSIS AND ATHEROSCLEROSIS?

Endometriosis affects younger women, whereas atherosclerosis is a disease of "old age." In fact, younger women are protected from coronary artery disease. These two diseases, although seemingly unrelated, are remarkably alike. Both have tissue macrophages that express scavenger receptors and these macrophages are exposed to lipoproteins. More importantly, both atherosclerotic lesions and the PF of women with endometriosis are characterized by the presence of inflammatory cytokines, chemokines, and growth factors. For example, lipoproteins (LDL, HDL), macrophages, and cytokines derived from macrophages; T cells and cytokines derived from T cells; chemotactic factors for T cells and macrophages; growth factors; and mildly oxidized LDL have been noted both in the atherosclerotic lesion and in the PF of women with endometriosis. More importantly, these are suggested to play similar roles, for example, recruitment of monocytes, growth promotion, and generation of localized inflammation, at these sites.

LIPOPROTEINS IN THE PF

The PF is derived from follicular fluid and secretions from the cells of fallopian tubes, uterus, and the peritoneal wall and fluid.[100] Follicular fluid lipoproteins have been well studied.[101–103] Follicular fluid is rich in HDL and very little, if any, LDL and VLDL are present. Liver and intestine are the major lipoprotein-producing organs and it is very unlikely that VLDL and LDL are generated by the cells of the uterus, fallopian tubes, or PC. We recently observed that the PF of endometriosis subjects contains substantial quantities of LDL, suggesting the infiltration of plasma components into the PC, thus mimicking components that are present in inflammatory, interstitial fluid. Very little, if any, LDL was present in the PF of control subjects. The PF lipoproteins are distinct from the plasma in having several major nutrients depleted during their passage through the endothelial cell barrier of the blood vessels. Besides, large lipoprotein (VLDL and chylomicrons) cellular components of blood do not cross the endothelial barrier.

OXIDIZED LDL

The importance of oxidative modifications of LDL (Ox-LDL) in the pathogenesis of atherosclerosis is now well recognized[104–106] and treatments based on antioxidant properties are already in clinical trials. The general properties of Ox-LDL have been reviewed in a number of publications and we will briefly review information pertaining to the current application. Its detection primarily involves marginal increases in electrophoretic mobility and bioassay for the induction of MCP-1 and M-CSF genes, as well as the chemical identification of peroxidized phospholipids.

OXIDIZED LDL AND MACROPHAGES

The presence of an increased number of monocytes/macrophages in the PF of endometriosis subjects as compared to normal women has been well documented.[31,75,81,110] There is a growing body of evidence suggesting that the presence of activated macrophages and LDL together may lead to oxidation.[108–111] Specific enzymatic oxidations of lipoproteins by 15-lipoxygenase and myeloperoxidase, by either direct interactions or seeding mechanisms, have been suggested.[55,111–113] Monocytes, which are precursors of macrophages, do not possess 15-lipoxygenase and readily express this enzyme upon differentiation into macrophages. Cytokines such as IL-4 and IL-13 activate this enzyme and the presence of this enzyme activity has been observed only in mouse peritoneal and tissue macrophages.[114–116] We reported the presence of this enzyme in mouse peritoneal macrophages,[117] suggesting that PF macrophages, at least in this animal, are present in an already differentiated form. Two important diseases, atherosclerosis and endometriosis, with no obvious connections to each other, represent conditions that would place activated macrophages and lipoproteins together. In both diseases, the commonalities include recruitment and retention of monocytes/macrophages, differentiation and growth of monocytes and smooth muscle cells (or endometrial cells), activation of inflammatory genes, and cytotoxicity.[55,118]

IS THERE ANY EVIDENCE TO SUGGEST THAT THE FACTORS THAT MAY BE INVOLVED IN ENDOMETRIOSIS MAY BE INDUCED BY AN OXIDATIVE STRESS?

A number of components have been identified to be present at increased levels in the PF of endometriosis subjects. Some of these may or may not play a role in endometriosis. As mentioned earlier, the factors that influence and induce the expression of the genes for these proteins in the PF of endometriosis subjects are not known. However, these genes have been well studied in other diseases and it has now been recognized that oxidants may be responsible for the induction of these genes. Many of them have NFκB or AP-1 response elements in their genes, which are known to be associated with oxidative stress.[15,17,21,119] In TABLE 1, we present suggestions from literature that would imply that oxidized lipids and lipoproteins might enhance the formation of some of these components.

TABLE 1. Can oxidized lipids/lipoproteins induce components associated with endometriosis?

	Activators	
Component	Nonoxidant	Oxidant
MCP-1	IL-1, TNF-α, LPS	Oxidized phospholipids of mildly Ox-LDL
CSF-1, M-CSF	IL-1, TNF-α	Oxidized phospholipids of mildly Ox-LDL
IL-1	LPS	Lipid peroxides, products derived from lipid peroxides, Ox-LDL, oxidatively modified proteins
RANTES	IFN-γ, TNF-α	Contains NFκB-activated domains suggesting potential activation by oxidants
IL-6	Glycodelin	
PDGF, FGF		Ox-LDL, lyso-PC
Prostaglandins	LPS, innumerable cell activators	Innumerable cross-reactive PG-like products

IS THE PERITONEAL ENVIRONMENT IN THE PATIENT WITH ENDOMETRIOSIS CONDUCIVE TO AN OXIDATIVE PROINFLAMMATORY STATUS?

The presence of oxidized lipids and oxidatively modified proteins has been demonstrated in the atherosclerotic artery wherein macrophages and LDL interact to generate the foam cells of the fatty streak lesion. Studies by Mitchinson and coworkers[120,121] have also shown that the mere presence of macrophages with lipoproteins is sufficient to generate oxidized lipids and ceroid-like lipid-protein complexes. The PF is rich in lipoproteins, particularly LDL. Our studies show that the concentration of LDL can be as much as 40% of its plasma concentration. In fact, if one compares it to arterial LDL concentration, it can be severalfold higher. Considering the co-occurrence of activated macrophages and LDL in the PF, it is likely that oxidation is a major event in the peritoneum. Furthermore, the PF LDL may be already depleted of its antioxidants during its passage through the capillary endothelium, thus becoming increasingly susceptible to lipid peroxidation.

IS THERE ANY EVIDENCE TO SUGGEST THAT PF LIPOPROTEINS MAY REPRESENT OXIDIZED LIPOPROTEIN?

Raymond and colleagues have used a sponge implantation model to document the "oxidized nature" of the sponge-associated lipoproteins.[122–128] In this model, a sponge was implanted subcutaneously and, after some time, was taken out and squeezed to obtain the "inflammatory interstitial fluid". Lipoproteins of the atherosclerotic lesion have been well studied and characterized.[129–132] Studies from Hoff and coworkers and from others have provided evidence to suggest that LDL isolated from the interstitial fluid of lesions is different from plasma LDL. The lesion LDL showed characteristics of oxidized LDL,[105,110] showed evidence of aggregation and increased electrophoretic mobility, and cross-reacted with antibodies generated against oxidized LDL. Immunohistochemical evidence also has provided evidence documenting that modified lipid-protein adducts resembling those in oxidized LDL are present in the atherosclerotic artery and may be localized near the macrophage.[106,112,133] Metal ions have significantly enhanced lipid peroxidation.[134,135] Increased amounts of iron have been noted in the PF of women with endometriosis, perhaps indicative of the release from macrophages that took up damaged RBC.[97,99] The presence of increased amounts of iron in endometriotic tissue (with the characteristic rustic appearance) has been known for a long time. Despite these lines of indirect, circumstantial evidence, there has been no direct evidence for the occurrence of lipid peroxidation in the cul-de-sac fluid.[98] In fact, the TBARS assay (a test for the terminal, water-soluble degradation products of lipid peroxidation) failed to find any differences in their amounts in the PF of normal and endometriosis subjects.[98] This could be due to rapid removal of these products from the peritoneum, the poor sensitivity of the assay, or more importantly the presence of not extensively oxidized LDL, but mildly oxidized LDL in the PF. Such LDL does not possess increased levels of MDA or F_2-isoprostanes.

PF AND PROLIFERATION OF ENDOMETRIOSIS

It has been hypothesized that growth-promoting substances in PF may enhance the ectopic growth of endometrial cells.[76–78,136] However, little data are known about which factors within the PF compartment promote endometrial cell proliferation, which is presumed to be the essence of disease initiation and progression. Hammond *et al.* showed an increase in endometrial stromal cell proliferation with the addition of cell-free PF of endometriosis patients when compared to fertile controls with similar PF estradiol concentration.[92] Halme *et al.* have shown that conditioned media of activated macrophages of women with endometriosis can induce a significantly greater degree of fibroblast growth than fertile controls or infertile patients with tubal abnormalities.[75] This "macrophage-derived growth factor" has been shown to be distinct from IL-1 and may well be composed, at least partially, of PDGF and FGF. Furthermore, Olive has shown that macrophage-conditioned media from patients with endometriosis can function as a competence growth factor.[79] A competence factor confers on the cell the ability to respond to specific mitogens, and a progression factor causes a "competent" cell to progress through the G_1 phase to the S phase of cell growth. Macrophage-derived growth factors stimulate stromal growth in the presence of a known progression factor (insulin) in serum-free media, but cannot promote growth with insulin-free serum. Recently, the proliferation of endometrial cells in the presence of monocytes has been described.[80]

Products of lipid peroxidation have profound effects on cell growth. Recent studies have shown that lipid peroxides induce cellular oncogene expression and promote protein phosphorylation reactions involved in cell signaling and growth.[137,138] Ox-LDL promotes smooth muscle cell proliferation at low concentrations,[139] presumably as a result of induction of the PDGF gene. The biochemical mechanisms involved in Ox-LDL-mediated proliferation of smooth muscle may involve the presence of lyso-PC.[139] Both m-LDL and Ox-LDL have increased levels of lyso-PC. The incubation of aortic endothelial cells with Ox-LDL results in a sevenfold increase in the secretion of GM-CSF and a severalfold increase in mRNA and protein levels of bFGF.[139] The induction of the latter has also been attributed to the presence of lyso-PC. The role of lipid peroxidation products in promoting proliferation of endometrial cells is unexplored.

While the above discussion presents an intriguing picture, the question of whether promotion of macrophage adhesion and prevention of inflammatory response would alleviate pain and infertility associated with endometriosis cannot be answered easily. More basic research into the factors that prevent macrophage adhesion and endometrial cell growth is needed to generate criteria that can be used to further test the hypothesis.

ACKNOWLEDGMENTS

This work was supported by NIH Grant No. PO1 HD5276 and by generous funds from the Department of Gynecology and Obstetrics of the Emory University School of Medicine. We thank John A. Rock for his continued support.

REFERENCES

1. HALME, J., M.G. HAMMOND, J.F. HULKA *et al.* 1984. Retrograde menstruation in healthy women and in patients with endometriosis. Obstet. Gynecol. **64:** 151–154.
2. HALME, J., S. BECKER, M.G. HAMMOND & S. RAJ. 1982. Pelvic macrophages in normal and infertile women: the role of patent tubes. Am. J. Obstet. Gynecol. **142:** 890–895.
3. D'HOOGHE, T.M., C.S. BAMBRA, B.M. RAEYMAEKERS & P.R. KONINCKX. 1996. Increased prevalence and recurrence of retrograde menstruation in baboons with spontaneous endometriosis. Hum. Reprod. **11:** 2022–2025.
4. KRUITWAGEN, R.F. 1993. Menstruation as the pelvic aggressor. Bailliere's Clin. Obstet. Gynaecol. **7:** 687–700.
5. DARROW, S.L., J.E. VENA, R.E. BATT *et al.* 1993. Menstrual cycle characteristics and the risk of endometriosis. Epidemiology **4:** 135–142.
6. BARTOSIK, D., S.L. JACOBS & L.J. KELLY. 1986. Endometrial tissue in peritoneal fluid. Fertil. Steril. **46:** 796–800.
7. VAN DER WEIDEN, R.M., P.W. ARENTZ & M. VESELIC. 1992. Endometrial cells in the peritoneal cavity after laparoscopy and chromotubation. J. R. Soc. Med. **85:** 397–398.
8. KRUITWAGEN, R.F., L.G. POELS, W.N. WILLEMSEN *et al.* 1991. Retrograde seeding of endometrial epithelial cells by uterine-tubal flushing. Fertil. Steril. **56:** 414–420.
9. BADAWY, S.Z., V. CUENCA, A. STITZEL & D. TICE. 1987. Immune rosettes of T and B lymphocytes in infertile women with endometriosis. J. Reprod. Med. **32:** 194–197.
10. VINATIER, D., P. DUFOUR & D. SUBTIL. 1996. Apoptosis: a programmed cell death involved in ovarian and uterine physiology. Eur. J. Obstet. Gynecol. Reprod. Biol. **67:** 85–102.
11. SPENCER, S.J., N.A. CATALDO & R.B. JAFFE. 1996. Apoptosis in the human female reproductive tract. Obstet. Gynecol. Surv. **51:** 314–323.
12. MCLAREN, J., A. PRENTICE, D.S. CHARNOCK-JONES *et al.* 1997. Immunolocalization of the apoptosis regulating proteins Bcl-2 and Bax in human endometrium and isolated peritoneal fluid macrophages in endometriosis. Hum. Reprod. **12:** 146–152.
13. WATANABE, H., H. KANZAKI, S. NARUKAWA *et al.* 1997. Bcl-2 and Fas expression in eutopic and ectopic human endometrium during the menstrual cycle in relation to endometrial cell apoptosis. Am. J. Obstet. Gynecol. **176:** 360–368.
14. KOKAWA, K., T. SHIKONE & R. NAKANO. 1996. Apoptosis in the human uterine endometrium during the menstrual cycle. J. Clin. Endocrinol. Metab. **81:** 4144–4147.
15. SANDSTROM, P.A., D. PARDI, P.W. TEBBEY *et al.* 1995. Lipid hydroperoxide-induced apoptosis: lack of inhibition by Bcl-2 over-expression. FEBS Lett. **365:** 66–70.

16. KORSMEYER, S.J., J.R. SHUTTER, D.J. VEIS *et al.* 1993. Bcl-2/Bax: a rheostat that regulates an anti-oxidant pathway and cell death. Semin. Cancer Biol. **4:** 327–332.
17. HOCKENBERY, D.M., Z.N. OLTVAI, X.M. YIN *et al.* 1993. Bcl-2 functions in an antioxidant pathway to prevent apoptosis. Cell **75:** 241–251.
18. SLATER, A.F., C.S. NOBEL, E. MAELLARO *et al.* 1995. Nitrone spin traps and a nitroxide antioxidant inhibit a common pathway of thymocyte apoptosis. Biochem. J. **306:** 771–778.
19. GREENSPAN, H.C. & O.I. ARUOMA. 1994. Oxidative stress and apoptosis in HIV infection: a role for plant-derived metabolites with synergistic antioxidant activity. Immunol. Today **15:** 209–213.
20. HAWKINS, C.J. & D.L. VAUX. 1994. Analysis of the role of bcl-2 in apoptosis. Immunol. Rev. **142:** 127–139.
21. BESSHO, R., K. MATSUBARA, M. KUBOTA *et al.* 1994. Pyrrolidine dithiocarbamate, a potent inhibitor of nuclear factor kappa B (NF-kappa B) activation, prevents apoptosis in human promyelocytic leukemia HL-60 cells and thymocytes. Biochem. Pharmacol. **48:** 1883–1889.
22. FARLIE, P.G., R. DRINGEN, S.M. REES *et al.* 1995. Bcl-2 transgene expression can protect neurons against developmental and induced cell death. Proc. Natl. Acad. Sci. U.S.A. **92:** 4397–4401.
23. PRUIMBOOM, W.M., A.P. VAN DIJK, C.J. TAK *et al.* 1994. Production of inflammatory mediators by human macrophages obtained from ascites. Prostaglandins Leukotrienes Essent. Fatty Acids **50:** 183–192.
24. BROWNLOW, M.A. 1982. Mononuclear phagocytes of peritoneal fluid. Equine Vet. J. **14:** 325–328.
25. KUBICKA, U., W.L. OLSZEWSKI, W. TARNOWSKI *et al.* 1996. Normal human immune peritoneal cells: subpopulations and functional characteristics. Scand. J. Immunol. **44:** 157–163.
26. BERKE, G. & B. SCHICK. 1980. Tumor immunity in the peritoneal cavity. Contemp. Top. Immunobiol. **10:** 297–315.
27. HALME, J., S. BECKER & R. WING. 1984. Accentuated cyclic activation of peritoneal macrophages in patients with endometriosis. Am. J. Obstet. Gynecol. **148:** 85–90.
28. HALME, J., S. BECKER, M.G. HAMMOND *et al.* 1983. Increased activation of pelvic macrophages in infertile women with mild endometriosis. Am. J. Obstet. Gynecol. **145:** 333–337.
29. HANEY, A.F. 1993. Endometriosis, macrophages, and adhesions. Prog. Clin. Biol. Res. **81:** 19–44.
30. HALME, J., S. BECKER & S. HASKILL. 1987. Altered maturation and function of peritoneal macrophages: possible role in pathogenesis of endometriosis. Am. J. Obstet. Gynecol. **156:** 783–789.
31. UEKI, M., T. TSURUNAGA, T. USHIROYAMA & M. UEDA. 1994. Macrophage activation factors and cytokines in peritoneal fluid from patients with endometriosis. Asia Oceania J. Obstet. Gynaecol. **20:** 427–431.
32. DUNSELMAN, G.A., M.G. HENDRIX, P.X. BOUCKAERT & J.L. EVERS. 1988. Functional aspects of peritoneal macrophages in endometriosis of women. J. Reprod. Fertil. **82:** 707–710.
33. COLACURCI, N., F. ZULLO, C. CARRAVETTA *et al.* 1991. Immune system and endometriosis. Acta Eur. Fertil. **22:** 161–162.
34. BONATZ, G., M.L. HANSMANN, F. BUCHHOLZ *et al.* 1992. Macrophage- and lymphocyte-subtypes in the endometrium during different phases of the ovarian cycle. Int. J. Gynaecol. Obstet. **37:** 29–36.
35. LEA, R.G. & D.A. CLARK. 1991. Macrophages and migratory cells in endometrium relevant to implantation. Bailliere's Clin. Obstet. Gynaecol. **5:** 25–59.
36. STARKEY, P.M., L.M. CLOVER & M.C. REES. 1991. Variation during the menstrual cycle of immune cell populations in human endometrium. Eur. J. Obstet. Gynecol. Reprod. Biol. **39:** 203–207.
37. WEIL, S.J., S. WANG, M.C. PEREZ & C.R. LYTTLE. 1997. Chemotaxis of macrophages by a peritoneal fluid protein in women with endometriosis. Fertil. Steril. **67:** 865–869.

38. ARICI, A., E. ORAL, E. ATTAR *et al.* 1997. Monocyte chemotactic protein-1 concentration in peritoneal fluid of women with endometriosis and its modulation of expression in mesothelial cells. Fertil. Steril. **67:** 1065–1072.
39. KHORRAM, O., R.N. TAYLOR, I.P. RYAN *et al.* 1993. Peritoneal fluid concentrations of the cytokine RANTES correlate with the severity of endometriosis. Am. J. Obstet. Gynecol. **169:** 1545–1549.
40. AKOUM, A., A. LEMAY, S.R. MCCOLL *et al.* 1996. Increased monocyte chemotactic protein-1 level and activity in the peripheral blood of women with endometriosis. Am. J. Obstet. Gynecol. **175:** 1620–1625.
41. HORNUNG, D., I.P. RYAN, V.A. CHAO *et al.* 1997. Immunolocalization and regulation of the chemokine RANTES in human endometrial and endometriosis tissues and cells. J. Clin. Endocrinol. Metab. **82:** 1621–1628.
42. MURPHY, A.A., N. SANTANAM, A.J. MORALES & S. PARTHASARATHY. 1998. Lysophosphatidylcholine, a chemotactic factor for monocytes/T-lymphocytes, is elevated in endometriosis. J. Clin. Endocrinol. Metab. **83:** 2110–2113.
43. VERCELLOTTI, G.M., G. BALLA, J. BALLA *et al.* 1994. Heme and the vasculature: an oxidative hazard that induces antioxidant defenses in the endothelium. Artif. Cells Blood Substit. Immobil. Biotechnol. **22:** 207–213.
44. BALLA, G., H.S. JACOB, J.W. EATON *et al.* 1991. Hemin: a possible physiological mediator of low density lipoprotein oxidation and endothelial injury. Arterioscler. Thromb. **11:** 1700–1711.
45. CONNOR, J. & A.J. SCHROIT. 1989. Transbilayer movement of phosphatidylserine in nonhuman erythrocytes: evidence that the aminophospholipid transporter is a ubiquitous membrane protein. Biochemistry **28:** 9680–9685.
46. CONNOR, J. & A.J. SCHROIT. 1991. Transbilayer movement of phosphatidylserine in erythrocytes: inhibitors of aminophospholipid transport block the association of photolabeled lipid to its transporter. Biochim. Biophys. Acta **1066:** 37–42.
47. RAMPRASAD, M.P., W. FISCHER, J.L. WITZTUM *et al.* 1995. The 94- to 97-kDa mouse macrophage membrane protein that recognizes oxidized low density lipoprotein and phosphatidylserine-rich liposomes is identical to macrosialin, the mouse homologue of human CD68. Proc. Natl. Acad. Sci. U.S.A. **92:** 9580–9584.
48. STANTON, L.W., R.T. WHITE, C.M. BRYANT *et al.* 1992. A macrophage Fc receptor for IgG is also a receptor for oxidized low density lipoprotein. J. Biol. Chem. **267:** 22446–22451.
49. ENDEMANN, G., L.W. STANTON, K.S. MADDEN *et al.* 1993. CD36 is a receptor for oxidized low density lipoprotein. J. Biol. Chem. **268:** 11811–11816.
50. BROWN, M.S., S.K. BASU, J.R. FALCK *et al.* 1980. The scavenger cell pathway for lipoprotein degradation: specificity of the binding site that mediates the uptake of negatively-charged LDL by macrophages. J. Supramol. Struct. **13:** 67–81.
51. OTTNAD, E., S. PARTHASARATHY, G.R. SAMBRANO *et al.* 1995. A macrophage receptor for oxidized low density lipoprotein distinct from the receptor for acetyl low density lipoprotein: partial purification and role in recognition of oxidatively damaged cells. Proc. Natl. Acad. Sci. U.S.A. **92:** 1391–1395.
52. NICHOLSON, A.C., S. FRIEDA, A. PEARCE & R.L. SILVERSTEIN. 1995. Oxidized LDL binds to CD36 on human monocyte-derived macrophages and transfected cell lines: evidence implicating the lipid moiety of the lipoprotein as the binding site. Arterioscler. Thromb. Vasc. Biol. **15:** 269–275.
53. KODAMA, T., P. REDDY, C. KISHIMOTO & M. KRIEGER. 1988. Purification and characterization of a bovine acetyl low density lipoprotein receptor. Proc. Natl. Acad. Sci. U.S.A. **85:** 9238–9242.
54. STEINBERG, D., S. PARTHASARATHY, T.E. CAREW *et al.* 1989. Beyond cholesterol: modifications of low-density lipoprotein that increase its atherogenicity. N. Engl. J. Med. **320:** 915–924.
55. PARTHASARATHY, S. 1994. Modified Lipoproteins in the Pathogenesis of Atherosclerosis. R. G. Landes Co. Austin, TX.
56. MOULTON, K.S., H. WU, J. BARNETT *et al.* 1992. Regulated expression of the human acetylated low density lipoprotein receptor gene and isolation of promoter sequences. Proc. Natl. Acad. Sci. U.S.A. **89:** 8102–8106.

57. Wu, H., K. Moulton, A. Horvai *et al.* 1994. Combinatorial interactions between AP-1 and ets domain proteins contribute to the developmental regulation of the macrophage scavenger receptor gene. Mol. Cell. Biol. **14:** 2129–2139.
58. Geng, Y.J. & G.K. Hansson. 1992. Interferon-gamma inhibits scavenger receptor expression and foam cell formation in human monocyte-derived macrophages. J. Clin. Invest. **89:** 1322–1330.
59. Bottalico, L.A., R.E. Wager, L.B. Agellon *et al.* 1991. Transforming growth factor-beta 1 inhibits scavenger receptor activity in THP-1 human macrophages. J. Biol. Chem. **266:** 22866–22871.
60. Fong, L.G. 1996. Modulation of macrophage scavenger receptor transport by protein phosphorylation. J. Lipid Res. **37:** 574–587.
61. Hara, H., H. Tanishita, S. Yokoyama *et al.* 1987. Induction of acetylated low density lipoprotein receptor and suppression of low density lipoprotein receptor on the cells of human monocytic leukemia cell line (THP-1 cell). Biochem. Biophys. Res. Commun. **146:** 802–808.
62. Tabas, I., G.C. Boykow & A.R. Tall. 1987. Foam cell–forming J774 macrophages have markedly elevated acyl coenzyme A:cholesterol acyl transferase activity compared with mouse peritoneal macrophages in the presence of low density lipoprotein (LDL) despite similar LDL receptor activity. J. Clin. Invest. **79:** 418–426.
63. Hirsch, L.J. & T. Mazzone. 1986. Dexamethasone modulates lipoprotein metabolism in cultured human monocyte-derived macrophages: stimulation of scavenger receptor activity. J. Clin. Invest. **77:** 485–490.
64. van Lenten, B.J. & A.M. Fogelman. 1992. Lipopolysaccharide-induced inhibition of scavenger receptor expression in human monocyte-macrophages is mediated through tumor necrosis factor-alpha. J. Immunol. **148:** 112–116.
65. Fong, L.G., T.A. Fong & A.D. Cooper. 1990. Inhibition of mouse macrophage degradation of acetyl–low density lipoprotein by interferon-gamma. J. Biol. Chem. **265:** 11751–11760.
66. de Villiers, W.J., I.P. Fraser, D.A. Hughes *et al.* 1994. Macrophage-colony-stimulating factor selectively enhances macrophage scavenger receptor expression and function. J. Exp. Med. **180:** 705–709.
67. Hughes, D.A., I.P. Fraser & S. Gordon. 1995. Murine macrophage scavenger receptor: *in vivo* expression and function as receptor for macrophage adhesion in lymphoid and non-lymphoid organs. Eur. J. Immunol. **25:** 466–473.
68. Fraser, I., D. Hughes & S. Gordon. 1993. Divalent cation–independent macrophage adhesion inhibited by monoclonal antibody to murine scavenger receptor. Nature **364:** 343–346.
69. Hughes, D.A., I.P. Fraser & S. Gordon. 1994. Murine M phi scavenger receptor: adhesion function and expression. Immunol. Lett. **43:** 7–14.
70. Kim, J.G., C. Keshava, A.A. Murphy *et al.* 1997. Fresh mouse peritoneal macrophages have low scavenger receptor activity. J. Lipid Res. **38:** 2207–2215.
71. Krieger, M. & J. Herz. 1994. Structures and functions of multiligand lipoprotein receptors: macrophage scavenger receptors and LDL receptor–related protein (LRP). Annu. Rev. Biochem. **63:** 601–637.
72. Lessey, B.A., A.J. Castelbaum, S.W. Sawin *et al.* 1994. Aberrant integrin expression in the endometrium of women with endometriosis. J. Clin. Endocrinol. Metab. **79:** 643–649.
73. Lessey, B.A. & A.J. Castelbaum. 1995. Integrins in the endometrium of women with endometriosis. Br. J. Obstet. Gynaecol. **102:** 347–348.
74. Oral, E. & A. Arici. 1996. Peritoneal growth factors and endometriosis. Semin. Reprod. Endocrinol. **14:** 257–267.
75. Halme, J., C. White, S. Kauma *et al.* 1988. Peritoneal macrophages from patients with endometriosis release growth factor activity *in vitro*. J. Clin. Endocrinol. Metab. **66:** 1044–1049.
76. McLaren, J., A. Prentice, D.S. Charnock-Jones & S.K. Smith. 1996. Vascular endothelial growth factor (VEGF) concentrations are elevated in peritoneal fluid of women with endometriosis. Hum. Reprod. **11:** 220–223.

77. McLaren, J., A. Prentice, D.S. Charnock-Jones *et al.* 1996. Vascular endothelial growth factor is produced by peritoneal fluid macrophages in endometriosis and is regulated by ovarian steroids. J. Clin. Invest. **98:** 482–489.
78. Ferriani, R.A., D.S. Charnock-Jones, A. Prentice *et al.* 1993. Immunohistochemical localization of acidic and basic fibroblast growth factors in normal human endometrium and endometriosis and the detection of their mRNA by polymerase chain reaction. Hum. Reprod. **8:** 11–16.
79. Olive, D.L., I. Montoya, R.M. Riehl & R.S. Schenken. 1991. Macrophage-conditioned media enhance endometrial stromal cell proliferation *in vitro*. Am. J. Obstet. Gynecol. **164:** 953–958.
80. Braun, D.P., A. Muriana, H. Gebel *et al.* 1994. Monocyte-mediated enhancement of endometrial cell proliferation in women with endometriosis. Fertil. Steril. **61:** 78–84.
81. Taketani, Y., T.M. Kuo & M. Mizuno. 1992. Comparison of cytokine levels and embryo toxicity in peritoneal fluid in infertile women with untreated or treated endometriosis. Am. J. Obstet. Gynecol. **167:** 265–270.
82. Skrzypczak, J., P. Jedrzejczak, M. Kasprzak *et al.* 1995. Inflammatory cytokines in peritoneal fluid of women with endometriosis. Ann. N.Y. Acad. Sci. **762:** 496–498.
83. Koutsilieris, M., E. Lavergne & A. Lemay. 1997. Association of protease activity against IGFBP-3 with peritoneal fluid mitogens: possible implications for the ectopic growth of endometrial cells in women with endometriosis. Anticancer Res. **17:** 1239–1244.
84. Taskin, O., L. Giudice, R. Mangal *et al.* 1996. Insulin-like growth factor binding proteins in peritoneal fluid of women with minimal and mild endometriosis. Hum. Reprod. **11:** 1741–1746.
85. Overton, C., S. Fernandez-Shaw, B. Hicks *et al.* 1996. Peritoneal fluid cytokines and the relationship with endometriosis and pain. Hum. Reprod. **11:** 380–386.
86. Croxtall, J.D., A. Jamil, M. Ayub *et al.* 1992. TGF-beta stimulation of endometrial and breast-cancer cell growth. Int. J. Cancer **50:** 822–827.
87. Ryan, I.P., J.F. Tseng, E.D. Schriock *et al.* 1995. Interleukin-8 concentrations are elevated in peritoneal fluid of women with endometriosis. Fertil. Steril. **63:** 929–932.
88. Keenan, J.A., T.T. Chen, N.L. Chadwell *et al.* 1994. Interferon-gamma (IFN-gamma) and interleukin-6 (IL-6) in peritoneal fluid and macrophage-conditioned media of women with endometriosis. Am. J. Reprod. Immunol. **32:** 180–183.
89. Koninckx, P.R., L. Riittinen, M. Seppala & F.J. Cornillie. 1992. CA-125 and placental protein 14 concentrations in plasma and peritoneal fluid of women with deeply infiltrating pelvic endometriosis. Fertil. Steril. **57:** 523–530.
90. Braun, D.P., A. Muriana, H. Gebel *et al.* 1994. Monocyte-mediated enhancement of endometrial cell proliferation in women with endometriosis. Fertil. Steril. **61:** 78–84.
91. Koutsilieris, M., W. Niklinski, G. Frenette & A. Lemay. 1993. Heparin-sepharose binding growth factors in peritoneal fluid of women with endometriosis. Fertil. Steril. **59:** 93–97.
92. Hammond, M.G., S.T. Oh, J. Anners *et al.* 1993. The effect of growth factors on the proliferation of human endometrial stromal cells in culture. Am. J. Obstet. Gynecol. **168:** 1131–1136.
93. Whitworth, C.M., J. Mulholland, R.C. Dunn & S.R. Glasser. 1994. Growth factor effects on endometrial epithelial cell differentiation and protein synthesis *in vitro*. Fertil. Steril. **61:** 91–96.
94. Surrey, E.S. & J. Halme. 1991. Effect of platelet-derived growth factor on endometrial stromal cell proliferation *in vitro*: a model for endometriosis? Fertil. Steril. **56:** 672–679.
95. Giudice, L.C., B.A. Dsupin, S.E. Gargosky *et al.* 1994. The insulin-like growth factor system in human peritoneal fluid: its effects on endometrial stromal cells and its potential relevance to endometriosis. J. Clin. Endocrinol. Metab. **79:** 1284–1293.
96. Simms, J.S., N. Chegini, R.S. Williams *et al.* 1991. Identification of epidermal growth factor, transforming growth factor-alpha, and epidermal growth factor receptor in surgically induced endometriosis in rats. Obstet. Gynecol. **78:** 850–857.
97. Arumugam, K. & Y.C. Yip. 1995. *De novo* formation of adhesions in endometriosis: the role of iron and free radical reactions. Fertil. Steril. **64:** 62–64.

98. ARUMUGAM, K. & Y.C. YIP. 1995. Endometriosis and infertility: the role of exogenous lipid peroxides in the peritoneal fluid. Fertil. Steril. **63:** 198–199.
99. ARUMUGAM, K. 1994. Endometriosis and infertility: raised iron concentration in the peritoneal fluid and its effect on the acrosome reaction. Hum. Reprod. **9:** 1153–1157.
100. HUANG, J.C., C. PAPASAKELARIOU & M.Y. DAWOOD. 1996. Epidermal growth factor and basic fibroblast growth factor in peritoneal fluid of women with endometriosis. Fertil. Steril. **65:** 931–934.
101. NAGY, B., T. PULAY, G. SZARKA & S. CSOMOR. 1989. The serum protein content of human follicular fluid and its correlation with the maturity of oocytes. Acta Physiol. Hung. **73:** 71–75.
102. LE GOFF, D. 1994. Follicular fluid lipoproteins in the mare: evaluation of HDL transfer from plasma to follicular fluid. Biochim. Biophys. Acta **1210:** 226–232.
103. VOLPE, A., G. COUKOS, E. UCCELLI *et al.* 1991. Follicular fluid lipoproteins in preovulatory period and their relationship with follicular maturation and progesterone production by human granulosa-luteal cells *in vivo* and *in vitro*. J. Endocrinol. Invest. **14:** 737–742.
104. PALINSKI, W., M.E. ROSENFELD, S. YLA HERTTUALA *et al.* 1989. Low density lipoprotein undergoes oxidative modification *in vivo*. Proc. Natl. Acad. Sci. U.S.A. **86:** 1372–1376.
105. YLA HERTTUALA, S., W. PALINSKI, M.E. ROSENFELD *et al.* 1989. Evidence for the presence of oxidatively modified low density lipoprotein in atherosclerotic lesions of rabbit and man. J. Clin. Invest. **84:** 1086–1095.
106. STEINBRECHER, U.P., H.F. ZHANG & M. LOUGHEED. 1990. Role of oxidatively modified LDL in atherosclerosis. Free Radical Biol. Med. **9:** 155–168.
107. OLIVE, D.L., J.B. WEINBERG & A.F. HANEY. 1985. Peritoneal macrophages and infertility: the association between cell number and pelvic pathology. Fertil. Steril. **44:** 772.
108. BALL, R.Y., J.P. BINDMAN, K.L. CARPENTER & M.J. MITCHINSON. 1986. Oxidized low density lipoprotein induces ceroid accumulation by murine peritoneal macrophages *in vitro*. Atherosclerosis **60:** 173–181.
109. MORTON, R.E., G.A. WEST & H.F. HOFF. 1986. A low density lipoprotein–sized particle isolated from human atherosclerotic lesions is internalized by macrophages via a non-scavenger-receptor mechanism. J. Lipid Res. **27:** 1124–1134.
110. HOFF, H.F., T.E. WHITAKER & J. O'NEIL. 1992. Oxidation of low density lipoprotein leads to particle aggregation and altered macrophage recognition. J. Biol. Chem. **267:** 602–609.
111. YLA HERTTUALA, S., M.E. ROSENFELD, S. PARTHASARATHY *et al.* 1991. Gene expression in macrophage-rich human atherosclerotic lesions: 15-lipoxygenase and acetyl low density lipoprotein receptor messenger RNA colocalize with oxidation specific lipid-protein adducts. J. Clin. Invest. **87:** 1146–1152.
112. YLA HERTTUALA, S., M.E. ROSENFELD, S. PARTHASARATHY *et al.* 1990. Colocalization of 15-lipoxygenase mRNA and protein with epitopes of oxidized low density lipoprotein in macrophage-rich areas of atherosclerotic lesions. Proc. Natl. Acad. Sci. U.S.A. **87:** 6959–6963.
113. DERIAN, C.K. & D.F. LEWIS. 1992. Activation of 15-lipoxygenase by low density lipoprotein in vascular endothelial cells: relationship to the oxidative modification of low density lipoprotein. Prostaglandins Leukotrienes Essent. Fatty Acids **45:** 49–57.
114. SIGAL, E., D.L. SLOANE & D.J. CONRAD. 1993. Human 15-lipoxygenase: induction by interleukin-4 and insights into positional specificity. J. Lipid Mediators **6:** 75–88.
115. CONRAD, D.J., H. KUHN, M. MULKINS *et al.* 1992. Specific inflammatory cytokines regulate the expression of human monocyte 15-lipoxygenase. Proc. Natl. Acad. Sci. U.S.A. **89:** 217–221.
116. NASSAR, G.M., J.D. MORROW, L.J. ROBERTS *et al.* 1994. Induction of 15-lipoxygenase by interleukin-13 in human blood monocytes. J. Biol. Chem. **269:** 27631–27634.
117. RANKIN, S.M., S. PARTHASARATHY & D. STEINBERG. 1991. Evidence for a dominant role of lipoxygenase(s) in the oxidation of LDL by mouse peritoneal macrophages. J. Lipid Res. **32:** 449–456.
118. LIBBY, P. & Z.S. GALIS. 1995. Cytokines regulate genes involved in atherogenesis. Ann. N.Y. Acad. Sci. **748:** 158–168; 168–170 (discussion).

119. KORSMEYER, S.J., J.R. SHUTTER, D.J. VEIS *et al.* 1993. Bcl-2/Bax: a rheostat that regulates an anti-oxidant pathway and cell death. Semin. Cancer Biol. **4:** 327–332.
120. CARPENTER, K.L., R.Y. BALL, N.P. CARTER *et al.* 1989. Modulation of ceroid accumulation in macrophages *in vitro*. Adv. Exp. Med. Biol. **266:** 333–343.
121. CARPENTER, K.L., G.M. WILKINS, B. FUSSELL *et al.* 1994. Production of oxidized lipids during modification of low-density lipoprotein by macrophages or copper. Biochem. J. **304:** 625–633.
122. RAYMOND, T.L., S.A. REYNOLDS & J.A. SWANSON. 1986. Turnover of low-density lipoprotein isolated from interstitial inflammatory fluid of the rabbit. Inflammation **10:** 93–98.
123. RAYMOND, T.L. & S.A. REYNOLDS. 1983. Lipoprotein metabolism in the extravascular space: cyclophosphamide inhibits modification of low-density lipoproteins in interstitial inflammatory fluid of the rabbit. Inflammation **7:** 241–246.
124. RAYMOND, T.L. & S.A. REYNOLDS. 1984. Direct modification of plasma low-density lipoproteins in interstitial inflammatory fluid of the rabbit. Inflammation **8:** 337–342.
125. RAYMOND, T.L. & S.A. REYNOLDS. 1984. Effect of cholesterol feeding on lipoprotein distribution in interstitial inflammatory fluid of the rabbit. Atherosclerosis **52:** 175–183.
126. RAYMOND, T.L. & S.A. REYNOLDS. 1983. Lipoproteins of the extravascular space: alterations in low density lipoproteins of interstitial inflammatory fluid. J. Lipid Res. **24:** 113–119.
127. RAYMOND, T.L. & S.A. REYNOLDS. 1982. Circulating phospholipids in interstitial inflammatory fluid of the rabbit. Inflammation **6:** 285–289.
128. RAYMOND, T.L., S.A. REYNOLDS & J.A. SWANSON. 1985. Lipoproteins of the extravascular space: enhanced macrophage degradation of low density lipoproteins from interstitial inflammatory fluid. J. Lipid Res. **26:** 1356–1362.
129. SMITH, E.B. & C. ASHALL. 1983. Variability of the electrophoretic mobility of low density lipoprotein: comparison of interstitial fluid from human aortic intima and serum. Atherosclerosis **49:** 89–98.
130. SMITH, E.B. 1986. Plasma macromolecules in interstitial fluid from normal and atherosclerotic human aorta. Monogr. Atheroscler. **14:** 179–183.
131. SMITH, E.B. & C. ASHALL. 1983. Low-density lipoprotein concentration in interstitial fluid from human atherosclerotic lesions: relation to theories of endothelial damage and lipoprotein binding. Biochim. Biophys. Acta **754:** 249–257.
132. SMITH, E.B. & E.M. STAPLES. 1982. Plasma protein concentrations in interstitial fluid from human aortas. Proc. R. Soc. Lond. Ser. B: Biol. Sci. **217:** 59–75.
133. ROSENFELD, M.E., W. PALINSKI, S. YLA HERTTUALA *et al.* 1990. Distribution of oxidation specific lipid-protein adducts and apolipoprotein B in atherosclerotic lesions of varying severity from WHHL rabbits. Arteriosclerosis **10:** 336–349.
134. HEINECKE, J.W., H. ROSEN & A. CHAIT. 1984. Iron and copper promote modification of low density lipoprotein by human arterial smooth muscle cells in culture. J. Clin. Invest. **74:** 1890–1894.
135. STEINBRECHER, U.P., S. PARTHASARATHY, D.S. LEAKE *et al.* 1984. Modification of low density lipoprotein by endothelial cells involves lipid peroxidation and degradation of low density lipoprotein phospholipids. Proc. Natl. Acad. Sci. U.S.A. **81:** 3883–3887.
136. RAO, G.N., R.W. ALEXANDER & M.S. RUNGE. 1996. Linoleic acid and its metabolites, hydroperoxyoctadecadienoic acids, stimulate c-Fos, c-Jun, and c-Myc mRNA expression, mitogen-activated protein kinase activation, and growth in rat aortic smooth muscle cells. J. Clin. Invest. **96:** 842–847.
137. FUNK, C.D. & G.A. FITZGERALD. 1991. Eicosanoid forming enzyme mRNA in human tissues: analysis by quantitative polymerase chain reaction. J. Biol. Chem. **266:** 12508–12513.
138. HOFF, H.F. & R.E. MORTON. 1985. Lipoproteins containing apo B extracted from human aortas: structure and function. Ann. N.Y. Acad. Sci. **454:** 183–194.
139. CHAI, Y.C., P.H. HOWE, P.E. DICORLETO & G.M. CHISOLM. 1996. Oxidized low density lipoprotein and lysophosphatidylcholine stimulate cell cycle entry in vascular smooth muscle cells: evidence for release of fibroblast growth factor-2. J. Biol. Chem. **271:** 17791–17797.

Panel Discussion (Part V)

A.T. FAZLEABAS (*University of Illinois, Chicago, IL*): Dr. Sidell, can you try to resolve what Sam Parthasarathy presented and what you presented? His hypothesis was that you have got these nonadherent macrophages that are capable of producing growth factors to stimulate stromal cell and epithelial cell development, yet prevent them from being degraded. You presented an idea that retinoic acid can actually stimulate a receptor on these nonadherent monocytes to allow for scavenger function. I am trying to resolve these two issues in terms of how both of you think about this whole process.

N. SIDELL (*Emory University, Atlanta, GA*): The answer is a simple one. We are talking only in the context of endometriosis and not in the development of the endometrium after menstruation. Sam's hypothesis suggests that these nonadherent macrophages in the peritoneal cavity do not scavenge the endometrial debris coming from retrograde menstruation and, in addition, might contribute to endometriosis by generating growth-promoting activity. My hypothesis complements his by suggesting that, if we make the macrophages express scavenger receptor(s), they might scavenge these menstrual components and there wouldn't be any cells to grow. From my standpoint, what I am trying to do is change immunological parameters in a way that will be beneficial to the immune system and detrimental to the growth of endometrial cells. That is clear. One way would be to try to induce scavenger receptors on nonadherent monocyte macrophages. This is what retinoic acid seems to be able to do. Now, it might do other things in terms of cytokine regulation; in addition to reducing IL-6, it will undoubtedly do other types of things to other cytokines that might favor endometrial growth. We just have to go through the list one by one and determine exactly what it does. At the same time, we have to compare that knowledge with our developing understanding of what is really important in the growth of endometriosis and see if we can distinguish the good from the bad.

FAZLEABAS: I have a follow-up question. Experimentally, can you take these cells, for example, these nonadherent macrophages and monocyte macrophages, stimulate the scavenger receptor on them, and then put them in an *in vitro* bioassay to see if there is a differential function when you stimulate them with retinoic acid as opposed to the other ones?

SIDELL: That is a good idea. Those experiments are planned.

C.R. LYTTLE (*Wyeth Ayerst Research, Radnor, PA*): A question for Dr. Sidell. In your NFκB mechanism, you propose that there were changes in the concentration of NFκB. Have you examined the concentration or association of IκB with NFκB and the phosphorylation of that?

SIDELL: No. The assay simply measures the binding of the NFκB-binding element to nuclear protein. We have not yet determined whether there is an increase or decrease of the NFκB protein itself or changes in IκB.

K. CHWALISZ (*TAP Pharmaceutical Products, Lake Forest, IL*): Dr. Sidell, you presented the interesting hypothesis that RU486 may act on endometriosis as an antioxidant and showed that ZK112,993 was a similar compound. Just for your information, we did a census study some years ago with Gary Hodgen using that K compound in monkeys and also showed that, in animal models for endometriosis, it was very effective in blocking endometrial growth. Therefore, the effect *in vivo* might be more complex. It might include the effect of the vessels on the ovarian seclusiveness. There may be an additional factor, but again ZK112,993 showed very strong antiproliferative effects on the endometrium in monkeys.

QUESTION: Sam Parthasarathy told us that patients with endometriosis have more cardiovascular disease than normal females. These patients usually are very complex. They go under a lot of stress. They undergo a lot of surgical treatments, medical treatments that cause hypoestrogenia, and then many of them undergo castration at a very young age that might cause increased cardiovascular morbidity.

K.L. SHARPE-TIMMS (*University of Missouri, Columbia, MO*): This question is for Dr. Parthasarathy. We have looked at *de novo* synthesized endometriotic haptoglobin and found that it reduces macrophage adherence at the same time, while activating macrophages as measured by increased production of IL-6. Have you compared macrophages from women with and without endometriosis and seen any difference in the adherence level? Do you know of any molecules that may be contributing to those effects you noted?

S. PARTHASARATHY (*Emory University, Atlanta, GA*): That is an excellent question. So far, we have just simply compared the number of macrophages in the peritoneal cavity at the time of surgery. The cells from control subjects are few in number and are more monocyte-like in nature, while those from endometriosis are abundant and more similar to macrophages. It is attractive to speculate that cells that are macrophage-like from control subjects are adherent and have effectively performed their scavenging function. Maybe we could try to isolate these adherent cells from normal by lavaging with EDTA or some other agent. We do not know the resident time of these macrophages, so we are planning to do such studies at least in animal models.

QUESTION: The lipid peroxidation is augmented by the presence of iron. With iron present in this disease, have you explored either ferrosoferric or transferrin?

PARTHASARATHY: That is an excellent question. So far, we cannot distinguish between various types of lesions to see if those containing iron would have more lipid peroxidation or less. We have just used endometriosis as such without making those distinctions. However, by the end of this study, we hope to have enough samples to make that kind of comparison. I should point out that the level of oxidation that we suggest in the peritoneal cavity is not "optimal oxidation". For example, you will find very little, if any, increase in thiobarbituric acid products. The type of oxidation or the extent of oxidation that these lipoproteins undergo in the peritoneal cavity is what Fogelman and others call mildly oxidized or minimally oxidized lipoproteins.

The Potential Role of Exposure to Environmental Toxicants in the Pathophysiology of Endometriosis

SHERRY E. RIER

Department of Obstetrics and Gynecology, Vanderbilt University Medical Center, Nashville, Tennessee 37232, USA

ABSTRACT: Humans and animals are exposed daily to a complex mixture of polyhalogenated aromatic hydrocarbons (PHAHs). Previous work has shown that exposure to 2,3,7,8-tetrachlorodibenzo-*p*-dioxin (TCDD) is associated with a dose-dependent increase in the incidence and severity of endometriosis in the rhesus monkey. Dioxin-like chemicals can also exert effects in combination with TCDD via the aryl hydrocarbon receptor. Using a rhesus model of chronic TCDD exposure and endometriosis, serum concentrations of TCDD and 19 dioxin-like PHAHs were quantified 13 years after termination of exposure to TCDD. In additional studies, the immune status of TCDD-exposed monkeys was evaluated. For TCDD-exposed and unexposed animals, TCDD exposure correlated with an increased serum TCDD concentration. Furthermore, TCDD exposure and an elevated serum TCDD concentration were associated with increased serum levels of triglycerides, 1,2,3,6,7,8-hexachlorodibenzofuran (HxCDF), PCB77, and PCB126. Importantly, the animals with elevated serum levels of PCB77 and PCB126 and increased total serum TCDD equivalents (TEQs) had a high prevalence of endometriosis, and the severity of disease correlated with the serum concentration of PCB77. In immune studies, TCDD exposure correlated with increased tumor necrosis factor alpha (TNFα) production by peripheral blood mononuclear cells (PBMC) in response to stimulation by T cell mitogen and decreased NK cytolytic activity. Elevated serum concentrations of TCDD, 1,2,3,6,7,8-HxCDF, and PCB126 correlated with increased numbers of CD3+/CD25– and CD3–/CD25+ leukocytes and enhanced secretion of TNFα by mitogen-stimulated PBMC. This evidence suggests that TCDD exposure and endometriosis in the rhesus monkey may be associated with increased serum concentrations of specific coplanar PCB compounds and long-term alterations in systemic immunity. Furthermore, the data suggest a potential involvement of an increased body burden of PCB compounds in the etiology of endometriosis in the rhesus. Recent advances in the detection and assay of individual PHAH congeners in biological samples have made it possible to assess total PHAH body burden in humans and animals. Future studies are expected to exploit this advance to assess the health impact of PHAH body burdens in both exposed individuals and the general population. Serum PHAH concentrations and TEQs in TCDD-exposed monkeys with endometriosis are similar to or lower than blood levels in the general human population; thus, it is important to consider the implications of these findings for human health and the prevalence of endometriosis in humans. Additional

Address for correspondence: Sherry E. Rier, Department of Obstetrics and Gynecology, Vanderbilt University Medical Center, B-1100 Medical Center North, Nashville, TN 37232. Voice: 615-322-4196; fax: 615-343-7913.
sherry.rier@mcmail.vanderbilt.edu

studies are warranted, particularly in human subjects, to explore the potential implications of these data.

KEYWORDS: **endometriosis; environmental toxicants; dioxin; TCDD; PCBs; dioxin-like chemicals; rhesus monkey**

INTRODUCTION

2,3,7,8-Tetrachlorodibenzo-*p*-dioxin (TCDD) and structurally related polyhalogenated aromatic hydrocarbon chemicals (PHAHs) are ubiquitous environmental contaminants worldwide. TCDD is a potent chemical toxicant that serves as a reference compound for a large class of PHAHs.[1] Evidence indicates that the actions of TCDD are mediated by the aryl hydrocarbon receptor (AhR). The AhR is an orphan nuclear receptor whose natural ligand is not known. Similar to the steroid hormone receptor family of proteins, the AhR acts as a signal transducer and transcription factor. Following receptor activation, the receptor-ligand complex is translocated to the nucleus via the AhR nuclear translocator (ARNT) where DNA binding occurs, resulting in transcriptional activation. Target genes include cytochrome P-450 and genes involved in cellular growth, differentiation, and inflammation.[2,3] Other polychlorinated dibenzo-*p*-dioxins (PCDDs) and dibenzofurans (PCDFs) substituted in the 2,3,7,8-lateral positions also have high binding affinity for the AhR and elicit toxic effects similar to TCDD.[4] Moreover, non-ortho- and mono-ortho-polychlorinated biphenyls (PCBs) are AhR agonists and contribute significantly to the toxicity of complex mixtures of environmental PHAHs.[5,6] Studies have shown that the potency of PCDDs, PCDFs, and PCBs relates to the affinity of individual congeners for the AhR.[4,5] TCDD and dioxin-like PHAHs are classified as "dioxins" and are associated with a spectrum of toxic effects on the reproductive, immune, and endocrine systems.[7] In addition, certain non-coplanar PCBs can elicit toxic effects independent of the AhR, including disruption of estrogen activity.[5,8]

Dioxin, PCDDs, and PCDFs are produced as unwanted contaminants during incineration, pulp and paper processing, petroleum refining, and chemical manufacturing processes, whereas PCBs have been used extensively in a broad range of commercial applications.[4,5] These chemicals are resistant to degradation and, due to their lipophilic nature, bioaccumulate and biomagnify at higher trophic levels of the food chain. TCDD and related PHAH congeners are found in serum and accumulate in tissues of exposed individuals and the general population.[4,7,9–11] In the general population, ingestion of contaminated foods is the most likely source of TCDD and other PHAHs, but accidental exposure has also occurred in the workplace, during wartime, and as a result of industrial accidents.[4,5,7] In industrialized countries, exposure to environmental PHAHs has led to serum TCDD levels of 1 to 5 lipid-adjusted parts per trillion (PPT-LIPID) and body burdens estimated at 25 TCDD equivalents (TEQs) PPT-LIPID in individuals with no overt exposure.[12] Although the toxic effects of TCDD in animals are unequivocal, its effect in humans is less clear. However, studies indicate that humans exhibit many of the biological effects of dioxins observed in animals, and sensitive individuals may respond to dioxin exposures with cancer and noncancer endpoints at doses close to background exposure.[13] It has been postulated that increased concentrations of TCDD and dioxin-like chemicals in blood and tissues participate in disease pathogenesis via disruption of endocrine and immune responses in susceptible humans and animals.[7,14]

Endometriosis is classically defined as the growth of endometrial glands and stroma at extrauterine sites. Often accompanied by chronic pelvic pain, infertility, and adhesion formation, it is a prevalent gynecologic disorder that may be present in 10% of reproductive-aged women.[15] Disease pathogenesis may involve endocrine and immune dysregulation since uterine endometrial growth is regulated by sex hormones in concert with bioactive mediators produced by uterine immune and endocrine cells, including the matrix metalloproteinases (MMPs)[16] and cytokines.[17] The aberrant expression of hormonally regulated MMPs and cytokines is associated with numerous disease states that involve invasive processes, including endometriosis and tumorigenesis.[17,18] Thus, exposure to environmental toxicants that disrupt endocrine and immune responses potentially may impact the development and progression of endometriosis.

Endometriosis occurs exclusively in menstruating species, including humans and nonhuman primates, with spontaneous development in rhesus monkeys closely resembling human disease.[19] Thus, the monkey is the most appropriate, yet expensive, animal model for the study of disease pathogenesis. In animal models, disease can be surgically induced by the implantation of autologous endometrial tissue at ectopic sites.[20,21] Since spontaneous endometriosis in monkeys appears to develop over a period of 7 to 10 years, surgical induction of disease has been employed utilizing three methods in the rhesus, baboon, or cynomolgus monkey: (1) suturing fragments of endometrial tissue to the peritoneal cavity or to subcutaneous locations on the abdomen, (2) diverting the cervix from the vagina to the peritoneal cavity, and (3) seeding the peritoneal cavity with minced fragments of endometrium. In addition, rodent and rabbit models of disease have been employed utilizing surgical autotransplantation of endometrium[20] or injection of human endometrial tissue into the peritoneal cavity of athymic nude mice.[22]

MONKEY MODELS OF EXPOSURE TO DIOXINS AND ENDOMETRIOSIS

We provided the first report of an association between chronic TCDD exposure and endometriosis in the rhesus monkey.[23] Animals were exposed to 0, 5, or 25 PPT TCDD via their feed for approximately 4 years. Spontaneous endometriosis was assessed at surgical laparoscopy 10 years after termination of TCDD treatment. This study demonstrated a significant dose-dependent increase in the incidence and severity of endometriosis in TCDD-exposed monkeys. In a recent study, Yang *et al.*[24] utilized a model of surgically induced endometriosis in the cynomolgus monkey to investigate the effects of TCDD exposure on the survival and growth of ectopic endometrium. Fragments of endometrium were autotransplanted to the pelvic cavity of animals dosed 5 days a week with 0, 1, 5, or 25 PPT TCDD for 1 year. The growth and survival of implants was assessed by laparoscopy at 1, 3, and 6 months, and at 1 year during autopsy performed in the luteal phase of the menstrual cycle. The size and survival of implants were similar among animal groups at 1, 3, or 6 months. Consistent with previous work in the rhesus monkey,[23] exposure to 5 or 25 PPT TCDD for 1 year resulted in a higher survival rate of implants, as well as an increased implant size in animals fed 25 PPT TCDD. In contrast, the implant size was decreased in animals fed 1 PPT TCDD. Therefore, this group found that TCDD facilitates the survival of endometrial implants and exerts a bimodal effect on endometrial implant growth.

Dioxin-like PCBs contribute significantly to the toxicity of commercial mixtures of PCBs.[4] Campbell *et al.*[25] initially observed a possible link between PCB exposure and aggressive intestinal endometriosis in the rhesus monkey exposed to Aroclor 1254. No evidence of increased endometriosis was found in this colony of PCB-exposed animals at 6 years after initiation of toxin treatment.[26] However, this study may have been terminated before endometriosis was clinically apparent in all PCB-treated animals since spontaneous disease appears to develop in the rhesus at approximately 7 years following exposure to TCDD[23] or radiation.[19]

RODENT MODELS OF EXPOSURE TO DIOXINS AND ENDOMETRIOSIS

Rodent studies demonstrate that treatment with TCDD at doses of 1 or 3 μg/kg or the dioxin-like furan chemical, 2,3,4,7,8-pentachlorodifuran, at 100 μg/kg over a period of 12 weeks produces a dose-dependent increase in the size of surgically induced endometrial lesions utilizing an estrogen-responsive model of endometriosis.[27,28] In contrast, treatment of mice with non-dioxin-like compounds has no effect on the growth of endometriotic sites,[28] providing preliminary evidence that PHAH-promoted endometriosis may be AhR-mediated. In addition, perinatal plus adult exposure to TCDD in this mouse model increases the size of endometriotic lesions.[29] TCDD treatment prior to surgical induction of disease, subacute dosing, the estrogen level in the animal, and an adequate time between exposure and disease development appear to be important to the PHAH-mediated effects in this model. Regression of endometrial implants has been observed in a variation of this model when mice are treated with TCDD and high levels of exogenous estrogen after surgical induction of disease, and implant size is evaluated at time points less than 9 weeks[30] or when TCDD dose (≥10 μg/kg) is toxic to the ovaries.[31]

Recent work has shown that TCDD promotes the establishment of ectopic lesions of human endometrium in a nude mouse model of disease by disrupting progesterone regulation of matrilysin expression, an MMP involved in tumorigenic invasive processes and tissue remodeling during endometrial proliferation and menstruation.[22,32,33] This model offers several advantages: (1) it uses human endometrium; (2) it allows hormonal and chemical modulation of the explants prior to implantation; and (3) it enables the correlation of parallel *in vitro* biochemical analyses of the explants with *in vivo* measurements of disease severity so that experimental disease can be related to potential biochemical mechanisms. In this model, treatment of cultured human endometrial explants with estradiol maintains both stromal- and epithelial-specific MMP secretion *in vitro* and spontaneously promotes the establishment of ectopic peritoneal lesions *in vivo* when the explants are injected into recipient animals. In contrast, treatment with progesterone (P4) in conjunction with estradiol suppresses both *in vitro* MMP secretion and *in vivo* lesion formation.[22] This suppression is coordinately regulated by both P4 and transforming growth factor beta (TGFβ). Additional studies have shown that suppression of MMP activity inhibits the establishment of disease in this model.[32] Treatment with TCDD plus estradiol increased both the number and size of the lesions compared to treatment with estrogen alone, and treatment with TCDD in the presence of estradiol and P4 disrupted the ability of P4 to block lesion formation and metalloproteinase expression.[33] These results provide mechanistic evidence linking the steroidal regulation of MMP secretion in human endometrial tissue with the establishment of an endometriosis-like disease in the nude mouse and demonstrate the ability of TCDD to disrupt this regulation. The aberrant expression of MMPs induced by dioxins could mediate peritoneal and organ invasion, required for establishment of ectopic sites of growth.

HUMAN STUDIES ON EXPOSURE TO DIOXINS AND ENDOMETRIOSIS

Although no direct evidence exists for a relationship between exposure to dioxins and the development of endometriosis in human populations, evidence is beginning to accumulate. In Belgium, Koninckx noted that the prevalence of endometriosis in women presenting at clinics with infertility is 60% to 80%,[34] and TCDD concentrations in breast milk in this country are among the highest in the world.[35] Consistent with this notion, Pauwels *et al.*[36] conducted a case-controlled study of women in Belgium and found that an increased risk of endometriosis is associated with an elevated total serum TEQ derived from dioxins. In Israel, Mayani and colleagues[37] reported that an increased proportion of infertile women with endometriosis have a detectable serum TCDD level (18%) as compared to infertile controls without disease (3%). A comprehensive study on reproductive health and the prevalence of endometriosis in a human population exposed to TCDD in Seveso, Italy, is under way.[38] In a mostly German population, an association between exposure to non-dioxin-like PCBs and endometriosis is suggested by a report finding increased total serum levels of higher chlorinated non-coplanar (non-dioxin-like) PCBs (PCB138, PCB153, and PCB180) in women with endometriosis.[39,40] A Canadian study showed that serum levels of individual non-coplanar PCB congeners are similar in women with and without disease.[41] The discrepancy in these findings may arise from differences in comparison of individual versus groups of PCB congeners or quantification methods, such as assay sensitivity or lipid adjustment. Evaluation of the body burden of TCDD and dioxin-like chemicals (concentrations and TEQs) in animals and humans, rather than non-dioxin-like congeners alone, is important in establishing an association between exposure to dioxins and an increased prevalence of endometriosis.

COMPARISON OF SERUM DIOXINS IN TCDD-EXPOSED MONKEYS AND THE HUMAN GENERAL POPULATION

In recent work, serum concentrations of TCDD, 19 dioxin-like PHAH congeners, and lipids were determined in the colony of TCDD-exposed rhesus monkeys at 13 years after termination of TCDD exposure.[42] Similar to the human general population, TCDD-treated and control animals were exposed to a mixture of dioxin-like chemicals via their diet and other environmental sources. Data on serum PHAHs and lipids in these animals were analyzed for an association with the presence and

TABLE 1. Increased serum PHAH and lipid concentrations in TCDD-treated animals

Congener/lipid	0 PPT	5 PPT	25 PPT	All TCDD
TCDD	4.6	18.9	154[a]	23.6[a]
1,2,3,6,7,8-HxCDF	4.4	10.9	14.3[a]	11.1[a]
PCB77	ND	984	1584	1584[a]
PCB126	96.7	295[a]	532[a]	296[a]
Triglycerides	118	337[b]	497[a]	351[b]

NOTE: Results are expressed as median serum analyte concentration in parts per quadrillion (PPQ) or median lipid concentration per dL blood in TCDD-treated (n = 9) and unexposed (n = 6) animals. Significant differences between groups were determined using Wilcoxon's rank sum test. ND = not detected.

[a]Significantly different compared with corresponding value for 0 PPT TCDD group; $p < 0.05$.

[b]Significantly different compared with corresponding value for 0 PPT TCDD group; $p < 0.01$.

severity of endometriosis. This study[42] found that TCDD exposure in the rhesus directly correlates with a long-term increase in the serum levels of triglycerides, TCDD, 1,2,3,6,7,8-hexachlorodifuran (HxCDF), PCB 77, and PCB 126 (TABLE 1). Importantly, the animals in this study with elevated serum levels of PCB77 and PCB126 and an increased total serum TEQ had a high prevalence of endometriosis (TABLE 2). The severity of the disease correlates with the serum concentration of PCB77, but not the serum TCDD level. These data suggest a potential involvement of an increased body burden of PCB compounds in the etiology of endometriosis in rhesus monkeys. Serum concentrations and TEQs of TCDD and dioxin-like PCBs in TCDD-treated animals[42] are similar to or lower than blood levels in the general human population.[4,5,9,10,43,44] Thus, it is important to consider the implications of these findings for human health, particularly with regard to the average body burden of dioxins and the prevalence of endometriosis.

The burden of PCDDs, PCDFs, and total PHAH compounds is higher in the general human population than in the TCDD-treated monkeys (PCDDs: 8- to 20-fold higher; PCDFs and total PHAHs: 2- to 6-fold higher). The magnitude of this difference is not precisely known since the lipid-adjusted values used for comparing human and monkey PHAH levels may underestimate the PHAH concentration in the treated monkeys by as much as 2-fold. The following PHAH values evaluated in this study have been reported in blood samples from the general human population: 500 to 1360 PPT-LIPID, PCDDs; 30 to 60 PPT-LIPID, PCDFs; 100 to 190 PPT-LIPID, PCBs; 700 to 1500 PPT-LIPID, all PHAHs.[4,5,9,10,43,44] In contrast, serum from TCDD-treated monkeys contained the following total concentrations: 65 PPT-LIPID, PCDDs; 11 PPT-LIPID, PCDFs; 322 PPT-LIPID, all PHAHs. A significant degree of variation is observed in the amounts of PCB compounds in human samples. The following ranges of values have been reported for the PCB congeners of interest in this study in human blood and milk: 8–490 PPT-LIPID, PCB77; 40–90 PPT-LIPID, PCB126. In human adipose tissue, concentrations of each of these PCB compounds range from 30 to 800 PPT-LIPID.[9,43,44] In TCDD-treated animals, serum contained 241 PPT-LIPID, PCB77, and 40 PPT-LIPID, PCB126, similar to human serum and milk in some geographic locations. The total TEQ for all PHAH compounds in

TABLE 2. Increased serum PCB levels in TCDD-treated animals with endometriosis

	0 PPT TCDD		All TCDD	
Congener/lipid	No EM	With EM	No EM	With EM
TCDD	5.5	4.6	247	22.1
1,2,3,6,7,8-HxCDF	ND	13.1	9.4	11.1
PCB77	ND	ND	ND	1969[a]
PCB126	114	95.2	437[a]	295[a]
Triglycerides	116	128	423[b]	323[b]

NOTE: Results are expressed as median serum analyte concentration in parts per quadrillion (PPQ) or median lipid concentration per dL blood in TCDD-treated (n = 9) and unexposed (n = 6) animals. Significant differences between groups were determined using Wilcoxon's rank sum test. ND = not detected.

[a]Significantly different compared with –TCDD groups; $p < 0.05$.

[b]Significantly different compared with –TCDD groups; $p < 0.01$.

human blood is also higher than in the TCDD-treated animals in this study (25 PPT-LIPID, human blood; 10 PPT-LIPID, TCDD-treated monkeys). In Japan, Yoshida *et al.*[45] reported that margin-of-exposure (MOE) values for endometriosis are not sufficiently high to guarantee safety against endometriosis for local residents living near a solid-waste incinerator, heavy fish consumers and their infants, and populations exposed to higher concentrations than the general population. In the most recent risk characterization of dioxin and related compounds by the U.S. EPA, endometriosis is considered a low-dose biological effect of dioxins occurring at or near human background levels.[12]

IMMUNE AND ENDOCRINE FINDINGS IN TCDD-EXPOSED RHESUS MONKEYS WITH ENDOMETRIOSIS

TCDD-exposed animals with endometriosis also exhibit immune and endocrine alterations. Thirteen years after exposure, the phenotypic distribution and function of peripheral blood leukocytes in TCDD-treated animals were examined.[46] The data were analyzed for an association with endometriosis and elevated serum levels of TCDD and dioxin-like PHAHs. For all animals, TCDD exposure correlates with increased peripheral blood leukocyte secretion of tumor necrosis factor alpha (TNFα) in response to T cell stimulation and decreased natural killer (NK) cytolytic activity.[46] Elevated serum concentrations of TCDD, 1,2,3,6,7,8-HxCDF, and PCB126 correlate with increased numbers of nonactivated T cells (CD3+/CD25–) and activated NK cells (CD3–/CD25+) and enhanced secretion of TNFα by mitogen-stimulated leukocytes. In TCDD-exposed animals with endometriosis, serum estradiol concentrations are decreased, whereas serum levels of cortisol are increased relative to unexposed controls without disease.[47] Decreased serum estradiol levels correlate with increased serum levels of TCDD and PCB126. Testosterone is detected exclusively in serum from TCDD-treated animals without endometriosis. A trend in increased serum insulin was observed in TCDD-exposed animals, suggestive of altered glucose tolerance reported in recent epidemiological studies in TCDD-exposed humans.[48,49] At autopsy, TCDD-exposed animals exhibited disseminated endometriosis with sites of invasion including the intestines, liver, spleen, bladder, ureters, and lung.[47] These findings suggest that TCDD exposure may be associated with severe disseminated endometriosis and an altered immune and endocrine profile in the rhesus monkey; also, endogenous serum testosterone may protect exposed animals from disease development.

PERSPECTIVE ON ANIMAL MODELS FOR DISEASE PATHOGENESIS

Studies in humans and nonhuman primates have shown that endometriosis is a dynamic disease with periods of development, progression, and regression.[21,50] Lesions change in appearance during remodeling processes over time and disappear at some sites, while other lesions progress in severity. D'Hooghe *et al.*[21] observed the spontaneous evolution of moderately progressive endometriosis in baboons. After 10 months, the mean number of endometriotic lesions was significantly higher than at initial laparoscopy, although 55% of the initial implants had disappeared. This finding resulted from the high proportion of new lesions (82%) in these animals. This is comparable to observations of progression, regression, stabilization, and remodeling of endometriotic lesions in women with endometriosis.[50] When designing studies to investigate the role of dioxins in the pathogenesis of endometriosis, it is important to utilize animal models that most closely resemble human disease. Since spontaneous endometriosis appears to develop approximately 7 years following exposure to TCDD[23] or radiation,[19] surgically induced endometriosis in nonhuman primates and rodents is the most practical model of disease. However, disease induction by peritoneal seeding of endometrial tissue in the monkey and the nude mouse model,[22] rather than autotransplantation of endometrium, may be critical to mimic the human disease process. As described by Yang and colleagues,[24] lesions of autotransplanted endometrium regress over time in control and TCDD-treated animals. Therefore, these studies may document the effect of toxicant exposure on a modulation of "normal" growth inhibition at ectopic sites. Thus, studies that employ surgical induction by autotransplantation of endometrium in monkeys and rodents may be limited in scope since they test the effect of dioxins on established disease only, not the capacity to form and remodel lesions. The microenvironment at the ectopic site that receives the endometrial tissue must be considered. TCDD may increase inflammation at these sites via leukocyte infiltration and activation, priming the site for acceptance or rejection of endometrial tissue. In addition, one cannot investigate the effect of dioxins on biochemical mechanisms active in the disease process in rodents with surgically induced lesions since menstruation and endometriosis do not occur in these animals.

FUTURE STUDIES AND DATA GAPS

Recent advances in the detection and assay of individual PHAH congeners in biological samples have made it possible to assess total PHAH body burden in humans and animals. Future studies are expected to exploit this advance to assess the health impact of PHAH body burdens in exposed cohorts and the general population. However, long-term prospective studies in human populations must be carefully designed and will be severely hampered until the development of (1) a blood biomarker for endometriosis and (2) biomarkers of human exposure to dioxins. Progress in this area of research would greatly strengthen our ability to investigate the relationship between exposure to dioxins and an increased prevalence of endometriosis in humans. Mechanistic studies must be designed in the most appropriate animal models to test the effect of dioxins on pathogenic processes active in endometriosis. Biological assays must be developed to assess the effect of dioxins on the disease process of endometriosis. Although preliminary work suggests a potential involvement of exposure to dioxins and PCBs in the pathogenesis of endometriosis, much work remains to clearly define cause and effect and to understand the potential mechanism of toxicity leading to new therapeutic strategies.

CONCLUSIONS

This generation of young women reaching reproductive age is the first to be exposed to complex mixtures of chemicals in the womb. Coinciding with the worldwide contamination with dioxins, the prevalence of endometriosis appears to be on the rise and this increase in prevalence can only partially be explained by better physician awareness and diagnosis.[51] The evidence presented indicates that endometriosis may be associated with exposure to TCDD and PCBs in monkey models. These findings are relevant to human endometriosis since the serum levels of these environmental chemicals in TCDD-exposed animals are similar to concentrations reported in serum, milk, and tissues from the general human population. Preliminary studies in rodent models of endometriosis and in humans also suggest that exposure to dioxins may be associated with increased endometriosis. Additional studies in humans and animals are warranted to investigate the potential role of environmental dioxins in the etiology of this disease.

ACKNOWLEDGMENTS

This work was supported by The Endometriosis Association, Tracy H. Dickinson, The Fairleigh Dickinson Jr. Foundation, Inc., and by Grant No. ES08545-01 from the National Institute of Environmental Health Sciences (NIH). Sherry E. Rier is the Tracy H. Dickinson Research Chair of The Endometriosis Association.

REFERENCES

1. POLAND, A. & J.C. KNUTSON. 1982. 2,3,7,8-Tetrachlorodibenzo-*p*-dioxin and related halogenated aromatic hydrocarbons: examination of the mechanism of toxicity. Annu. Rev. Pharmacol. Toxicol. **22:** 517–554.
2. WHITLOCK, J.P. 1990. Genetic and molecular aspects of 2,3,7,8-tetrachlorodibenzo-*p*-dioxin action. Annu. Rev. Pharmacol. **30:** 251–277.
3. SUTTER, T.R. *et al.* 1991. Targets for dioxin: genes for plasminogen activator inhibitor-2 and interleukin-1-beta. Science **254:** 55–64.

4. SAFE, S. 1990. Polychlorinated biphenyls (PCBs), dibenzo-*p*-dioxins (PCDDs), dibenzofurans (PCDFs), and related compounds: environmental and mechanistic considerations which support the development of toxic equivalency factors (TEFs). Crit. Rev. Toxicol. **21:** 51–88.
5. SAFE, S. 1994. Polychlorinated biphenyls (PCBs): environmental impact, biochemical and toxic responses, and implications for risk assessment. Crit. Rev. Toxicol. **24:** 87–149.
6. VAN DEN BERG, M. *et al.* 1998. Toxic equivalency factors (TEFs) for PCBs, PCDDs, and PCDFs for humans and wildlife. Environ. Health Perspect. **106:** 775–792.
7. DEVITO, M.J. *et al.* 1995. Comparisons of estimated human body burdens of dioxinlike chemicals and TCDD body burdens in experimentally exposed animals. Environ. Health Perspect. **103:** 820–831.
8. WHITLOCK, J.P. 1994. The aromatic hydrocarbon receptor, dioxin action, and endocrine homeostasis. Trends Endocrinol. Metab. **5:** 183–188.
9. SCHECTER, A. *et al.* 1994. Polychlorinated biphenyl levels in the tissues of exposed and nonexposed humans. Environ. Health Perspect. **102:** 149–158.
10. SCHECTER, A. *et al.* 1994. Chlorinated dioxins and dibenzofurans in human tissue from general populations: a selective review. Environ. Health Perspect. **102:** 159–171.
11. VAN DEN HEUVEL, J.P. *et al.* 1994. Accumulation of polychlorinated dibenzo-*p*-dioxins and dibenzofurans in liver of control laboratory rats. Fundam. Appl. Toxicol. **23:** 465–469.
12. FARLAND, W. *et al.* 2000. USEPA's risk characterization of dioxin and related compounds. Organohalogen Comp. **48:** 248–251.
13. BIRNBAUM, L.S. 2000. Health effects of dioxins: people are animals and vice versa! Organohalogen Comp. **49:** 101–103.
14. CLARK, G. *et al.* 1992. Integrated approach for evaluating species and interindividual differences in responsiveness to dioxins and structural analogs. Environ. Health Perspect. **98:** 125–132.
15. WHEELER, J.M. 1992. Epidemiology and prevalence of endometriosis. Infertil. Reprod. Med. Clin. North Am. **3:** 545–549.
16. RODGERS, W.H. *et al.* 1994. Patterns of matrix metalloproteinase expression in cycling endometrium imply differential functions and regulation by steroids. Gynecol. Obstet. Invest. **48:** 45–56.
17. RIER, S.E. & G.R. YEAMAN. 1997. Immune aspects of endometriosis: relevance of the uterine mucosal immune system. Semin. Reprod. Endocrinol. **15:** 209–220.
18. OSTEEN, K.G. *et al.* 1996. Steroid and growth factor regulation of matrix metalloproteinase expression and endometriosis. Semin. Reprod. Endocrinol. **14:** 247–255.
19. FANTON, J.W. & J.G. GOLDEN. 1991. Radiation-induced endometriosis in *Macaca mulatta*. Radiat. Res. **126:** 141–146.
20. VERNON, M.W. 1992. Animal models in endometriosis research. Infertil. Reprod. Med. Clin. North Am. **3:** 565–581.
21. D'HOOGHE, T.M. *et al.* 1992. Evolution of spontaneous endometriosis in the baboon (*Papio anubis, Papio cynocephalus*) over a 12-month period. Fertil. Steril. **58:** 409–412.
22. BRUNER, K.L. *et al.* 1995. Transforming growth factor-β mediates the progesterone suppression of an epithelial metalloproteinase by adjacent stroma. Proc. Natl. Acad. Sci. U.S.A. **92:** 7362–7366.
23. RIER, S.E. *et al.* 1993. Endometriosis in rhesus monkeys (*Macaca mulatta*) following chronic exposure to 2,3,7,8-tetrachlorodibenzo-*p*-dioxin [see comments]. Fundam. Appl. Toxicol. **21:** 433–441.
24. YANG, J.Z. *et al.* 2000. Subchronic exposure to 2,3,7,8-tetrachlorodibenzo-*p*-dioxin modulates the pathophysiology of endometriosis in the cynomolgus monkey. Toxicol. Sci. **56:** 374–381.
25. CAMPBELL, J.S. *et al.* 1985. Is simian endometriosis an effect of immunotoxicity? Presented at the Forty-eighth Annual Meeting of the Ontario Association of Pathology, London, Ontario, Canada.
26. ARNOLD, D.L. *et al.* 1996. Prevalence of endometriosis in rhesus (*Macaca mulatta*) monkeys ingesting PCB (Aroclor 1254): review and evaluation. Fundam. Appl. Toxicol. **31:** 42–55.

27. CUMMINGS, A.M. *et al.* 1996. Promotion of endometriosis by 2,3,7,8-tetrachlorodibenzo-*p*-dioxin in rats and mice: time-dose dependence and species comparison. Toxicol. Appl. Pharmacol. **138:** 131–139.
28. JOHNSON, K.L. *et al.* 1997. Promotion of endometriosis in mice by polychlorinated dibenzo-*p*-dioxins, dibenzofurans, and biphenyls. Environ. Health Perspect. **105:** 750–755.
29. CUMMINGS, A.M. *et al.* 1999. Effect of prenatal exposure to TCDD on the promotion of endometriotic lesion growth by TCDD in adult female rats and mice. Toxicol. Sci. **52:** 45–49.
30. YANG, J.Z. & W.G. FOSTER. 1997. Continuous exposure to 2,3,7,8-tetrachlorodibenzo-*p*-dioxin inhibits the growth of surgically induced endometriosis in the ovariectomized mouse treated with high dose estradiol. Toxicol. Ind. Health **13:** 15–25.
31. MATSUI, K.A. *et al.* 2000. Effects of 2,3,7,8-tetrachlorodibenzo-*p*-dioxin on surgically induced endometriosis in mice and the role of Ah receptor. Organohalogen Comp. **49:** 345–348.
32. BRUNER, K.L. *et al.* 1997. Suppression of matrix metalloproteinases inhibits establishment of ectopic lesions by human tissue in nude mice. J. Clin. Invest. **99:** 2851–2857.
33. BRUNER-TRAN, K. *et al.* 1999. The potential role of environmental toxins in the pathophysiology of endometriosis. Gynecol. Obstet. Invest. **48:** 45–56.
34. KONINCKX, P.R. *et al.* 1994. Dioxin pollution and endometriosis in Belgium [see comments]. Hum. Reprod. **9:** 1001–1002.
35. WHO. 1989. Levels of PCBs, PCDDs, and PCDFs in breast milk: result of WHO coordinated interlaboratory quality control studies and analytical field studies. WHO Environmental Series.
36. PAUWELS, A. *et al.* 2000. The risk of endometriosis associated with the exposure to dioxins and related compounds: a case control study. Abstract presented at the Seventh Biennial World Endometriosis Congress, London.
37. MAYANI, A. *et al.* 1997. Dioxin concentrations in women with endometriosis. Hum. Reprod. **12:** 373–375.
38. ESKENAZI, B. *et al.* 2000. Seveso Women's Health Study: a study of the effects of 2,3,7,8,-tetrachlorodibenzo-*p*-dioxin on reproductive health. Chemosphere **40:** 1247–1253.
39. GERHARD, I. & B. RUNNEBAUM. 1992. Limits of hormone substitution in the case of exposure to harmful substances and fertility disturbances. Zentralbl. Gynaekol. **114:** 593–602.
40. GERHARD, I. *et al.* 1999. Chlorinated hydrocarbons in infertile women. Environ. Res. **80:** 299–310.
41. LEBEL, G. *et al.* 1998. Organochlorine exposure and the risk of endometriosis. Fertil. Steril. **69:** 221–228.
42. RIER, S.E. *et al.* 2001. Serum levels of TCDD and dioxinlike chemicals in rhesus monkeys chronically exposed to dioxin: correlation of increased serum PCB levels with endometriosis. Toxicol. Sci. **59:** 147–159.
43. KAHN, P.C. *et al.* 1988. Dioxins and dibenzofurans in blood and adipose tissue of Agent Orange–exposed Vietnam veterans and matched controls. JAMA **259:** 1661–1667.
44. WATANBE, S. *et al.* 2000. Health effects of chronic exposure to polychlorinated dibenzo-*p*-dioxins, dibenzofurans, and coplanar PCB around municipal waste incinerators. Organohalogen Comp. **48:** 199–202.
45. YOSHIDA, K. *et al.* 2000. Assessment of human health risk of dioxins in Japan. Chemosphere **40:** 177–185.
46. RIER, S.E. *et al.* 2001. Increased tumor necrosis factor alpha by peripheral blood leukocytes from TCDD-exposed rhesus monkeys. Toxicol. Sci. In press.
47. RIER, S.E. *et al.* 2000. TCDD-exposed rhesus monkeys exhibit disseminated endometriosis, decreased serum estradiol, and increased serum cortisol levels. Abstract presented at the Seventh Biennial World Endometriosis Congress, London.
48. MICHALEK, J.E. *et al.* 1999. Serum dioxin, insulin, fasting glucose, and sex hormone–binding globulin in veterans of Operation Ranch Hand. J. Clin. Endocrinol. Metab. **84:** 1540–1543.
49. CALVERT, G.M. *et al.* 1999. Evaluation of diabetes mellitus, serum glucose, and thyroid function among United States workers exposed to 2,3,7,8,-tetrachlorodibenzo-*p*-dioxin. Occup. Environ. Med. **56:** 270–276.

50. REDWINE, D.B. 1987. Age-related evolution in color appearance of endometriosis. Fertil. Steril. **48:** 1062–1063.
51. MOLPUS, K.L. 1995. Pathophysiology and management of prior or current endometriosis in the perimenopausal woman. *In* Infertility and Reproductive Clinics of North America, pp. 805–828. Saunders. Philadelphia.

Environmental Contaminants and Dietary Factors in Endometriosis

WARREN G. FOSTER AND SANJAY K. AGARWAL

Department of Obstetrics and Gynecology, Cedars-Sinai Medical Center, Los Angeles, California, USA

ABSTRACT: Endometriosis is an estrogen-dependent disease characterized by the presence of endometrial glands and stroma outside the uterine cavity. The etiology of this disease remains elusive, but is clearly influenced by genetic, immune, and endocrine factors. Exposure to environmental contaminants has recently been added to the list of potential factors that contribute to the pathogenesis of endometriosis. The objective of this paper is to review the weight of the evidence from hospital-based case-control studies and animal experiments for an association between exposure to environmental contaminants and endometriosis.

KEYWORDS: endometriosis; animal models; toxicology; monkeys; TCDD

INTRODUCTION

Endometriosis is an estrogen-dependent disease characterized by the presence of endometrial glands and stroma outside the uterine cavity. The etiology of this disease remains elusive, but is clearly influenced by genetic, immune, and endocrine factors. Retrograde menstruation or bleeding into the peritoneal cavity during menstruation is widely accepted as a major contributing factor in the pathogenesis of this disease. However, backflow of menstrual materials through the fallopian tubes to the pelvic cavity is a common phenomenon even in women without endometriosis.[1] Hence, factors other than retrograde menstruation such as hormonal stimulation or impaired immune function are thought to contribute to the development and progression of endometriosis. Exposure to environmental contaminants has recently been added to the list of potential factors that contribute to the pathogenesis of endometriosis. This view is supported by a number of lines of evidence. Specifically, exposure to various environmental contaminants has been demonstrated through the detection of chemical contaminants in the serum and ovarian follicular fluid of women attending fertility clinics.[2] Further, estrogenic activity for numerous environmental contaminants, together with the estrogen dependence of endometriosis, leads us to speculate that environmental contaminants can play a role in the pathophysiology of endometriosis. The association between exposure to environmental contaminants and endometriosis has previously been reviewed.[3–5] Thus, the objective of this paper

Address for correspondence: Warren G. Foster, Ph.D., Director, Reproductive Biology, Department of Obstetrics and Gynecology, HSC-3N52, McMaster University, 1200 Main Street West, Hamilton, Ontario, Canada L8N 3Z5. Voice: 905-525-9140, ext. 22822; fax: 905-524-2911.
fosterw@mcmaster.ca

is to review the weight of the evidence from hospital-based case-control studies and animal experiments for an association between exposure to environmental contaminants and endometriosis. While it is concluded that the evidence at present neither supports nor refutes the hypothesis that environmental contaminants are associated with endometriosis, cause for continued investigation remains. New animal models for endometriosis research promise to provide useful tools to explore the etiology and pathophysiology of endometriosis.

ENVIRONMENTAL CONTAMINANTS AND ENDOMETRIOSIS

Evidence from Case-Control Human Studies

Endometriosis is a complex disease characterized by estrogen dependence and impairment of immune function. Dependence upon estrogen is shown by occurrence of endometriosis in (1) men treated with high levels of estrogen and (2) women with active menstrual cycles and by (3) regression of endometriotic lesions in women treated with GnRH analogues or an aromatase inhibitor, all of which result in lower serum estradiol concentrations. Moreover, endometriosis is more common among obese women[6] and those that consume alcohol,[7,8] both of which favor increased circulating levels of estrogens. Since estrogens play a central role in the pathobiology of endometriosis, a number of investigators have sought to determine the association between endometriosis and exposures to environmental contaminants, some of which act as environmental estrogens.

A small number of hospital-based case-control studies have been conducted in which exposure of women with endometriosis to environmental contaminants has been investigated (TABLE 1). Exposure to polychlorinated biphenyls (PCBs)[9] and dioxins[10] has been loosely linked with endometriosis. In the former study,[9] serum levels of PCBs 138, 153, and 180 were elevated compared to women without endometriosis. In a letter to the editor, Koninckx and colleagues[10] noted that the levels of dioxins in Belgium are among the highest in the world and the incidence of endometriosis is also higher in this country than elsewhere. A positive association between endometriosis and dioxin (2,3,7,8-tetrachlorodibenzo-*p*-dioxin, TCDD) exposure was reported in a single case-control study in which 44 women with endometriosis were compared with 35 age-matched women with tubal infertility.[11] In this study, 1 control subject had a detectable level of TCDD, whereas 8 women of 44 had detectable levels. While an odds ratio (OR) of 7.6 was obtained, the 95% confidence interval (CI) included unity (0.87–169.7); thus, it cannot be concluded that dioxin exposure alone is associated with endometriosis, but other chemical contaminants that migrate with dioxin or act through a common mechanistic pathway may be involved. A weakness of this study is the failure to control for obstetrical history. Since a full-term pregnancy and breast-feeding are thought to decrease body burdens of lipophilic environmental contaminants, it is not possible to determine if prior pregnancies may have accounted for the low number of detections observed in this study. In an ongoing study,[12] the association between endometriosis and exposure to dioxin has been investigated in women living in Seveso, Italy. Preliminary results of the Seveso Women's Health Study (SWHS) reveal a nonsignificant doubling of risk.[13]

TABLE 1. Summary of exposures and outcomes in five epidemiological studies designed to investigate the association between exposure to persistent organic pollutants and endometriosis

Authors	Cases vs. controls	Exposure	Tissue	Outcome
Gerhard and Runnebaum, 1992[9]	28/441	PCB congeners, heavy metals, and chlorinated pesticides	S	Positive association for PCBs (138, 153, and 180).
Boyd *et al.*, 1995[15]	15/15	Dioxins and furans	S	No relationship.
Mayani *et al.*, 1997[11]	44/35	Dioxin	B	Positive association for TCDD; 8 of 44 cases (18%) had detectable levels of TCDD compared to 1 of 35 controls (3%). Concentration of TCDD was low, ranging between 0.4 and 1.2 ppt.
Lebel *et al.*, 1998[14]	86/70	PCB congeners and chlorinated pesticides	P	No relationship.
Eskenazi *et al.*, 2001[13]	82/307	Dioxin	S	Nonsignificant doubling of risk.

NOTE: PCB = polychlorinated biphenyls; S = serum; B = blood; P = plasma.

In another study, no association between endometriosis and PCB-specific congeners and organochlorine pesticide concentrations could be found in a case-control study of 86 women with endometriosis and 70 controls matched for the indication of laparoscopy.[14] In this study, congener-specific PCB analysis was conducted as a surrogate for TCDD, which is thought to comigrate with the PCBs. While the exposure assessment taken in this study permitted a broader assessment of the exposures that could influence the pathogenesis of endometriosis, the absence of a truly unexposed control population and sample size limitations are both limiting factors that may have prevented detection of an association between endometriosis and exposure. Similarly, Boyd and coworkers[15] were unable to find an association between endometriosis and exposure to dioxins and furans in a study involving 15 control subjects and 15 cases.

All of the case-control studies described in the literature to date are relatively small and thus may not have the statistical power to detect differences if they were indeed present. Hence, the human data at present neither confirm nor refute the hypothesis that environmental contaminants play a role in the pathobiology of endometriosis.

TABLE 2. Summary of exposures and outcomes in several nonhuman primate studies designed to investigate the association between exposure to hormonally active environmental contaminants and endometriosis

Authors	Animal model	*N*	Exposure	Outcome
Rier *et al.*, 1993[16]	Rhesus monkey	7	0, 5, and 25 ppt TCDD in diet	Dose-related increase in incidence and severity of endometriosis.
Arnold *et al.*, 1996[18]	Rhesus monkey	16	Aroclor 1254, oral capsule	No association between treatments and endometriosis.
Yang *et al.*, 2000[19]	Cynomolgus monkey	6	0, 1, 5, and 25 ng TCDD/kg/day, oral capsule	Inhibition of endometriotic implant growth by low dose and facilitated growth by medium and high doses. Regression of implants over time, which was retarded in medium- and high-dose groups.
Rier *et al.*, 2001[17]	Rhesus monkey	7	TCDD, PCB congener-specific analysis, and lead	3,3′,4,4′-Tetrachlorobiphenyl, 3,3′,4,4′,5-hexachlorobiphenyl associated with presence of endometriosis and severity, respectively.

Evidence from Animal Studies

An association between endometriosis and exposure to environmental contaminants has been explored in nonhuman primate studies (TABLE 2). The notion that environmental contaminants are involved in the pathophysiology of endometriosis gained momentum with the demonstration that the incidence and severity of spontaneous endometriosis were increased in rhesus monkeys following treatment with 5 or 25 ppt TCDD.[16] In this reproductive/developmental toxicology study, monkeys were treated with TCDD for 4 years and, approximately 6 years later, laparoscopies were performed to investigate the relationship between TCDD treatment and endometriosis. A dose-dependent increase in the incidence and severity of endometriosis was found at laparoscopy in this study. However, Rier and coworkers[17] have subsequently reported the results of residue analysis of the serum for TCDD and PCB-specific congeners from the monkeys involved in the original endometriosis study[16] and discovered that the incidence and severity of endometriosis were not correlated with serum TCDD levels. Elevated serum levels of 3,3′,4,4′-tetrachlorobiphenyl (TCB) and 3,3′,4,4′,5–pentachlorobiphenyl (PnCB) and an increased total serum TEQ were associated with a higher prevalence of endometriosis, whereas the severity of endometriosis was correlated with the serum concentration of 3,3′,4,4′-TCB. Both of these coplanar PCBs are believed to act through the aryl hydrocarbon receptor (AhR). The toxic effects of TCDD are thought to be mediated through the AhR. Consequently, we propose that AhR ligands together with or in addition to TCDD are important in the pathophysiology of endometriosis.

Rhesus monkeys treated with a commercial PCB mixture, Aroclor 1254, however, failed to show any relationship between the incidence and/or severity of endometriosis and PCB dose.[18] In this reproductive/developmental toxicology study, monkeys were exposed to the PCB mixture over a 5-year period before being examined by either laparoscopy (control and high-dose monkeys) or necropsy for evidence of endometriosis and adenomyosis. Both the Rier *et al.*[16] and the Arnold *et al.*[18] studies employed feral rhesus monkeys with varied clinical backgrounds. However, monkeys in the latter study, although still menstruating, likely were in the perimenopausal to menopausal age range and consequently may have affected endometriotic implant survival. Alternatively, we propose that the PCB mixture used in this study[18] possesses low dioxin-like activity and thus would not be expected to have similar effects to TCDD.

In another study,[19] the effect of TCDD on surgically induced endometriosis was investigated. The doses of TCDD employed in this study were selected to be equivalent to those used by Rier and colleagues[16] and expanded to include one lower dose level. Interestingly, this study revealed a bimodal effect of TCDD on the maximum and minimum implant diameter. Maximum and minimum diameters of the lesions were significantly greater in the 25-ppt dose group compared to controls and reduced in the 1-ppt group compared to controls. Over the course of the study, implants were found to regress in all treatment groups, but significant differences were not found until the completion of the study at 1-year postimplantation. Second, the implant site was found to affect survival, with the ovary being a preferential site. Survival of ectopic endometrial implants was also affected by TCDD treatment, with survival being significantly enhanced at the 5- and 25-ppt level compared to the controls. Consequently, this study supports and extends the findings of the earlier study in rhesus monkeys.[16] Furthermore, these data suggest that the duration of exposure to TCDD and by implication other AhR ligands must be lengthy before effects on endometrial implant survival and proliferation can be discerned.

Surgical induction of endometriosis in rodents has been used to investigate the effect of environmental contaminants on the establishment of endometrial implants, survival of existing implants, and the mechanism of contaminant action (TABLE 3). In two separate studies[20,21] involving mice and rats, autologous uterine implants were found to be estrogen-dependent and responsive to an estrogenic contaminant, methoxychlor. In another study, ovariectomized mice with autotransplanted uterine strips were used to demonstrate that administration of 4-chlorodiphenyl ether, an estrogenic compound, could facilitate implant growth.[22] These studies thus reveal that estrogenic contaminants affect the survival and proliferation of autologous uterine implants in rodent models, making these suitable models for testing chemical contaminants for potential activity in this disease. Accordingly, these models have been used to explore the effect of TCDD on the growth of uterine implants. TCDD treatment enhanced the growth of implants.[23] In these studies, administration of 0, 3, or 10 μg TCDD/kg on gestational day 8 and then again 3 weeks before surgical induction of endometriosis in both the rat and the mouse resulted in an increase in implant size.[23] In another study in mice, endometriosis was surgically induced and the animals were treated with 0, 1, 3, or 10 μg TCDD/kg; 3 or 30 mg PCB 153; 100, 300, or 1000 μg PCB 126/kg; 10, 30, or 100 μg 4-PeCDF/kg; or 2 or 20 mg 1,3,6,8-TCDD by gavage, five times at 3 weeks apart. Following necropsy 3 weeks after the final dose, 2,3,7,8-TCDD and 4-PeCDF significantly enhanced the growth of endo-

TABLE 3. Summary of exposures and outcomes in several rodent studies designed to investigate the association between exposure to hormonally active environmental contaminants and endometriosis

Authors	Animal model	*N*	Exposure	Outcome
Cummings and Metcalf, 1995[20]	Rats	6	Intact, OVX, and OVX + 0.5 μg/day estrone	Showed estrogen dependence of implants.
Cummings and Metcalf, 1995[21]	Rats	10	250 mg MXC/kg, gavage; 1 μg estrone/rat, sc	MXC maintained endometriotic implant size in ovariectomized rats equal to estrone.
Cummings *et al.*, 1996[23]	Rats and mice	8	0, 3, or 10 μg TCDD/kg on GD 8 and then again 3 weeks before surgery	Increase in implant diameter.
Johnson *et al.*, 1997[24]	Mice	10	0, 1, 3, or 10 μg TCDD/kg; 3 or 30 mg PCB 153; 100, 300, or 1000 μg PCB 126/kg; 10, 30, or 100 μg 4-PeCDF/kg; or 2 or 20 mg 1,3,6,8-TCDD by gavage, five times at 3 weeks apart	Endometriosis was surgically induced during the week of the second dosing. Following necropsy 3 weeks after the final dose, 2,3,7,8-TCDD and 4-PeCDF significantly enhanced the growth of endometrial lesions. PCB 126 and the highest dose of TCDD were without effect on growth of the endometrial lesions. The nondioxin-like compounds were without effect on lesion growth.
Cummings *et al.*, 1999	Rats and mice	12	0, 1, or 3 μg TCDD/kg on GD 8 and then again 3 weeks before surgery	In mice, a significant increase in lesion diameter. No effect in rats.
Yang *et al.*, 1997[22]	Mice	8	0, 10, 75, or 150 mg 4-CDE/kg, gavage	Dose-related increase in implant survival.
Yang and Foster, 1997[25]	Mice	8	0, 10, 50, or 100 ng TCDD/kg, gavage	Regression of implants.

NOTE: OVX = ovariectomy; MXC = methoxychlor; TCDD = 2,3,7,8-tetrachlorodibenzo-*p*-dioxin; 4-PeCDF = 2,3,4,7,8-pentachlorodibenzofuran; 4-CDE = chlorodiphenyl ether; sc = subcutaneous.

metrial lesions, whereas PCB 126 and the highest dose of TCDD were without effect on the growth of endometrial lesions. Moreover, the nondioxin-like compounds were without effect on lesion growth. These data therefore suggest that it is the dioxin-like compounds that possess the ability to modulate the pathophysiology of endometriosis. In contrast to these findings, ovariectomized and estrogen-replaced mice, treated with 10, 50, and 100 ng TCDD/kg/day, resulted in inhibited growth of previously established implants.[25] Taken together, these data suggest that the dose of TCDD and the length of time that the implants are exposed to TCDD are also important in the outcome.

Rodent models of endometriosis are fraught with a number of significant limitations. The estrous cycle in rodents is significantly shorter than in humans and is characterized by endocrinological differences such as an abbreviated luteal phase compared to humans. While rodents do not go through a process of menstruation, they do possess a process of reorganization of the uterine epithelium. Moreover, circulating levels of estradiol in rodents are markedly lower than in humans. Rodents do however offer significant advantages over other animal models or humans. Since endometriosis is already well established by the time a diagnosis is made, investigation of the factors important in the pathogenesis of this disease in humans is not practical. In addition, rodents are significantly less expensive than primates, smaller, and easier to handle. Thus, animal models continue to be important for the study of the pathobiology of endometriosis.

FUTURE DIRECTIONS

Animal Models

The demonstration that heterotransplants of animal and human tumors maintain their tumorigenicity, morphology,[26–30] and hormone responsiveness, as in the case of endometrial adenocarcinoma,[31] in immune-deficient mice, such as the athymic nude mouse and severe combined immune-deficient mice (SCID), suggests that these animals may prove to be useful models to study human endometriosis. Several teams of investigators have examined immune-deficient mice, either athymic nude mice[32–36] or SCID mice,[37,38] as short-term models of endometriosis (TABLE 4). Low natural killer cell activity has been postulated to play a role in the pathogenesis of endometriosis.[39,40] It has been argued[37] that nude mice are inappropriate for heterotransplantation of human endometrial tissue for studies of 1 to 3 months because nude mice have compensatory high natural killer cell activity that results in spontaneous regression of implants. SCID mice are deficient in T and B lymphocyte function and have been used previously as recipients of 2-mm cubes of human eutopic endometrium transplanted into subcutaneous pockets.[37] Heterotransplantation was successful and implants were still present at the conclusion of the study 10 weeks later. Histologically, the implants resembled endometriotic lesions. Therefore, we suggest that immune-compromised mouse models bearing human eutopic and ectopic endometrium will provide advantages over previous rodent models that will generate results that are more readily generalizable to humans.

TABLE 4. Immune-compromised mouse models of endometriosis, treatments, and experimental outcomes

Authors	Model	Source of tissue and treatments	Transplantation site and outcome
Bergqvist *et al.*, 1985[33,34]	Nude	Eutopic and ectopic endometrium fragments, polyestradiol phosphate, medroxyprogesterone acetate, danazol, control.	Subcutaneous; histologically the implants reacted in a similar manner to treatments as eutopic endometrium.
Zamah *et al.*, 1984[32]	Nude	Proliferative and secretory phase eutopic and ectopic endometrium. Control or 30 μg estradiol cyprionate/kg weekly, intramuscularly.	Subcutaneous; implants of proliferative endometrium became undetectable between 24 and 32 days, whereas ectopic endometrium was detectable for up to 70 days and resembled intraperitoneal endometriotic lesions.
Aoki *et al.*, 1994[37]	SCID and nude	Eutopic endometrium fragments obtained by hysterectomy and samples were from the proliferative, late proliferative, and early secretory phase. Danazol (10–100 mg/kg/day, oral), buserelin (0.01 mg/kg/day, subcutaneous), or estradiol (0.5 mg/kg/day, intraperitoneal).	Subcutaneous; heterotransplantation of endometrial tissue was successful in 100% of SCID and only 40% of nude mice at 10 weeks after transplantation.
Bruner *et al.*, 1997[35]	Nude	Eutopic endometrium fragments from the proliferative interval of the menstrual cycle. Twenty-four-hour organ culture with estradiol or estradiol plus progesterone. Ovariectomized mice bearing endometrial implants received estradiol or progesterone via subcutaneous capsules.	Intraperitoneal injection of 8–10 endometrial fragments; suppression of matrix metalloproteinases with progesterone treatment inhibits formation of ectopic endometrial lesions.
Awwad *et al.*, 1999[38]	SCID	Minced cells from the secretory phase eutopic endometrium. Estradiol (30 μg/kg) and estradiol plus progesterone (10 mg/kg).	Intraperitoneal by injection. Tissue successfully implanted in 96.5% of animals. Estradiol plus progesterone favored larger and multiple implants.
Nisolle *et al.*, 2000[36]	Nude	Menstruated endometrium, fragments.	Intraperitoneal by laparotomy. Implants detected in all 10 mice and increase in proliferation of glandular cells and VEGF score of stroma seen at 5 days postimplantation.

Environmental and Dietary Factors in the Pathophysiology of Endometriosis

Investigation of the association between exposure to environmental contaminants and endometriosis has focused exclusively on persistent organic pollutants (POPs) and has previously been reviewed.[4,5] While the pathophysiology of endometriosis is both complex and incompletely understood, we do know that this disease involves processes of attachment of endometrial cells to pelvic structures, implantation, revascularization, proliferation, and remodeling of implants. It is thus conceivable that many chemical contaminants and possibly dietary factors can affect one or more of these processes and thus impact the pathogenesis of endometriosis via multiple mechanisms. Therefore, we speculate that there are potentially a large number of environmental contaminants that modulate the pathophysiology of endometriosis due to estrogenic action, immune suppression, effects on angiogenesis and attachment of endometrial cells to pelvic structures, or dysregulation of enzymes involved in the synthesis or metabolism of endogenous steroids. Furthermore, we propose that dietary factors with biological activity such as the phytoestrogens and glucosinolates should not be overlooked as potential modifying factors in endometriosis.

AhR Ligands

The AhR is a high-affinity, low-capacity protein that binds chemicals such as glucosinolates, TCDD, constituents of cigarette smoke such as benzo[*a*]pyrene, and other polynuclear aromatic hydrocarbons[41,42] to which the American population is exposed. This receptor is present in many tissues, such as placenta,[43] eutopic and ectopic endometrium,[44] and various tumor cells including those from breast[45,46] and cervix.[47] There are no known endogenous ligands for this receptor, although metabolites of tryptophan, namely tryptamine, have been shown to bind to and activate the AhR in culture.[48]

TCDD is a ubiquitous contaminant produced during the manufacture of chlorophenols and phenoxy herbicides,[49,50] waste incineration,[51,52] and the bleaching of pulp for paper. The mean adipose tissue level for the American population has been reported[53–55] to be between 5.2 and 5.4 ng/kg. Adipose tissue levels in individuals exposed either through the workplace or as a result of accidental exposure range between 10 and 141 ng/kg.[55] In women with both endometriosis and measurable levels of TCDD in whole blood, the nonlipid-adjusted concentration of TCDD was between 0.7 and 1.2 ng/kg.[11]

TCDD and other AhR agonists may modulate the endometriosis via a number of independent processes. AhR ligand binding affects a number of genes that are potentially important in the pathobiology of endometriosis. In particular, AhR ligand binding regulates epidermal growth factor (EGF), IL-1β, TGF-α, and TGF-β.[56–58] Furthermore, in the rat, TCDD treatment inhibited the 17β-estradiol-induced increase in uterine wet weight[59] and, in mice, the 17β-estradiol-induced increase in uterine EGF mRNA levels. Contradictory reports have appeared in the literature concerning the effect of TCDD on uterine estrogen receptor levels: TCDD-induced suppression in rats has been reported by some,[60,61] whereas others found no effect in mice.[62] However, decreased expression of estrogen receptor mRNA in the ovaries and uteri of TCDD-treated mice has recently been demonstrated.[63] The effect of TCDD on ERβ expression in rodents and human ERα and ERβ expression has not been studied previously. Recently, progesterone-induced suppression of matrix metalloproteinase expression was impaired by TCDD treatment in an experimental model of endometriosis.[64] TCDD-induced dysregulation of IL-6 has also been demonstrated in both spontaneous and experimentally induced endometriosis in the monkey.[16,19]

ER Ligands

Estrogenic environmental compounds are much less potent than either DES or estradiol as revealed by their poor affinity for the estrogen receptor[65] and weak induction of MCF-7 cell proliferation *in vitro.*[66,67] Because man-made chemicals with estrogenic activity are weak hormone mimics and are less potent than the endogenous estrogens, it has been suggested that they are unlikely to pose a threat to human health.[68] However, the potential for these compounds to act in an additive manner has not been explored. Moreover, detection of estrogenic chemicals in human ovarian follicular fluid and serum[2] raises the possibility that these chemicals may be present in sufficient concentration to reach target tissue at stages critical in the pathogenesis of endometriosis, such as attachment of endometrial cells to pelvic structures, angiogenesis, invasion, and proliferation. Examples of estrogenic contaminants that could affect endometrial implant proliferation include insecticides such as endosulfan I and II, methoxychlor, toxaphene, dieldrin, Kepone, lindane, DDT, *o,p′*-DDT, and *o,p′*-DDE. Industrial chemicals that have been shown to be estrogenic include the PCB congeners and their hydroxylated metabolites.[69] A number of plasticizers have also been identified as estrogenic and include bisphenol A, benzylbutylphthalate, and dibutylphthalate. However, to our knowledge, the association between endometriosis and exposure to estrogenic contaminants has not been investigated to any appreciable degree.

Unlike man-made chemical contaminants, the dietary phytoestrogens are much more potent, ranging from 1/10,000th to 1/100th the potency of estradiol. Phytoestrogens are naturally occurring plant estrogens that are present in greater than 300 different plants from more than 16 different families.[70] While isoflavones are found mainly in legumes such as soy, lentils, beans, and chickpeas, lignins and flavones are found in most cereals and fruits. The major phytoestrogens of soybeans are the isoflavones, genistein (GEN) and daidzein (DAZ), whereas naringenin (NAR), a flavanone, is derived from foods such as citrus fruits. Other isoflavones include coumestrol, formononetin, and biochanin A.

Although phytoestrogens are relatively weak estrogens, there is evidence in the literature that suggests that these chemicals exert biologically relevant effects on the human reproductive tract. Altered reproductive function in women[71] decreased serum estrogen levels, and increased levels of sex hormone binding globulin[72,73] have been reported in women with high consumption of soy-rich diets. Menstrual disturbances have also been reported in vegetarian women compared to age-matched nonvegetarians.[74] Adverse effects of phytoestrogens in rodents have also been reported,[75] although at much higher dose levels (approximately 50 mg/kg/day) than used in studies in which GEN (approximately 15 mg/kg/day) has inhibited endometrial proliferation.[76] Human data have been brought forward in the literature indicating that lower levels of dietary isoflavones protect from endometrial proliferation, as shown by a decreased incidence of endometrial cancer in Japanese and American (Hawaiian) women consuming isoflavone-rich diets.[77] Specifically, high consumption of soy products and other legumes was associated with a decreased risk of endometrial cancer (p for trend = 0.01; OR = 0.46; 95% CI = 0.26–0.83) for the highest compared with the lowest quartile of soy intake. Others have demonstrated that soy isoflavones inhibit estradiol-mediated endometrial proliferation in macaque monkeys.[76] While beneficial effects of dietary phytoestrogens on the eutopic endometrium have been reported, no data are available regarding the impact of isoflavones or flavones on human endometriotic tissue. For the most part, dietary exposure to phytoestrogens is assumed to be safe because, despite years of use and the substantial contribution of these agents to Asian diets, no adverse effects have been reported. However, an association between endometriosis and dietary phytoestrogen intake has not been conducted and comparative data on the prevalence of endometriosis in Japan versus North America are not available. Hence, it is not possible to conclude at this stage that phytoestrogens have either a beneficial or adverse effect in this disease.

There are a number of reasons why phytoestrogens are thought to modulate the pathophysiology of endometriosis. Phytoestrogens possess both estrogenic and anti-estrogenic activities that are both organ-specific[78] and dose-dependent.[79] Moreover, these agents exhibit both receptor- and nonreceptor-mediated activities. Given the evidence that, relative to estradiol binding to ERα and ERβ, the isoflavone GEN has one-twentieth the affinity at ERα, but one-third the affinity at ERβ, we should consider GEN to be a preferential ERβ ligand. The predominant estrogen receptor in the uterus is ERα,[80] although ERβ mRNA is also expressed in human endometrial stroma and epithelial cells of endometrial glands.[81] In knockout mice failing to express ERα (ERKO), no response to estrogen could be demonstrated, although these mice do express ERβ.[82,83] Consequently, ERβ is thought to modulate estrogenic action at ERα and thus dietary phytoestrogens can disrupt estrogen signaling in the endometrium depending upon preferential binding with ERα or ERβ. Moreover, in some studies, isoflavones have been shown to inhibit both estrogen-dependent and estrogen-independent cell proliferation.[84] The isoflavone phytoestrogens, GEN and DAZ, inhibit steroid-metabolizing enzymes[85] and GEN inhibits protein tyrosine kinases.[86] Recently, the aromatase inhibitory activity of various isoflavones and one flavanone, NAR, was investigated in traditional binding studies and computer modeling.[87] In this study, both GEN and NAR inhibited aromatase, but NAR was a much more potent aromatase inhibitor. However, the *in vivo* efficacy of these compounds has not been determined. Therefore, we speculate that dietary phytoestrogens possess the potential to modulate estrogen action in the endometrium and suppress aromatase activity of ectopic endometrium in women with endometriosis.

Steroidogenic Enzyme Modulators

$P450_{AROM}$ is an enzyme that catalyzes the conversion of androgens or C19 steroids (androstenedione and testosterone) to estrone and subsequently estrone to estradiol. Expression of $P450_{AROM}$ has been demonstrated for a number of reproductive tissues, including ovarian granulosa cells,[88] Leydig cells,[89] and placenta.[90] This enzyme is also expressed in nonreproductive tissues such as adipose tissue,[91] breast cancer tissue,[92] and the brain.[93] Normal endometrium and myometrium do not contain $P450_{AROM}$ transcripts and thus do not express this enzyme.[94] However, $P450_{AROM}$ expression has been demonstrated in endometriotic tissue, but was not detectable in normal endometrium from women with endometriosis or in nonendometriotic pelvic tissues from women with endometriosis.[95] These data therefore indicate that endometriotic tissue possesses the capacity for *de novo* synthesis of estradiol. Recently, the triazine herbicides (atrazine, simazine, and propazine) were shown to increase aromatase activity in the H295R human adrenocortical carcinoma cell line.[96] We thus suggest that it is plausible for environmental contaminants to affect aromatase activity in human tissues, thereby representing a novel pathway for endocrine disruption.

SUMMARY AND CONCLUSIONS

While the human case-control studies fail to provide a compelling case for an association between endometriosis and exposure to environmental contaminants, various animal studies involving both spontaneous and surgically induced endometriosis provide evidence that supports the hypothesis that AhR ligands or dioxin-like compounds modulate the pathophysiology of this disease. Sample size, control of confounding factors, selection of appropriate control or reference populations, and analytes to be examined are all factors that must be considered and they must receive particular attention in future epidemiological studies.

It is now evident that eutopic and ectopic endometrium are biochemically distinct and thus the effects of cytokines and exogenous factors on the eutopic endometrium cannot be extrapolated to ectopic endometrium. Of the multitude of chemical contaminants to which the population is exposed, the dioxin-like compounds have been consistently shown in nonhuman primate and rodent studies to modulate the pathophysiology of endometriosis. However, the mechanism of action of TCDD and related compounds remains unclear. Insight into TCDD dose-response characteristics and duration of exposure require investigation. Such studies can be expected to advance our understanding of the potential adverse effects of dioxin and related compounds in endometriosis, as well as offering insight into potential novel therapeutic interventions that might be derived from various dietary factors such as the glucosinolates. Potential effects of environmental contaminants and dietary isoflavones on aromatase activity in ectopic endometrium represent another interesting avenue of inquiry that has yet to be explored. Furthermore, to better appreciate the potential for exogenous factors to modulate the pathophysiology of endometriosis, a better understanding of the basic mechanisms underlying this disease will be essential. For example, examination of genetic polymorphisms for the AhR, ER, and progesterone receptors in endometriosis is needed, as is clarification of the role of ERβ in human eutopic and ectopic endometrium. The uses of gene knockout and gene knockdown animal models together with immune-compromised mouse models of endometriosis all promise to yield valuable results concerning the initiation and temporal changes in the pathophysiology of this disease.

REFERENCES

1. HALME, J., M.G. HAMMOND & J.F. HULKA. 1984. Retrograde menstruation in healthy women and in patients with endometriosis. Obstet. Gynecol. **64:** 151–154.
2. JARRELL, J., D. VILLENEUVE, C. FRANKLIN *et al.* 1993. Contamination of human ovarian follicular fluid and serum by chlorinated organic compounds in three Canadian cities. Can. Med. Assoc. J. **148:** 1321–1327.

3. AHLBORG, U.G., L. LIPWORTH, L. TITUS-ERNSTOFF *et al.* 1995. Organochlorine compounds in relation to breast cancer, endometrial cancer, and endometriosis: an assessment of the biological and epidemiological evidence. Crit. Rev. Toxicol. **25:** 463–531.
4. RIER, S.E., D.C. MARTIN, R.E. BOWMAN & J.L. BECKER. 1995. Immunoresponsiveness in endometriosis: implications of estrogenic toxicants. Environ. Health Perspect. **103**(suppl. 7)**:** 151–156.
5. ZEYNELOGLU, H.B., A. ARICI & D.L. OLIVE. 1997. Environmental toxins and endometriosis. Obstet. Gynecol. Clin. North Am. **24:** 307–329.
6. BERUBE, S., S. MARCOUX, M. LANGEVIN & R. MAHEUX. 1998. Fecundity of infertile women with minimal or mild endometriosis and women with unexplained infertility: The Canadian Collaborative Group on Endometriosis. Fertil. Steril. **69:** 1034–1041.
7. PERPER, M.M., L.J. BREITKOPF, R. BREITSTEIN *et al.* 1993. MAST scores, alcohol consumption, and gynecological symptoms in endometriosis patients. Alcohol Clin. Exp. Res. **17:** 272–278.
8. GRODSTEIN, F., M.B. GOLDMAN & D.W. CRAMER. 1994. Infertility in women and moderate alcohol use. Am. J. Public Health **84:** 1429–1432.
9. GERHARD, I. & B. RUNNEBAUM. 1992. Fertility disorders may result from heavy metal and pesticide contamination which limits effectiveness of hormone therapy. Zentralbl. Gynaekol. **114:** 593–602.
10. KONINCKX, P.R., P. BRAET, S.H. KENNEDY & D.H. BARLOW. 1994. Dioxin pollution and endometriosis in Belgium. Hum. Reprod. **9:** 1001–1002.
11. MAYANI, A., S. BAREL, S. SOBACK & M. ALMAGOR. 1997. Dioxin concentration in women with endometriosis. Hum. Reprod. **12:** 373–375.
12. ESKENAZI, B., P. MOCARELLI, M. WARNER *et al.* 2000. Seveso Women's Health Study: a study of the effects of 2,3,7,8-tetrachlorodibenzo-*p*-dioxin on reproductive health. Chemosphere **40:** 1247–1253.
13. ESKENAZI, B. *et al.* 2001. http://es.epa.gov/nserqa/final/grants/95/human/eskenazi//.
14. LEBEL, G., S. DODIN, P. AYOTTE *et al.* 1998. Organochlorine exposure and the risk of endometriosis. Fertil. Steril. **69:** 221–228.
15. BOYD, J.A., G.C. CLARK, D.K. WALMER *et al.* 1995. Endometriosis and the environment: biomarkers of toxin exposure. Presented at the Conference on Endometriosis 2000 (May 15–17, 1995), National Institutes of Health, Bethesda.
16. RIER, S.E., D.C. MARTIN, R.E. BOWMAN *et al.* 1993. Endometriosis in rhesus monkeys (*Macaca mulatta*) following chronic exposure to tetrachlorodibenzo-*p*-dioxin. Fundam. Appl. Toxicol. **21:** 433–441.
17. RIER, S.E., W.E. TURNER, D.C. MARTIN *et al.* 2001. Serum levels of TCDD and dioxin-like chemicals in rhesus monkeys chronically exposed to dioxin: correlation of increased serum PCB levels with endometriosis. Toxicol. Sci. **59:** 147–159.
18. ARNOLD, D.L., E.A. NERA, R. STAPLEY *et al.* 1996. Prevalence of endometriosis in rhesus (*Macaca mulatta*) monkeys ingesting PCB (Aroclor 1254): review and evaluation. Fundam. Appl. Toxicol. **31:** 42–55.
19. YANG, J.Z., S.K. AGARWAL & W.G. FOSTER. 2000. Subchronic exposure to 2,3,7,8-tetrachlorodibenzo-*p*-dioxin modulates the pathophysiology of endometriosis in the cynomolgus monkey. Toxicol. Sci. **56:** 374–381.
20. CUMMINGS, A.M. & J.L. METCALF. 1995. Induction of endometriosis in mice: a new model sensitive to estrogen. Reprod. Toxicol. **9:** 233–238.
21. CUMMINGS, A.M. & J.L. METCALF. 1995. Effects of estrogen, progesterone, and methoxychlor on surgically induced endometriosis in rats. Fundam. Appl. Toxicol. **27:** 287–290.
22. YANG, J.Z., A. YAGMINAS & W.G. FOSTER. 1997. Stimulating effects of 4-chlorodiphenyl ether on surgically induced endometriosis in the mouse. Reprod. Toxicol. **11:** 69–75.
23. CUMMINGS, A.M., J.L. METCALF & L. BIRNBAUM. 1996. Promotion of endometriosis by 2,3,7,8-tetrachlorodibenzo-*p*-dioxin in rats and mice: time-dose dependence and species comparison. Toxicol. Appl. Pharmacol. **138:** 131–139.
24. JOHNSON, K.L., A.M. CUMMINGS & L.S. BIRNBAUM. 1997. Promotion of endometriosis in mice by polychlorinated dibenzo-*p*-dioxins, dibenzofurans, and biphenyls. Environ. Health Perspect. **105:** 750–755.

25. YANG, J.Z. & W.G. FOSTER. 1997. Continuous exposure to 2,3,7,8-tetrachlorodibenzo-*p*-dioxin inhibits the growth of surgically-induced endometriosis in the ovariectomized mouse treated with high dose estradiol. Toxicol. Ind. Health **13:** 15–25.
26. POVLSEN, C.O., P.J. FIALKOW, E. KLEIN *et al.* 1973. Growth and antigenic properties of a biopsy derived Burkitt's lymphoma in thymus-less (nude) mice. Int. J. Cancer **11:** 30–39.
27. POVLSEN, C.O., N.E. SKAKKEBAEK, J. RYGAARD & G. JENSEN. 1974. Heterotransplantation of human foetal organs to the mouse mutant nude. Nature **248:** 247–249.
28. MERENDA, C., B. SORDAT, J.P. MACH & S. CARREL. 1975. Human endometrial carcinomas serially transplanted in nude mice and established in continuous cell lines. Int. J. Cancer **16:** 559–570.
29. STILES, C.D., W. DESMOND, L.M. CHUMAN *et al.* 1976. Growth control of heterologous tissue culture cells in the congenitally athymic nude mouse. Cancer Res. **36:** 1353.
30. FOGH, J., J.M. FOGH & T. ORFED. 1977. One hundred and twenty-seven cultured human tumor cell lines producing tumors in nude mice. J. Natl. Cancer Inst. **59:** 221–226.
31. SATYASWAROOP, P.G., R.J. ZAINO & R. MORTEL. 1983. Human endometrial adenocarcinoma transplanted into nude mice: growth regulation by estradiol. Science **219:** 58–60.
32. ZAMAH, N.M., M.G. DODSON, L.C. STEPHENS *et al.* 1984. Transplantation of normal and ectopic human endometrial tissue into athymic nude mice. Am. J. Obstet. Gynecol. **149:** 591–597.
33. BERGQVIST, A., S. JEPPSSON, S. KULLANDER & O. LJUNGBERG. 1985. Human endometrium transplanted into nude mice: histological effects of various steroid hormones. Am. J. Pathol. **119:** 336–344.
34. BERGQVIST, A., S. JEPPSSON, S. KULLANDER & O. LJUNGBERG. 1985. Human uterine endometrium and endometriotic tissue transplanted into nude mice. Am. J. Pathol. **121:** 337–341.
35. BRUNER, K.L., L.M. MATRISIAN, W.H. RODGERS *et al.* 1997. Suppression of matrix metalloproteinases inhibits establishment of ectopic lesions by human endometrium in nude mice. J. Clin. Invest. **99:** 2851–2857.
36. NISOLLE, M., F. CASANAS-ROUX & J. DONNEZ. 2000. Early-stage endometriosis: adhesion and growth of human menstrual endometrium in nude mice. Fertil. Steril. **74:** 306–312.
37. AOKI, D., Y. KATSUKI, A. SHIMIZU *et al.* 1994. Successful heterotransplantation of human endometrium in SCID mice. Obstet. Gynecol. **83:** 220–228.
38. AWWAD, J.T., R.A. SAYEGH & X.J. TAO. 1999. The SCID mouse: an experimental model for endometriosis. Hum. Reprod. **14:** 3107–3111.
39. OOSTERLYNCK, D.J., F.J. CORNILLIE, M. WAER *et al.* 1991. Women with endometriosis show a defect in natural killer cell activity resulting in a decreased cytotoxicity to autologous endometrium. Fertil. Steril. **56:** 45–51.
40. WILSON, T., P. HERTZOG *et al.* 1994. Decreased natural killer cell activity in endometriosis patients: relationship to disease pathogenesis. Fertil. Steril. **62:** 1086–1088.
41. FARRELL, K.L., L. SAFE & S. SAFE. 1987. Synthesis and Ah receptor binding properties of radiolabeled polychlorinated dibenzofuran congeners. Arch. Biochem. Biophys. **259:** 185–195.
42. OKEY, A.B., G.P. BONDY, M.E. MASON *et al.* 1980. Temperature-dependent cytosol-to-nucleus translocation of the Ah receptor for 2,3,7,8-tetrachlorodibenzo-*p*-dioxin in continuous cell culture lines. J. Biol. Chem. **255:** 11415–11422.
43. MANCHESTER, D.K., S.K. GORDON, C.L. GOLAS *et al.* 1987. Ah receptor in human placenta: stabilization by molybdate and characterization of binding of 2,3,7,8-tetrachlorodibenzo-*p*-dioxin, 3-methylcolanthrene, and benzo[*a*]pyrene. Cancer Res. **47:** 4861–4868.
44. IGARASHI, T., U. OSUGA, O. TSUTSUMI *et al.* 1999. Expression of Ah receptor and dioxin-related genes in human uterine endometrium in women with or without endometriosis. Endocr. J. **46:** 765–772.
45. HARRIS, M., J. PISKORSKA-PLISZCZNSKA, T. ZACHAREWSKI *et al.* 1989. Structure-dependent induction of aryl hydrocarbon hydroxylase in human breast cancer cell lines and characterization of the Ah receptor. Cancer Res. **49:** 4531–4535.

46. THOMSEN, J.S., L. NISSEN, S.N. STACEY *et al.* 1991. Differences in 2,3,7,8-tetrachlorodibenzo-*p*-dioxin-inducible CYP1A1 expression in human breast carcinoma cell lines involve altered *trans*-acting factors. Eur. J. Biochem. **197:** 577–582.
47. WANG, X., R. ROSENGREN, V. MORRISON *et al.* 1992. Characterization of the aryl hydrocarbon receptor in the human C-4II cervical squamous carcinoma cell line. Biochem. Pharmacol. **43:** 1635–1642.
48. HEATH-PAGLIUSO, S., W.J. ROGERS, K. TULLIS *et al.* 1998. Activation of the Ah receptor by tryptophan and tryptophan metabolites. Biochemistry **37:** 11508–11515.
49. FIRESTONE, D., J. RESS, N.L. BROWN *et al.* 1972. Determination of polychlorodibenzo-*p*-dioxin and related compounds in commercial chlorophenols. J. Assoc. Anal. Chem. **55:** 85–92.
50. LILIEFIELD, D.E. & M.A. GALLO. 1989. 2,4-D, 2,4,5-T, and 2,3,7,8-TCDD: an overview. Epidemiol. Rev. **11:** 28–58.
51. ALEXANDROU, N. & J. PAWLISZYN. 1989. Superficial fluid extraction for the rapid determination of polychlorinated dibenzo-*p*-dioxins and dibenzofurans in municipal incinerator fly ash. Anal. Chem. **61:** 2770–2776.
52. RAPPE, C., M. NYGREN & G. GUSTAFFSON. 1983. Human exposure to polychlorinated dibenzo-*p*-dioxins and dibenzofurans. *In* Chlorinated Dioxins and Dibenzofurans in the Total Environment. Vol. 1, pp. 355–365. Butterworths. London.
53. ORBAN, J.E., J.S. STANLEY, J.G. SCHWENBERGER & J.C. REMMERS. 1994. Dioxins and dibenzofurans in adipose tissue of the general U.S. population and selected subpopulations. Am. J. Public Health **84:** 439–445.
54. SCHECTER, A., P. FURST, C. FURST *et al.* 1994. Chlorinated dioxins and dibenzofurans in human tissue from general populations: a selective review. Environ. Health Perspect. Suppl. **102:** 159–171.
55. SCHECTER, A., J.J. RYAN, Y. MASUDA *et al.* 1994. Chlorinated and brominated dioxins and dibenzofurans in human tissue following exposure. Environ. Health Perspect. Suppl. **102:** 135–147.
56. GAIDO, K.W., S.C. MANESS, L.S. LEONARD & W.F. GREENLEE. 1992. 2,3,7,8-Tetrachlorodibenzo-*p*-dioxin-dependent regulation of transforming growth factor-α and β_2 in a human keratinocyte cell line involves both transcriptional and post-transcriptional control. J. Biol. Chem. **267:** 24591–24595.
57. MADHUKAR, B.V., D.W. BREWSTER & F. MATSUMURA. 1984. Effects of *in vivo* administration of 2,3,7,8-tetrachlorodibenzo-*p*-dioxin on receptor binding of epidermal growth factor in the hepatic plasma membrane of rat, guinea pig, mouse, and hamster. Proc. Natl. Acad. Sci. U.S.A. **81:** 7407–7411.
58. SUTTER, T.R., K. GUZMAN, K.M. DOLD & W.F. GREENLEE. 1991. Targets for dioxin: genes for plasminogen activator inhibitor-2 and interleukin-1β. Science **254:** 415–418.
59. GALLO, M.A., E.J. HESSE, G.J. MACDONALD & T.H. UMBREIT. 1986. Interactive effects of estradiol and 2,3,7,8-tetrachlorodibenzo-*p*-dioxin on hepatic cytochrome P-450 and mouse uterus. Toxicol. Lett. **32:** 123–132.
60. ASTROFF, B., C. ROWLANDS, R. DICKERSON & S. SAFE. 1990. 2,3,7,8-Tetrachlorodibenzo-*p*-dioxin inhibition of 17β-estradiol-induced increase in rat uterine EGF receptor binding activity and gene expression. Mol. Cell. Endocrinol. **72:** 247–252.
61. ROMKES, M., J. PISKORSKA-PLISZCZYNSKA & S. SAFE. 1987. Effects of 2,3,7,8-tetrachlorodibenzo-*p*-dioxin on hepatic and uterine estrogen receptor levels in rats. Toxicol. Appl. Pharmacol. **87:** 306–314.
62. DE VITO, M.J., X. MA, J.G. BABISH *et al.* 1994. Dose-response relationships in mice following subchronic exposure to 2,3,7,8-tetrachlorodibenzo-*p*-dioxin: CYP1A1, CYP1A2, estrogen receptor, and protein tyrosine phosphorylation. Toxicol. Appl. Pharmacol. **124:** 82–90.
63. TIAN, Y., S. KE, T. THOMAS *et al.* 1998. Transcriptional suppression of estrogen receptor gene expression by 2,3,7,8-tetrachlorodibenzo-*p*-dioxin (TCDD). J. Steroid Biochem. Mol. Biol. **67:** 17–24.
64. BRUNER-TRAN, K.L., S.E. RIER, E. EISENBERG & K.G. OSTEEN. 1999. The potential role of environmental toxins in the pathophysiology of endometriosis. Gynecol. Obstet. Invest. **48**(suppl. 1): 15–46.

65. WADE, M.G., D. DESAULNIERS, K. LEINGARTNERE & W.G. FOSTER. 1997. Interactions between endosulfan and dieldrin on estrogen-mediated processes *in vitro* and *in vivo*. Reprod. Toxicol. **11:** 791–798.
66. SOTO, A.M., K.L. CHUNG & C. SONNENSCHEIN. 1994. The pesticides endosulfan, toxaphene, and dieldrin have estrogenic effects on human estrogen-sensitive cells. Environ. Health Perspect. **102:** 380–383.
67. DESAULNIERS, D., K. LEINGARTNERE, M. WADE *et al.* 1999. Effects of acute exposure to PCB 126 and 153 on anterior pituitary and thyroid hormones and FSH isoforms in adult Sprague Dawley male rats. Toxicol. Sci. **47:** 158–169.
68. SAFE, S.H. 1995. Do environmental estrogens play a role in development of breast cancer in women and male reproductive problems? Hum. Ecol. Risk Assessment **1:** 17–23.
69. SOTO, A.M. & C. SONNENSCHEIN. 1999. Estrogens, xenoestrogens, and the development of neoplasms. *In* Endocrine Disruptor Effects on Male and Female Reproductive Systems, pp. 125–163. CRC Press. New York.
70. FARNSWORTH, N.R., A.S. BINGEL, G.S. CORDELL *et al.* 1975. Potential value of plants as sources of new antifertility agents: II. J. Pharm. Sci. **64:** 717–754.
71. CASSIDY, A., S. BINGHAM & K. SETCHELL. 1994. Biological effects of a diet of soy protein rich in isoflavones on the menstrual cycle of premenopausal women. Am. J. Clin. Nutr. **60:** 333–340.
72. ALDERCREUTZ, H., K. HÖCKERSTEDT, C. BANNWART *et al.* 1987. Effect of dietary components, including lignins and phytoestrogens, on enterhepatic circulation and liver metabolism of estrogens and on sex hormone binding globulin (SHBG). J. Steroid Biochem. **27:** 1135–1144.
73. ALDERCREUTZ, H., Y. MOUSAVI, J. CLARK *et al.* 1992. Dietary phytoestrogens and cancer: *in vitro* and *in vivo* studies. J. Steroid Biochem. **41:** 331–337.
74. PEDERSEN, A.B., M. BARTHOLOMEW, L.A. DOLENCE *et al.* 1991. Menstrual differences due to vegetarian and nonvegetarian diets. Am. J. Clin. Nutr. **53:** 879–885.
75. AWONIYI, C.A., D. ROBERTS, D.N. VEERAMACHANENI *et al.* 1994. Reproductive sequelae in female rats after *in utero* and neonatal exposure to the phytoestrogen genistein. Fertil. Steril. **70:** 440–447.
76. FOTH, D. & J.M. CLINE. 1998. Effects of mammalian and plant estrogens on mammary glands and uteri of macaques. Am. J. Clin. Nutr. **68:** 1413S–1417S.
77. GOODMAN, M.T., L.R. WILKENS, J.H. HANKIN *et al.* 1997. Association of soy and fiber consumption with the risk of endometrial cancer. Am. J. Epidemiol. **146:** 294–306.
78. SETCHELL, K.D.R. 1985. Naturally occurring nonsteroidal estrogens of dietary origin. *In* Estrogens in the Environment, pp. 69–85. Elsevier. Amsterdam/New York.
79. FOLMAN, Y. & G.S. POPE. 1966. The interaction in the immature mouse of potent estrogens with coumestrol, genistein, and other uterovaginotropic compounds of low potency. J. Endocrinol. **34:** 215–225.
80. KUIPER, G.J.M., B. CARLSSON & K. GRANDIEN. 1997. Comparison of the ligand binding specificity and transcript distribution of estrogenic receptors α and β. Endocrinology **138:** 863–870.
81. MATSUZAKI, S., T. FUKAYA, T. SUZUKI *et al.* 1999. Oestrogen receptor α and β mRNA expression in human endometrium throughout the menstrual cycle. Mol. Hum. Reprod. **5:** 559–564.
82. COUSE, J.F., S.W. CURTIS, T.F. WASHBURN *et al.* 1995. Analysis of transcription and estrogen insensitivity in the female mouse after targeted disruption of the estrogen receptor gene. Mol. Endocrinol. **9:** 1441–1454.
83. COUSE, J.F., J. LINDZEY, K. GRANDIEN *et al.* 1997. Tissue disruption and quantitative analysis of estrogen receptor α (ERα) and estrogen receptor β (ERβ) messenger ribonucleic acid in the wild-type and ER-knockout mouse. Endocrinology **138:** 4613–4621.
84. PETERSEN, T.G. & S. BARNES. 1991. Genistein inhibition of the growth of human breast cancer cells: independence from estrogen receptors and the multidrug resistance gene. Biochem. Biophys. Res. Commun. **179:** 661–667.
85. BAKER, M.E. 1991. Origins of regulation of gene transcription by steroid, retinoid, and thyroid hormones. *In* The New Biology of Steroid Hormones, pp. 187–202. Raven Press. New York.

86. AKIYAMA, T., J. ISHIDA, S. NAKAGAWA *et al.* 1987. Genistein, a specific inhibitor of tyrosine-specific protein kinases. J. Biol. Chem. **262:** 5592–5595.
87. KAO, Y-C., C. ZHOU, M. SHERMAN *et al.* 1998. Molecular basis of the inhibition of human aromatase (estrogen synthetase) by flavone and isoflavone phytoestrogens: a site directed mutagenesis study. Environ. Health Perspect. **106:** 85–92.
88. FITZPATRICK, S.L. & J.S. RICHARDS. 1991. Regulation of cytochrome P450 aromatase messenger ribonucleic acid and activity by steroids and gonadotropins in rat granulosa cells. Endocrinology **129:** 1452–1462.
89. BERKOWITZ, G.D., T. BISAT & K.M. CARTER. 1989. Aromatase activity in microsomal preparations of human genital skin fibroblasts: influence of glucocorticoids. J. Steroid Biochem. **33:** 341–347.
90. RYAN, K.J. 1959. Biological aromatization of steroids. J. Biol. Chem. **234:** 268–272.
91. ACKERMAN, G.E., M.E. SMITH, C.R. MENDELSON *et al.* 1981. Aromatization of androstenedione by human adipose tissue stromal cells in monolayer culture. J. Clin. Endocrinol. Metab. **53:** 412–417.
92. REED, M.J., A.M. OWEN, L.C. LAI *et al.* 1989. *In situ* oestrone synthesis in normal breast tissue and breast tumor tissue: effect of treatment with 4-hydroxyandrostenedione. Int. J. Cancer. **44:** 233–237.
93. PRICE, T., J. AITKEN & E.R. SIMPSON. 1992. Relative expression of aromatase cytochrome P450 in human fetal tissues as determined by competitive polymerase chain reactor (PCR) amplification. J. Clin. Endocrinol. Metab. **74:** 879–883.
94. BULUN, S.E., M.S. MAHENDROO & E.R. SIMPSON. 1993. Polymerase chain reaction amplification fails to detect aromatase cytochrome P450 transcripts in normal human endometrium or decidua. J. Clin. Endocrinol. Metab. **76:** 1458–1463.
95. NOBLE, L.S., E.R. SIMPSON, A. JOHNS & S.E. BULUN. 1996. Aromatase expression in endometriosis. J. Clin. Endocrinol. Metab. **81:** 174–179.
96. SANDERSON, J.T., W. SEINEN, J.P. GIESY & M. VAN DEN BERG. 2000. 2-Chloro-*s*-triazine herbicides induce aromatase (CYP19) activity in H295R human adrenocortical carcinoma cells: a novel mechanism for estrogenicity. Toxicol. Sci. **54:** 121–127.

Panel Discussion (Part VI)

S.E. BULUN (*University of Illinois, Chicago, IL*): I have a question for Warren Foster. How different are these levels or the doses of dioxin that you use compared with the levels of dioxin in humans in contaminated areas? Would you put that in a perspective?

W.G. FOSTER (*McMaster University, Hamilton, Ontario, Canada*): The levels that we have used, the 5 and 25 parts per trillion, are equivalent to the doses used in the rhesus monkey study by Rier *et al.* These doses can be considered to be reflective of a high exposure that might occur with accidental exposure, such as that occurred in Seveso, Italy, and elsewhere. The 1 part per trillion, the lowest dose used in our study, is considered to be a dose representative of human exposure in the general population.

J. JARRELL (*University of Calgary, Calgary, Canada*): I have a question for Sherry Rier. One of the biggest predictors of organochlorines in humans is the presence of weight loss. I was wondering if any of your monkeys are losing weight prior to having their blood taken.

S.E. RIER (*Vanderbilt University Medical Center, Nashville, TN*): Well, we were quite interested in that as well. We were concerned about animals who were ill or wasting and that is also of concern if you are measuring serum levels of these compounds. In this case, interestingly, none of these animals were losing weight. The ones that lost weight had intestinal blockages and died of disease earlier on, and the wasting was probably due to nutritional imbalances. There are some studies showing that you can have TCDD exposure without weight loss. We did not see weight loss in these animals without intestinal obstruction.

S.H. KENNEDY (*University of Oxford, Oxford, United Kingdom*): Could I ask you two quick questions? First, was disease severity assessed at laparoscopy or at necropsy?

RIER: In the case of these studies, disease was assessed at laparoscopy. As you know, these studies are ongoing and ongoing. Disease was also assessed at human sacrifice of the animals in the following year after the present studies. At sacrifice, we cycled the animals on estrogen and progesterone, so they had similar levels of hormones since they were perimenopausal. The present studies were done when they were not cycled, prior to necropsy.

KENNEDY: Second, you mentioned that levels had been measured in animals that were not part of the original study to give you some idea of what the background level might be in the colony, but you did not present any of those data.

RIER: I did not present these data here because it gets quite complicated and we did not have much time. It is in the publication that is out now (2001. *Toxicol. Sci.* **59:** 147–159). We had difficulty finding animals that had no other exposures. We needed feral animals that had been at the facility because there are concerns about possible contamination from other sources. The only animals that were available were lead-treated animals that were feral and had resided at the facility for the same length of time as the TCDD-treated colony. Lead-treated animals had similar serum

PCB levels as TCDD-treated monkeys, and 75% of those animals also had endometriosis, which is a story in and of itself. I do have data on many animals at Harlow. It appears that during the 1980s especially that there were PCB levels in a lot of animals. Perhaps, without a hit, an environmental hit, they were able to metabolize them. However, if they had a hit of TCDD or lead, they were not able to. The source of the PCBs was most likely in the fish meal component of the Purina Monkey Chow. Like the fish eaters around the Great Lakes, they were getting their load of PCBs.

QUESTION: This is for anyone on the panel. When you are talking about the TEFs of these various congeners, one of the assumptions that you are making with the exposure to many of them is that there is an additive effect. Do we actually know that? It seems that many of them could actually be acting as weak agonists and even antagonists in some cases, all binding to the same Ah receptor. Have we done any experimental work to determine if mixtures of these congeners are actually additive?

RIER: You are absolutely right. The truth is that we have many of these compounds in our blood and tissues. We know that there are synergistic and antagonistic interactions and we do not know, of that mix of chemicals, what might be important and what might not be important to disease processes. In this case, the rhesus model unexpectedly has provided some potential clues as to what might be important to endometriosis. However, we always have to keep in mind that we are exposed to a mix of chemicals and we must find ways to study it and to find models specific to the disease process of endometriosis. Thus far, data have been accumulated, but in other model systems and specific to other biological activities. Does that answer your question?

QUESTION: I think so. By narrowing down the important congeners, at least in endometriosis, this allows us to experimentally mix these congeners and see what the actual effect is.

RIER: Exactly. Out of 202 different PCB congeners, for example, there are certainly a whole range of non-coplanar PCBs that are potential interrupters of estrogen-like activity. It is a way of finding candidates to try in model systems.

QUESTION: I was wondering if you looked at the aerohydrocarbon receptor polymorphisms among the TCDD-treated animals because some got endometriosis and some did not.

RIER: We have not. I think that is an extremely interesting point. I have always been fascinated by the two animals that were treated with TCDD that did not get disease. We have tissues stored and there are probably many studies to be done on these animals. We do know that those two animals that escaped disease have circulating testosterone levels, while the TCDD-treated animals with endometriosis did not. There are also differences in circulating hormones in these animals, particularly increased cortisol levels and some modulation of insulin levels in the animals. There were actually decreased circulating estrogen levels in TCDD-treated animals, so this demonstrates that there is a complexity here that needs to be explored and we must not focus only on estrogenic activity.

R.M. BRENNER (*Oregon Regional Primate Research Center, Beaverton, OR*): I have a question for Warren Foster. You mentioned that your big pool of animals had about 1% endometriosis and your research pool had about 35%. What do you attribute that big difference to?

FOSTER: The monkeys in our breeding pool are regularly producing babies or they are assigned to the research pool. Since they are pregnant or lactating, the majority of the time they do not have a chance to establish lengthy intervals of menstruation uninterrupted by a pregnancy. With so few menstrual cycles, any backflow of menstrual contents to the pelvic cavity is limited. Thus, even if endometriosis does establish, it is mild and does not come to the attention of the handlers. On the other hand, once monkeys come into the research pool, they are individually housed, preventing any chance of pregnancy. These monkeys start menstruating regularly then, with regular 28- to 32-day cycles. It could be a number of years before the animals are assigned to a research study. With repeated menstrual cycles uninterrupted by pregnancy, there is an increased opportunity for menstrual contents that have entered the pelvic cavity to implant and for endometriosis to become established. Over time, the disease progresses with the result that animal handlers familiar with the monkey begin to see behavioral indications of pain that prompts investigation. Increased awareness that endometriosis is an issue among the animals in the research pool has lead to an increase in detection and thus we have seen an increase in the incidence of endometriosis.

BRENNER: Do you think it is really due to retrograde menstruation in these primates? I do not think that this has ever been clearly demonstrated.

FOSTER: I do not think it has been clearly demonstrated at all. It is only indirect evidence that leads us to suspect that retrograde menstruation is the most likely contributing factor.

QUESTION: I have a question for Dr. McLachlan. You mentioned that the early exposure to estrogens may, in fact, affect DNA methylation and thus gene imprinting and it may affect later gene expression in individuals. How concerned should pregnant mothers be nowadays?

J.A. MCLACHLAN (*Tulane University, New Orleans, LA*): I have no idea how concerned pregnant mothers should be nowadays. I do think it is the case that both natural and exogenous hormones have to play some role in setting the programs in cells that we call differentiation. There are numerous studies looking at diseases and disorders of pregnancy for which there are high or low levels of estradiol and estrone that are associated with later increased risk for breast cancer. We did a study showing that there is an association with Torkettism. Thus, one could imagine a variety of different sets of signals that get put in place. This is a question that comes up over and over again in terms of what do you do and how do you avoid what is becoming almost a ubiquitous environmental factor. I really do not have an answer for that.

J. HEINDEL (*National Institute of Environmental Health Sciences, NIH, Research Triangle Park, NC*): Thus, the bottom line is that we are at a very early stage here of trying to figure out the environmental component of endometriosis, but there are some interesting leads.

The Genetic Epidemiology of Spontaneous Endometriosis in the Rhesus Monkey

KRINA ZONDERVAN,[a] LON CARDON,[a] RONALD DESROSIERS,[b] DALLAS HYDE,[c] JOSEPH KEMNITZ,[d] KEITH MANSFIELD,[b] JEFF ROBERTS,[c] JOAN SCHEFFLER,[d] DANIEL E. WEEKS,[e] AND STEPHEN KENNEDY[f]

[a]*Wellcome Trust Centre for Human Genetics, University of Oxford, Oxford, United Kingdom*

[b]*New England Regional Primate Research Center, Harvard Medical School, Boston, Massachusetts, USA*

[c]*California Regional Primate Research Center, University of California at Davis, Davis, California, USA*

[d]*Wisconsin Regional Primate Research Center, University of Wisconsin–Madison, Madison, Wisconsin, USA*

[e]*Department of Human Genetics, University of Pittsburgh, Pittsburgh, Pennsylvania, USA*

[f]*Nuffield Department of Obstetrics and Gynaecology, University of Oxford, Oxford, United Kingdom*

ABSTRACT: The etiology of endometriosis is uncertain, but there is increasing evidence that it is inherited as a complex genetic trait like diabetes or asthma. In such complex traits, multiple gene loci conferring susceptibility to the disease interact with each other and the environment to produce the phenotype. The study of such interactions in humans can be problematic. Thus, the availability of an animal model, which shares many aspects of anatomy and physiology with humans, is potentially a valuable tool for investigating the genetic epidemiology of the disease. Since endometriosis develops spontaneously in the rhesus monkey (*Macaca mulatta*) and the tissue is morphologically identical to its human counterpart, this population provides a unique opportunity to conduct such studies in this condition.

KEYWORDS: endometriosis; genetics; epidemiology; rhesus monkey

ENDOMETRIOSIS

Endometriosis is a major women's health-care problem that affects an estimated 1% to 2% of women of reproductive age.[1] Accurate population-based prevalence data, however, are difficult to obtain because surgery is required to make a definitive diagnosis. The main clinical manifestations are painful periods, pain during inter-

Address for correspondence: Stephen Kennedy, Nuffield Department of Obstetrics and Gynaecology, University of Oxford, John Radcliffe Hospital, Oxford OX3 9DU, United Kingdom. Voice: +44 1865 221013; fax: +44 1865 769141.
skennedy@molbiol.ox.ac.uk

course, chronic pelvic pain, and subfertility. The treatment options are limited because the cause of the disease is unclear. They include the use of hormonal drugs to suppress the menstrual cycle, surgical ablation of endometriotic lesions, and (if necessary) removal of the pelvic organs.

The disease is defined as the presence of tissue resembling endometrium in sites outside the uterine cavity, such as the peritoneal surface and ovaries, where cyst formation is common. It is generally accepted that retrograde menstruation is a permissive factor in the etiology of the disease. The formation of a lesion is likely therefore to involve the dissemination of uterine endometrium into the peritoneal cavity at the time of menstruation, and the attachment of the endometrial cells to the peritoneal surface. An alternative explanation is that endometriosis occurs because of *in situ* metaplasia. In either model, there is proliferation and differentiation, and subsequent invasion into the underlying tissue.[2]

There is increasing evidence that genetic predisposition plays a role in disease etiology,[3] which raises the possibility that molecular genetic studies can be used to discover disease mechanisms independently of previously hypothesis-driven research. The principal evidence for a genetic basis comes from a large twin study, in which 51% of the variance of susceptibility to endometriosis was attributed to genetic factors,[4] and from three case-control studies showing that the first-degree relatives of affected women are at 6–9 times increased risk of developing the disease compared to first-degree relatives of controls.[5–7] In addition, polymorphisms and null mutations in a number of functional candidate genes, for example, genes involved in the detoxification of environmental pollutants (*GTSM1*, *GSTT1*, and *NAT2*), have been reported to be more frequent in affected women than controls (see references 8 and 9).

The mode of inheritance is unknown, but it is likely that endometriosis is inherited as a complex trait such as diabetes, asthma, or hypertension, in which multiple genes interact with each other and the environment to produce the disease phenotype. Studies investigating environmental risk factors for endometriosis in humans have generally focused on the effect of prolonged and heavy menstruation and factors that increase exposure to estrogen.[10] However, both genetic and epidemiological studies have been limited in terms of their number, scope, choice of study populations, and sample sizes. They have consequently left many unanswered questions as to the relative influence of genetic versus environmental factors and possible gene-environment interaction. Given the large number of different environmental factors that women may be exposed to, up to and during their reproductive years, studying such interactions in humans can be problematic. An animal model, in which exposures are carefully controlled and recorded, would thus be a valuable tool to investigate the etiology of endometriosis. The advantage of nonhuman primates is that they have many anatomical and physiological features in common with humans, and spontaneous endometriosis has been described in several species both in captivity and in the wild.

THE RHESUS MONKEY AS AN ANIMAL MODEL

The rhesus monkey (*Macaca mulatta*) is the nonhuman primate species that has been most extensively studied in the field of reproductive medicine. Menarche in the rhesus monkey occurs at ~3 years of age, the length of the menstrual cycle is ~28 days, and menstrual bleeding lasts for ~4 days. The first pregnancy typically occurs at 3–5 years of age; gestational age is ~165 days and infants are weaned at 7 to 14 months. Ovarian function diminishes from the age of ~25 years onwards, at which point menstrual cycles start to become irregular, but few animals become menopausal. The rhesus monkey is a seasonal breeder in the wild and in captivity when kept outdoors.[11] However, this seasonality may disappear in indoor-housed animals maintained on a constant light/dark and temperature/humidity regimen. The average life span is 29 years, but some animals live to 40 years of age.[12]

Endometriosis develops spontaneously in the rhesus monkey and the tissue is morphologically identical to its human counterpart.[13] Clinical manifestations include abdominal distension due to a pelvic mass and altered behavior, especially at menstruation, which may be related to discomfort. There is a tendency for full-thickness bowel involvement with endometriosis, resulting in cachexia and death if no intervention occurs. Risk factors for the development of the disease include age, hysterotomy and estradiol treatment,[14] chronic exposure to 2,3,7,8-tetrachloro-dibenzo-*p*-dioxin,[15] and ionizing radiation.[16]

UNIQUE DATA HELD BY PRIMATE CENTERS

The Nuffield Department of Obstetrics and Gynaecology, University of Oxford, which has an extensive program aimed at identifying disease susceptibility genes in humans using a positional cloning approach, has been collaborating for 5 years with the Wisconsin Regional Primate Research Center (WRPRC), University of Wisconsin–Madison, in a study investigating the genetic epidemiology of endometriosis in a large colony of rhesus monkeys. The WRPRC is one of eight federally supported (NIH–NCRR) primate centers in the United States and it has consistently maintained a population of ~1000 rhesus macaques since 1971 for research and breeding. Most of the monkeys have lived in a controlled indoor environment (12 h on/off lighting, constant temperature). Those assigned to experimental protocols have been utilized mainly in the field of reproductive medicine (e.g., laparoscopy studies to observe ovarian folliculogenesis; hysterotomy during pregnancy for fetal experiments; and estradiol treatment to investigate follicular atresia). Comprehensive records of the animals' experimental and environmental history, including all familial relationships, are available. Paternity is known for ~90% of the animals; however, some of the animals in the colony are of feral origin and therefore neither parent is known. The WRPRC has a strict policy to avoid inbreeding.

In 1996, a case-control study was conducted to investigate the effect of several risk factors on endometriosis in the WRPRC colony.[14] The necropsy records of all female rhesus monkeys ($n = 399$) that died aged ≥4 years old between 1980 and 1995 were examined for evidence of endometriosis. Disease status could only be reliably determined through necropsy records as the surgical records at laparoscopies performed for experimental purposes rarely contained information about whether endometriosis was present. Only necropsy records of animals that died aged ≥4 years old were examined as the rhesus monkey does not reach sexual maturity and cannot therefore develop endometriosis until this age. The necropsies were nearly all performed by the same pathologist (Hideo Uno), who routinely recorded macroscopic evidence of endometriosis, including the site, extent of disease, and presence of adhesions. Endometriosis cases were defined as those with macroscopic evidence of endometriosis; histological confirmation was also available in most cases. The severity of disease was assessed retrospectively from the records using an adapted version of the revised American Fertility Society (rAFS) classification system.[17] Eighty-one (20%) of the animals had endometriosis and, of these, 63 (78%) had the equivalent of rAFS stage III–IV (moderate-severe) disease, often affecting the whole abdominal cavity and involving bowel in two-thirds of the cases. Of the 81 affected animals, 41% were related to at least 1 other affected animal.

Since age was an important risk factor for endometriosis (no animals were found to be affected under the age of 10), 62 of the 81 affected animals were matched to unaffected controls for age at death (to within 1 year) and year of death (to within 2 years). The effect of several experimental factors on the development of endometriosis was determined using conditional logistic regression.[14] Exposures to three or more estradiol implants and one or more hysterotomies were both significant risk factors, with estimated relative risks of 9.7 (95% CI 2.5–37.2) and 5.8 (95% CI 1.6–20.2), respectively. Animals that had been exposed to one or more laparoscopies showed no increased risk for developing endometriosis.

In addition to the 81 affected animals identified at necropsy for the case-control study, 2 more animals were identified through surgical records. To explore the familial characteristics of these animals, magnetic resonance imaging (MRI) was performed on 113 living descendants of the 83 affected animals. Only animals that were ≥9 years old were chosen for MRI as no animal that was <10 years old was affected in the original necropsy study. The monkeys had MRI scans of the pelvis and lower abdominal region with fat presaturation. Disease was suspected radiologically in 22 out of 113 animals (19%) as peritoneal or ovarian lesions > 3 cm in diameter ($n = 5$), as peritoneal or ovarian lesions 1–3 cm in diameter ($n = 3$), or as equivocal findings ($n = 14$).[18]

Of the 103 cases diagnosed at necropsy, surgery, and MRI, 68 (66%) were related to at least 1 other affected animal; together, these formed 12 distinct family groups. Within these groups, there were 2 full-sibling pairs, 11 mother-daughter pairs, and 64 half-sibling pairs. A larger pedigree of 1806 animals was then constructed by including all animals related to the affected animals in the 12 family groups (unpublished data). This was achieved by working backwards to the feral, founding ancestors of the affected animals and including all descendants of these ancestors in the database. The disease status of females in the pedigree since 1996 is currently being updated, and the mode of inheritance within the pedigree is being studied using complex segregation analysis.

The collaboration has recently been extended to include the New England RPRC, at Harvard Medical School, and the California RPRC, at the University of California at Davis. At the New England center, 40 of the 227 animals (18%), ≥9 years of age, that died in the last 12 years had endometriosis. Parental identities are known in ~70% of the cases and the records of ~3000 animals are being examined to determine whether there is a familial tendency in this colony. At the California center, 121 of the 1459 animals (8.3%), ≥4 years of age, that died between 1982 and 1996 had endometriosis. Among the colony records of ~10,000 animals, the 121 affected animals fall into 12 paternal half-sib pairs, 2 maternal half-sib pairs, 1 full-sib pair, and 3 half-aunt/niece pairs. The attempt to construct larger pedigrees has been hampered by difficulty in determining paternity in many cases because animals are mostly housed outdoors, as opposed to indoors at the New England and Wisconsin centers. However, recently acquired DNA marker data have increased the number of known paternities, which will facilitate further analysis of the familial tendency.

The collaborative project represents a unique resource to study the interaction between genetic and environmental factors that predispose animals to develop disease with different prevalence rates in the three colonies. Detailed nutritional, experimental, menstrual, and reproductive histories that were prospectively acquired are available to evaluate the influence of risk factors in a more reliable way than is possible in humans. The future availability of more microsatellite markers for use in the rhesus monkey will allow functional and positional candidate genes to be studied and a genome-wide screen to be performed for linkage analysis.

As a preliminary step towards developing a linkage mapping set in the rhesus monkey, 400 primers to human polymorphic microsatellite markers from the ABI (Applied Biosystems) linkage mapping set 2 (10-cM resolution) were tested without optimization, using DNA obtained from 9 unrelated female rhesus monkeys kept at the University of Oxford's rhesus breeding facility. Samples were run on an ABI prism 377 automated sequencer (Applied Biosystems) and the results were analyzed using Genescan™ and Genotyper™ software (Applied Biosystems). Of 400 markers tested, 76 (19%) gave rise to PCR products in or close to the expected range for products arising from human DNA that exhibited polymorphism and some heterozygosity across the 9 monkeys tested. The mean heterozygosity for these 76 markers in humans is 0.80, compared with 0.65 for the 9 rhesus monkeys tested. The average number of alleles per marker was 9.1 for human DNA and 4.9 for rhesus monkey DNA. The modal allele size in humans and the 9 rhesus monkeys tested showed a strong correlation ($r = 0.97$, $p < 0.0001$) between the most frequent allele size for human and rhesus monkey microsatellites.[19]

In summary, the availability of an animal model, which shares many aspects of anatomy and physiology with humans, is potentially an extremely valuable tool to investigate the genetic epidemiology of a disease. The existence of well-characterized populations of rhesus monkeys with endometriosis provides a unique opportunity to conduct such studies in this condition. The collaborative group aims to (i) further investigate the effect of environmental factors (data about which have been prospectively collected) on the risk of developing spontaneous endometriosis in the rhesus monkey, (ii) conduct association studies with functional candidate genes and positional candidates derived from linkage studies in humans and investigate their effect combined with that of environmental factors, and (iii) perform a genome-wide scan once a marker set specific to the rhesus macaque is available. We predict that the findings will greatly speed up the search for, and help validate the identification of, susceptibility genes in humans.

REFERENCES

1. Moen, M.H. & B. Schei. 1997. Epidemiology of endometriosis in a Norwegian county. Acta Obstet. Gynecol. Scand. **76:** 559–562.
2. Koninckx, P.R., D.H. Barlow & S.H. Kennedy. 1999. Implantation versus infiltration: the Sampson versus the endometriotic disease theory. Gynecol. Obstet. Invest. **47**(suppl. 1)**:** 3–9.

3. KENNEDY, S.H. 1999. The genetics of endometriosis. Eur. J. Obstet. Gynecol. Reprod. Biol. **82:** 129–133.
4. TRELOAR, S.A., D.T. O'CONNOR, V.M. O'CONNOR & N.G. MARTIN. 1999. Genetic influences on endometriosis in an Australian twin sample. Fertil. Steril. **71:** 701–710.
5. COXHEAD, D. & E.J. THOMAS. 1993. Familial inheritance of endometriosis in a British population: a case control study. J. Obstet. Gynaecol. **13:** 42–44.
6. MOEN, M.H. & P. MAGNUS. 1993. The familial risk of endometriosis. Acta Obstet. Gynecol. Scand. **72:** 560–564.
7. SIMPSON, J.L., S. ELIAS, L.R. MALINAK & J. BUTTRAM. 1980. Heritable aspects of endometriosis: I. Genetic studies. Am. J. Obstet. Gynecol. **137:** 327–331.
8. ZONDERVAN, K.T., L.R. CARDON & S.H. KENNEDY. 2001. The genetic basis of endometriosis. Curr. Opin. Obstet. Gynecol. **13:** 309–314.
9. KENNEDY, S.H., S.T. BENNETT & D.E. WEEKS. 2001. Affected sib-pair analysis in endometriosis. Hum. Reprod. Update **7:** 411–418.
10. ESKENAZI, B. & M.L. WARNER. 1997. Epidemiology of endometriosis. Obstet. Gynecol. Clin. North Am. **24:** 235–258.
11. CATCHPOLE, H.R. & G. VAN WAGENEN. 1975. Reproduction in the rhesus monkey, *Macaca mulatta*. *In* The Rhesus Monkey, pp. 117–140. Academic Press. New York.
12. COLMAN, R. & J.W. KEMNITZ. 1998. Aging experiments using nonhuman primates. *In* Methods in Aging Research, pp. 249–267. CRC Press. Boca Raton, FL.
13. MACKENZIE, W.F. & H.W. CASEY. 1975. Animal model of human disease: endometriosis in rhesus monkeys. Am. J. Pathol. **80:** 341–344.
14. HADFIELD, R.M., P.L. YUDKIN, C.L. COE *et al.* 1997. Risk factors for endometriosis in the rhesus monkey (*Macaca mulatta*): a case-control study. Hum. Reprod. Update **3:** 109–115.
15. RIER, S.E., D.C. MARTIN, R.E. BOWMAN *et al.* 1993. Endometriosis in rhesus monkeys (*Macaca mulatta*) following chronic exposure to 2,3,7,8-tetrachlorodibenzo-*p*-dioxin. Fundam. Appl. Toxicol. **21:** 433–441.
16. WOOD, D.H., M.G. YOCHMOWITZ, Y.L. SALMON *et al.* 1983. Proton irradiation and endometriosis. Aviat. Space Environ. Med. **54:** 718–724.
17. AMERICAN FERTILITY SOCIETY. 1985. Revised American Fertility Society classification of endometriosis. Fertil. Steril. **43:** 351–352.
18. HADFIELD, R.M., R. COLMAN, J. SCHEFFLER *et al.* 2001. MRI scanning in a pedigree of rhesus monkeys with spontaneous endometriosis. Submitted.
19. HADFIELD, R.M., J.G. PULLEN, K.F. DAVIES *et al.* 2001. Towards developing a genome-wide microsatellite marker set for linkage analysis in the rhesus macaque (*Macaca mulatta*): identification of 76 polymorphic markers. Am. J. Primatol. **54:** 223–231.

Heritability and Molecular Genetic Studies of Endometriosis

JOE LEIGH SIMPSON AND FARIDEH Z. BISCHOFF

Department of Obstetrics and Gynecology, Baylor College of Medicine, Houston, Texas 77030, USA

ABSTRACT: Endometriosis is well established as a condition showing heritable tendencies. Polygenic/multifactorial etiology appears far more likely to be the etiology than Mendelian inheritance. The current task is to determine the number and location of genes responsible for endometriosis. This paper shall review the basis for concluding that endometriosis is a genetic disorder of polygenic/multifactorial inheritance and outline selected strategies for identifying the number and location of causative genes. It shall also illustrate our approach to testing the hypothesis that endometriosis bears similarity to neoplasia and, hence, is a multistep phenomenon of clonal origin.

KEYWORDS: heritability; polygenic; quantitative linkage analysis; oncogenes; gene expression; endometriosis

INTRODUCTION

Endometriosis is well established as a condition showing heritable tendencies. Case reports of familial aggregates date from the 1940s, and the overall recurrence risk for relatives has long been accepted as increased.[1,2] Polygenic/multifactorial etiology appears far more likely to be the etiology than Mendelian inheritance. This parallels etiology of most adult-onset conditions, including many familiar to physicians in reproductive medicine (e.g., polycystic ovarian disease, leiomyomata, pelvic cancer). The current task is to determine the number and location of genes responsible for endometriosis.

In this communication, we shall review the basis for concluding that endometriosis is a genetic disorder of polygenic/multifactorial inheritance and outline selected strategies for identifying the number and location of causative genes. Finally, we shall illustrate our approach to testing the hypothesis that endometriosis bears similarity to neoplasia and, hence, is a multistep phenomenon of clonal origin.

FAMILIAL AGGREGATES AND HERITABILITY TENDENCIES

Following several prior case reports and one questionnaire study, Simpson *et al.*[3] conducted the first formal genetic study in 1980. A total of 123 probands with histo-

Address for correspondence: Joe Leigh Simpson, Department of Obstetrics and Gynecology, Baylor College of Medicine, 6550 Fannin, Suite 901, Houston, TX 77030. Voice: 713-798-8360; fax: 713-798-8410.

jsimpson@bcm.tmc.edu

TABLE 1. Incidence of endometriosis among proband's first-degree relatives as compared with controls

		Proband's first-degree relatives			
Reference	Venue	Mothers	Sisters	Overall	Controls
Simpson *et al.*[3]	United States	5.9%	8.1%	6.9% (19/276)	0.9% (2/211)
Lamb *et al.*[5]	United States	6.2%	3.8%	4.9%	2.0%
Moen and Magnus[6]	Norway	3.9%	4.8%	4.3% (45/1038)	0.6% (2/318)
Coxhead and Thomas[8]	United Kingdom			5.5% (7/127)	0.8% (2/258)

logically verified endometriosis were identified. Nine of 153 (5.9%) female sibs older than 18 years had endometriosis; 10 (8.1%) of their 23 mothers were affected. Only 1% of the patient's husband's first-degree relatives (controls) had endometriosis. Of two sets of monozygotic (MZ) twins, one was concordantly affected. Women with an affected sib or parent proved more likely to have severe than mild or moderate endometriosis,[4] with severe endometriosis being present in 11 of the 18 probands (61%) having an affected first-degree relative. Severe endometriosis was present in only 25 of 105 (23%) of the affected probands having no affected first-degree relative.

Later studies by other groups have been consistent with these initial observations (TABLE 1). Lamb *et al.*[5] used questionnaires from 491 members of the Endometriosis Association, a United States–based support and research organization. Positive family history was reported by 18% of respondents. Sixty-six women were evaluated in greater detail, with 43 returning a detailed questionnaire completed as well by a friend (control). Endometriosis was present in 6.2% of mothers of probands and 3.8% of sisters; endometriosis was reported in less than 1% of first-degree relatives of friends. The frequency in second-degree relatives was 0.4% in grandmothers and 3.1% in aunts. In this study, most (93%) affected relatives were in the maternal lineage. A pitfall was that no attempts were made to confirm the diagnosis in relatives said to be affected; however, Endometriosis Association members can be assumed to be highly knowledgeable concerning the disorder.

In Norway, Moen and Magnus[6] conducted a study similar to that of Simpson *et al.*[3] Among 522 informative cases, 3.9% of mothers and 4.8% of sisters had endometriosis; only 0.6% of sisters of women not having endometriosis were affected. These controls underwent laparoscopy for other reasons. In this study, either endometriosis or adenomyosis sufficed as the basis for diagnosis. Affected mothers were far more likely to have adenomyosis than affected sisters. As in the United States study of Simpson *et al.*[3] and Malinak *et al.*,[4] familial cases in Norway proved more likely to show severe endometriosis than did sporadic cases. In another report from the same Norwegian center, 8 MZ twins were observed among 515 endometriosis cases.[7] Six of the 8 sets were concordant, and 3 mothers were also affected.

In the United Kingdom, Coxhead and Thomas[8] reported a sixfold increase in frequency of endometriosis among first-degree relatives. From Brazil, dos Reis *et al.*[9] reported that 8.6% of 81 Brazilian probands had first-degree relatives compared to none in 43 controls.

Higher concordance for monozygotic (MZ) than dizygotic (DZ) twins has consistently been observed.[7,10,11] In addition, endometriosis detected in the context of surgical menopause is more highly correlated in MZ twins than in DZ twins ($r = 0.52$ vs. 0.19).[11]

No associations have been identified between HLA antigens and endometriosis.[7,12,13] This may subsequently prove germane. Neoplasias rarely show HLA association, in contrast to adult-onset disorders of immunologic basis (e.g., diabetes mellitus). The latter may show HLA associations in linkage disequilibrium.

POLYGENIC/MULTIFACTORIAL INHERITANCE

Data reviewed above show endometriosis is clearly heritable, with the increased risk being 5% to 8% for first-degree relatives. Recurrence risks of this magnitude are most consistent with polygenic/multifactorial etiology. Actually, the observed recurrence risk is higher than the 2% to 5% expected in general for polygenic/multifactorial inheritance, and the frequency of affected relatives might be even higher if one could directly measure a gene product (or products). Still, a single Mendelian mechanism seems unlikely. That severity is greater in familial cases than in nonfamilial (sporadic) cases is consistent with predictions based on a polygenic model. This model predicts that the greater the severity, the greater the underlying genetic liability and, hence, the greater the proportion of affected relatives. That endometriosis is more severe in familial cases also lessens the likelihood that existence of one affected family member led to the identification of an affected relative merely because of a higher index of clinical suspicion. Also supporting polygenic inheritance is the earlier age of onset for familial versus nonfamilial cases, and similar age of onset among affected relatives.[14]

The other formal explanation, not inconsistent with polygenic etiology, is that not all cases of endometriosis represent the same disorder—that is, etiologic heterogeneity exists. One or more forms of endometriosis might be Mendelian, but the larger proportion could be nongenetic or polygenic/multifactorial. The latter has proved to be the likely explanation for many other adult-onset disorders.

Of considerable significance is that only a few genes, or conversely only a few alleles at a single locus, can produce enough different genotypes to yield continuous genotypic and, hence, phenotypic variation in the population. Suppose there exists 2 genes, each with 2 alleles. Nine genotypes exist in the population if each of the genes has 2 alleles: A,a or B,b. The following genotypes are possible: AABB, AABb, AAbb, AaBB, AaBb, Aabb, aaBB, aaBb, aabb. There will be 9 phenotypes if the phenotypic contributions of the 4 alleles are different. If contributions are equal (i.e., A = B or a = b), there could be only 5 phenotypes in the population. If 3 genes influence a trait, each existing in 2 allelic forms, 27 different genotypes would exist in the population ($3^3 = 27$). The general formula is thus 3^n, where n equals the number of genes, each with 2 allelic forms. If more than 2 alleles exist, often the case, the number of different genotypes would further increase per locus. These examples do not take into account the possibility of parental imprinting. If imprinting exists for one of the genes (i.e., $A^m \neq A^p$, where m and p connote maternal and paternal origin), the number of genotypes and phenotypes would be even greater.

The overall significance is that only a small number of genes and relatively few polymorphic alleles are necessary to generate a Gaussian distribution in the population. Identifying one or two genes of major effect could explain most cases of a disorder inherited in polygenic/multifactorial fashion.

STRATEGIES FOR IDENTIFYING MULTIPLE CAUSATIVE GENES

Given that endometriosis is heritable and presumably polygenic/multifactorial in etiology, the task is to determine the number of genes responsible and their chromosomal location(s). This can be approached in three general ways. Two require no knowledge of the nature of the causative genes; the third requires candidate gene hypotheses.

The first approach is to use genome-wide quantitative linkage analysis (QTL), searching throughout the genome with no prior expectation that a given gene or chromosomal region is causally involved. This approach has become practical within the past decade now that informative DNA polymorphic markers have been identified throughout the genome. Dinucleotide and trinucleotide repeats are most commonly used. Single nucleotide polymorphisms (SNPs) are spaced 1:1000 nucleotides apart. Many of these loci are highly polymorphic, multiple alleles existing at a given locus. This assures that informative segregations are likely to exist in a given family.

A second genome-wide approach is to search for altered gene expression, comparing endometriosis and normal (nonendometriosis) cells. The comparison could be between individuals (affected, unaffected) or between different tissues from the same individual (endometriosis, nonendometriosis). Either approach is based upon the hypothesis that differentially expressed genes connote or pinpoint causality. A pitfall of this approach is that the true causative gene may not be expressed at the point in time when the tissue was studied. Conversely, genes expressed may have little to do with causality or disease progression. Nonetheless, this approach is likely to become highly popular in the next few years as microarray technology becomes widely available for testing.

The third approach is less omnibus and more focused, depending upon the arguable strategy of exploiting candidate genes. Which candidate genes seem plausibly related to endometriosis? Do these necessarily reflect cellular mechanisms known to be perturbed in these disorders? Several obvious examples have been discussed already at this meeting—aromatase, calhedrin, estrogen receptor (ER), and GALT. Unfortunately, identifying altered biologic processes in endometriosis does not necessarily imply that genes responsible for these processes were pivotal to the initiation of the disorder. Rather, cellular processes could have become perturbed secondarily (epiphenomena) or be restricted to progression or maintenance of the pathology. Therefore, one can expect many frustrations. Prior to the availability of genome-wide QTL and gene expression technologies (e.g., microarrays), the candidate gene approach was the only one available. Now this approach complements the two more general approaches.

In the following sections, we shall explore the progress and potential in each of these three approaches.

GENOME-WIDE QTL

QTL across the whole genome is being pursued by several groups. All seek to localize the genes paramount to the etiology of endometriosis. This approach is predicated on the assumption that any region could encode gene(s) of importance. The method usually used is the sib-pair method, based on the thesis that affected relatives inherit identical copies of any given allele (identify by descent; IBD) more often than expected by chance alone. If the same locus shows allele sharing in different families of affected individuals, a pivotal gene could be identified. Sib-pair methods for QTL do not depend on specifying a specific mode of inheritance because IBD sharing at a given locus is compared with the random expectation of 0.5 for first-degree relatives. Excess IBD sharing can be detected in affected relatives irrespective of (incomplete) penetrance, phenocopy, or genetic heterogeneity. No information is necessary concerning candidate genes or chromosomal regions. QTL has been used successfully in the identifying of genes in such complex traits as asthma or hypertension.

The longest standing QTL project involving endometriosis is being conducted at Oxford. Sib-pair analysis is performed using polymorphic DNA markers and fluorescence-based automated analysis.[10,15] Several regions of exclusion have been noted, but no linkages published.

A genome-wide linkage approach is also being pursued in Iceland. A genome-wide scan of 15 families, with a total of 33 individuals affected with endometriosis and 23 relatives, was carried out using markers 5 cM apart. A suggestive locus was found on 9q, albeit not in the region of the *GALT* gene, which is on the short arm of chromosome 9.[16]

Limits and pitfalls abound in QTL. For success, large numbers of families need to be ascertained with accurate diagnosis of affected and unaffected individuals. Special difficulties exist in ascertaining sufficient numbers of extended multi-generational families and in confirming absence of disease in ostensibly unaffected individuals. Another problem is difficulty in demonstrating linkage using the traditional genetic criteria of a logarithm of the odds (LOD) score of 3.0. Given the log scale, the LOD score of 3 corresponds to 10^3 or accepting only 1:1000 likelihood that the purported linkage is not truly valid. This high bar is considered necessary given false assignments being a known problem in linkage analysis. Relaxing statistical requirements is genetically almost heretical. Another pitfall is disease misclassification, a problem in disorders like endometriosis that are plagued by clinical mimicry and are thus not always easy to detect clinically with certainty. Misclassification adversely affects statistical power, already tenuous given requirements for an LOD score of 3.0.

Another potentially major limitation is interaction between loci. The consequence is that detecting linkage for polygenic traits becomes more difficult as the number of key genes is increased. This can be shown by considering λ_s, the general term used to designate total genetic variation of a trait. Variation attributable to individual genes is termed λ_i, such that there can exist $\lambda_{i1}, \lambda_{i2}, \ldots, \lambda_{i(n-1)}, \lambda_{in}$. If more than one locus exists (the situation by definition for polygenic traits) and if these loci interact (rather than sum), then the total genetic variation (λ_s) equals the *product* of all individual locus variation. If λ_s is high and the number of λ_i low, this interaction is of relatively little consequence. For example, if $\lambda_s = 25$ and there are two loci of equal variation, $\lambda_{i1} = \lambda_{i2} = 5$ because $\lambda_{i1} \cdot \lambda_{i2}$ must equal 25. In endometriosis, λ_s is defined as the risk to a relative of the proband/risk in the general population such that, for monogenic conditions, $\lambda - 1$ decreases by 2 with each decreasing degree in relationship (i.e., first-degree to second-degree to third-degree relative). In endometriosis, λ_s is approximately 5% to 7% (see TABLE 1). Suppose heuristically that $\lambda_s = 8$ and there exist only 3 major loci. Further assume simplistically that all λ_i are equal in importance; thus, $\lambda_s = \lambda_{i1} \cdot \lambda_{i2} \cdot \lambda_{i3}$. The third root of 8 is 2 ($2^n = 8$). Not only is the individual contribution of each gene low ($\lambda_i = 2$), but the interaction further adversely affects power.

ALTERED GENE EXPRESSION (MICROARRAYS)

Early work in this area involved differences between gene products expressed in endometriosis and controls as assessed by immunocytochemical studies. High protein levels were found for various proto-oncogenes, compared to levels in normal endometrium: *c-myc*, *c-fms*, *c-erbB-1/2*, and *ras*.[17,18] Data suggested that altered proto-oncogene expression may be involved in disregulated growth and differentiation of endometriotic cells. Monoclonal cell expansion in endometriosis has also been observed.[19,20] Using an established endometriosis cell line, overexpression of oncogenes *c-myc* and *c-erbB-1* and *-2* has been observed by Gogusev *et al.*[21]

Another search involved the *bcl-2* gene, a member of the Bcl-2 gene family. Overexpression leads to a decreased rate of cell death.[22] This gene plays a role in the normal endometrium cycle by regulating cellular homeostasis and apoptosis; increased expression is detected in the proliferative endometrial phase, but not in the secretory phase.[23] Several studies have examined expression of *bcl-2* in endometrial carcinomas and hyperplasia, with controversial results.[24] In one study, *bcl-2* overexpression in ectopic endometrial lesions by immunohistochemical staining was reported, indicating that endometriotic cells fail to undergo apoptosis.[25] Using a cell death detection enzyme-linked immunosorbent assay (ELISA), Dmowski *et al.*[26] demonstrated that apoptosis is significantly decreased in eutopic endometrium of women with endometriosis, compared with fertile controls.

Recent advances in molecular biology and the development of microarray technology now make possible large-scale gene expression profiling. Rather than examine the expression of single genes of putative importance one by one, many and possibly all relevant genes can be tested simultaneously. Production of high-density oligonucleotide or cDNA arrays has been described.[27,28] In the development of oligonucleotide arrays, 16,000 to more than 65,000 different 20-mer oligonucleotides of defined sequence (referred to as probes) are synthesized directly onto derivatized glass slides using photolithography and oligonucleotide chemistry. Surface-bound oligonucleotides or probes subsequently bind or hybridize to labeled mRNA. RNAs of frequency 1:300,000 are unambiguously detected in a quantitative manner. Use of synthetic oligonucleotides allows for the use of the growing body of sequence information and for evaluation of large numbers of tens to thousands of genes. Selection of appropriate control tissues and proper RNA standards is crucial.

A caveat is that overexpressed genes need not necessarily be those involved in initiation (etiology). The converse also holds true. Finally, pure endometriosis tissue must be studied; admixtures encompassing contiguous (normal) endometrium or connective tissues could lead to spuriously negative results.

CANDIDATE GENES AND ALTERATIONS IN DNA

Loss of Heterozygosity (LOH) and Comparative Genome Hybridization (CGH)

The third general approach to uncovering genes pivotal to endometriosis is to search systematically for perturbations in selective candidate genes or chromosomal regions. An advantage is that loci need not be expressed at the time that tissue is obtained, unlike requirements for the expression assays discussed in the previous section. A disadvantage is that the correct gene or region must be selected and that perturbation must be detectable by the method chosen. In addition, any observed changes in DNA may or may not parallel any changes found in expression patterns (messenger RNA or protein) using techniques in the previous section. Theoretically, DNA-based approaches should more closely approximate causality. However, the risk of uninformative or fruitless studies is considerable. Irrespective of whether a candidate gene or chromosomal region is sought, the principle involves searching for loss or gain of either alleles at a given locus (loss of heterozygosity, LOH) or for an entire chromosomal region (comparative genome hybridization, CGH).

Initial work was disappointing. Failure to find nonrandom cytogenetic abnormalities in any of 42 endometrial implants was reported by Dangel *et al.*[29] Another group failed to find mutations in the Ras oncogene or p53 tumor suppressor gene in ectopic and eutopic endometrial tissue from 10 women with severe endometriosis.[30] Given the benefit of subsequent knowledge, the likely explanation for these negative studies was that unwittingly normal tissue (fibrous tissue or decidua) was analyzed rather than endometriotic tissue per se.

More recent studies have been more fruitful. Significant findings were made in a human endometriosis–derived permanent cell line (FbEM-1) established and characterized by Bouquet de Joliniere *et al.*[31] Chromosomal studies (R-banding) showed numerous chromosomal aberrations: monosomy X; 4q+, 5q+; trisomy 7, 8, and 10; tetrasomy for chromosomes 17, 18, 19, and 20. CGH was later used to identify somatic chromosomal alterations in DNA both from this cell line as well as from endometriotic lesions ($n = 9$).[21] CGH revealed these chromosome abnormalities in the FbEM-1 line: 1q+, 4q–, 11p–, 13q–; loss of 9, 12, and 18; and amplification of 6p. However, these changes were not consistent with previous cytogenetic results, suggesting that the cultured cells may be unstable and, hence, genetically heterogeneous. Chromosomal alterations were observed in only 4 of the 9 endometriotic tissue samples, with unbalanced aberrations involving gain on 1q, 4q, 11p, 17, and 20. Failure to find genetic imbalance among the remaining five cases may have been due to the presence of contaminating normal DNA.

Selected Candidate Genes in Endometriosis

There is no shortage of specific candidate genes, as noted already. Obvious examples include genes governing immunology, cell adhesion, or steroidogenesis, processes that have been the subject of presentations at this meeting. The first steps usually involved studies in which association was sought between endometriosis and normal individuals for selected genes (or polymorphisms at these loci). To date, results are disappointing.

One candidate gene is galactose-1-phosphate uridyl transferase (GALT), specifically an adenine to guanine change (polymorphism) in exon 10 that results in substitution of aspartate for asparagine (N314D). This polymorphism was found to be associated with endometriosis by Cramer *et al.*,[32] but not confirmed by Morland *et al.*[33] or Hadfield *et al.*[34] The latter found frequencies of N314D to be 15.8% (9/57) and 14.3% (13/91) in familial and sporadic endometriosis cases, respectively, versus 11.3% (6/53) in female controls and 13.7% (13/95) in male controls.

Another attractive candidate gene is aromatase, expressed in endometriotic tissue and stimulated by prostaglandin E_2 (PGE_2). (See Bulun *et al.* elsewhere in this volume.) Local production of estrogen and further induction of PGE_2, in turn, establish a positive feedback cycle. 17β-Hydroxysteroid dehydrogenase type II expression has also been shown to be deficient in endometriosis, leading to impaired inactivation of estradiol (E_2) to estrone. Collectively, these molecular aberrations favor accumulation of increasing quantities of E_2 and PGE_2 in endometriosis.[35]

An estrogen receptor gene polymorphism that can be detected by the PvuII restriction endonuclease was reported by Georgiou *et al.*[36] Homozygosity or heterozygosity was found in 72% (82/114) of endometriosis subjects versus 49% (56/114) of controls.

Increased frequency for the null (deletion) allele of glutathione-S-transferase M1 (GSTm1) was reported by Baranova *et al.*:[37] 86% (43/50) in endometriosis subjects versus 46% (33/72) in controls.

In addition to their studies on GSTm1, Baranova *et al.*[37] reported increased frequency of the slow acetylation allele of arylamine *N*-acetyltransferase 2 (NAT2). The potential significance of pharmacogenetic susceptibility involving this locus has been discussed elsewhere by us.[1]

Oncogenes and Tumor Suppressor Genes in Endometriosis

Our own hypothesis is that the pattern of chromosomal aberrations combined with the invasive nature of endometriosis suggested parallels between the latter and neoplasia.[1] Recall that we have already observed monoclonal cell expansion in endometriosis.[20,38] Overexpression of certain oncogenes (*c-myc*, *c-erbB-1* and -2) as well as 6p DNA amplification have been noted.[21]

Pathogenesis of neoplasia is accepted as involving clonal origin of a progenitor cell that is conferred selective advantage. By this scenario, two "hits" (mutational events) are necessary; either both mutations may be somatic or one may be germline and the other somatic. In the former (sporadic cases), heritability is low. This simplistic (two-hit) model should probably be amended to a more complicated multihit hypothesis, but irrespective the concept remains that two or more genes are necessary to initiate neoplasia and, by analogy, endometriosis. Additional mutations may be needed or yet more could result in secondary changes in the disease process. These latter genes might be important in the progression, but not necessarily the initiation, of endometriosis.

We first turned for candidates to the genes or chromosomal regions involved in ovarian endometrioid and endometrial cancer, even while realizing that less than 1%

TABLE 2. Common chromosomal regions and genes associated with ovarian endometrioid and endometrial cancers

Chromosomal region	Genes mapped	Gene function
2p16	MSH2	DNA mismatch repair protein
2p16	MSH6 (GTBP)	DNA mismatch (G/T) binding protein
2q31-q33	PMS1	DNA mismatch repair protein
3p21	MLH1	DNA mismatch repair protein
5q11-q12	MSH3	DNA mismatch repair protein
7p22	PMS2	DNA mismatch repair
9p21	p16/CDKN2	Negative regulator of cell-cycle progression; cyclin-dependent kinase inhibitor
10q23.3	PTEN	Cell adhesion; signal transduction
16q22.1	E-cadherin	Cell adhesion molecule
17p13.1	TP53	Transcription factor; cell-death/-cycle regulator at G_1 checkpoint of cell cycle
17q11.2-q12	HER-2/neu	Oncogene; transmembrane tyrosine kinase receptor; member of EGFR family
17q21	BRCA1	Tumor suppressor; may act directly or indirectly in transcription-coupled repair of oxidative DNA damage
18q22.1	DCC	Putative tumor suppressor with homology to cell adhesion molecules
18q21	bcl-2	Inhibitor of apoptosis (expression inhibits cell death)
Xq	Unknown	Ovarian development/function

of endometriosis undergoes neoplastic transformation. TABLE 2 shows some genes known to be involved in the above cancers. Support for the hypothesis that ovarian endometrioid cancers arise through malignant transformation of endometriotic lesions stems from recent evaluation of DNA alterations among subtypes of epithelial ovarian cancers. Mutations in the tumor suppressor *PTEN* gene on chromosome 10q23 have been reported in endometrioid, but in neither serous nor mucinous epithelial ovarian tumors.[39] Although LOH was common among the endometrioid (43%) and serous (28%) tumors, somatic mutations involving *PTEN* in the remaining allele were observed only in the endometrioid (21%) tumors. These results demonstrate that the developmental pathways of the three epithelial ovarian cancer subtypes (serous, mucinous, endometrioid) appear to be different and that somatic mutations in *PTEN* may represent early events in the transformation of benign endometriotic cells to malignancy. The *PTEN* protein is believed to function as a tyrosine phosphatase and to play a role in signal transduction. Interestingly, other studies have shown *PTEN* mutations to be common in endometrial cancers when microsatellite instability is detected.[40,41] Clearly, the role of *PTEN* in the pathogenesis of endometriosis should be pursued in the near future.

LOH studies, which assess the extent and variation of allele loss, were first employed in endometriosis by Jiang *et al.*[42] LOH was sought in late-stage endometriosis, using microdissection to separate endometriotic glands and stroma from fixed archival tissue. Evidence for LOH involving chromosomes 9p, 11q, and 22q was found, compared with matched normal genomic DNA. In a subsequent study, the same authors demonstrated common genetic alterations in 9 of 11 cases in which ovarian carcinoma had arisen within, or adjacent to, endometriosis.[43] Alterations in chromosomal regions 5q, 6q, 9p, 11q, and 22q were observed in 25% to 30% of the cases involving endometriosis with associated carcinoma. In one endometriosis sample, mutation in the p53 gene at codon 220 (Tyr to Cys) was detected.

Before beginning our own work in earnest, we first addressed the issue of assuring that we were sampling genuine endometriotic tissue. Indeed, we now have greater confidence that our data are derived from endometriosis tissue rather than normal tissue. We use fresh tissue touch preparations of endometriotic tissues, which permit direct placement of cells from select tissue areas onto slides, thus reducing the number of potentially contaminating cells. We can also examine single cells, using chromosome-specific probes with fluorescent *in situ* hybridization (FISH). We have also developed a modified microwave-enhanced FISH method for use in studying fixed archival tissue.[44] Overall, this approach enables cytogenetic analysis of specimens whose histology can be verified in mirror-image serial tissue section.

We first reported nonrandom chromosome alterations that included trisomy 11, monosomy 16, and monosomy 17 in late-stage disease.[45] Undisrupted cells from endometriotic tissue were placed onto the surface of a slide and 80% of the nuclei were shown to be monosomy 16. Such studies provided evidence that acquired chromosome-specific alterations may be involved in endometriosis, presumably reflecting clonal expansion of chromosomally abnormal cells. That candidate tumor suppressor genes and oncogenes have been mapped to these chromosomes further makes attractive the hypothesis that chromosomal loss or gain plays a role in the development and/or progression of endometriosis.

Using a two-color FISH approach with probes specific to the p53 locus (17p13) and 17-centromere, we further observed a significantly greater frequency of chromosome 17 aneuploidy in the endometriotic specimens ($n = 8$, mean 65%), compared with matched normal endometrial cells (mean 25%). Moreover, we found significant ($p < 0.0001$) differences between the distribution of FISH signals among various endometriosis samples, implying a high degree of heterogeneity involving chromosome 17 aneuploidy. We also observed a high incidence of monosomy p53 (only one signal detected): 18% to 28% of cells scored in 4 of 8 cases. These findings support a multistep pathway involving somatic genetic alterations in the development and progression of endometriosis. Specifically, these data suggest that p53 may be involved in the pathogenesis of endometriosis.

Findings of chromosome 11, 16, and 17 aneuploidy are consistent with genetic alterations observed in endometrial cancers (TABLE 2). Results of LOH involving the long arm of chromosome 17[46] and increased heterogeneity involving chromosome 17 aneuploidy in endometriosis further suggest that genomic instability and chromosome 17 alterations may be involved in late-stage disease.[44]

Given our initial work showing a relationship between perturbations of chromosome 17 and p53, we are now sequencing the entire p53 gene in endometriosis.

Direct automated DNA sequencing for high-throughput analysis of all 10 p53 exons in affected and matched control tissues is currently under way. To date, exons 2–10 have been amplified in 10 patients. No mutations have yet been identified.[47]

ACKNOWLEDGMENTS

This investigation was supported by the National Institute of Child Health and Development, the Endometriosis Association, and the Women's Fund for HER.

REFERENCES

1. Bischoff, F. & J.L. Simpson. 2000. Heritability and molecular genetic studies of endometriosis. Hum. Reprod. Update **6:** 37–44.
2. Simpson, J.L. 2001. Genetic factors in common disorders of female infertility. Reprod. Med. Rev. **8:** 173–202.
3. Simpson, J., S. Elias, L. Malinak *et al.* 1980. Heritable aspects of endometriosis: 1. Genetic studies. Am. J. Obstet. Gynecol. **137:** 327–331.
4. Malinak, L.R., V.C. Buttram, S. Elias *et al.* 1980. Heritable aspects of endometriosis: II. Clinical characteristics of familial endometriosis. Am. J. Obstet. Gynecol. **137:** 332–337.
5. Lamb, K., R.G. Hoffmann & T.R. Nichols. 1986. Family trait analysis: a case-control study of 43 women with endometriosis and their best friends. Am. J. Obstet. Gynecol. **154:** 596–601.
6. Moen, M.H. & P. Magnus. 1993. The familial risk of endometriosis. Acta Obstet. Gynecol. Scand. **72:** 560–564.
7. Moen, M.H. 1994. Endometriosis in monozygotic twins. Acta Obstet. Gynecol. Scand. **73:** 59–62.
8. Coxhead, D. & E.J. Thomas. 1993. Familial inheritance of endometriosis in a British population: a case control study. J. Obstet. Gynecol. **13:** 42–44.
9. dos Reis, R.M., M.F. de Sa, M.D. de Moura *et al.* 1999. Familial risk among patients with endometriosis. J. Assist. Reprod. Genet. **16:** 500–503.
10. Kennedy, S.H., H.J. Mardon & D.H. Barlow. 1995. Familial endometriosis. J. Assist. Reprod. Genet. **12:** 32–34.
11. Treloar, S., N. Martin & A. Health. 1998. Longitudinal genetic analysis of menstrual flow, pain, and limitation in a sample of Australian twins. Behav. Genet. **28:** 107–116.
12. Simpson, J.L., L.R. Malinak, S. Elias *et al.* 1984. HLA associations in endometriosis. Am. J. Obstet. Gynecol. **148:** 395–397.
13. Maxwell, C., D.C. Kilpatrick, R. Haining *et al.* 1989. No HLA-DR specificity is associated with endometriosis. Tissue Antigens **34:** 145–147.
14. Kennedy, S., R. Hadfield, H. Mardon *et al.* 1996. Age of onset of pain symptoms in non-twin sisters concordant for endometriosis. Hum. Reprod. **11:** 403–405.
15. Kennedy, S.H. 1998. The genetics of endometriosis. J. Reprod. Med. **43:** 263–268.
16. Stefansson, H., R.T. Geirsson, G.A. Guanason *et al.* 1998. A genome-wide search for endometriosis genes in Icelandic patients [abstract]. Am. J. Hum. Genet. **63:** 311.
17. Bergqvist, A., A. Borg & O. Ljungberg. 1991. Proto-oncogenes in endometriotic and endometrial tissue. Ann. N.Y. Acad. Sci. **626:** 276–283.
18. Schenken, R.S., J.V. Johnson & R.N. Riehl. 1991. C-myc proto-oncogene polypeptide expression in endometriosis. Am. J. Obstet. Gynecol. **164:** 1031–1037.
19. Nibert, M., T. Pejovic, N. Mandahl *et al.* 1995. Monoclonal origin of endometriosis cysts. Int. J. Gynecol. Cancer **5:** 61–63.
20. Jimbo, H., Y. Hitomi, H. Yoshikawa *et al.* 1997. Evidence for monoclonal expansion of epithelial cells in ovarian endometrial cysts. Am. J. Pathol. **150:** 1173–1178.

21. GOGUSEV, J., J. BOUQUET DE JOLINIERE, M. DOUSSAU *et al.* 1998. Detection of genetic abnormalities in human endometriosis by comparative genomic hybridization. Presented at the American Society for Reproductive Medicine, Toronto, Canada.
22. YANG, E. & S. KORSMEYER. 1996. Molecular thanatopsis: a discourse on the BCL2 family and cell death. Blood **88:** 386–401.
23. LU, O.L., R. POULSOM, L. WONG *et al.* 1993. Bcl-2 expression in adult and embryonic non-hematopoietic tissues. J. Pathol. **169:** 431–437.
24. HENDERSON, G., K. BROWN, S. PERKINS *et al.* 1996. Bcl-2 is down-regulated in atypical endometrial hyperplasia and adenocarcinoma. Mod. Pathol. **9:** 430–438.
25. WATANABE, H., H. KANZAKI, S. NARUKAWA *et al.* 1997. Bcl-2 and Fas expression in eutopic and ectopic human endometrium during the menstrual cycle in relation to endometrial cell apoptosis. Am. J. Obstet. Gynecol. **176:** 360–368.
26. DMOWSKI, W., H. GEBEL & D.P. BRAUN. 1998. Decreased apoptosis and sensitivity to macrophage mediated cytolysis of endometrial cells in endometriosis. Hum. Reprod. Update **4:** 696–701.
27. LOCKHART, D.J., H. DONG, M.C. BYRNE *et al.* 1996. Expression monitoring by hybridization to high-density oligonucleotide arrays. Nat. Biotechnol. **14:** 1675–1680.
28. SCHENA, M., D. SHALON, R.W. DAVIS *et al.* 1995. Quantitative monitoring of gene expression patterns with a complementary DNA microarray. Science **270:** 467–470.
29. DANGEL, A., M. MEDCHILL, G. DAVIS *et al.* 1994. Cytogenetic studies in endometriosis tissue. Cancer Genet. Cytogenet. **78:** 172–174.
30. VERCELLINI, P., D. TRECCA, S. OLDANI *et al.* 1994. Analysis of p53 and ras gene mutations in endometriosis. Gynecol. Obstet. Invest. **38:** 70–71.
31. BOUQUET DE JOLINIERE, J., P. VALIDIRE, M. CANIS *et al.* 1997. Human endometriosis–derived permanent cell line (FbEM-1): establishment and characterization. Hum. Reprod. Update **3:** 117–123.
32. CRAMER, D.W., M.D. HORNSTEIN, W.G. NG *et al.* 1996. Endometriosis associated with the N314D mutation of galactose-1-phosphate uridyl transferase (GALT). Mol. Hum. Reprod. **2:** 149–152.
33. MORLAND, S.J., X. JIANG, A. HITCHCOCK *et al.* 1998. Mutation of galactose-1-phosphate uridyl transferase and its association with ovarian cancer and endometriosis. Int. J. Cancer **77:** 825–827.
34. HADFIELD, R.M., S. MANEK, S. NAKAGO *et al.* 1999. Absence of a relationship between endometriosis and the N314D polymorphism of galactose-1-phosphate uridyl transferase in a UK population. Mol. Hum. Reprod. **5:** 990–993.
35. BULUN, S.E., K.M. ZEITOUN, H. SASANO *et al.* 2000. Estrogen biosynthesis in endometriosis: molecular basis and clinical relevance. J. Mol. Endocrinol. **25:** 35–42.
36. GEORGIOU, I., M. SYRROU, I. BOUBA *et al.* 1999. Association of estrogen receptor gene polymorphisms with endometriosis. Fertil. Steril. **72:** 164–166.
37. BARANOVA, H., R. BOTHORISHVILLI, M. CANIS *et al.* 1997. Glutathione S-transferase M1 gene polymorphism and susceptibility to endometriosis in a French population. Mol. Hum. Reprod. **3:** 775–780.
38. TAMURA, M., T. FUKAYA, T. MURAKAMI *et al.* 1998. Analysis of clonality in human endometriotic cysts based on evaluation of X chromosome inactivation in archival formalin-fixed, paraffin-embedded tissue. Lab. Invest. **78:** 213–218.
39. OBATA, K., S.J. MORLAND, R.H. WATSON *et al.* 1998. Frequent PTEN/MMAC mutations in endometrioid, but not serous or mucinous epithelial ovarian tumors. Cancer Res. **58:** 2095–2097.
40. PEIFFER, K., T. HERZOG, D. TRIBUNE *et al.* 1995. Allelic loss of sequences from the long arm of chromosome 10 and replication errors in endometrial cancers. Cancer Res. **55:** 1922–1926.
41. TASHIRO, H., M.S. BLAZES, R. WU *et al.* 1997. Mutations in PTEN are frequent in endometrial carcinoma, but rare in other common gynecological malignancies. Cancer Res. **57:** 3935–3940.
42. JIANG, X., A. HITCHCOCK, E. BRYAN *et al.* 1996. Microsatellite analysis of endometriosis reveals loss of heterozygosity at candidate ovarian tumor suppressor gene loci. Cancer Res. **56:** 3534–3537.

43. JIANG, X., S.J. MORLAND, A. HITCHCOCK *et al.* 1998. Allelotyping of endometriosis with adjacent ovarian carcinoma reveals evidence of a common lineage. Cancer Res. **58:** 1707–1711.
44. KOSUGI, Y., S. ELIAS, L.R. MALINAK *et al.* 1999. Increased heterogeneity of chromosome 17 aneuploidy in endometriosis. Am. J. Obstet. Gynecol. **180:** 792–797.
45. SHIN, J.C., H.L. ROSS, S. ELIAS *et al.* 1997. Detection of chromosomal aneuploidy in endometriosis by multi-color fluorescence *in situ* hybridization (FISH). Hum. Genet. **100:** 401–406.
46. BISCHOFF, F.Z., H.L. ROSS, D. NGUYEN *et al.* 1997. Loss of heterozygosity for chromosome 17 (p53) in endometriosis by molecular genetic and two-color FISH analysis [abstract]. J. Soc. Gynecol. Invest. (Suppl.) **4:** 205.
47. HEARD, M.J., D. NGUYEN, D. MARQUEZ *et al.* 2001. Genetic analysis of p53 tumor suppressor gene in endometriosis [abstract]. J. Soc. Gynecol. Invest. (Suppl.) **8:** 173.

The Molecular Basis for Implantation Failure in Endometriosis

On the Road to Discovery

LINDA C. GIUDICE, TRACEY L. TELLES, SHALINI LOBO, AND LEE KAO

Center for Research on Women's Health and Reproductive Medicine, Division of Reproductive Endocrinology and Infertility, Department of Gynecology and Obstetrics, Stanford University Medical Center, Stanford, California 94305, USA

ABSTRACT: Endometriosis is a benign gynecologic disorder associated with pelvic pain and infertility, with the latter being due, in part, to failure of embryonic implantation in the maternal endometrium. Adequacy of the endometrium for fertility has been classically investigated by histologic evaluation of a mid-late luteal phase biopsy and, historically, normal histology has been reassuring. However, recent studies demonstrate histologically normal, but biochemically abnormal, endometrium during the window of implantation in some women with endometriosis. In the pregenomic era, a "one-by-one" approach has been adopted to investigate proteins and genes expressed in the window of implantation, and several genes or gene products have been found to be aberrantly expressed in endometrium of women with endometriosis either during the implantation window or at other times of the cycle. Some of these are related to failure of implantation, while others likely contribute to the establishment and growth of endometriotic lesions. The time has come for a genome-wide approach to evaluate uterine endometrium for embryonic implantation. Knowing the biochemical mechanisms underlying normal implantation and the abnormalities in endometriosis will facilitate development of new diagnostic criteria beyond histologic evaluation and will permit identification and validation of molecular targets for future drug discovery. This monograph reviews (a) some of the evidence of compromised fertility in women with endometriosis and treatments targeted to improve their fertility; (b) the concept of the window of implantation; (c) genes/gene products aberrantly expressed in endometrium during the window of implantation or other times of the cycle in women with endometriosis; and (d) the use of microarray technology to investigate endometrial gene expression in human endometrial stromal cells and preliminary data resulting from a collaborative consortium effort of a genome-wide investigation of gene expression in the window of implantation of women with versus without endometriosis.

KEYWORDS: endometriosis; infertility; microarray; genomics; genes

Address for correspondence: Linda C. Giudice, Center for Research on Women's Health and Reproductive Medicine, Division of Reproductive Endocrinology and Infertility, Department of Gynecology and Obstetrics, Stanford University Medical Center, 300 Pasteur Drive, Stanford, CA 94305. Voice: 650-723-6175; fax: 650-498-4320.

giudice@stanford.edu

ENDOMETRIOSIS: CURRENT CONCEPTS ON ETIOLOGY AND FERTILITY COMPROMISE AND THERAPIES

Endometriosis is a benign gynecologic disorder and, as is evident from the proceedings of this workshop, the pathophysiology of endometriosis is not well understood. However, in the majority of women with the disorder, pelvic and peritoneal disease are believed to result from retrograde menstruation, in the setting of undefined genetic, environmental, and/or immunologic influences. The origins of pelvic pain and infertility associated with endometriosis are complex and also are not well understood. With regard to infertility, animal models[1–4] and some clinical studies,[5] but not others,[6,7] support an adverse effect of endometriosis on pregnancy rates. While several studies from assisted reproduction have variably supported decreased pregnancy rates among women with versus without endometriosis, a recent meta-analysis of most of the Assisted Reproduction Technology (ART) studies to date demonstrates a pregnancy rate in women with endometriosis to be about 50% of the pregnancy rate of women with tubal factor infertility, once confounding factors are controlled.[8] With regard to therapies and their effects on pregnancy, two meta-analyses found no benefit of surgical or medical therapy,[9,10] whereas two large-scale studies support surgical ablation of minimal and mild disease to improve fertility rates.[11,12] Since the underlying mechanisms contributing to decreased fecundity in women with endometriosis have been poorly understood, to date most therapies have been empiric. Furthermore, since endometriosis is a heterogeneous disorder, it is not unexpected that prescribed therapies may be beneficial for some, but not others.

POTENTIAL MECHANISMS UNDERLYING INFERTILITY IN WOMEN WITH ENDOMETRIOSIS

It is well established that peritoneal fluid in women with endometriosis has increased levels of cytokines, growth factors, and activated macrophages, likely a result of endometriosis tissue being in an abnormal location and the normal immune response to this ectopic tissue.[13] This fluid has been demonstrated to be toxic to sperm function and exhibits an adverse effect on embryo survival.[14–17] In addition, peritoneal fluid from women with endometriosis reduces implantation rates in rabbits,[1] mice,[18] and hamsters.[4] There is an evolving literature supporting abnormal eutopic endometrium and implantation failure in some women with endometriosis as an underlying cause of infertility in this population. In addition, evidence is accumulating to support the idea that aberrant gene and gene product expression in eutopic endometrium at other times of the cycle in women with endometriosis may be related to infertility or to the establishment of the disease. These are considered herein, after a brief description of the window of implantation.

THE WINDOW OF IMPLANTATION

The endometrium is receptive to embryonic implantation during a defined "window" that is temporally and spatially restricted. Evidence supporting this concept comes from hysterectomy specimens containing early gestations, from scanning electron microscopy of human endometrium throughout the secretory phase, and from the clinical practice of assisted reproduction. Early studies by Hertig and Rock[19] suggested that the window of implantation in human endometrium resided in the mid-secretory phase. Embryos identified in secretory phase hysterectomy specimens were all free-floating before day 20 of the cycle and all were attached or had invaded into the endometrial stroma when specimens were obtained after day 20. Definition of the window of implantation has received substantial support from the appearance of domelike structures involving the luminal epithelium. These structures, called pinopods (Greek: pino = drink; podia = feet), are believed to be important for water and solute transport across the epithelium and for embryonic attachment. Scanning electron microscopy demonstrates that 78% of endometrial biopsies obtained from normally cycling women on postovulatory day (POD) 6 have pinopods, compared to rare pinopods visualized on POD 2 or 9.[20–22] Pinopods form briefly and last for 1 to 2 days, and their numbers positively correlate with implantation sites.[23] In natural cycles, there is up to 5 days variation in the days postovulation in which pinopods form.[24] Additional support for the implantation window derives from assisted reproductive cycles. For example, Navot *et al.*[25] tested the window of endometrial receptivity by performing embryo transfers between days 16 and 24 of hormonally and histologically defined cycles. For transfers within cycle days 17–19, 40.5% conceptions occurred; in contrast, in cycles in which embryos were transferred on or after day 20, no conceptions occurred. Furthermore, Wilcox *et al.*[26] reported a high success of continuing pregnancy for embryos that implanted between POD 8 and 10 (84%), compared to 18% when implantation occurred 11 days or more after ovulation. There are striking data demonstrating limited plasticity of the implantation window, with advancing of the window to POD 5–6 in clomiphene- or gonadotropin-stimulated cycles[27] and delaying of the window to POD 9–10 in steroid hormone replacement cycles for donor recipients.[28] These observations collectively support a distinct and narrow period of endometrial specialization that coincides with the window of implantation (FIG. 1).

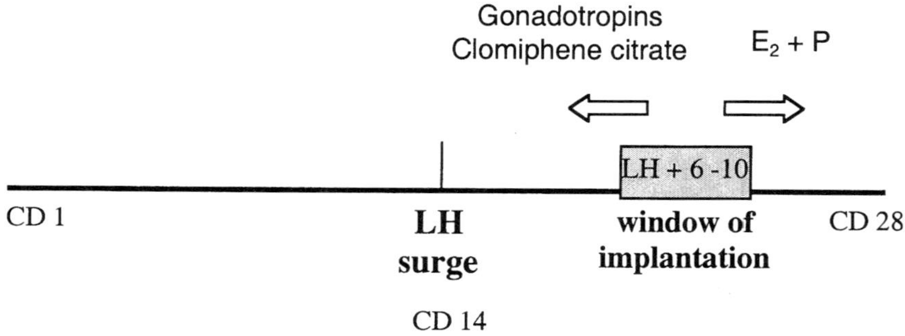

FIGURE 1. Schematic of the implantation window (see text).

TABLE 1. Genes and gene products aberrantly expressed in endometrium from women with endometriosis

Aromatase
Endometrial bleeding factor
Hepatocyte growth factor
17β-Hydroxysteroid dehydrogenase
HoxA-10
HoxA-11
Leukemia inhibitory factor
Matrix metalloproteinase-7, -11
Progesterone receptors

GENE PRODUCTS ABERRANTLY EXPRESSED IN ENDOMETRIUM FROM WOMEN WITH ENDOMETRIOSIS

TABLE 1 shows the genes currently known to be aberrantly expressed during the window of implantation and at other times of the cycle in women with versus without endometriosis. These include integrins (e.g., $\alpha_v\beta_3$), matrix metalloproteinases (e.g., MMP-7 and -11), transcription factors (e.g., hepatocyte nuclear factor), endometrial bleeding factor, enzymes involved in steroid hormone metabolism (e.g., aromatase, 17β-hydroxysteroid dehydrogenase), leukemia inhibitory factor, Hox genes, and progesterone receptor isoforms. Lessey and colleagues have demonstrated that, concomitant with the loss of progesterone receptors in endometrial epithelium, the window of implantation is opened by epithelial $\alpha_v\beta_3$ integrin expression.[29] The finding of Lessey and colleagues of histologically normal endometrium, but lacking expression of a marker of uterine receptivity, the $\alpha_v\beta_3$ integrin, during the window of implantation in women with endometriosis versus those who are disease-free,[29] is a seminal contribution that has challenged the fundamental paradigm that secretory phase endometrial histology is sufficient for fertility. While the secretory phase endometrial biopsy has been the "gold standard" for evaluating endometrial adequacy,[30] the concept of endometrial abnormalities not reflected by altered histology has raised the question of occult deficiencies leading to failure of embryonic implantation that are not diagnosable by classic diagnostic testing. Indeed, Lessey and colleagues[31] have suggested a classification of two types of endometrial defects: the "type I defect", reflecting lack of endometrial expression of $\alpha_v\beta_3$ integrin associated with histologic delay (i.e., classical luteal phase defect); and the "type II defect", in which the endometrium is histologically normal (i.e., without histologic delay), but associated with the absence of expression of this marker of uterine receptivity. The latter suggests an intrinsic defect in endometrial function and is found largely in women with minimal or mild endometriosis[32] and in women with hydrosalpinges,[33] unexplained infertility,[31] and polycystic ovarian syndrome.[34] Since regulation of $\alpha_v\beta_3$ is not precisely defined, pharmacologic correction of this defect is empiric, although ovarian suppression with GnRH agonists[35] or laparoscopic ablation of pelvic endometriosis may restore $\alpha_v\beta_3$ expression in the eutopic endometrium.[36]

Several other endometrial gene products are aberrantly expressed in endometrium of women with endometriosis. Leukemia inhibitory factor (LIF) has been shown in a knockout mouse model to be important in embryonic attachment to the epithelium and also for endometrial decidualization.[37] In humans, LIF is expressed in endometrium and decidua.[38–40] LIF mRNA is preferentially expressed in the secretory, compared to the proliferative, phase and is expressed threefold higher in glandular epithelium, compared to stroma. LIF acts on human cytotrophoblasts, diverting them to differentiate to the anchoring phenotype by increasing synthesis of fibronectin and decreasing hCG production[41] and differentiating along the invasive pathway.[42] Thus, LIF may also play a role in trophoblast differentiation. Recently, Lessey, Stewart, and colleagues reported that mice treated with peritoneal fluid from infertile women with endometriosis had decreased fertility and a reduction in endometrial LIF expression.[18] Whether peritoneal fluid in women with pelvic endometriosis promotes decreased LIF expression in eutopic endometrium in women with disease remains to be determined.

Hepatocyte growth factor (HGF) is a mitogen, derived from endometrial stromal cells, that stimulates proliferation of endometrial epithelial cells and is a morphogen for these cells *in vitro*.[43] Endometrial stromal cells from patients with endometriosis demonstrate a marked increase in HGF secretion when cultured *in vitro*, suggesting glandular abnormalities in women with endometriosis.[43] Endometrial bleeding factor (ebaf), a member of the TGF-β superfamily, is expressed in late secretory endometrium and during menses, and is downregulated in the window of implantation. It is a marker for uterine nonreceptivity and is abundantly expressed in the window of implantation in women with endometriosis and infertility.[44] Homeobox (Hox) genes mediate embryonic development and are important in regulating endometrial development. HoxA-10 and HoxA-11 are upregulated in the window of implantation in human endometrium and are both downregulated during this period in women with endometriosis.[45] Matrix metalloproteinases are enzymes that degrade extracellular matrix components. MMP-7 and MMP-11 are normally expressed in endometrium during menstrual breakdown and subsequent estrogen-mediated endometrial growth, and are suppressed by progesterone during the secretory phase.[46] However, in women with endometriosis, there appears to be a resistance to progesterone action.[29,47] Indeed, there is persistent expression of these two MMPs during the secretory phase, likely due to complex interactions between progesterone and local cytokines that may affect MMP expression during the development of endometriosis.[46] Whether there is aberrant expression of these enzymes in the implantation window and such effects on implantation await further investigation.

Aromatase expression is also aberrant in some women with endometriosis. This enzyme catalyzes conversion of androstenedione and testosterone, derived from ovarian and adrenal sources, to estrone and estradiol, respectively. Aromatase is normally expressed in ovarian granulosa cells, placental syncytiotrophoblasts, adipose tissue, skin fibroblasts, and the brain, and is normally absent in the endometrium.[48] Regulation of aromatase expression is via the inhibitory transcription factor, chicken ovalbumin upstream promoter transcription factor (COUP-TF), which is ubiquitously expressed in both eutopic endometrium and endometriosis.[49] In contrast, steroidogenic factor-1 (SF-1), competing for the same binding site in the aromatase promoter II as COUP-TF, acts as a stimulatory transcription factor.[49] SF-1 has been shown to be expressed in endometriosis, but absent in eutopic endometrium.[49] When SF-1 is present, it binds to the aromatase promoter with greater affinity than COUP-TF, causing increased aromatase activity and, thus, increased conversion of androstenedione to estrone.[48] This estrone, which is weakly estrogenic, is subsequently converted to the more potent estrogen, estradiol, by 17β-hydroxysteroid dehydrogenase-1 (17β-HSD-1). Inactivation of estradiol is completed by 17β-HSD-2, normally present in endometrial glandular cells. However, endometriotic glandular cells lack this enzyme, which impairs inactivation of estradiol and leads to increased local concentrations of estradiol.[50] These increased concentrations of estradiol are known to stimulate production of prostaglandins, specifically PGE_2, which further stimulates activity of aromatase.[51] Therefore, it is the increased activity of aromatase, due to the binding of SF-1, that eventually leads to increased concentrations of estradiol, coupled with the decreased ability of the glandular cells to inactivate estradiol, due to the absence of 17β-HSD-2, that collectively results in growth of endometriosis. A more recent approach to the treatment of endometriosis has been the use of aromatase inhibitors.[52–54] Preliminary evidence suggests that these aromatase inhibitors may have success in eradicating endometriotic lesions when other medical therapies, such as GnRH agonists, have failed.[48]

During the luteal phase, endometrial decidualization is induced by progesterone, through the mediation of its receptors that act as ligand-activated transcription factors. The human progesterone receptor (PR) is expressed as PR-A and PR-B isoforms, which differ functionally. While progesterone action on target genes is conferred primarily by PR-B homodimers, the truncated PR-A acts as a repressor of PR-B function. By immunohistochemistry, both isoforms are present throughout the mid-to-late proliferative phase of the menstrual cycle, and both are expressed in the endometrial glands, prior to subnuclear vacuole formation. Persistence of PR-B into the mid-secretory phase suggests its role in glandular secretion. In the stroma, PR-A predominates throughout the cycle, implicating its role for postovulatory events.[55,56] Normal endometrial receptivity has been associated with the timely downregulation of epithelial PR content, and histological delay is associated with a failure of such PR downregulation.[57] In patients with endometriosis, both PR-A and PR-B transcripts are readily detectable in eutopic endometrium and appear to be dysregulated; in endometriotic implants, only the PR-A transcript is present. The presence of the inhibitory isoform, PR-A, and the absence of the stimulatory isoform, PR-B, provide a possible explanation for progesterone resistance of endometriotic implants.[58]

A lack of proper immune surveillance in the peritoneum is considered one of the causes of endometriosis. An immune cell that shows decreased activity leading to impaired immune surveillance is the natural killer (NK) cell. These cells are cytolytic in function, including lysis of endometrial cells in the peritoneal cavity. NK cell activity may be deficient in women with endometriosis,[59,60] thereby resulting in decreased cytotoxicity towards ectopic lesions. IL-12, previously known as natural killer cell stimulatory factor (NKSF), is a cytokine known to stimulate NK cell activity.[61] Therefore, IL-12, acting through NK cells, may be important in the pathogenesis of the disease. IL-12 is a heterodimer composed of a p40 and a p35 subunit. IL-12 in its heterodimeric form does not seem to show any change that correlates with endometriosis.[62,63] However, higher levels of the p40 subunit are present in the peritoneal fluid of women with endometriosis. The ratio of IL-12 + free p40/IL-12 increases with the severity of the disease.[64] Interestingly, in a mouse model for endometriosis, intraperitoneal injections of IL-12 were able to abrogate lesions.[65] Given that IL-12 has potent antitumor, antimetastatic, and antiangiogenic activity and is under study for treatment in human cancer, it may be potentially important for endometriosis, both in diagnosis and in treatment.

Once endometriotic lesions are formed, they secrete a number of proinflammatory molecules. Cytokines[66] like IL-1, IL-8, TNF-α, and IFN-λ act on chemotactic factors that, in turn, recruit macrophages and T lymphocytes to the peritoneum. These immune cells then mediate the inflammatory reaction associated with endometriosis. RANTES (regulated on activation, normal T expressed and secreted) is a potent chemoattractant for monocytes and T lymphocytes. Its concentration in the peritoneal fluid is increased in endometriosis and correlates with the severity of the disease.[67] MCP-1 (monocyte chemoattractant protein-1) is another chemotactic protein found to be increased in the peritoneal fluid of patients that could account for the increased number of activated macrophages in the peritoneum of women with endometriosis.[68] Cytokines in endometriosis have recently been reviewed.[66]

GENOMIC APPROACH TO ENDOMETRIAL GENE EXPRESSION

From the discussion above, it is evident that a limited number of molecules have been identified to be dysregulated in endometrium from women with endometriosis. In the pregenomic era, a "one-by-one" approach has been adopted to investigate proteins and genes expressed in the window of implantation. Genome-wide approaches using microarray technologies are extensively being employed to evaluate global gene expression in a variety of systems from bacteria to primates. We and others have begun investigation into gene expression in human endometrium on a global scale, compared to the more classical "one-by-one" approach.

Microarrays come in various types, including cDNAs spotted onto filters (e.g., Clontech) or oligonucleotides spotted onto glass or other matrices (Affymetrix). We have used both approaches to investigate gene expression in human endometrium. Since decidualization of endometrial stromal cells is effected by progesterone (P) and cAMP, we investigated genes differentially expressed in human endometrial stromal cells decidualized *in vitro* in response to P or cAMP, compared to non-decidualized cells. Total RNA was isolated and reverse-transcribed to synthesize ^{32}P-labeled cDNA probes using primers corresponding to genes represented on the Clontech Human Atlas cDNA Expression Array. After hybridization, signals were quantified by phosphoimaging densitometry and were normalized to GAPDH and ubiquitin. Of the 588 genes screened, marked upregulation (TABLES 2 and 3) was observed for cytokines, growth factors, members of the RAR/RXR family, Hox genes, and mediators of the cAMP signal transduction pathways.[69] Expression of previously unrecognized genes upregulated in decidualized human endometrial stromal cells (e.g., inhibin subunits and neuromodulators and neurotransmitter receptors) suggests mechanisms not yet appreciated in the endometrium during decidualization. In addition, marked upregulation of cytokines, chemokines, growth factors, and their receptors in decidualized stromal cells supports a major role for paracrine interactions between the stroma and other endogenous and transient cell populations within the endometrium and during early pregnancy.

TABLE 2. mRNAs encoding growth factors, cytokines, chemokines, receptors, and binding proteins in P and cAMP decidualized vs. nondecidualized human endometrial stromal cells

	patient 1		patient 2	
	P	cAMP	P	cAMP
IL-5	30.6	4.9	3.7	1.6
IL-6	8.3	1.6	34.8	4.9
IL-7	4.9	2.7	2.6	1.7
IL-8	24.0	3.5	27.1	6.8
IL-10	4.7	1.8	3.2	14.8
IL-11	6.0	3.6	3.1	1.9
IL-13	125.6	13.7	7.4	3.5
IL-14	29.1	5.7	2.4	2.7
IGFBP-1	3.2	10.4	4.4	15.4
IGFBP-3	3.3	2.6	10.4	3.1
insulin R	3.3	3.1	3.1	2.9
prorelaxin H2	7.9	2.4	3.0	3.3
EGF	9.7	3.8	1.8	1.9
EGF R	9.9	3.9	3.0	1.5
amphiregulin	1.4	4.9	1.7	5.8

	patient 1		patient 2	
	P	cAMP	P	cAMP
GM-CSF	5.1	2.8	1.7	2.3
endothelin-2	2.6	1.5	3.0	2.6
endothelin R type B	1.9	3.0	1.5	8.7
VEGF	1.3	3.6	1.6	4.1
VEGFR-3 (FLT-4)	3.3	2.4	9.5	1.6
VEGF R/KDR	2.4	4.0	2.3	2.6
FLT 3 ligand	6.4	3.6	2.8	1.4
TGF-β2	8.4	9.0	2.2	2.0
TGF β R type III	6.9	3.2	1.7	1.5
MCP-1	2.1	15.2	2.1	11.5
INF-α	4.9	1.7	4.8	13.7
INF-β	8.3	5.2	8.2	4.3
TNF-α	5.5	1.2	3.2	1.4
TNF receptor-1	5.5	4.2	4.0	2.0

	patient 1		patient 2	
	P	cAMP	P	cAMP
neurotrophin-3	7.8	2.9	2.8	1.4
neuromodulin	1.3	3.1	0.8	2.7
neurotrophin-4	4.9	2.2	2.0	3.1
α-adrenergic R 2A	2.1	1.4	3.5	4.2
angiotensin II-1A R	3.1	1.0	2.8	1.8
renin-binding protein	6.0	2.8	2.6	3.7
acyl Co-A BP	3.2	2.2	5.1	1.5
glucagon precursor	6.6	2.8	2.6	3.8
inhibin α subunit	8.7	2.9	3.6	2.9
inhibin/activin $β_A$ subunit	5.0	2.8	2.8	1.6
FSH R	5.8	2.3	2.8	1.5
placental-like GF 1 & 2	3.5	1.9	7.1	1.8
estrogen sulfotransferase	4.1	1.1	2.4	1.9

R = receptor; BP = binding protein; GF = growth factor.

TABLE 3. mRNAs encoding cell cycle regulators, intracellular signaling, apoptosis, DNA synthesis, repair, and transcription factors in P and cAMP decidualized vs. nondecidualized endometrial stromal cells

	patient 1		patient 2	
	P	cAMP	P	cAMP
Oncogenes, cell cycle regulators				
c-myc	3.3	2.1	8.2	5.0
c-fms (CSF-1-R)	4.9	2.8	2.0	1.3
c-fer	3.9	3.2	1.9	3.3
c-src kinase	3.1	2.1	3.0	1.9
CDK N1C	1.5	3.0	1.9	3.4
colorectal ca* supp	3.6	7.9	1.4	3.6
bullous pemphigoid Ag*	1.0	3.0	2.0	3.1
G1/S-cyclin E	2.8	3.9	1.5	8.7
cyclin 4 inhibitor 2B	4.7	1.5	3.0	2.2

	patient 1		patient 2	
	P	cAMP	P	cAMP
Apoptosis, DNA synthesis, repair				
GADD45	3.1	3.3	3.1	2.7
RAR-ε	8.9	4.2	4.1	1.2
RAR-β	2.6	1.3	6.6	2.9
Microsomal GT	3.0	1.9	7.8	1.4
TRAIL*	2.8	2.9	2.7	4.1
Intracellular signaling				
cAMP PDE4A6	4.8	1.5	2.5	1.9
SCDF* 1R	3.8	5.2	4.3	2.6
guanine nucleotide BP*	3.7	1.4	3.3	2.5
CDK-activating kinase	2.5	2.7	1.0	3.2

	patient 1		patient 2	
	P	cAMP	P	cAMP
Transcription factors, DNA BPs				
TATA-box factor	2.4	1.7	3.4	2.0
Hox 2A	4.0	3.1	3.7	4.1
HoxD-3; Hox 4A	3.6	2.5	2.2	2.2
Hox 11	1.8	2.6	2.1	4.6
brain-specific Hox	1.8	3.1	2.1	4.4
homeobox hLim1	4.5	2.5	15.4	2.4
NF-ATc	3.1	2.9	3.2	4.2
colorectal ca mut pro	2.5	9.1	5.3	7.4
gf-inducible np* 475	3.8	2.4	2.3	8.0
NF-90	1.8	3.7	4.0	1.4
forkhead TF AFX	3.4	4.5	3.9	3.0

*Ca = cancer; Ag = antigen; SCDF = stromal cell-derived factor; BP = binding protein; nf = nuclear factor; np = nuclear protein; TF = transcription factor; GT = glutathione transferase; TRAIL = TNF-related apoptosis inducing ligand

We recently investigated genes expressed in human endometrium during the window of implantation, compared to the proliferative phase, using the Affymetrix Hu95A microarray with probe sets for more than 12,000 full-length human genes and ESTs.[70] These data suggest that, in women with endometriosis, there is down-regulation of gene expression for some of the known secretory proteins as well as other gene families. These observations are consistent with reports on women with endometriosis failing to respond to progestins, possibly resulting from an insensitivity to progesterone[71] via altered progesterone receptor isoforms[58] or from modification of progesterone action by cytokines or other factors.[46] Given the global profiling approach in endometrial biopsies taken during the window of implantation and with subsequent evaluation of such in women with implantation disorders (e.g., endometriosis), we envision that the stage will be set for development of diagnostic tools for screening such abnormalities and for development of targeted drug therapies to correct these disorders.

ACKNOWLEDGMENTS

This work was supported, in part, by the National Institutes of Health Specialized Cooperative Centers Program in Reproductive Research (Grant No. HD 31398 to L. C. Giudice), the National Institutes of Health Office of Women's Health Research (to L. C. Giudice), and the National Institutes of Health Women's Reproductive Health Research Career Development Award (to L. Kao). Special thanks are also extended to the Endometriosis Association for their help in subject recruitment.

REFERENCES

1. HAHN, D.W., R.P. CARRAHER, R.G. FOLDESY & J.L. MCGUIRE. 1986. Experimental evidence for failure to implant as a mechanism of infertility associated with endometriosis. Am. J. Obstet. Gynecol. **155:** 1109–1113.
2. SCHENKEN, R.S. & R.H. ASCH. 1980. Surgical induction of endometriosis in the rabbit: effects on fertility and concentration of peritoneal fluid prostaglandins. Fertil. Steril. **34:** 581–587.
3. VERNON, M.W. & E.A. WILSON. 1985. Studies on the surgical induction of endometriosis in the rat. Fertil. Steril. **44:** 684–694.
4. STEINLEITNER, A., H. LAMBERT, C. KAZENSKY & P. DANKS. 1990. Peritoneal fluid from endometriosis patients affects reproductive outcome in an *in vivo* model. Fertil. Steril. **53:** 926–929.
5. JANSEN, R.P. 1986. Minimal endometriosis and reduced fecundability: prospective evidence from an artificial insemination by donor program. Fertil. Steril. **46:** 141–143.
6. EVERS, J.L. 1989. The pregnancy rate of the no-treatment group in randomized clinical trials of endometriosis therapy. Fertil. Steril. **52:** 906–907.
7. PAULSON, J.D., P. ASMAR & D.S. SAFFAN. 1991. Mild and moderate endometriosis: comparison of treatment modalities for infertile couples. J. Reprod. Med. **36:** 151–155.
8. BARNHART, K.T., R. DUNSMOOR & C. COUTIFARIS. 2000. The effect of endometriosis on IVF outcome. Fertil. Steril. **74:** 576–584.
9. HUGHES, E.G., D.M. FEDORKOW & J.A. COLLINS. 1993. A quantitative overview of controlled trials in endometriosis-associated infertility. Fertil. Steril. **59:** 963–970.
10. ADAMSON, G.D. & D.J. PASTA. 1994. Surgical treatment of endometriosis-associated infertility: meta-analysis compared with survival analysis. Am. J. Obstet. Gynecol. **171:** 1488–1505.

11. NOWROOZI, K., J.S. CHASE, J.H. CHECK & C.H. WU. 1987. The importance of laparoscopic coagulation of mild endometriosis in infertile women. Int. J. Fertil. **32:** 442–444.
12. MARCOUX, S., R. MAHEUX, E.S. BERUB *et al.* 1997. Laparoscopic surgery in infertile women with minimal or mild endometriosis. N. Engl. J. Med. **337:** 217–222.
13. GIUDICE, L.C., S.T. TAZUKE & L. SWIERSZ. 1998. Current update on research in endometriosis. J. Reprod. Med. **43:** 252–262.
14. AEBY, T.C., T. HUANG & R.T. NAKAYAMA. 1996. The effect of peritoneal fluid from patients with endometriosis on human sperm function *in vitro*. Am. J. Obstet. Gynecol. **174:** 1779–1783.
15. MORCOS, R.N., W.E. GIBBONS & W.E. FINDLEY. 1986. Effect of peritoneal fluid on *in vitro* cleavage of 2-cell mouse embryos: possible role in infertility associated with endometriosis. Fertil. Steril. **44:** 678–683.
16. ORAL, E., A. ARICI, D.L. OLIVE & G. HUSZAR. 1996. Peritoneal fluid from women with moderate or severe endometriosis inhibits sperm motility: the role of seminal fluid components. Fertil. Steril. **66:** 787–792.
17. TAKETANI, Y., T.M. KUO & M. MIZUNO. 1992. Comparison of cytokine levels and embryo toxicity in peritoneal fluid in infertile women with untreated or treated endometriosis. Am. J. Obstet. Gynecol. **167:** 265–270.
18. ILLERA, M.J., L. YUAN, C.L. STEWART & B.D. LESSEY. 2000. Effect of peritoneal fluid from women with endometriosis on implantation in the mouse model. Fertil. Steril. **74:** 41–48.
19. HERTIG, A. & J.A. ROCK. 1956. A description of 34 human ova within the first 17 days of development. Am. J. Anat. **98:** 435–494.
20. MARTEL, D., R. FRYDMAN, M. GLISSANT *et al.* 1987. Scanning electron microscopy of postovulatory human endometrium in spontaneous cycles and cycles stimulated by hormone treatment. J. Endocrinol. **114:** 319–324.
21. MARTEL, D., C. MALET, J.P. GAUTRAY & A. PSYCHOYOS. 1987. Surface changes of the luminal uterine epithelium during human menstrual cycle: a scanning electron microscopic study. *In* The Endometrium—Hormonal Impacts, pp. 15–29. Plenum. New York.
22. MARTEL, D., M.N. MONIER, D. ROICHE & A. PSYCHOYOS. 1991. Hormonal dependence of pinopod formation at the uterine luminal surface. Hum. Reprod. **6:** 597–603.
23. NIKAS, G. 1999. Cell surface morphological events relevant to human implantation. Hum. Reprod. **14**(suppl. 2)**:** 37–44.
24. NIKAS, G., A. MAKRIGIANNAKIS, O. HOVATTA & H.W. JONES, JR. 2000. Surface morphology of the human endometrium: basic and clinical aspects. Ann. N.Y. Acad. Sci. **900:** 316–324.
25. NAVOT, D., R.T. SCOTT, K. DROESCH *et al.* 1991. The window of embryo transfer and the efficiency of human conception *in vitro*. Fertil. Steril. **55:** 114–118.
26. WILCOX, A.J., D.D. BAIRD & C.R. WEINBERG. 1999. Time of implantation of the conceptus and loss of pregnancy. N. Engl. J. Med. **340:** 1796–1799.
27. NIKAS, G., O.H. DEVELIOGLU, J.P. TONER & H.W. JONES, JR. 1999. Endometrial pinopods indicate a shift in the window of receptivity in IVF cycles. Hum Reprod. **14:** 787–792.
28. DEVELIOGLU, O.H., J.G. HSIU, G. NIKAS *et al.* 1999. Endometrial estrogen and progesterone receptor and pinopod expression in stimulated cycles in oocyte donation. Fertil. Steril. **71:** 1040–1047.
29. LESSEY, B.A., L. DAMJANOVICH, C. COUTIFARIS *et al.* 1992. Integrin adhesion molecules in the human endometrium: correlation with the normal and abnormal menstrual cycle. J. Clin. Invest. **90:** 188–195.
30. NOYES, R.W., A.I. HERTIG & J. ROCK. 1950. Dating the endometrial biopsy. Fertil. Steril. **1:** 3–25.
31. LESSEY, B.A., A.J. CASTLEBAUM, S.J. SAWIN *et al.* 1995. Integrins as markers of uterine receptivity in women with primary unexplained infertility. Fertil. Steril. **63:** 535–542.
32. LESSEY, B.A., A.J. CASTLEBAUM, S.J. SAWIN *et al.* 1994. Aberrant integrin expression in the endometrium of women with endometriosis. J. Clin. Endocrinol. Metab. **79:** 643–649.

33. MEYER, W.R., A.J. CASTELBAUM, S. SOMKUTI *et al.* 1997. Hydrosalpinges adversely affect markers of endometrial receptivity. Hum. Reprod. **12:** 1393–1398.
34. LESSEY, B.A., A.J. CASTLEBAUM, J. HARRIS *et al.* 2000. Use of integrins to date the endometrium. Fertil. Steril. **73:** 779–787.
35. LESSEY, B.A., K.B.C. APPA RAO, L.P. LOVELY & Y. GUI. 2001. Elevated endometrial androgen receptor expression in women with polycystic ovarian syndrome (PCOS). Biol. Reprod. In press.
36. CASTLEBAUM, A.J. & B.A. LESSEY. 2001. Infertility and implantation defects. Infertil. Reprod. Med. Clin. North Am. **12:** 427–446.
37. STEWART, C.L. 1994. Leukemia inhibitory factor and the regulation of pre-implantation development of the mammalian embryo. Mol. Reprod. Dev. **39:** 233–238.
38. CHARNOCK-JONES, D.S., A.M. SHARKEY, P. FENWICK & S.K. SMITH. 1994. Leukaemia inhibitory factor mRNA concentration peaks in human endometrium at the time of implantation and the blastocyst contains mRNA for the receptor at this time. J. Reprod. Fertil. **101:** 421–426.
39. KOJIMA, K., H. KANZAKI, M. IWAI *et al.* 1994. Expression of leukemia inhibitory factor in human endometrium and placenta. Biol. Reprod. **50:** 882–887.
…., S.J. ABBONDANZO, P.S. ANDERSON *et al.* 1996. Leukemia inhibitory … and LIF receptor expression in human endometrium suggest a potential …racrine function in regulating embryo implantation. Proc. Natl. Acad. …3: 3115–3120.
…M.J., H.J. KLIMAN, R.F. FEINBERG *et al.* 1996. The effect of leukemia …ctor on trophoblast differentiation: a potential role in human implantation. …ocrinol. Metab. **81:** 801–806.
…. HAENGGELI & A. CAMPANA. 1995. Effect of leukemia inhibitory factor …totrophoblast differentiation along the invasive pathway. Am. J. Reprod. …: 225–230.
…, T. FUKAYA, T. MURAKAMI *et al.* 1997. Increased secretion of hepatocyte …or by eutopic endometrial stromal cells in women with endometriosis. Fertil. Steril. **68:** 468–472.
44. TABIBZADEH, S., J.M. MASON, W. SHEA *et al.* 2000. Dysregulated expression of ebaf, an occult and novel molecular defect in the endometria of patients with infertility. J. Clin. Endocrinol. Metab. **85:** 2526–2536.
45. TAYLOR, H.S., C. BAGOT, A. KARDANA *et al.* 1999. HOX gene expression is altered in the endometrium of women with endometriosis. Hum. Reprod. **14:** 1328–1331.
46. OSTEEN, K.G., N.R. KELLER, F.A. FELTUS & M.H. MEINER. 1999. Paracrine regulation of matrix metalloproteinase expression in normal human endometrium. Gynecol. Obstet. Invest. **48**(suppl. 1)**:** 2–13.
47. BERQVIST, A. & M. FERNO. 1993. Oestrogen and progesterone receptors in endometriotic tissue and endometrium: comparison of different cycle phases and ages. Hum. Reprod. **8:** 2211–2217.
48. ZEITOUN, K.M. & S.E. BULUN. 1999. Aromatase: a key molecule in the pathophysiology of endometriosis and a therapeutic target. Fertil. Steril. **72:** 961–969.
49. ZEITOUN, K., K. TAKAYAMA, M.D. MICHAEL & S.E. BULUN. 1999. Stimulation of aromatase P450 promoter (II) activity in endometriosis and its inhibition in endometrium are regulated by competitive binding of steroidogenic factor-1 and chicken ovalbumin upstream promoter transcription factor to the same *cis*-acting element. Mol. Endocrinol. **13:** 239–253.
50. ZEITOUN, K.M., K. TAKAYAMA, H. SASANO *et al.* 1998. Deficient 17β-hydroxysteroid dehydrogenase type 2 expression in endometriosis: failure to metabolize 17β-estradiol. J. Clin. Endocrinol. Metab. **83:** 4474–4480.
51. NOBLE, L.S. *et al.* 1997. Prostaglandin E2 stimulates aromatase expression in endometriosis-derived stromal cells. J. Clin. Endocrinol. Metab. **82:** 600–606.
52. TAKAYAMA, K., K. ZEITOUN, R.T. GUNBY *et al.* 1998. Treatment of severe post-menopausal endometriosis with an aromatase inhibitor. Fertil. Steril. **69:** 709–713.
53. BULUN, S.E., K.M. ZEITOUN, K. TAKAYAMA *et al.* 2000. Aromatase as a therapeutic target in endometriosis. Trends Endocrinol. Metab. **11:** 22–27.

54. BULUN, S.E., K.M. ZEITOUN, K. TAKAYAMA & H. SASANO. 2000. Molecular basis for treating endometriosis with aromatase inhibitors. Hum. Reprod. Update **6:** 413–418.
55. MOTE, P.A., R.L. BALLEINE, E.M. MCGOWAN & C.L. CLARKE. 2000. Heterogeneity of progesterone receptors A and B expression in human endometrial glands and stroma. Hum. Reprod. **15**(suppl. 3)**:** 48–56.
56. MOTE, P.A., R.L. BALLEINE, E.M. MCGOWAN & C.L. CLARKE. 1999. Co-localization of progesterone receptors A and B by dual immunofluorescent histochemistry in human endometrium during the menstrual cycle. J. Clin. Endocrinol. Metab. **84:** 2963–2971.
57. LESSEY, B.A., I. YEH, A.J. CASTELBAUM *et al.* 1996. Endometrial progesterone receptors and markers of uterine receptivity in the window of implantation. Fertil. Steril. **65:** 477–483.
58. ATTIA, G.R., K. ZEITOUN, D. EDWARDS *et al.* 2000. Progesterone receptor isoform A, but not B is expressed in endometriosis. J. Clin. Endocrinol. Metab. **85:** 2897–2902.
59. OOSTERLYNCK, D.J., C. MEULEMAN, M. WAER *et al.* 1992. The natural killer activity of peritoneal fluid lymphocytes is decreased in women with endometriosis. Fertil. Steril. **58:** 290–295.
60. WU, M.Y., J.H. YANG, K.H. CHAO *et al.* 2000. Increase in the expression of killer cell inhibitory receptors on peritoneal natural killer cells in women with endometriosis Fertil. Steril. **74:** 1187–1191.
61. TRINCHIERI, G. 1998. Immunobiology of interleukin-12. Immunol. Res. **17:** 269–278.
62. ZEYNELOGLU, H.B., L.M. SENTURK, E. SELI *et al.* 1998. The peritoneal fluid levels of interleukin-12 in women with endometriosis. Am. J. Reprod. Immunol. **39:** 152–156.
63. GAZVANI, R., M. BATES, G. VINCE *et al.* 2001. Concentration of interleukin-12 in the peritoneal fluid is not influenced by the presence of endometriosis, its stage, or the phase of the menstrual cycle. Acta Obstet. Gynecol. Scand. **80:** 175–178.
64. MAZZEO, D., A.M. VIGANO, A.M. DI BLASIO *et al.* 1998. Interleukin-12 and its free p40 subunit regulate immune recognition of endometrial cells: potential role in endometriosis. J. Clin. Endocrinol. Metab. **83:** 911–916.
65. SOMIGLIANA, E., P. VIGANO, G. ROSSI *et al.* 1999. Endometrial ability to implant in ectopic sites can be prevented by interleukin-12 in a murine model of endometriosis. Hum. Reprod. **14**(12)**:** 2944–2950.
66. LEBOVIC, D.I., M.D. MUELLER & R.N. TAYLOR. 2001. Immunobiology of endometriosis. Fertil. Steril. **75**(1)**:** 1–10.
67. KHORRAM, O., R.N. TAYLOR, I.P. RYAN *et al.* 1993. Peritoneal fluid concentrations of the cytokine RANTES correlate with the severity of endometriosis. Am. J. Obstet. Gynecol. **169**(6)**:** 1545–1549.
68. AKOUM, A., A. LEMAY, S. MCCOLL *et al.* 1996. Elevated concentration and biologic activity of monocyte chemotactic protein-1 in the peritoneal fluid of patients with endometriosis. Fertil. Steril. **66**(1)**:** 17–23.
69. POPOVICI, R.M., L.C. KAO & L.C. GIUDICE. 2000. Discovery of new inducible genes in *in vitro* decidualized human endometrial stromal cells using microarray technology. Endocrinology **41:** 3510–3513.
70. KAO, L.C., J-P. YANG, S. TULAC *et al.* 2001. Global gene analysis during the implantation window suggests an endometrial basis for infertility in women with endometriosis. Endocr. Soc. Abstr. In press.
71. LESSEY, B.A., D.A. METZGER, A.F. HANEY & K.S. MCCARTY, Jr. 1989. Immunohistochemical analysis of estrogen and progesterone receptors in endometriosis: comparison with normal endometrium during the menstrual cycle and the effect of medical therapy. Fertil. Steril. **49:** 229–235.

Implantation Defects in Infertile Women with Endometriosis

BRUCE A. LESSEY

Division of Reproductive Endocrinology, Department of Obstetrics and Gynecology, University of North Carolina at Chapel Hill, Chapel Hill, North Carolina 27599, USA

ABSTRACT: The endometrium undergoes characteristic histologic changes during the menstrual cycle as it prepares for embryo implantation. Historic and current data suggest the presence of a defined period of maximal uterine receptivity during the mid-secretory phase occurring between days 7 and 10 post-ovulation. In recent years, we and others have sought to define biochemical markers of receptivity that might be used to better understand this time of endometrial differentiation. Based on the work with cell adhesion molecules, we have discovered three different integrins that are only coexpressed during this time in the cycle when embryos will successfully implant. By studying the regulation of one of these, the αvβ3 integrin, and its extracellular matrix ligand, osteopontin (OPN), we have defined two separate regulatory pathways that may regulate endometrial receptivity. While αvβ3 expression appears to be stimulated by EGF or heparin-binding EGF, osteopontin is stimulated by progesterone. We now believe the former pathway is a paracrine-mediated signal, while the latter is a direct effect of progesterone on the estrogen-primed endometrial epithelium. In women with endometriosis, it appears that αvβ3 expression is reduced, while OPN expression is unaffected. Interestingly, binding of OPN to the surface epithelium appears quite limited when αvβ3 expression is lacking. Such evidence continues to reinforce the notion that endometrium from some women with endometriosis is dysfunctional and may account for the reduction in cycle fecundity noted in this group of patients.

KEYWORDS: integrins; endometrium; implantation; infertility; contraception; osteopontin

INTRODUCTION

The endometrium serves as a selective barrier to embryo implantation during much of the menstrual cycle, assuring synchrony between embryo, endometrium, and corpus luteum. Historically, implantation was thought to occur after cycle day 20,[1] consistent with recent evidence from Assisted Reproductive Technology (ART) cycles supporting the concept of a "window of implantation".[2,3] Very recent clinical evidence further underscores the importance of this control over the timing of implantation.[4] In this study of the timing of implantation, Wilcox and coworkers

Address for correspondence: Bruce A. Lessey, Ph.D., M.D., Division of Reproductive Endocrinology, Department of Obstetrics and Gynecology, University of North Carolina at Chapel Hill, Chapel Hill, NC 27599. Voice: 919-966-5288; fax: 919-966-5214.
lessey@med.unc.edu

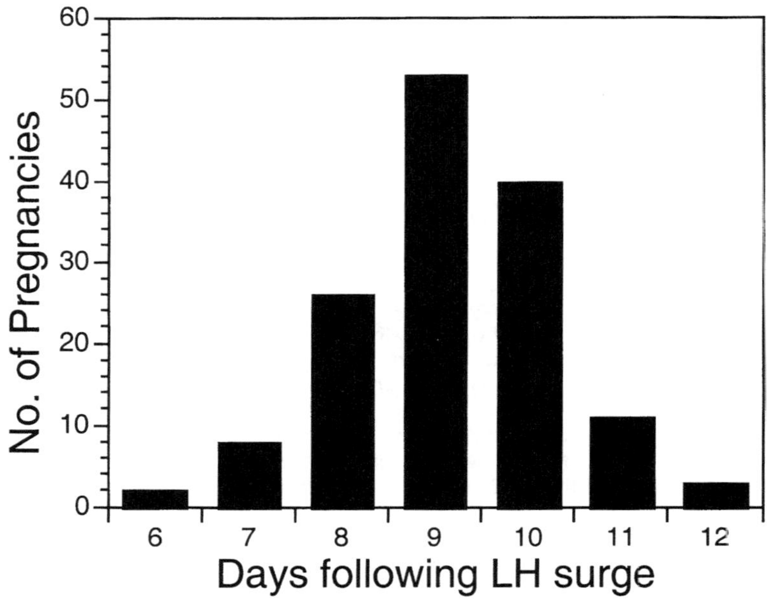

FIGURE 1. The timing of implantation in naturally occurring pregnancies. Adapted from Wilcox *et al.*[4]

demonstrated that most successful pregnancies begin during a narrow period of time between postovulatory day 21 and 24 (FIG. 1).

In certain infertility states, endometrial dysfunction may be secondary to delayed histologic maturation[5] or due to biochemical disturbances.[6,7] The latter types of defects may be occult since they are not necessarily accompanied by histologic delay.[8] Clinical evidence suggests that such defects are relatively common and account for a significant percentage of infertility and/or recurrent pregnancy loss.[9] Given the complex and cell-specific interactions between the embryo and endometrium, it may not be surprising that the mechanics of implantation occasionally malfunction. This chapter reviews the role of the endometrium in embryo attachment and early implantation with a focus on the effects of endometriosis on this process. Using two sentinel endometrial proteins with patterns of expression that originate during this period of maximal receptivity ($\alpha v\beta 3$ and osteopontin), we demonstrated that two distinct pathways of regulation exist in the endometrium.[10] Disruption of one of these two pathways occurs in some women with endometriosis and infertility.[6] Since these two proteins normally interact during the window of implantation, we were interested to examine the consequences if one of these two proteins failed to be expressed, as occurs sometimes in women with endometriosis.

THE ENDOMETRIUM AND A DEFINED WINDOW OF IMPLANTATION

The endometrium is normally a barrier to implantation. In fact, in contrast to most tissues, the endometrium is one into which the embryo will not implant, except for a narrow period of receptivity. It has previously been shown that embryos placed in other locations in the body can readily grow and invade,[11,12] while the surface epithelium of the endometrium of most species represents a barrier. In the mouse, Cowell showed that the luminal surface provided a gatekeeper role, allowing implantation only during certain times after mating. Once the luminal surface was removed, embryos could attach and invade at times other than the usual day 4.5 of pregnancy.[13] In the human, the endometrium undergoes a precise progression of developmental changes that have been well defined by the Noyes criteria of histologic dating.[14] After menses, the *proliferative phase* represents a period of growth of the glandular epithelium under the direction of estradiol (E2) from the developing follicle. With ovulation, the endometrium is transformed into a secretory tissue by progesterone (P4) derived from the corpus luteum.[15]

Essentially all of the important events of endometrial growth during the menstrual cycle are controlled by estrogen and progesterone. These two ovarian steroids act through their respective steroid receptors, ER and PR, to mediate these changes.[16,17] We have been interested in the regulation of these steroid receptors during the menstrual cycle. In humans, as well as most species studied, both ERs and PRs appear to decline in the epithelial cells, but persist in the stromal compartment at the opening of the window of implantation.[17–20] Such downregulation appears to be progesterone-dependent[21] and can be delayed when hormone level or response is reduced, as seen in luteal phase defect (LPD).[22]

The rise in P4 during the secretory phase is responsible for the expression of a myriad of proteins, many of which are critical for normal implantation. This effect may be direct (acting through PR in the epithelial cell) or indirect by stimulation of a stromal (paracrine) factor that, in turn, induces specific epithelial gene products.[23] Such mechanisms are in keeping with the studies of Cunha and colleagues, who demonstrated that *stromal* ER and PR can regulate epithelial responsiveness to ovarian steroids in the endometrium.[24,25] To study this issue further, we have focused on two proteins that fortuitously are coexpressed during this period of maximal uterine receptivity. One is the integrin $\alpha v\beta 3$ and the other is its ligand, an extracellular protein named osteopontin (OPN).

BIOMARKERS OF ENDOMETRIAL RECEPTIVITY

We and others have been working toward identification of marker proteins that are expressed only during the "receptive" versus "nonreceptive" endometrium.[26] Candidate biomarkers include progesterone-induced proteins such as insulin-like growth factor binding protein-1 (IGF-BP1)[27] and glycodelin (formerly known as PP-14).[28] Together, these two proteins account for a majority of the total endometrial proteins expressed in the mid-to-late secretory phase and both have been suggested as useful for the study of endometrial growth, development,[29,30] and function.[31–33] Recent evidence suggests that IGF-BP1 may interact with the invading cytotrophoblast to limit trophoblast invasiveness,[27] while glycodelin has been shown to reduce sperm binding to the zona pellucida[34] and may have regulatory roles on the immune system.[35] Both proteins appear to play a greater role after pregnancy has been established.

More recently, as molecular biology techniques have advanced, there has been an explosion in the number of implantation-specific gene products that may serve as biomarkers of endometrial receptivity. The classic example was leukemia inhibitory factor (LIF).[36] LIF was originally shown to induce differentiation of a myeloid leukemia cell line, M1,[37] but gained attention by the observation of Stewart that LIF is present in the mouse uterus with maximal expression on day 4 of pregnancy, corresponding to the day that embryos implant in the mouse.[38] Using the delayed implantation model, Stewart showed that female homozygotes lacking a functional LIF gene were infertile, while similar homozygous males were unaffected. The female null mutants had normal-appearing blastocytes within their uteri, but failed to implant, unless transferred to a wild-type female, suggesting a defect in endometrial receptivity.[39] Further studies have been carried out on LIF in the human, demonstrating that LIF is produced by the receptive phase endometrium in women.[40–43] Cullinan *et al.* noted a decreased level of LIF expression in some women with infertility[43] and Danielsson *et al.* showed reduced immunostaining for LIF after treatment with the antiprogestin, mifepristone.[44] Together, these data suggest that LIF is an essential endometrial gene product that plays a major role in implantation in most mammalian species studied.

HB-EGF and the other EGF-like molecules have recently been shown to be expressed during the time of implantation in the mouse,[45–47] along with EGF receptors.[48] Mouse embryos adhere to the transmembrane form of endometrium HB-EGF[49] and such interaction has been suggested to be independent of the EGF receptor.[50] In the human, HB-EGF was shown to be expressed during the time of maximal endometrial receptivity.[51,52] One function of the EGF family of growth factors may be the stimulation of embryo development. Machida *et al.* demonstrated that EGF and TGFα significantly stimulated trophoblast outgrowth *in vitro.*[53] This is consistent with the finding of others who demonstrated EGF receptors present in the placenta[54,55] and preimplantation embryo.[56,57] Based on recent studies, it is tempting to think that HB-EGF maintains a role in both adhesion and development in the embryo.[49,58] HB-EGF has been shown to improve the development[59] or quality of human embryos *in vitro.*[60]

Our group has been interested in a family of cell adhesion molecules called integrins.[61,62] Using immunohistochemical assessment of the endometrium throughout the cycle, we and others found both constitutive and cycle-dependent patterns of integrin expression.[61–64] The integrins are now perhaps the best characterized of the immunohistochemical markers of uterine receptivity.[65] There has been increasing interest in integrins and the reproductive tract and significant data to suggest their involvement in both fertilization and placentation.[66,67] Integrins are glycoproteins that serve as receptors for ECM ligands and act as modulators of cellular function. We described three integrins that are expressed by the endometrium with a pattern that coincides well with the window of implantation: $\alpha1\beta1$, $\alpha4\beta1$, and $\alpha v\beta3$ are co-expressed on glandular epithelium only during cycle days 20 to 24, corresponding to the putative window of implantation (FIG. 2). The apical surface of the luminal epithelium expresses the $\alpha v\beta3$ integrin[68] and localizes to the bulbous projects that have

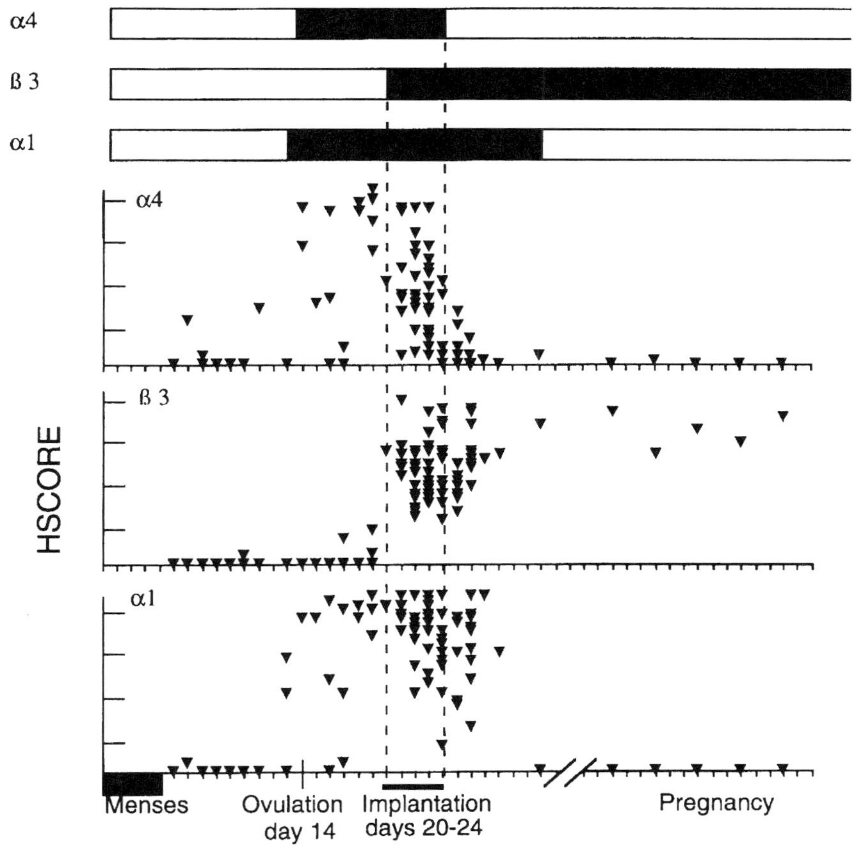

FIGURE 2. Relative intensity of staining for the epithelial α4, β3, and α1 integrin subunits throughout the menstrual cycle and in early pregnancy. Immunohistochemical staining was assessed by a blinded observer using the semiquantitative HSCORE (ranging from 0 to 4) and correlated to the estimate of histological dating based on pathologic criteria or by LMP in patients undergoing therapeutic pregnancy termination. The negative staining (open bars) was shown for immunostaining of an average HSCORE ≤ 0.7, for each of the three integrin subunits. Positive staining for all three integrin subunits was seen only during a 4-day interval, corresponding to cycle days 20–24, based on histologic dating criteria of Noyes *et al.*[14] This interval of integrin coexpression corresponds to the putative window of implantation. Of the three, only the αvβ3 integrin was seen in the epithelium of pregnant endometrium. Used with permission from the American Society for Reproductive Medicine.[62]

been referred to as pinopods.[69] This localization to the apical pole of the luminal epithelium suggests a role for this integrin in initial embryo-endometrial interaction.[68,70] Decidualized endometrial stromal cells also display alteration of integrins at the time of implantation.[62,71]

The αvβ3 integrin recognizes many different extracellular matrix ligands and interacts with these through their three-amino-acid sequence, Arg-Gly-Asp (RDG).

This sequence has been implicated in trophoblast attachment and outgrowth,[72,73] and blockade of either the integrin or its ligand binding sequence reduces implantation in the mouse[74] and rabbit.[75] Possible roles include signaling the embryo through fibronectin motifs[76,77] or stimulating the invasive phenotype of the embryo or placental cytotrophoblast cells.[78]

One of the RGD-containing ligands for $\alpha v\beta 3$ is the glycoprotein, osteopontin (OPN). OPN is a 70-kDa secreted glycosylated phosphoprotein that was originally isolated from bone matrix.[79] It is also found in a wide variety of tissues and body fluids, including milk and urine, uterus, placenta, kidney, leukocytes, smooth muscle cells, and some tumors.[80–83] Young demonstrated that the expression of OPN is elevated in the secretory phase endometrium and in the decidua of pregnancy in women.[81] Recent studies have demonstrated the presence of OPN in uterine flushings from pregnant ewes between days 11 and 17,[84] a period that corresponds to the adherence and attachment phase of early implantation in this species. Further, the presence of OPN mRNA in glands and protein secretions into the lumen was also demonstrated, the expression of which is regulated by progesterone.[85] We recently demonstrated that this ligand is precisely coexpressed with $\alpha v\beta 3$ in human endometrium, yet the regulation of each was different.[10] It now appears that $\alpha v\beta 3$ is regulated by a stromal factor, HB-EGF,[86] while OPN is directly regulated by P4 acting through the PR-B isoform of the progesterone receptor.[87] The immunohistochemical appearance of endometrium before and after onset of OPN expression is shown in FIGURES 3A and 3B, respectively.

ENDOMETRIUM FROM WOMEN WITH INFERTILITY AND ENDOMETRIOSIS

The diagnosis of "unexplained" infertility is given to 20% to 37% of infertile couples.[88] The past decade has seen new insights into the underlying pathology of many of these patients. Day-3 FSH levels and clomiphene citrate challenge testing have identified apparently normal ovulatory women who have significantly diminished egg number and/or quality. Similarly, new markers of uterine receptivity, beyond Noyes' conventional histology, have been identified. Endometrial proteins including integrins,[61,62] endometrial bleeding associated factor (ebaf),[89] LIF,[43] and HOXA10[90,91] have advanced our understanding of uterine receptivity and endometrial maturation. In women with endometriosis and otherwise unexplained infertility, it now appears that many of these proteins are aberrantly expressed.[43,90–92]

Integrins are a ubiquitous class of cell membrane bound proteins critical for cell-cell and cell-substratum adhesion. They comprise two components, an alpha subunit and a beta subunit. Over 22 different integrins have been identified and are present in all human cells, except for erythrocytes. Integrins are among the best-described markers of uterine receptivity[43,61,62] and they have been implicated in many aspects of reproduction, including fertilization and implantation.[66,67]

Endometrial integrins are expressed in both epithelium and stroma, as well as on the vascular endothelium. While most integrins are constitutively expressed in the endometrium, we and others have identified several cycle-dependent integrins, including the $\alpha 1$, $\alpha 4$, $\beta 3$, and $\beta 5$ integrin subunits.[61,62,68] These patterns have since

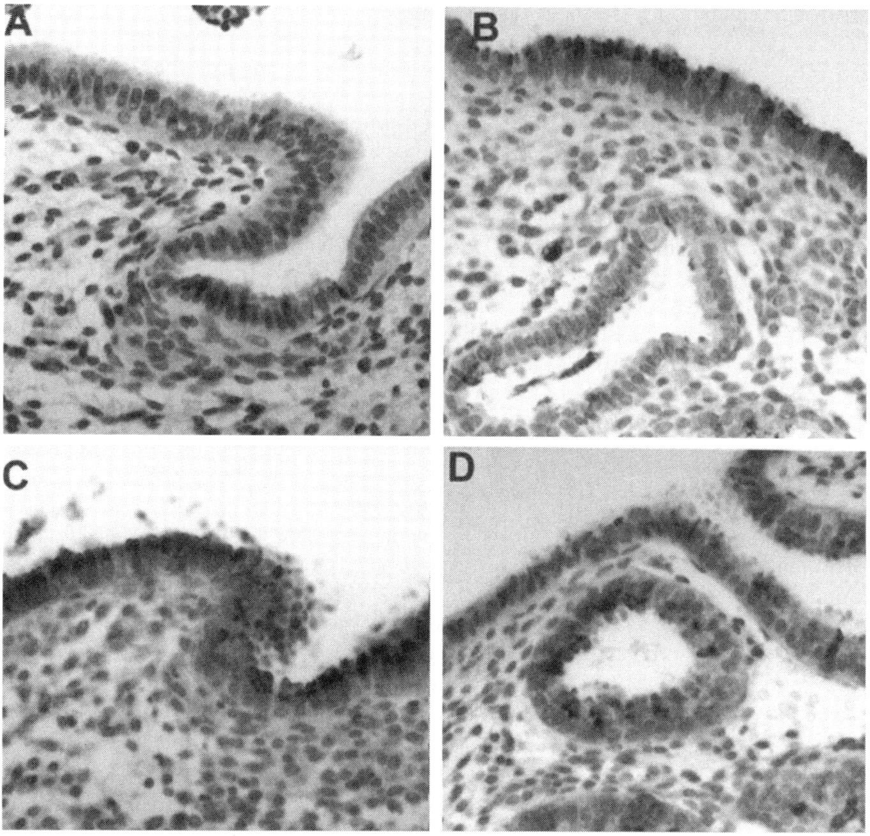

FIGURE 3. Photomicrographs of immunostaining results using the mab53 monoclonal antibody against osteopontin in human endometrium from prereceptive (**A**) and receptive (**B**) endometrium from healthy volunteers. In women with endometriosis, the endometrium from the receptive phase stains differently in women who express the αvβ3 integrin (**C**) compared to endometrium from women who exhibit aberrant lack of this integrin (**D**). Note the loss of luminal (surface epithelial) staining in panel D compared to panels B and C. This observation suggests that glandular osteopontin is secreted and binds to the luminal surface via apically distributed αvβ3 integrin. Loss of this integrin in some women with infertility may have functional consequences as shown here. Magnification: ×200. [Figure reduced to 95%.]

been confirmed by various techniques, including flow cytometry and PCR evaluation,[93,94] and recently by *in situ* hybridization.[10] The reproducibility of integrin expression in the endometrium allows a complementary approach to histologic dating for the evaluation of uterine receptivity.[43]

Most interest has been focused on the αvβ3 integrin since this integrin appears in endometrial glands and luminal surfaces on cycle days 20 to 21, coincident with the opening of the window of implantation.[62] Women with maturational delay of the endometrium (LPD) fail to express the αvβ3 integrin when biopsied during the window of implantation.[61] We have termed this form of αvβ3 deficiency as a "type I" defect. The lack of αvβ3 in cycles with retarded development is quite reliable, as recently demonstrated.[43,95] The vast majority of these patients, when treated with supplemental progesterone, have a return to normal histologic endometrial maturation and normal αvβ3 expression.[8] Interestingly, many infertile women with "in-phase" endometrium also fail to express the αvβ3 integrin. These women have what must be considered occult uterine receptivity defects, given that the pathologist finds these samples to be histologically normal. We have termed this as a "type II" defect, which has now been described among women with endometriosis,[6] hydrosalpinges,[7] and recurrent pregnancy loss,[96] and recently in some women with polycystic ovarian disease.[97] In a prospective study of 87 women with primary unexplained infertility, type I defects were noted in 26% and type II defects in 39% of patients. Of note, in each case, we identified only a subset that was affected, suggesting that such a method for determining uterine receptivity may help unravel some of the controversy surrounding the association between certain diagnoses and infertility.[98]

While only 2% to 5% of the general population are thought to have endometriosis, the prevalence in an infertile population may approach 40%.[99,100] Controversy surrounding the relationship between infertility and minimal or mild forms of endometriosis has arisen primarily because of the lack of data demonstrating efficacy of treatment protocols on cycle fecundity in women with this disorder.[101,102] While animal models[103–106] and some clinical studies[107] have supported an adverse effect of endometriosis on pregnancy rates, others fail to reveal this association.[108,109] Results from *in vitro* fertilization with embryo transfer (IVF-ET) have also been divergent in their conclusions.[110,111] A recent meta-analysis of most of the IVF studies to date reveals what many of us suspected: when confounding factors are controlled, subjects with endometriosis have a pregnancy rate that is almost half of that of subjects with tubal factor infertility.[9] Most of the underlying data are suspect, however, since it is unclear how the endometriosis was treated prior to IVF-ET and how protracted treatment with GnRH agonist affects IVF outcome.[98]

Since many patients with minimal or mild endometriosis can conceive without further therapy,[108] many researchers in the field have concluded that endometriosis does not cause infertility or that treatment is not beneficial. Two meta-analyses have found no benefit of surgical or medical therapy.[101,102] Isolated studies, including the recent prospective, randomized Canadian trial, support the use of ablative surgery for the treatment of infertility and minimal and mild endometriosis.[112,113] In the former paper,[112] selection criteria included an 8-month delay in initiation of therapy that effectively preselected for a group of women who would not conceive by expectant management alone. In the latter Canadian study,[113] population size may have been large enough to detect a positive effect of surgery, despite the inclusion of a heterogeneous group of responders. In a recent review of medical treatment of endometriosis and infertility, we point out that medical treatment may help as many patients as it hurts because half of the patients with endometriosis appear to conceive without therapy. While pregnancy may be facilitated in some women, pregnancy is delayed in others. Analysis of the results will frequently demonstrate no effect, even though some women with this disorder may see improvement in their pregnancy rates.[98]

Other studies have also demonstrated differences in the endometrium[114–116] or peritoneal fluid (PF)[117] of women with endometriosis. We have predicted that specific biomarkers, such as the endometrial integrins or OPN, may be useful in predicting pregnancy outcome or response to therapy for this disease. In a prospective, longitudinal follow-up of women who underwent nonrandomly assigned treatments for endometriosis, we found surprising differences in outcome that may suggest strategies to identify those women with endometriosis who are least likely to conceive with expectant management alone.[118]

We[6] and others[119,120] have observed that subsets of infertile women with endometriosis can be identified on the basis of biomarker endometrial proteins. On the basis of endometrial integrin expression, we found that some women with minimal or mild disease appear to have dysfunctional endometrium when compared to women without this disorder.[68] If $\alpha v\beta 3$ is aberrantly expressed in some women with endometriosis, we wondered if OPN binding would be affected. As shown in FIGURES 3C and 3D, OPN binding to the luminal epithelium appears to be reduced in the absence of the $\alpha v\beta 3$ integrin (panel C), while copious luminal binding is observed when this integrin is present (panel D). Such observations suggest that there are functional consequences of the loss of this integrin during the implantation window. If $\alpha v\beta 3$ or OPN is involved in the attachment phase of the human embryo, the loss of both biomarkers from the luminal surface may have a cumulative effect.

The mechanism by which endometriosis may alter cycle fecundity remains unsettled. Possibilities include acquired endometrial defects[116–118] or toxic effects on sperm function and embryo survival.[121–124] Evidence from rabbits has suggested that the PF of endometriosis possesses transferable factors that alter implantation.[105] We have recently shown that PF from women with endometriosis reduces implantation rates in the mouse,[125] similar to that shown for hamsters.[106] In our study, two critical biomarkers of uterine receptivity (LIF and $\alpha v\beta 3$) were specifically disrupted by PF injections from a woman with endometriosis, suggesting that there is, in fact, a direct effect exerted on the endometrium by factors contained within the PF of women with this disease. Taken together, it appears that subsets of women with endometriosis exhibit defects in uterine receptivity that are apparent using available or new biomarkers. It is obvious that further study is warranted in this area of reproductive biology.

SUMMARY AND FUTURE STUDIES

Endometriosis is associated with a decrease in cycle fecundity, and the prevalence of endometriosis is increased in infertile women. The study of endometrium in women with endometriosis continues to yield interesting differences when compared to women without this disease. The greatest obstacle to understanding how endometriosis alters fertility is the heterogeneity of this disorder. In addition, in lieu of biomarkers that predict the presence of endometriosis in the general population, our control groups may also contain confounding and occult disease that limits our ability to study this disorder. Biomarkers of uterine receptivity may provide a key to both of these questions. If we can develop markers that predict all endometriosis, we will be able to ascertain the true prevalence of this disease. If we find endometrial biomarkers that predict potential for pregnancy, then studies to examine the effect of endometriosis on fertility will likely have greater concordance. We also predict that studies to examine the effect of medical treatment will demonstrate efficacy in select populations of women. Further research into the use of such biomarkers holds the key to our future successes in these areas.

ACKNOWLEDGMENTS

This work was supported in part by the NIH through Cooperative Agreement No. U54 HD-35041 as part of the Specialized Cooperative Centers Program in Reproduction Research and by the National Cooperative Program on Markers of Uterine Receptivity for Blastocyst Implantation (No. HD-34824).

REFERENCES

1. HERTIG, A.T., J. ROCK & E.C. ADAMS. 1956. A description of 34 human ova within the first 17 days of development. Am. J. Anat. **98:** 435–493.
2. NAVOT, D. & P. BERGH. 1991. Preparation of the human endometrium for implantation. Ann. N.Y. Acad. Sci. **622:** 212–219.
3. NAVOT, D., P.A. BERGH, M. WILLIAMS *et al.* 1991. An insight into early reproductive processes through the *in vivo* model of ovum donation. J. Clin. Endocrinol. Metab. **72:** 408–414.
4. WILCOX, A.J., D.D. BAIRD & C.R. WENBERG. 1999. Time of implantation of the conceptus and loss of pregnancy. N. Engl. J. Med. **340:** 1796–1799.
5. FRITZ, M.A. & B.A. LESSEY. 1998. Defective luteal function. *In* Estrogens and Progestogens in Clinical Practice, pp. 437–494. Churchill Livingstone. London.
6. LESSEY, B.A., A.J. CASTELBAUM, S.J. SAWIN *et al.* 1994. Aberrant integrin expression in the endometrium of women with endometriosis. J. Clin. Endocrinol. Metab. **79:** 643–649.
7. MEYER, W.R., A.J. CASTELBAUM, S. SOMKUTI *et al.* 1997. Hydrosalpinges adversely affect markers of endometrial receptivity. Hum. Reprod. **12:** 1393–1398.
8. LESSEY, B.A., A.J. CASTELBAUM, S.J. SAWIN & J. SUN. 1995. Integrins as markers of uterine receptivity in women with primary unexplained infertility. Fertil. Steril. **63:** 535–542.
9. BARNHART, K.T., R. DUNSMOOR & C. COUTIFARIS. 2000. The effect of endometriosis on IVF outcome [abstract]. Am. Soc. Reprod. Med. Annu. Meet.
10. APPARAO, K.B.C., J. ZHANG, P. TRUONG & B.A. LESSEY. 2001. Osteopontin expression during the menstrual cycle in women: regulation and binding to the endometrial $\alpha v\beta 3$ integrin. J. Clin. Endocrinol. Metab. **86:** 4991–5000.
11. FAWCETT, D.W. 1950. The development of mouse ova under the capsule of the kidney. Anat. Rec. **108:** 71–91.
12. KIRBY, D.R. 1963. The development of mouse blastocysts transplanted to the scrotal and cryptorchid testis. J. Anat. **97:** 119–130.
13. COWELL, T.P. 1969. Implantation and development of mouse eggs transferred to the uterus of non-progestational mice. J. Reprod. Fertil. **19:** 239–245.
14. NOYES, R.W., A.I. HERTIG & J. ROCK. 1950. Dating the endometrial biopsy. Fertil. Steril. **1:** 3–25.
15. BRENNER, R.M. & N.B. WEST. 1975. Hormonal regulation of the reproductive tract in female mammals. Annu. Rev. Physiol. **37:** 273–302.
16. BRENNER, R.M., N.B. WEST & M.C. MCCLELLAN. 1990. Estrogen and progestin receptors in the reproductive tract of male and female primates. Biol. Reprod. **42:** 11–19.
17. LESSEY, B.A., A.P. KILLAM, D.A. METZGER *et al.* 1988. Immunohistochemical analysis of human uterine estrogen and progesterone receptors throughout the menstrual cycle. J. Clin. Endocrinol. Metab. **67:** 334–340.

18. GARCIA, E., P. BOUCHARD, J. DE BRUX *et al.* 1988. Use of immunocytochemistry of progesterone and estrogen receptors for endometrial dating. J. Clin. Endocrinol. Metab. **67:** 80–87.
19. PRESS, M.F., N.A. NOUSEK GOEBL, M. BUR & G.L. GREENE. 1986. Estrogen receptor localization in the female genital tract. Am. J. Pathol. **123:** 280–292.
20. PRESS, M.F., J.A. UDOVE & G.L. GREENE. 1988. Progesterone receptor distribution in the human endometrium: analysis using monoclonal antibodies to the human progesterone receptor. Am. J. Pathol. **131:** 112–124.
21. SLAYDEN, O.D., M.B. ZELINSKI-WOOTEN, K. CHWALISZ *et al.* 1998. Chronic treatment of cycling rhesus monkeys with low doses of the antiprogestin ZK 137 316: morphometric assessment of the uterus and oviduct. Hum. Reprod. **13:** 269–277.
22. LESSEY, B.A., I.T. YEH, A.J. CASTELBAUM *et al.* 1996. Endometrial progesterone receptors and markers of uterine receptivity in the window of implantation. Fertil. Steril. **65:** 477–483.
23. LESSEY, B.A. & J.T. ARNOLD. 1998. Paracrine signaling in the endometrium: integrins and the establishment of uterine receptivity. J. Reprod. Immunol. **39:** 105–116.
24. COOKE, P.S., D.L. BUCHANAN, P. YOUNG *et al.* 1997. Stromal estrogen receptors mediate mitogenic effects of estradiol on uterine epithelium. Proc. Natl. Acad. Sci. U.S.A. **94:** 6535–6540.
25. KURITA, T., P. YOUNG, J.R. BRODY *et al.* 1998. Stromal progesterone receptors mediate the inhibitory effects of progesterone on estrogen-induced uterine epithelial cell deoxyribonucleic acid synthesis. Endocrinology **139:** 4708–4713.
26. ILESANMI, A.O., D.A. HAWKINS & B.A. LESSEY. 1993. Immunohistochemical markers of uterine receptivity in the human endometrium. Microsc. Res. Tech. **25:** 208–222.
27. GIUDICE, L.C. 1997. Multifaceted roles for IGFBP-1 in human endometrium during implantation and pregnancy. Ann. N.Y. Acad. Sci. **828:** 146–156.
28. RUTANEN, E.M. & M. SEPPALA. 1992. Insulin-like growth factor binding protein-1 in female reproductive functions. Int. J. Gynaecol. Obstet. **39:** 3–9.
29. JULKUNEN, M., R. KOISTINEN, J. SJOBERG *et al.* 1986. Secretory endometrium synthesizes placental protein 14. Endocrinology **118:** 1782–1786.
30. SUHONEN, S., M. HAUKKAMAA, T. HOLMSTRÖM *et al.* 1996. Endometrial response to hormone replacement therapy as assessed by expression of insulin-like growth factor–binding protein-1 in the endometrium. Fertil. Steril. **65:** 776–782.
31. WANG, H-S., J-D. LEE & Y-K. SOONG. 1995. Serum levels of insulin-like growth factor I and insulin-like growth factor–binding protein-1 and -3 in women with regular menstrual cycles. Fertil. Steril. **63:** 1204–1209.
32. TULPPALA, M., M. JULKUNEN, A. TIITINEN *et al.* 1995. Habitual abortion is accompanied by low serum levels of placental protein 14 in the luteal phase of the fertile cycle. Fertil. Steril. **63:** 792–795.
33. WESTERGAARD, L.G., N. WIBERG, C. YDING *et al.* 1998. Circulating concentrations of placenta protein 14 during the natural menstrual cycle in women significantly reflect endometrial receptivity to implantation and pregnancy during successive assisted reproduction cycles. Hum. Reprod. **13:** 2612–2619.
34. OEHNINGER, S., C.C. CODDINGTON, G.D. HODGEN & M. SEPPALA. 1995. Factors affecting fertilization: endometrial placental protein 14 reduces the capacity of human spermatozoa to bind to the human zona pellucida. Fertil. Steril. **63:** 377–383.
35. CLARK, G.F., S. OEHNINGER, M.S. PATANKAR *et al.* 1996. A role for glycoconjugates in human development: the human feto-embryonic defence system hypothesis. Hum. Reprod. **11:** 467–473.
36. STEWART, C.L. 1994. The role of leukemia inhibitory factor (LIF) and other cytokines in regulating implantation in mammals. Ann. N.Y. Acad. Sci. **734:** 157–165.
37. HILTON, D.J. & N.M. GOUGH. 1991. Leukemia inhibitory factor: a biological perspective. J. Cell. Biochem. **46:** 21–26.
38. BHATT, H., L.J. BRUNET & C.L. STEWART. 1991. Uterine expression of leukemia inhibitory factor coincides with the onset of blastocyst implantation. Proc. Natl. Acad. Sci. U.S.A. **88:** 11408–11412.
39. STEWART, C.L., P. KASPAR, L.J. BRUNET *et al.* 1992. Blastocyst implantation depends on maternal expression of leukaemia inhibitory factor. Nature **359:** 76–79.

40. CHEN, D., R. HILSENRATH, Z. YANG *et al.* 1995. Leukaemia inhibitory factor in human endometrium during the menstrual cycle: cellular origin and action on production of glandular epithelial cell prostaglandin *in vitro*. Hum. Reprod. **10:** 911–918.
41. SAWAI, K., C. AZUMA, M. KOYAMA *et al.* 1995. Leukemia inhibitory factor (LIF) enhances trophoblast differentiation mediated by human chorionic gonadotropin (hCG). Biochem. Biophys. Res. Commun. **211:** 137–143.
42. KOJIMA, K., H. KANZAKI, M. IWAI *et al.* 1994. Expression of leukemia inhibitory factor in human endometrium and placenta. Biol. Reprod. **50:** 882–887.
43. CULLINAN, E.B., S.J. ABBONDANZO, P.S. ANDERSON *et al.* 1996. Leukemia inhibitory factor (LIF) and LIF receptor expression in human endometrium suggest a potential autocrine paracrine function in regulating embryo implantation. Proc. Natl. Acad. Sci. U.S.A. **93:** 3115–3120.
44. DANIELSSON, K.G., M.L. SWAHN & M. BYGDEMAN. 1997. The effect of various doses of mifepristone on endometrial leukaemia inhibitory factor expression in the midluteal phase—an immunohistochemical study. Hum. Reprod. **12:** 1293–1297.
45. DAS, S.K., X-N. WANG, B.C. PARIA *et al.* 1994. Heparin-binding EGF-like growth factor gene is induced in the mouse uterus temporally by the blastocyst solely at the site of its apposition: a possible ligand for interaction with blastocyst EGF-receptor in implantation. Development **120:** 1071–1083.
46. DAS, S.K., I. CHAKRABORTY, B.C. PARIA *et al.* 1995. Amphiregulin is an implantation-specific and progesterone-regulated gene in the mouse uterus. Mol. Endocrinol. **9:** 691–705.
47. DAS, S.K., N. DAS, J. WANG *et al.* 1997. Expression of betacellulin and epiregulin genes in the mouse uterus temporally by the blastocyst solely at the site of its apposition is coincident with the "window" of implantation. Dev. Biol. **190:** 178–190.
48. LIM, H., S.K. DAS & S.K. DEY. 1998. *erbB* genes in the mouse uterus: cell-specific signaling by epidermal growth factor (EGF) family of growth factors during implantation. Dev. Biol. **204:** 97–110.
49. RAAB, G., K. KOVER, B.C. PARIA *et al.* 1996. Mouse preimplantation blastocysts adhere to cells expressing the transmembrane form of heparin-binding EGF-like growth factor. Development **122:** 637–645.
50. PARIA, B.C., K. ELENIUS, M. KLAGSBRUN & S.K. DEY. 1999. Heparin-binding EGF-like growth factor interacts with mouse blastocysts independently of ErbB1: a possible role for heparan sulfate proteoglycans and ErbB4 in blastocyst implantation. Development **126:** 1997–2005.
51. YOO, H.J., D.H. BARLOW & H.J. MARDON. 1997. Temporal and spatial regulation of expression of heparin-binding epidermal growth factor–like growth factor in the human endometrium: a possible role in blastocyst implantation. Dev. Genet. **21:** 102–108.
52. BIRDSALL, M.A., J.F. HOPKISSON, K.E. GRANT *et al.* 1996. Expression of heparin-binding epidermal growth factor messenger RNA in the human endometrium. Mol. Hum. Reprod. **2:** 31–34.
53. MACHIDA, T., M. TAGA & H. MINAGUCHI. 1995. Effects of epidermal growth factor and transforming growth factor alpha on the mouse trophoblast outgrowth *in vitro*. Eur. J. Endocrinol. **133:** 741–746.
54. DUELLO, T.M., P.J. BERTICS, D.L. FULGHAM & P.J. VAN ESS. 1994. Localization of epidermal growth factor receptors in first- and third-trimester human placentas. J. Histochem. Cytochem. **42:** 907–915.
55. MARUO, T., H. MATSUO, T. OTANI & M. MOCHIZUKI. 1995. Role of epidermal growth factor (EGF) and its receptor in the development of the human placenta. Reprod. Fertil. Dev. **7:** 1465–1470.
56. PARIA, B.C., S.K. DAS, R.A. MEAD & S.K. DEY. 1994. Expression of epidermal growth factor receptor in the preimplantation uterus and blastocyst of the western spotted skunk. Biol. Reprod. **51:** 205–213.
57. WILEY, L.M., J.X. WU, I. HARARI & E.D. ADAMSON. 1992. Epidermal growth factor receptor mRNA and protein increase after the four-cell preimplantation stage in murine development. Dev. Biol. **149:** 247–260.

58. TAMADA, H., C. HIGASHIYAMA, H. TAKANO *et al.* 1999. The effects of heparin-binding epidermal growth factor–like growth factor on preimplantation-embryo development and implantation in the rat. Life Sci. **64:** 1967–1973.
59. SARGENT, I.L., K.L. MARTIN & D.H. BARLOW. 1998. The use of recombinant growth factors to promote human embryo development in serum-free medium. Hum. Reprod. **13**(suppl. 4)**:** 239–248.
60. MARTIN, K.L., D.H. BARLOW & I.L. SARGENT. 1998. Heparin-binding epidermal growth factor significantly improves human blastocyst development and hatching in serum-free medium. Hum. Reprod. **13:** 1645–1652.
61. LESSEY, B.A., L. DAMJANOVICH, C. COUTIFARIS *et al.* 1992. Integrin adhesion molecules in the human endometrium: correlation with the normal and abnormal menstrual cycle. J. Clin. Invest. **90:** 188–195.
62. LESSEY, B.A., A.J. CASTELBAUM, C.A. BUCK *et al.* 1994. Further characterization of endometrial integrins during the menstrual cycle and in pregnancy. Fertil. Steril. **62:** 497–506.
63. TABIBZADEH, S. 1992. Patterns of expression of integrin molecules in human endometrium throughout the menstrual cycle. Hum. Reprod. **7:** 876–882.
64. ALBERS, A., M. THIE, H.P. HOHN & H.W. DENKER. 1995. Differential expression and localization of integrins and CD44 in the membrane domains of human uterine epithelial cells during the menstrual cycle. Acta Anat. (Basel) **153:** 12–19.
65. LESSEY, B.A. 1998. Endometrial integrins and the establishment of uterine receptivity. Hum. Reprod. **13**(suppl. 3)**:** 247–258.
66. BRONSON, R.A. & F.M. FUSI. 1996. Integrins and human reproduction. Mol. Hum. Reprod. **2:** 153–168.
67. SUEOKA, K., S. SHIOKAWA, T. MIYAZAKI *et al.* 1997. Integrins and reproductive physiology: expression and modulation in fertilization, embryogenesis, and implantation. Fertil. Steril. **67:** 799–811.
68. APLIN, J.D., C. SPANSWICK, F. BEHZAD *et al.* 1996. Integrins β5, β3, αv are apically distributed in endometrial epithelium. Mol. Hum. Reprod. **2:** 527–534.
69. LESSEY, B.A., K.B.C. APPARAO, R.C. BAGNELL *et al.* 2001. Osteopontin normally localized to the apical surface of receptive endometrium is lacking in women with endometriosis with aberrant $\alpha_v\beta_3$ integrin expression. Fertil. Steril. **76**(35)**:** 560.
70. LESSEY, B.A., A.O. ILESANMI, J. SUN *et al.* 1996. Luminal and glandular endometrial epithelium express integrins differentially throughout the menstrual cycle: implications for implantation, contraception, and infertility. Am. J. Reprod. Immunol. **35:** 195–204.
71. RUCK, P., K. MARZUSCH, E. KAISERLING *et al.* 1994. Distribution of cell adhesion molecules in decidua of early human pregnancy: an immunohistochemical study. Lab. Invest. **71:** 94–101.
72. ARMANT, D.R., H.A. KAPLAN, H. MOVER & W.J. LENNARZ. 1986. The effect of hexapeptides on attachment and outgrowth of mouse blastocysts cultured *in vitro*: evidence for the involvement of the cell recognition tripeptide Arg-Gly-Asp. Proc. Natl. Acad. Sci. U.S.A. **83:** 6751–6755.
73. YELIAN, F.D., Y. YANG, J.D. HIRATA *et al.* 1995. Molecular interactions between fibronectin and integrins during mouse blastocyst outgrowth. Mol. Reprod. Dev. **41:** 435–448.
74. ILLERA, M.J., E. CULLINAN, Y.T. GUI *et al.* 2000. Blockade of the αvβ3 integrin adversely affects implantation in the mouse. Biol. Reprod. **62:** 1285–1290.
75. ILLERA, M.J., P.L. LORENZO, Y-T. GUI *et al.* 2001. The role of αvβ3 integrin during implantation in the rabbit. Biol. Reprod. In preparation.
76. TURPEENNIEMI-HUJANEN, T., R.F. FEINBERG, A. KAUPPILA & U. PUISTOLA. 1995. Extracellular matrix interactions in early human embryos: implications for normal implantation events. Fertil. Steril. **64:** 132–138.
77. SHIOKAWA, S., Y. YOSHIMURA, H. SAWA *et al.* 1999. Functional role of Arg-Gly-Asp (RGD)–binding sites on β_1 integrin in embryo implantation using mouse blastocysts and human decidua. Biol. Reprod. **60:** 1468–1474.
78. MURRAY, M.J. & B.A. LESSEY. 1999. Embryo implantation and tumor metastasis: common pathways of invasion and angiogenesis. Semin. Reprod. Endocrinol. **17:** 275–290.

79. BUTLER, W.T. 1989. The nature and significance of osteopontin. Connect. Tissue Res. **23:** 123–136.
80. BROWN, L.F., B. BERSE, L. VAN DE WATER *et al.* 1992. Expression and distribution of osteopontin in human tissues: widespread association with luminal epithelial surfaces. Mol. Biol. Cell **3:** 1169–1180.
81. YOUNG, M.F., J.M. KERR, J.D. TERMINE *et al.* 1990. cDNA cloning, mRNA distribution and heterogeneity, chromosomal location, and RFLP analysis of human osteopontin (OPN). Genomics **7:** 491–502.
82. KHORI, K., S. NOMURA, Y. KITAMURA *et al.* 1993. Structure and expression of the mRNA encoding urinary stone protein (osteopontin). J. Biol. Chem. **268:** 15180–15184.
83. DENHARDT, D.T. & X. GUO. 1993. Osteopontin: a protein with diverse functions. FASEB J. **7:** 1475–1482.
84. JOHNSON, G.A., R.C. BURGHARDT, T.E. SPENCER *et al.* 1999. Ovine osteopontin: II. Osteopontin and αvβ3 integrin expression in the uterus and conceptus during the periimplantation period. Biol. Reprod. **61:** 892–899.
85. JOHNSON, G.A., T.E. SPENCER, R.C. BURGHARDT *et al.* 2000. Progesterone modulation of osteopontin gene expression in the ovine uterus. Biol. Reprod. **62:** 1315–1321.
86. LESSEY, B.A., Y. GUI, L. YUAN *et al.* 2001. Endometrial heparin binding epidermal growth factor (HB-EGF): a paracrine signal for uterine receptivity? Mol. Reprod. Dev. In press.
87. APPARAO, K.B.C., A.F. CHAMBERS & B.A. LESSEY. 2001. Progesterone receptor isoform-B modulates the expression of osteopontin in human endometrial epithelium during the window of implantation. Annu. Meet. Soc. Gynecol. Invest. **43:** 60A.
88. KIM, H.H. & M.D. HORNSTEIN. 1997. Unexplained infertility: defining the problem and understanding study design. Infertil. Reprod. Med. Clin. North Am. **8:** 487–499.
89. TABIBZADEH, S., J.M. MASON, W. SHEA *et al.* 2000. Dysregulated expression of ebaf, an occult and novel molecular defect in the endometria of patients with infertility. J. Clin. Endocrinol. Metab. **85:** 2526–2536.
90. GUI, Y-T., J. ZHANG, L. YUAN & B.A. LESSEY. 1999. Regulation of HoxA-10 and its expression in normal and abnormal endometrium. Mol. Hum. Reprod. **5:** 866–873.
91. TAYLOR, H.S., C. BAGOT, A. KARDANA *et al.* 1999. *HOX* gene expression is altered in the endometrium of women with endometriosis. Hum. Reprod. **14:** 1328–1331.
92. TABIBZADEH, S., J.M. MASON, W. SHEA *et al.* 2000. Dysregulated expression of *ebaf*, a novel molecular defect in the endometria of patients with infertility. J. Clin. Endocrinol. Metab. **85:** 2526–2536.
93. GONZALEZ, R.R., A. PALOMINO, A. BORIC *et al.* 1999. A quantitative evaluation of α1, α4, αv, and β3 endometrial integrins of fertile and unexplained infertile women during the menstrual cycle: a flow cytometric appraisal. Hum. Reprod. **14:** 2485–2492.
94. DOU, Q.C., R.S. WILLIAMS & N. CHEGINI. 1999. Expression of integrin messenger ribonucleic acid in human endometrium: a quantitative reverse transcription polymerase chain reaction study. Fertil. Steril. **71:** 347–353.
95. CREUS, M., J. BALASCH, J. ORDI *et al.* 1998. Integrin expression in normal and out-of-phase endometria. Hum. Reprod. **13:** 3460–3468.
96. LESSEY, B.A., A.J. CASTELBAUM, L. BELLARDO *et al.* 1995. Defective endometrial receptivity: an under-appreciated cause of recurrent pregnancy loss. Am. Fertil. Soc. Annu. Meet. **S26:** O-054.
97. LESSEY, B.A., K.B.C. APPARAO, L.P. LOVELY & Y. GUI. 2002. Elevated endometrial androgen receptor expression in women with polycystic ovarian syndrome (PCOS). Biol. Reprod. In press.
98. LESSEY, B.A. 2000. Medical management of endometriosis and infertility. Fertil. Steril. (Mod. Trends) **73:** 1089–1096.
99. STRATHY, J.H., C.A. MOLGAARD, C.B. COULAM & L.J. MELTON. 1982. Endometriosis and infertility: a laparoscopic study of endometriosis among fertile and infertile women. Fertil. Steril. **38:** 667–675.
100. VERKAUF, B.S. 1987. Incidence, symptoms, and signs of endometriosis in fertile and infertile women. J. Fla. Med. Assoc. **74:** 671–675.

101. HUGHES, E.G., D.M. FEDORKOW & J.A. COLLINS. 1993. A quantitative overview of controlled trials in endometriosis-associated infertility. Fertil. Steril. **59:** 963–970.
102. ADAMSON, G.D. & D.J. PASTA. 1994. Surgical treatment of endometriosis-associated infertility: meta-analysis compared with survival analysis. Am. J. Obstet. Gynecol. **171:** 1488–1505.
103. SCHENKEN, R.S. & R.H. ASCH. 1980. Surgical induction of endometriosis in the rabbit: effects on fertility and concentration of peritoneal fluid prostaglandins. Fertil. Steril. **34:** 581–587.
104. VERNON, M.W. & E.A. WILSON. 1985. Studies on the surgical induction of endometriosis in the rat. Fertil. Steril. **44:** 684–694.
105. HAHN, D.W., R.P. CARRAHER, R.G. FOLDESY & J.L. MCGUIRE. 1986. Experimental evidence for failure to implant as a mechanism of infertility associated with endometriosis. Am. J. Obstet. Gynecol. **155:** 1109–1113.
106. STEINLEITNER, A., H. LAMBERT, C. KAZENSKY & P. DANKS. 1990. Peritoneal fluid from endometriosis patients affects reproductive outcome in an *in vivo* model. Fertil. Steril. **53:** 926–929.
107. JANSEN, R.P. 1986. Minimal endometriosis and reduced fecundability: prospective evidence from an artificial insemination by donor program. Fertil. Steril. **46:** 141–143.
108. EVERS, J.L. 1989. The pregnancy rate of the no-treatment group in randomized clinical trials of endometriosis therapy. Fertil. Steril. **52:** 906–907.
109. PAULSON, J.D., P. ASMAR & D.S. SAFFAN. 1991. Mild and moderate endometriosis: comparison of treatment modalities for infertile couples. J. Reprod. Med. **36:** 151–155.
110. OLIVENNES, F., D. FELDBERG, H-C. LIU *et al.* 1995. Endometriosis: a stage by stage analysis—the role of *in vitro* fertilization. Fertil. Steril. **64:** 392–398.
111. ARICI, A., E. ORAL, O. BUKULMEZ *et al.* 1996. The effect of endometriosis on implantation: results from the Yale University *in vitro* fertilization and embryo transfer program. Fertil. Steril. **65:** 603–607.
112. TIMPL, R. 1989. Structure and biological activity of basement membrane proteins. Eur. J. Biochem. **180:** 487–502.
113. MARCOUX, S., R. MAHEUX, S. BÉRUBÉ *et al.* 1997. Laparoscopic surgery in infertile women with minimal or mild endometriosis. N. Engl. J. Med. **337:** 217–222.
114. SCHATZ, F., L. MARKIEWICZ, P. BARG & E. GURPIDE. 1986. *In vitro* inhibition with antiestrogens of estradiol effects on prostaglandin F2 alpha production by human endometrium and endometrial epithelial cells. Endocrinology **118:** 408–412.
115. ISAACSON, K.B., M. GALMAN, C. COUTIFARIS & C.R. LYTTLE. 1990. Endometrial synthesis and secretion of complement component-3 by patients with and without endometriosis. Fertil. Steril. **53:** 836–841.
116. OOSTERLYNCK, D.J., F.J. CORNILLIE, M. WAER *et al.* 1991. Women with endometriosis show a defect in natural killer activity resulting in a decreased cytotoxicity to autologous endometrium. Fertil. Steril. **56:** 45–51.
117. OVERTON, C., S. FERNANDEZ-SHAW, B. HICKS *et al.* 1996. Peritoneal fluid cytokines and the relationship with endometriosis and pain. Hum. Reprod. **11:** 380–386.
118. LESSEY, B.A., A.J. CASTELBAUM, S.G. SOMKUTI *et al.* 2001. Improvement in pregnancy rates with GnRH agonist in women with infertility, minimal or mild endometriosis, and aberrant $\alpha v\beta 3$ expression: a case-control study. Fertil. Steril. Submitted.
119. PITTAWAY, D.E., D. RONDINONE, K.A. MILLER & K. BARNES. 1995. Clinical evaluation of CA-125 concentrations as a prognostic factor for pregnancy in infertile women with surgically treated endometriosis. Fertil. Steril. **64:** 321–324.
120. DMOWSKI, W.P. 1995. Immunological aspects of endometriosis. Int. J. Gynecol. Obstet. **50**(suppl. 1)**:** S3–S10.
121. AEBY, T.C., T. HUANG & R.T. NAKAYAMA. 1996. The effect of peritoneal fluid from patients with endometriosis on human sperm function *in vitro*. Am. J. Obstet. Gynecol. **174:** 1779–1783.
122. ORAL, E., A. ARICI, D.L. OLIVE & G. HUSZAR. 1996. Peritoneal fluid from women with moderate or severe endometriosis inhibits sperm motility: the role of seminal fluid components. Fertil. Steril. **66:** 787–792.

123. TAKETANI, Y., T.M. KUO & M. MIZUNO. 1992. Comparison of cytokine levels and embryo toxicity in peritoneal fluid in infertile women with untreated or treated endometriosis. Am. J. Obstet. Gynecol. **167:** 265–270.
124. MORCOS, R.N., W.E. GIBBONS & W.E. FINDLEY. 1986. Effect of peritoneal fluid on *in vitro* cleavage of 2-cell mouse embryos: possible role in infertility associated with endometriosis. Fertil. Steril. **44:** 678–683.
125. ILLERA, M.J., L. YUAN, C.L. STEWART *et al.* 2000. Effect of peritoneal fluid from women with endometriosis on implantation in the mouse model. Fertil. Steril. **74:** 41–48.

Role of Endometriosis in Cancer and Tumor Development

LILLIAN MARIE SWIERSZ

Departments of Gynecology and Obstetrics and Radiation Biology, Stanford University, Stanford, California 94305, USA

ABSTRACT: **Endometriosis, like cancer, is characterized by cell invasion and unrestrained growth. Furthermore, endometriosis and cancer are similar in other aspects, such as the development of new blood vessels and a decrease in the number of cells undergoing apoptosis. In spite of these similarities, endometriosis is not considered a malignant disorder. The possibility that endometriosis could, however, transform and become cancer has been debated in the literature since 1925. Mutations in the genes that encode for metabolic and detoxification enzymes, such as GALT and GSTM, have been implicated in the pathogenesis of endometriosis and in the progression to carcinoma of the ovary. PTEN, a tumor suppressor commonly mutated (50%) in endometrial carcinoma, is found mutated in endometrioid carcinoma of the ovary, but not in other forms of ovarian cancer. A recent study has shown that somatic mutations in the PTEN gene were identified in 20% of endometrioid carcinomas and 20.6% of solitary endometrial cysts, suggesting that inactivation of the PTEN tumor suppressor gene is an early event in the development of ovarian endometrioid carcinoma. In addition to cancerous transformation at the site of endometriosis, there is recent evidence to indicate that having endometriosis itself may increase a woman's risk of developing non-Hodgkin's lymphoma, malignant melanoma, and breast cancer.**

KEYWORDS: **endometriosis; cancer; tumor development; melanoma**

BACKGROUND

Endometriosis is a disorder characterized by the growth of endometrial glands and stroma outside of the uterine cavity. Although endometriosis is not considered a malignant disorder, it does share common characteristics with malignant cells. For instance, endometriosis, like cancer, can be both locally and distantly metastatic; it attaches to other tissues, invades, and damages them. However, endometriosis does not create a cachectic or catabolic state and it is rarely fatal. For these reasons, endometriosis is commonly referred to as a "benign cancer". A malignant ovarian tumor has been documented to arise clinically in 0.3% to 1.6% of patients with endometriosis,[1] but the frequency of cancers originating in patients with pelvic endometriosis is less clear.

Address for correspondence: Lillian Marie Swiersz, Departments of Gynecology and Obstetrics and Radiation Biology, Stanford University, Stanford, CA 94305. Voice: 650-723-7439; fax: 650-723-7382.

lswiersz@leland.stanford.edu

Only one study has examined the risk of cancer after hospitalization for endometriosis.[2] The records of 20,686 women hospitalized with endometriosis during the period 1969–1983, as identified through the nationwide Swedish Inpatient Register, were linked against the National Swedish Cancer Registry through 1989 to identify all subsequent diagnoses of cancer. The study subjects were followed up for a mean of 11.4 years, with the cohort contributing 216,851 woman-years of follow-up. The standardized incidence ratio was defined as the ratio of the observed numbers of cancers to those expected. Since a high proportion of subjects had gynecologic operations (55.6%), evaluation of the risk of gynecologic cancers involved truncation of person-years at the time of any such operation. The overall cancer risk was 1.2 (95% confidence interval [CI]: 1.1 to 1.3). Significant excesses were observed for breast cancer (standardized incidence ratio = 1.3; 95% CI: 1.1 to 1.4), ovarian cancer (1.9; 1.3 to 2.8), and hematopoietic malignancies (1.4; 1.0 to 1.8); this latter excess was largely due to an excess risk of non-Hodgkin's lymphoma (1.8; 1.2 to 2.6).

The risk of ovarian cancer was particularly elevated among subjects with a long-standing history of ovarian endometriosis (4.2; 2.0 to 7.7). Ten of the 17 ovarian cancer cases occurred ≥ 10 years after follow-up, resulting in a standardized incidence ratio for this time period of 4.2 (95% CI: 2.0 to 7.7). These investigators also examined whether cancer risk varied by the method by which endometriosis was first diagnosed and classified patients according to the method of diagnosis—laparoscopy (34.9%), laparotomy (54.1%), or some other method (11%). Ovarian cancer risk was elevated in all three subgroups, although the excess was most striking and statistically significant only among those women whose endometriosis was detected through laparoscopy (standardized incidence ratio = 2.6; 95% CI: 1.2 to 4.9).

When the site of origin of endometriosis (ovary, pelvis, adenomyosis, or other site) was examined for cancer risk, no substantial variation was noted for all cancers combined. However, breast cancer risk was significantly elevated among patients with endometriosis arising in the pelvis or adenomyosis, with standardized incidence ratios of 1.79 and 1.39, respectively. Although the findings in this study must be interpreted with caution since the precise information regarding gynecological procedures and pathological reports were not available, the results do strongly suggest that women with endometriosis may experience elevated risks of certain types of cancers.[2] A large, multicenter, prospective study needs to be performed in order to address this question.

OVARIAN CANCER

In 1925, Sampson hypothesized that endometriosis sometimes undergoes malignant change.[3] Since that time, there have been many reports of an association between endometriosis and both clear cell and endometrioid cancer of the ovary. Mostoufizadeh and Scully published a large review paper quoting 31 case reports and series of patients with ovarian cancer starting as early as 1925.[4] They found low frequencies of endometriosis associated with serous and mucinous ovarian carcinomas, but clear cell and endometrioid carcinomas of the ovary were commonly associated with endometriosis. Also, women with endometrioid carcinoma of the ovary and endometriosis tended to be younger than the controls. They found 35 cases of extraovarian cancer, with 13 in the rectovaginal septum, 4 in the vagina, and 3 in the bladder. Adenocarcinoma was the most common type of extraovarian disease reported.[4]

In the 1990s, there were a number of large studies investigating the association between endometriosis and ovarian cancer. One study, consisting of 556 patients undergoing surgery for ovarian cancers, examined the frequency of concurrent endometriosis. The frequency of endometriosis ranged from 3.6% to 5.6% in serous, mucinous, and miscellaneous neoplasms versus 26.3%, 21.1%, and 22.2%, respectively, in endometrioid, clear cell, and mixed subtypes. The differences were statistically significant.[5] The incidence of ovarian atypical endometriosis and its association with malignant epithelial tumors were studied in a consecutive series of cases during the period 1987–1995 in Japan. Fifty-four (24.1%) of the 224 ovarian cancers were associated with ovarian endometriosis: 21 with typical and 33 with atypical endometriosis. Clear cell carcinomas and endometrioid carcinomas were most frequently associated with endometriosis, with 54% (27 of 50 cases) and 41.9% (13 of 31), respectively.[6]

An historical cohort study of all women with endometrioid adenocarcinoma of the ovary diagnosed between 1979 and 1991 at a number of university-based hospitals in the United States was undertaken to better understand the clinical presentation and biologic behavior of ovarian carcinomas arising in endometriosis. A review of pathology reports determined the presence or absence of coexisting endometriosis. Of 91 endometrioid ovarian carcinoma patients identified, 28 (31%) had endometriosis-associated endometrioid ovarian carcinoma. Significant differences between endometrioid cancer patients without endometriosis and with endometriosis existed for age at diagnosis (greater than 55 years; 56% vs. 32%, $p = 0.039$), nulliparity (19% vs. 46%, $p = 0.007$), stage (I and II combined; 37% vs. 70%, $p = 0.004$), and disease status at completion of primary surgery (complete tumor resection; 47% vs. 70%, $p = 0.04$). In conclusion, women with endometriosis associated with endometrioid ovarian cancer were significantly younger, presented with earlier stage disease, and had a longer disease-free survival than those with endometrioid cancer alone. These factors may reflect a more favorable biologic behavior of endometrioid cancer when arising in association with endometriosis.[7]

Another study sought to specifically look for malignancy arising in endometriosis. Seventy-nine patients with stage I epithelial ovarian cancer between 1975 and 1990 were identified retrospectively from the tumor registry and medical records. Pathological slides were evaluated for the presence of endometriosis, specifically looking for malignancy arising in endometriosis. Evidence of endometriosis was found in 22 of the 79 cases (28%). Endometrioid adenocarcinoma accounted for 41% of the tumors associated with endometriosis, clear cell carcinoma for 31%, mixed (endometrioid and/or clear cell types) for 18%, and other types for 9%. Among the 22 patients with associated endometriosis, 7 carcinomas (32%) arising in endometriosis were identified. In these 7 cases, a spectrum of benign and atypical endometriosis with a transition to clear cell or endometrioid adenocarcinoma could be identified. These premalignant changes were characterized by cytological atypia and architectural proliferation.[8]

In summary, these clinical studies suggest a correlation between endometriosis and endometrioid and clear cell cancer of the ovary. Also, some studies suggest that patients with endometriosis and ovarian cancer may be younger and have a better prognosis. Future research is needed to determine which patients with endometriosis will go on to develop ovarian cancer. Genetics rather than clinical data will likely allow us to make that determination.

GALT

Galactose is a common sugar found in dairy products and is metabolized by the enzyme, galactose-1-phosphate uridyltransferase (GALT). It is known that a hereditary form of galactosemia is associated with premature ovarian failure due to the buildup of metabolites. It was proposed that galactose consumption and metabolism may be risk factors for ovarian cancer based on evidence that galactose or its metabolites may contribute to premature ovarian failure[9] and ovarian cancer may arise in the setting of premature depletion of oocytes[10,11] in animal models. In order to determine if the development of galactosemia leads to ovarian cancer, a case-control study was performed in which the consumption of dairy food by 235 white women with epithelial cancer was compared with a control group of 239 women. Yogurt consumption was at least monthly by 49% of cases and 36% of controls and the mean transferase activity in women with ovarian cancer was significantly lower than that of controls. When the ratio of lactose consumption to transferase (L/T) was calculated, the cases had a mean L/T of 1.17 compared with 0.88 for controls, suggesting that women with ovarian cancer did not metabolize galactose as well as the controls. Based on these results, there may be both dietary and genetic risk factors for ovarian cancer.[12]

These authors went on to examine GALT activity in women with a family history of ovarian cancer to determine if low GALT activity occurs in women who are at risk for ovarian cancer, but in whom ovarian cancer has not yet developed. Specifically, 106 premenopausal women with 1 primary or 2 second-degree relatives with ovarian cancer were compared with 116 age-matched control subjects without a family history of ovarian cancer. All women completed questionnaires and had blood drawn to measure GALT activity and genotype. Mean erythrocyte GALT activity, in micromoles of hexose conversion per hour per gram of hemoglobin, was 21.5 in cases, significantly lower than the mean of 23.1 observed in controls ($p = 0.001$). In a subset of 87 patients and 113 control subjects for whom DNA was available, the allelic frequency of the N314D mutation of GALT was 15.5% among cases compared with 7.5% among control subjects ($p = 0.02$). Galactose consumption did not differ between cases and control subjects. In this study, galactose metabolism differed between women with and without a family history of ovarian cancer, suggesting that galactose metabolism may be a genetic risk factor for ovarian cancer, possibly mediated through oocyte toxicity from galactose metabolite.[13]

To explore a possible connection between endometriosis, Müllerian anomalies, and possession of the N314D allele, 33 women with endometriosis attending a fertility clinic were studied. Patients completed questionnaires, had DNA tested for the N314D mutation of GALT, and were compared to a general population of 111 women. Women with endometriosis were more likely to carry at least one N314D allele (30% vs. 14%) and more likely to report a medical history of scoliosis (21% vs. 2%) compared to general population controls, two features previously described in women with vaginal agenesis.[14] Compared with endometriosis cases without the N314D allele, those cases with the allele tended to have more advanced disease and a family history of endometriosis. The authors suggested that the relevance of the N314D mutation may derive from an association between abnormalities of galactose metabolism and vaginal agenesis.[15] A follow-up study by Cramer assessing the consumption of dairy products as well as biochemical and molecular genetic assessment of galactose metabolism in 563 women with newly diagnosed epithelial ovarian cancer and 523 control women was performed.[16] No significant differences between cases and controls in usual consumption of various types of dairy products or RBC activity of either GALT or galactokinase were found. The mean activity of uridine diphosphogalactose 4′-epimerase was significantly lower ($p = 0.005$) in cases compared with controls: 20.32 (0.31) versus 21.64 (0.36). Ovarian cancer cases were also more likely to carry the N314D polymorphism of the GALT gene, generally predisposing to lower GALT activity. The difference was most evident for endometrioid and clear cell types of ovarian cancer, in which 3.9% of cases were found to be homozygous for N314D compared with 0.4% of controls, yielding an odds ratio and 95% CI of 14.17 (2.62–76.60).[16]

Another group of authors examined paraffin-embedded tissues of histologically confirmed endometrium and endometriosis to look for allelic imbalance and alterations of the intensity of microsatellite alleles. Seventeen microsatellite markers were chosen: 1p31-p21, 1q21-q23, 1q42-q43, 2p22-p21, 2q21-q33, 3p24.2-p22, 9p22-p21, 9q31-q34, 17p13.1, and 17q11.2-q12. Specifically, 1q21 was chosen because it is commonly lost in ovarian neoplasms, 9p21 because it is associated with the tumor suppressor gene p16^{Ink4} and GALT, and 17p13.1 because it is associated with p53. Six of the 22 samples (27.3%) showed allelic imbalance on 9p21 compared with only 1 on locus 1q21-q23 (4.5%) and 1 on 17p13.1 (4.5%). Alterations at similar rates were observed among different patient age groups, but the rate increased 3-fold from stage II to III and IV of endometriosis, suggesting that allelic imbalance is independent of patient's age and accumulates during development of the disease.[17]

Although the studies discussed above suggest that mutations in GALT can lead to ovarian cancer and endometriosis, the mechanisms, which lead to disease progression, are still unclear. A large case-control study was conducted in three Australian states between 1990 and 1993. Approximately 800 histologically confirmed cases of ovarian cancer, 800 community controls, and 300 controls recruited through breast-screening clinics completed dietary questionnaires in order to understand dietary risk factors for ovarian cancer.[18] Approximately 100 cases and all breast-screening controls also provided a blood sample for analysis of GALT. Ovarian cancer risk was positively associated with increasing consumption of whole milk and other full-fat dairy foods, but was not associated with consumption of low-fat dairy foods and was inversely related to consumption of skim milk. There was no association between ovarian cancer and GALT, except among women with abnormally low GALT, who had a nonsignificant 2.5-fold increased risk of ovarian cancer. These results suggest that reported associations between milk consumption and ovarian cancer are due to the fat content of milk and not to lactose or galactose. An increased risk of ovarian cancer in women with abnormally low levels of GALT cannot, though, be ruled out by this study. However, a survey of 108 heterozygote women for the classic galactosemia gene, GALT, did not reveal that the carrier state was associated with premature ovarian failure or ovarian cancer. This survey did not support previous epidemiological studies suggesting an increased risk for ovarian dysfunction in women with deficiency of the GALT enzyme.[19] Since this study was addressing whether or not the carrier state was associated with a disease state, the authors needed to study more women in order to definitively state that there was no difference. Also, homozygous women were not studied and they may be more likely to be at risk for ovarian cancer.

GST

It is likely that heritable genetic factors contribute to the development of endometriosis, which is a putative precursor of the endometrioid and clear cell histological subtypes of ovarian cancer. The phase II glutathione S-transferases (GSTs) are a family of enzymes responsible for metabolism of a broad range of xenobiotics and carcinogens, and allelic variants of GSTs that have impaired detoxification function may increase the rate of certain cancers. One study addressed this by looking for homozygous gene deletions at the GSTM1 locus of genomic DNA from blood spots by PCR in a group of Slavic populations from the northwestern and central-eastern regions of European Russia and in patients with a variety of cancers and medical conditions. The frequencies of the GSTM1 0/0 genotype were 38.8% and 67.5% for both population groups, respectively. The proportion of the GSTM1 gene deletion genotype was estimated as significantly increased in endometriosis patients (81%) and the percentage was similar to lung cancer patients (81%). In this study, the high levels of GSTM1 0/0 genotypes in endometriosis patients favor the substantial contribution of certain environmental toxins in the pathogenesis of this widespread disease.[20] The genetic polymorphism of the GSTM1 gene was studied by PCR from the blood spots in patients with different stages of endometriosis ($n = 50$) and in controls ($n = 72$) of French origin. A total of 86.0% of patients appeared to lack GSTM1 enzyme activity due to the presence of an extended deletion (GSTM1 0/0 genotype), compared with 45.8% in a control group ($p = 0.0001$), which was consistent with the frequency of GSTM1 deletion in the French population. Moreover, the distribution of GSTM1-active genotypes was significantly different in patients and controls ($p = 0.0001$) as no patient with GSTM1A/B genotype, which is correlated with the highest activity of GSTM1 enzyme, has been found so far (18.1% in a control group). The unusually high frequency of homozygotes for the GSTM1 gene deletion among patients with endometriosis suggests a possible contribution of environmental toxins in the pathogenesis of this disease due to the absence or low activity of GSTM1 enzyme.[21] Next, a combined analysis of phase II detoxification system genes, arylamine *N*-acetyltransferase 2 (NAT2), and GSTM1 and GSTT1 was carried out in patients with minimal/mild (group I, $n = 36$) and moderate/severe endometriosis (group II, $n = 29$) and controls ($n = 72$) of French origin, using PCR and restriction fragment length polymorphism. The results show a significant difference between patients and controls with regard to NAT2 gene polymorphism ($p = 0.05$). This was mainly due to the high percentage of slow acetylator genotypes (SA) in patients compared with controls (60.0% vs. 38.9%; $p = 0.02$), with a distinct preponderance in subjects with minimal/mild endometriosis (69.4%; $p = 0.005$). Significantly increased proportions of GSTM1-deficient genotypes were found in both groups of patients in comparison with the controls (75.0% and 79.3% vs. 45.8%; $p = 0.0001$). These results suggest the involvement of both

NAT2 and GSTM1 detoxification system genes in the pathogenesis of endometriosis and the possible impact of NAT2 gene polymorphism in the development of different forms of this disease.[22]

Since the null genetic polymorphism in the gene encoding the GST class mu (GSTM1) enzyme has been reported to be significantly elevated in endometriosis, a study to determine the frequency of the GSTM1 null genotype was investigated in 84 cases of endometriosis, 293 cases of ovarian cancer, and 219 controls. All cases and controls were derived from women residing in southeast England. The frequency of the GSTM1 null allele was not overrepresented in the endometriosis patients (47.6%) compared with the controls (48.9%) ($p = 0.898$). In the ovarian cancer group, the GSTM1 null genotype was significantly elevated compared with controls (59.0% vs. 48.9%; $p = 0.025$). When stratified according to histological subtype, a significantly increased GSTM1 null genotype was only observed for the endometrioid (65.4%; $p = 0.013$) and the combined endometrioid/clear cell ovarian cancers (67.0%; $p = 0.004$). Based on these results, the GSTM1 null allele may not be an endometriosis susceptibility allele for endometriosis; however, it may predispose endometriotic lesions to malignant transformation to endometrioid and clear cell ovarian cancer.[23] Another group of investigators looked at the role of GST gene variants in ovarian cancer development. Here, 285 epithelial ovarian cancer cases and 299 unaffected controls were screened for the GSTT1 deletion (null) variant, the GSTM1 deletion (null) variant, and the GSTP1 codon 104 A→G Ile→Val amino acid substitution variant. There was a suggestion that ovarian cancers of the endometrioid or clear cell histological subtype had a higher frequency of the GSTT1 and GSTM1 deletion genotypes than other histological subgroups. The GSTT1, GSTM1, and GSTP1 genotype distributions did not differ significantly between unaffected controls and ovarian cancer cases (overall or invasive cancers only). However, the GSTM1 null genotype was associated with increased risk of endometrioid/clear cell invasive cancer [age-adjusted odds ratio (95% CI) = 2.04 (1.01–4.09); $p = 0.05$], suggesting that deletion of GSTM1 may increase the risk of ovarian cancer of these histological subtypes specifically.[24]

These studies are compelling, but not definitive, in showing that mutations in GST predispose to both endometriosis and ovarian cancer. Further studies are necessary to clarify the relationship between GST mutations and the development of endometriosis and/or ovarian cancer. Additionally, it may be that women with endometriosis and GST mutations are at an increased risk to develop clear cell or endometrioid carcinoma of the ovary.

PTEN

PTEN, a tumor suppressor located at chromosome 10q23,[25–27] is mutated in a variety of sporadic cancers[28,29] and in two autosomal dominant hamartoma syndromes.[30–32] PTEN is a phosphatase that dephosphorylates phosphatidylinositol (3,4,5)-triphosphate (PtdIns-3,4,5-P3), an important intracellular second messenger, lowering its level within the cell. By dephosphorylating PtdIns-3,4,5-P3, PTEN acts in opposition to phosphatidylinositol 3-kinase (PI3K), which has a pivotal role in the creation of PtdIns-3,4,5-P3. PtdIns-3,4,5-P3 is necessary for the activation of Akt, a serine/threonine kinase involved in cell growth and survival. By blocking the activation of Akt, PTEN regulates cellular processes such as cell cycling, translation, and apoptosis.[33,34] Data suggest that PTEN/MMAC1 is more commonly mutated than any other known gene in endometrial cancers.[29] In ovarian tumors, LOH of PTEN was common among the endometrioid (43%) and serous (28%) tumors, but was infrequent among the other histological subtypes. The majority of tumors with PTEN mutations were grade 1 and/or stage 1, suggesting that inactivation of PTEN is an early event in ovarian tumorigenesis.[35,36]

Since PTEN mutations are seen early in endometrioid ovarian carcinoma and endometrioid ovarian cancer is thought to arise from endometriosis, it has been proposed that somatic genetic alterations in the PTEN gene may be an early event in endometriotic cells.[37,38] A group investigating the potential role of the PTEN gene in the carcinogenesis of ovarian endometrioid carcinoma and its related subtype, clear cell carcinoma, found PTEN mutations in endometrial ovarian cysts. Twenty ovarian endometrioid carcinomas, 24 clear cell carcinomas, and 34 solitary endometrial cysts of the ovary were investigated for LOH at 10q23.3 and point mutations within the entire coding region of the PTEN gene. LOH was found in 8 of 19 ovarian endometrioid carcinomas (42.1%), 6 of 22 clear cell carcinomas (27.3%), and 13 of 23 solitary endometrial cysts (56.5%). In 5 endometrioid carcinomas synchronous with endometriosis, 3 cases displayed LOH events common to both the carcinoma and the endometriosis, 1 displayed an LOH event in only the carcinoma, and 1 displayed no LOH events in either lesion. In 7 clear cell carcinomas synchronous with endometriosis, 3 displayed LOH events common to both the carcinoma and the endometriosis, 1 displayed an LOH event in only the carcinoma, and 3 displayed no LOH events in either lesion. Somatic mutations in the PTEN gene were identified in 4 of 20 ovarian endometrioid carcinomas (20.0%), 2 of 24 clear cell carcinomas (8.3%), and 7 of 34 solitary endometrial cysts (20.6%).[39] These results along with previous results[35,36] indicate that inactivation of the PTEN tumor suppressor gene is an early event in the development of ovarian endometrioid carcinoma and clear cell carcinoma of the ovary. Additionally, these studies suggest a common pathway from endometriosis to ovarian cancer via a tumor suppressor gene, PTEN. Further molecular and transitional studies are necessary to clarify this relationship.

BREAST CANCER

Breast cancer is the most common female cancer in the United States and elevated levels of estrogens are suspected to increase the risk of this cancer. Endometriosis is also associated with altered hormonal levels and researchers have looked to see if endometriosis may influence breast cancer risk. The Brinton study[2] showed a significant excess for breast cancer (standardized incidence ratio = 1.3; 95% CI: 1.1 to 1.4) in women with a diagnosis of endometriosis. A study designed to examine breast cancer risk following a history of various medical procedures was done utilizing a population-based case-control study of young women in the United States: 2173 breast cancer cases and 1990 population-based controls under 55 years from three areas of the United States were administered a questionnaire including details of physician-diagnosed medical conditions. There was no significantly increased or decreased breast cancer risk associated with a history of thyroid disease, gallbladder disease, colorectal polyps, diabetes, high blood pressure, high cholesterol, or surgery for endometriosis. There was some evidence of an increased breast cancer risk associated with ovarian cysts among women who did not receive an oophorectomy (relative risk = 1.94; 95% CI: 1.0-3.9).[40] Since this study did not rely on medical records to confirm answers to the questionnaire, it may be that at least some of the women with surgery for ovarian cysts had endometriosis. A long-term prospective study needs to be done to further clarify this issue.

Risk of breast cancer was assessed in relationship to gynecologic operations using data from a record-linkage study involving 15,844 women in the Uppsala Health Care Region of Sweden, who underwent surgery between 1965 and 1983. Among women who were premenopausal at the time of operation, a bilateral oophorectomy before the age of 50 years was associated with a 50% reduction in the risk of breast cancer compared with the background population, a reduction in risk evident within 10 years of the operation. A bilateral oophorectomy after the age of 50 years in premenopausal women or after a natural menopause was not associated with any reduction in risk. The risk of breast cancer did not vary by indications for oophorectomy, including benign neoplasms and functional cysts, but endometriosis was associated with a nonsignificant increase in breast cancer risk. There were no reductions in risk associated with a unilateral oophorectomy or hysterectomy among women who were premenopausal at the time of operation. In fact, hysterectomy alone was associated with a slight increase in breast cancer risk when the operation was due to myomas, abnormal bleeding, and severe forms of endometriosis.[41]

These studies suggest that women with endometriosis may be at increased risk for breast cancer. Long-term prospective studies are needed to clarify the magnitude of the risk. Additionally, genetic and molecular studies of women with endometriosis are needed to determine who is at greatest risk for development of breast and other cancers. These studies can be facilitated through proteonomics, which is now being used to identify serum markers in ovarian and breast cancer.

MELANOMA

A group of investigators from Harvard University used data from 7559 female alumnae of 8 colleges and 2 universities who were sent detailed questionnaires regarding participation in athletics and detailed questions on medical history.[42] Previously, they reported that women who were college athletes had a decreased risk of breast and gynecological cancers, but there was no difference in the incidence of malignant melanomas and skin cancers. Next, they decided to investigate three groups of women: (1) women who reported melanomas of the skin; (2) women who reported cancer of the skin, but not melanomas; and (3) a sample that excluded women with melanoma or cancer of the skin. Four controls were selected for each of the 18 women reporting melanoma. The women were randomly selected with 5-year age groups and for whether the woman was a college athlete. The results showed that significantly more women with melanoma reported more procedures related to the reproductive system. The odds ratios comparing women with melanoma with those in the nonmelanoma skin cancer group and those in the random sample are 3.2% with 95% confidence limits (CL: 1.0, 10.1), $p = 0.049$, and 3.9% with 95% CL (1.2, 12.4), $p = 0.021$, respectively. The following procedures and diagnoses in the reproductive history were investigated: D & C, hysterectomy, endometriosis, benign tumor, and endometrial or other gynecological disorder.[42]

These investigators reported this association and went on to prospectively study a group of women attending the Pigmented Lesion Unit of Massachusetts General Hospital and who were asked detailed questions regarding reproductive history. The groups were patients with dysplastic nevi (n = 52), melanoma and dysplastic nevi (n = 83), and melanoma without dysplastic nevi (n = 71), and a random sample of women (n = 142). When compared to the random sample, patients with dysplastic nevi had an odds ratio of 16.5 for endometriosis. In addition, the dysplastic nevi group were the youngest of the patient groups (age: 35.1 ± 1.2 years) and overall had the largest number of significant differences from the random sample.[43] Next, this group of investigators looked prospectively at 139 women attending an infertility clinic. Study participants were administered a short questionnaire, which included specific questions about endometriosis and melanoma. All participants underwent an examination by the same dermatologist to determine the presence, number, and location of dysplastic nevi and melanomas. The odds ratio among all study subjects for the association between endometriosis and dysplastic nevi was 1.7 [95% CI: 0.7 to 4.3; p = 0.27]. Among those patients who were 32 years or younger, 41.0% of endometriosis patients had dysplastic nevi versus only 8.3% of controls (p = 0.038). Among women who were >32 years, 22.2% of endometriosis patients had dysplastic nevi versus 30.4% of controls (p = 0.514). Fourteen out of 49 patients (28.6%) with endometriosis had a family history of melanoma, while 3 of 30 nonendometriosis patients (p = 0.039) gave a similar history. These studies revealing a higher prevalence of dysplastic nevi, a known precursor and risk factor for melanoma in younger women with endometriosis and other gynecological disorders, suggest that these patients may be at higher risk for melanoma.[44] Other researchers have not confirmed the association between endometriosis and dysplastic nevi. Another investigation examining oral contraceptive use and reproductive factors was conducted in a population-based case-control study of patients who were diagnosed with melanoma during 1981–1986 and aged 25–59. These investigators did not find a difference in the risk between groups based on use and duration of oral contraception or history of miscarriage, induced abortion, or endometriosis.[45]

To summarize, these studies suggest that there is an association between dysplastic nevi and endometriosis in younger women. Although the explanation for the observed association between endometriosis and a premalignant skin condition is unknown, immune dysfunction is common to both conditions. Further clinical investigation by other groups is needed to corroborate these results, and ongoing basic research into the immune dysfunction associated with endometriosis will uncover mechanisms common to both diseases.

REFERENCES

1. SEIDMAN, J.D. 1996. Prognostic importance of hyperplasia and atypia in endometriosis. Int. J. Gynecol. Pathol. **15:** 1–9.
2. BRINTON, L.A., G. GRIDLEY, I. PERSSON *et al.* 1997. Cancer risk after a hospital discharge diagnosis of endometriosis. Am. J. Obstet. Gynecol. **176:** 572–579.
3. SAMPSON, J. 1925. Endometrial carcinoma of the ovary, arising in endometrial tissue in that organ. Arch. Surg. **10:** 1–72.

4. MOSTOUFIZADEH, M. & R.E. SCULLY. 1980. Malignant tumors arising in endometriosis. Clin. Obstet. Gynecol. **23:** 951–963.
5. VERCELLINI, P., F. PARAZZINI, G. BOLIS *et al.* 1993. Endometriosis and ovarian cancer. Am. J. Obstet. Gynecol. **169:** 181–182.
6. FUKUNAGA, M., K. NOMURA, E. ISHIKAWA & S. USHIGOME. 1997. Ovarian atypical endometriosis: its close association with malignant epithelial tumours. Histopathology **30:** 249–255.
7. MCMEEKIN, D.S., R.A. BURGER, A. MANETTA *et al.* 1995. Endometrioid adenocarcinoma of the ovary and its relationship to endometriosis. Gynecol. Oncol. **59:** 81–86.
8. SAINZ DE LA CUESTA, R., J.H. EICHHORN, L.W. RICE *et al.* 1996. Histologic transformation of benign endometriosis to early epithelial ovarian cancer. Gynecol. Oncol. **60:** 238–244.
9. CHEN, Y.T., D.R. MATTISON, L. FEIGENBAUM *et al.* 1981. Reduction in oocyte number following prenatal exposure to a diet high in galactose. Science **214:** 1145–1147.
10. FURTH, J. 1936. Neoplastic diseases occurring among mice subjected to general irradiation with X rays. Am. J. Cancer **28:** 66–95.
11. HOWELL, J.S. & J.W. ORR. 1954. The induction of ovarian tumors in mice with 9,10-dimethyl 1,2-benzanthracene. Br. J. Cancer **8:** 635–646.
12. CRAMER, D.W., B.L. HARLOW, W.C. WILLETT *et al.* 1989. Galactose consumption and metabolism in relation to the risk of ovarian cancer. Lancet **2:** 66–71.
13. CRAMER, D.W., M.G. MUTO, J.K. REICHARDT *et al.* 1994. Characteristics of women with a family history of ovarian cancer: I. Galactose consumption and metabolism. Cancer **74:** 1309–1317.
14. CRAMER, D.W., D.P. GOLDSTEIN, C. FRAER & J.K. REICHARDT. 1996. Vaginal agenesis (Mayer-Rokitansky-Küster-Hauser syndrome) associated with the N314D mutation of galactose-1-phosphate uridyl transferase (GALT). Mol. Hum. Reprod. **2:** 145–148.
15. CRAMER, D.W., M.D. HORNSTEIN, W.G. NG & R.L. BARBIERI. 1996. Endometriosis associated with the N314D mutation of galactose-1-phosphate uridyl transferase (GALT). Mol. Hum. Reprod. **2:** 149–152.
16. CRAMER, D.W., E.R. GREENBERG, L. TITUS-ERNSTOFF *et al.* 2000. A case-control study of galactose consumption and metabolism in relation to ovarian cancer. Cancer Epidemiol. Biomarkers Prev. **9:** 95–101.
17. GOUMENOU, A.G., D.A. ARVANITIS, I.M. MATALLIOTAKIS *et al.* 2001. Microsatellite DNA assays reveal an allelic imbalance in p16(Ink4), GALT, p53, and APOA2 loci in patients with endometriosis. Fertil. Steril. **75:** 160–165.
18. WEBB, P.M., C.J. BAIN, D.M. PURDIE *et al.* 1998. Milk consumption, galactose metabolism, and ovarian cancer (Australia). Cancer Causes Control **9:** 637–644.
19. KAUFMAN, F.R., S. DEVGAN & G.N. DONNELL. 1993. Results of a survey of carrier women for the galactosemia gene. Fertil. Steril. **60:** 727–728.
20. BARANOVA, V.S., T. IVASCHENKO, B. BAKAY *et al.* 1996. Proportion of the GSTM1 0/0 genotype in some Slavic populations and its correlation with cystic fibrosis and some multifactorial diseases. Hum. Genet. **97:** 516–520.
21. BARANOVA, H., R. BOTHORISHVILLI, M. CANIS *et al.* 1997. Glutathione S-transferase M1 gene polymorphism and susceptibility to endometriosis in a French population. Mol. Hum. Reprod. **3:** 775–780.
22. BARANOVA, H., M. CANIS, T. IVASCHENKO *et al.* 1999. Possible involvement of arylamine *N*-acetyltransferase 2, glutathione S-transferases M1 and T1 genes in the development of endometriosis. Mol. Hum. Reprod. **5:** 636–641.
23. BAXTER, S.W., E.J. THOMAS & I.G. CAMPBELL. 2001. GSTM1 null polymorphism and susceptibility to endometriosis and ovarian cancer. Carcinogenesis **22:** 63–65.
24. SPURDLE, A.B., P.M. WEBB, D.M. PURDIE *et al.* 2001. Polymorphisms at the glutathione S-transferase GSTM1, GSTT1, and GSTP1 loci: risk of ovarian cancer by histological subtype. Carcinogenesis **22:** 67–72.
25. LI, D.M. & H. SUN. 1997. TEP1, encoded by a candidate tumor suppressor locus, is a novel protein tyrosine phosphatase regulated by transforming growth factor beta. Cancer Res. **57:** 2124–2129.
26. LI, J., C. YEN, D. LIAW *et al.* 1997. PTEN, a putative protein tyrosine phosphatase gene mutated in human brain, breast, and prostate cancer. Science **275:** 1943–1947.

27. Steck, P.A., M.A. Pershouse, S.A. Jasser *et al.* 1997. Identification of a candidate tumour suppressor gene, MMAC1, at chromosome 10q23.3 that is mutated in multiple advanced cancers. Nat. Genet. **15:** 356–362.
28. Rasheed, B.K., T.T. Stenzel, R.E. McLendon *et al.* 1997. PTEN gene mutations are seen in high-grade, but not in low-grade gliomas. Cancer Res. **57:** 4187–4190.
29. Risinger, J.I., A.K. Hayes, A. Berchuck & J.C. Barrett. 1997. PTEN/MMAC1 mutations in endometrial cancers. Cancer Res. **57:** 4736–4738.
30. Nelen, M.R., W.C. van Staveren, E.A. Peeters *et al.* 1997. Germline mutations in the PTEN/MMAC1 gene in patients with Cowden disease. Hum. Mol. Genet. **6:** 1383–1387.
31. Liaw, D., D.J. Marsh, J. Li *et al.* 1997. Germline mutations of the PTEN gene in Cowden disease, an inherited breast and thyroid cancer syndrome. Nat. Genet. **16:** 64–67.
32. Marsh, D.J., P.L. Dahia, Z. Zheng *et al.* 1997. Germline mutations in PTEN are present in Bannayan-Zonana syndrome. Nat. Genet. **16:** 333–334.
33. Simpson, L. & R. Parsons. 2001. PTEN: life as a tumor suppressor. Exp. Cell Res. **264:** 29–41.
34. Di Cristofano, A. & P.P. Pandolfi. 2000. The multiple roles of PTEN in tumor suppression. Cell **100:** 387–390.
35. Obata, K., S.J. Morland, R.H. Watson *et al.* 1998. Frequent PTEN/MMAC mutations in endometrioid, but not serous or mucinous epithelial ovarian tumors. Cancer Res. **58:** 2095–2097.
36. Obata, K. & H. Hoshiai. 2000. Common genetic changes between endometriosis and ovarian cancer. Gynecol. Obstet. Invest. **50:** 39–43.
37. Bischoff, F.Z. & J.L. Simpson. 2000. Heritability and molecular genetic studies of endometriosis. Hum. Reprod. Update **6:** 37–44.
38. Thomas, E.J. & I.G. Campbell. 2000. Molecular genetic defects in endometriosis. Gynecol. Obstet. Invest. **50:** 44–50.
39. Sato, N., H. Tsunoda, M. Nishida *et al.* 2000. Loss of heterozygosity on 10q23.3 and mutation of the tumor suppressor gene PTEN in benign endometrial cyst of the ovary: possible sequence progression from benign endometrial cyst to endometrioid carcinoma and clear cell carcinoma of the ovary. Cancer Res. **60:** 7052–7056.
40. Weiss, H.A., L.A. Brinton, N.A. Potischman *et al.* 1999. Breast cancer risk in young women and history of selected medical conditions. Int. J. Epidemiol. **28:** 816–823.
41. Schairer, C., I. Persson, M. Falkeborn *et al.* 1997. Breast cancer risk associated with gynecologic surgery and indications for such surgery. Int. J. Cancer **70:** 150–154.
42. Wyshak, G., R.E. Frisch, N.L. Albright *et al.* 1989. Reproductive factors and melanoma of the skin among women. Int. J. Dermatol. **28:** 527–530.
43. Frisch, R.E., G. Wyshak, L.S. Albert & A.J. Sober. 1992. Dysplastic nevi, cutaneous melanoma, and gynecologic disorders. Int. J. Dermatol. **31:** 331–335.
44. Hornstein, M.D., P.P. Thomas, A.J. Sober *et al.* 1997. Association between endometriosis, dysplastic nevi, and history of melanoma in women of reproductive age. Hum. Reprod. **12:** 143–145.
45. Holly, E.A., R.D. Cress & D.K. Ahn. 1995. Cutaneous melanoma in women: III. Reproductive factors and oral contraceptive use. Am. J. Epidemiol. **141:** 943–950.

Panel Discussion (Part VII)

A. ARICI (*Yale University, New Haven, CT*): I have a comment for Lillian Swiersz and a question for Linda Giudice. My comment concerns the correlation between melanoma and endometriosis. It is interesting to note that, when first described, the first name given to IL-8 was MGSA, which stands for melanoma growth stimulatory activity. Thus, it will be interesting to see if there is any common path as far as IL-8 is concerned. It has been shown to stimulate melanoma cell growth. As for my question to Linda Giudice, I was very much impressed by the gene array showing that both IL-8 and MCP-1 are 24- and 27-fold higher in decidualized stromal cells. Were the control cells cultured over the same period of time without progesterone or without cAMP?

L.C. GIUDICE (*Stanford University, Stanford, CA*): Yes, they were.

ARICI: That is an impressive increase.

R.M. BRENNER (*Oregon Regional Primate Research Center, Beaverton, OR*): Dr. Simpson, in touch-tip method number one and concerning the chromosome errors that you detected, were they only glandular?

J.L. SIMPSON (*Baylor College of Medicine, Houston, TX*): No, not necessarily.

S. PARTHASARATHY (*Emory University, Atlanta, GA*): Could you take an endometrial biopsy at the time of severe pain versus control to see if pain-associated genes (e.g., COX2 and others) could be activated?

GIUDICE: The question was whether it is possible to take an endometrial biopsy during the time of dysmenorrhea or pelvic pain. It is possible. However, it would be difficult to recruit for a study like that. In these types of studies using gene arrays, we have to emphasize again that the subjects must be well characterized. To conduct a study such as this, it is really quite a request to ask women who have endometriosis to not be on nonsteroidals, oral contraceptives, danazol, or a GnRH agonist. I think they are quite heroic for giving us their endometrium.

P. HUGO (*Procrea Biosciences, Quebec, Canada*): I would like to discuss the usefulness of using gene arrays. From our own set of data, it is fairly easy to obtain results that appear to be meaningful at first glance. However, when you look at the reproducibility of those results over a large population scale, these very encouraging results tend to fade away. Thus, I would really encourage anyone doing that kind of study to use an *N* of at least 50 and over. I know it is very costly. Otherwise, you have very precise results on one set of patients: *N* equal to 10 or less. Those results usually represent individual differences rather than group differences. I am really concerned about the approach where we are averaging the results within the single group and after that comparing the means of controls versus endometriosis patients. This has not been a good approach and we have lost time.

GIUDICE: I think that is an excellent point. I hope the funding agency has heard that. The numbers, at least in the setting that we are in, are constrained by our ability to finance the purchasing of chips. However, you bring up an excellent point and that is the incredible data analysis that occurs and the statistical analysis that goes along with these large amounts of data. We are still mining and analyzing the data. To do it on behalf of 4 or 6 subjects, I agree with you. Of course, it is important to increase the *N*.

F.Z. BISCHOFF (*Baylor College of Medicine, Houston, TX*): I would like to comment on the analysis of allele frequencies with regard to the drug-metabolizing enzymes that have been studied and recorded in the literature. I think that the number of cases studied has to be considerably higher than what is being reported. In our own experience, when we have looked at GSTM1, we would run a set of samples (up to 50, say) and analyze the data, and then the results would change when we would add 20 more cases to our pool. Thus, in that respect, we need to do careful evaluations of our results. Concerning GSTM1, our group has not yet seen an association with endometriosis versus controls with regard to the null allele. However, for MAT2, we have preliminary results suggesting that there is some association, but again our case numbers are too small to make a significant statement at this time.

QUESTION: Dr. Lessey, have you noticed any change in biomarkers between each IVF attempt since you told us that each IVF attempt causes a pregnancy decrease? Are we doing something each time? Are we going in and out of the uterine cavity or is there an age effect?

B.A. LESSEY (*University of North Carolina, Chapel Hill, NC*): The data that I showed were adapted from Jacques Cohen's program and just represented that, in an IVF population, there are patients who seem to be recalcitrant to getting pregnant. We are collecting samples of women with recurrent IVF failure and are finding that they have a higher than expected incidence of implantation defects. However, we need to really have a collaborative project going to do that properly.

SIMPSON: The other possibility there, though, is a fundamental genetic defect. Recurrent aneuploidy as evidenced by chaotic embryos is known to be repetitive and could explain the same phenomenon—or, in particular, an unrecognized inversion or translocation. Now that we are starting to do preimplantation genetic diagnosis, we have had some astonishing results of people with reciprocal translocation that seem to have no ostensible relationship to the infertility. However, when you actually do the FISH analysis on the embryos, you find that something like 90% of all embryos are unbalanced as a result of an adjacent one and an adjacent two rather than alternate segregations. Thus, before you make too many overarching conclusions, you need to exclude the confounders in those data sets.

K. CHWALISZ (*TAP Pharmaceutical Products, Lake Forest, IL*): I would like to address some comments to Dr. Kennedy. You included monkeys who underwent biopsies, endometrial biopsies, and hysterotomies in your monkey population. This could theoretically reduce the power of your study. In a past collaboration with Gary Hodgen, who did multiple endometrial biopsy via hysterotomy in his monkeys, we observed that almost all the monkeys with multiple biopsies became endometriotic. Thus, endometrial biopsy represents a high risk factor to endometriosis that is independent probably of genetic factors.

S. KENNEDY (*University of Oxford, Oxford, United Kingdom*): I do not believe that the Wisconsin group was carrying out endometrial biopsies. The hysterotomies were to obtain fetuses, but clearly that is something that we need to look at.

BRENNER: Also, with the Oregon Primate Center colony, we thought that the incidence of endometriosis was related to the number of fetal surgeries. In previous times, a monkey might have four or five C-sections. In recent days, because of new animal policies, we are limited to three and the endometriosis rate is down.

J. McLACHLAN (*Tulane University, New Orleans, LA*): This is primarily for Dr. Simpson and it relates to genetics and epigenetics. One of the questions that I would like to raise is that those of us who have studied the pharmacology of the metabolism of estrogens have noticed that estrogens, not all, but some, including estradiol, tend to be spindle poisons and actually block polymerization of the spindle in *in vitro* and *in vivo* systems, leading to near diploidy/aneuploidy. I wonder if you could consider the possibility that some of the chromosomal abnormalities that are noticed in terms of aneuploidy could indeed be induced by the hormonal environment they are differentiating in.

SIMPSON: I certainly could consider it. There has been a lot of *in vitro* studies looking at hormones and their relationship to cytogenetics *in vitro* that really have not shown any consistent effects. This literature goes back for a long time, back when we used to fund contraceptive research in the United States. At that time, there was a lot of interest in breakage and other phenomena. This really has not been looked at with the modern technologies—that is, what we know about centromeric proteins and spindle proteins and the like—so a fresh look would be worthwhile. I would be surprised if it would be a major player in what we are talking about today because I would expect it to be a major player only if it had a unique effect on a selected subset of the population. To me, it does not quite fit the usual pharmacogenetic susceptibilities that are traditionally associated. I like the idea of pharmacosusceptibilities, as you have heard from Dr. Bischoff, but I am not sure that the mediator is going to be estrogen.

An *In Vitro* Model to Study the Pathogenesis of the Early Endometriosis Lesion

CRAIG A. WITZ,[a] HERVE DECHAUD,[a] IRIS A. MONTOYA-RODRIGUEZ,[a] MIKA R. THOMAS,[a] ANITHA S. NAIR,[a] VICTORIA E. CENTONZE,[b] AND ROBERT S. SCHENKEN[a]

[a]*Department of Obstetrics and Gynecology,* [b]*Department of Cellular and Structural Biology, The University of Texas Health Science Center at San Antonio, San Antonio, Texas 78229-3900, USA*

ABSTRACT: *Objective*—To determine if whole fragments of endometrium can adhere to peritoneum with intact mesothelium. *Design*—Tissue culture and immunohistochemical study. *Setting*—University Medical Center. *Patients*—Reproductive-age women undergoing surgery for benign conditions. *Interventions*—Whole explants of human peritoneum from the anterior abdominal wall and the posterior surface of the uterus were cultured with whole fragments of mechanically dispersed endometrium. *Main Outcome Measures*—Adhesion of endometrial fragments to the surface of the peritoneum was evaluated. Adherent fragments of endometrium were identified using the dissecting microscope and by performing serial sections of the peritoneum explants for light and confocal laser-scanning microscopy. Immunohistochemical staining of the mesothelium with antibodies to cytokeratin and vimentin was used to ensure an intact layer of mesothelium beneath the endometrial implants. Transmission electron microscopy was also used to evaluate the adhesion of endometrium to the mesothelium. *Results*—Endometrium was identified attached to the surface of the peritoneum. After 18–24 hours of culture, the majority of implants did not have identifiable mesothelium beneath them, but most had intact mesothelium running up to the point of attachment. Approximately 10% of the endometrial implants had intact mesothelium at the site of attachment. After 1 hour of culture, both endometrial stromal and epithelial cells were attached to intact mesothelium in nearly all cases. Early transmesothelial invasion involves endometrial stromal cells. *Conclusions*—Endometrial stromal and epithelial cells can attach to the intact mesothelial surface of the peritoneum. Endometrial stromal cell invasion through the mesothelium occurs in less than 18–24 hours.

KEYWORDS: endometriosis; endometrium; peritoneum; mesothelium; explant; cell adhesion; tissue culture

Address for correspondence: Robert S. Schenken, M.D., Professor, Department of Obstetrics and Gynecology, MSC 7836, The University of Texas Health Science Center at San Antonio, 7703 Floyd Curl Drive, San Antonio, TX 78229-3900. Voice: 210-567-4930; fax: 210-567-4958. schenken@uthscsa.edu

INTRODUCTION

The pathogenesis of endometriosis is poorly understood. A widely accepted theory is that of retrograde menstruation, introduced by Sampson in 1927.[1] According to this theory, fragments of endometrium are refluxed through the fallopian tubes into the peritoneal cavity and then attach and grow on peritoneal surfaces. The anatomic distribution of endometriosis supports this theory. Sites closest to the tubal fimbriae (i.e., ovary) and dependent portions of the pelvis are most commonly affected. Mobile structures such as the fallopian tubes are less commonly affected.[2]

Other data supporting Sampson's theory include the observation that almost all women (90%) with patent fallopian tubes have reflux menstruation into the peritoneal cavity.[3] The viability of sloughed endometrial cells in menstrual fluid has also been demonstrated, suggesting that these viable cells survive in peritoneal fluid.[4–6]

However, questions concerning the initial interaction of these viable endometrial cells with the peritoneum remain unsettled. It is not clear whether endometrial stroma or epithelium can attach to the peritoneum. Components of the peritoneum involved in the initial adhesion are also poorly defined. More specifically, it is unclear whether endometrial cells can attach to the mesothelium (i.e., the epithelium lining of the peritoneum). Some investigators propose that the mesothelium acts as a barrier to attachment of ectopic endometrium. They assert that exposure of the extracellular matrix via peritoneal damage is requisite to attachment of endometrium.[7]

The purpose of this manuscript is to summarize our preliminary studies on the attachment of endometrial cells to the peritoneum. A novel model of human explants of peritoneum cultured with mechanically dispersed endometrium is used to evaluate the role of the mesothelium and to determine which endometrial cells are involved in this process.

MATERIALS AND METHODS

The Institutional Review Board of the University of Texas Health Science Center at San Antonio granted approval for this study.

Peritoneum from the anterior abdominal wall (AP) (n = 19) and the posterior aspect of the uterine serosa (US) (n = 8) was obtained from reproductive-age women (n = 19) without endometriosis who were undergoing surgery for benign conditions. Surgery was performed during the proliferative (n = 11) and secretory (n = 8) phase of the cycle. The tissue was immediately placed in Dulbecco's Modified Eagle's Medium (DMEM) (Sigma, St. Louis, MO) plus 10% defined fetal calf serum (HyClone, Logan, UT) and transported to the laboratory. Care was taken to keep the tissue moist and to avoid abrasion of the mesothelial surface. Fat was carefully trimmed from the sections of AP, and smooth muscle was trimmed from sections of US. Peritoneal explants from both the AP and US were cut to approximately $6 \times 6\ mm^2$ and were placed in Millicell-CM 12-mm culture inserts (Millipore, Bedford, MA), which were placed in 24-well plates (Corning, Corning, NY) with the mesothelium facing upward. The explants were cultured in DMEM plus 10% defined fetal calf serum with antibiotic/antimycotic and L-glutamine (Sigma).

Endometrium was obtained by curettage or by aspiration biopsy using a Pipelle (Unimar Inc., Prodimed, Neuilly-en-Thelle, France). Endometrium was transported to the laboratory in DMEM plus 10% defined fetal calf serum. The endometrium was first mechanically dispersed with a scalpel and then by a series of gradually smaller hypodermic needles. Fifteen milligrams of endometrium (wet weight) was added to the culture inserts containing explants of AP and US. The explants were then cultured for 18–24 hours.

Endometrial Adhesion

Initially, combined cultures were incubated for 24–48 hours ($n = 15$). In subsequent studies, cultures were incubated for 1 hour ($n = 4$). The explants of AP and US were carefully removed from the culture insert and submerged in Hanks' balanced salt solution (Sigma) in a 6-cm petri dish (Becton Dickinson Labware, Lincoln Park, NJ). The explants were grasped with a fine tissue forceps beneath the mesothelial surface. The explants were rinsed and gently agitated in this media.

The explants were examined using a dissecting microscope at 60×. By continuously agitating the explant, buoyant fragments of endometrium could be identified that were attached to the explant.

Histology and Immunohistochemistry

The explants were then fixed in 4% formaldehyde and embedded in paraffin. Serial sections of 5-µm thickness were taken at 50-µm intervals. Sections were stained with hematoxylin and examined under the microscope. When fragments of endometrium were identified attached to the explants, serial 5-µm sections were taken through this area of attachment.

Slides revealing attached fragments of endometrium were stained with hematoxylin and eosin (H&E). To aid in identification of the mesothelium beneath an endometrial implant, immunohistochemistry was also performed using mouse monoclonal antibodies to cytokeratin (Oncogene Science, Uniondale, NY) and vimentin (Oncogene Science).[8] Slides were incubated with biotinylated horse antimouse secondary antibody followed by avidin-biotin peroxidase complex (Vectastain® Elite, Burlingame, CA). The slides were then reacted with diaminobenzidine (DAB) and hydrogen peroxide, yielding a brown reaction. Hematoxylin was used as a counterstain. For confocal laser-scanning microscopy (CLSM), immunohistochemistry was performed using a mouse monoclonal antibody to human cytokeratin 8 (clone 35µH11 Dako, Carpenteria, CA). Slides were then incubated with fluorescein-conjugated goat antimouse IgG (FITC) or rhodamine-conjugated goat antimouse IgG (TRITC) (Jackson ImmunoResearch Laboratories, West Grove, PA). Slides labeled with anticytokeratin antibodies were examined using CLSM. The endometrial cell type involved in the initial attachment to the mesothelium was then determined.

Confocal Laser-Scanning Microscopy (CLSM)

CLSM was performed using an Olympus IX70 inverted microscope and the Olympus Fluoview System (Nagano, Japan). Slides were examined with a 60× objective with a 1.2 N.A. water immersion lens. Fluorescein was excited with an argon laser at 488 nm (NEC, Nagano, Japan). Fluorescein emission was detected at 510–550 nm. Rhodamine was excited with a krypton laser (Omnichrome, Chino,

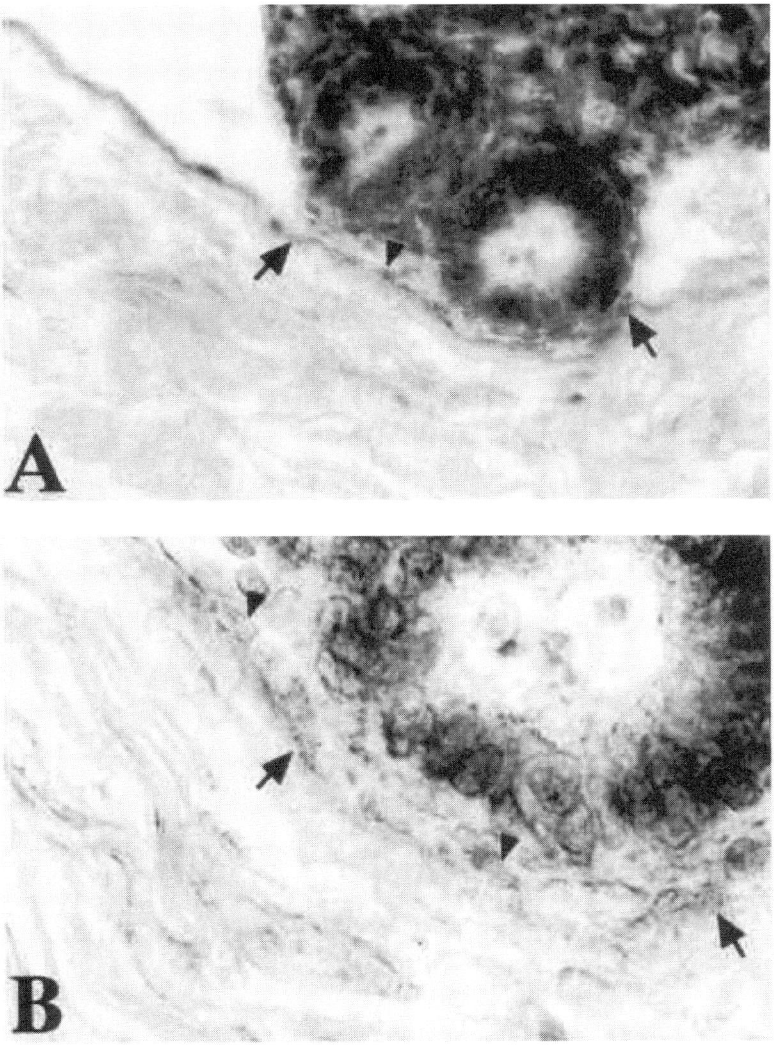

FIGURE 1. Endometrial fragment attached to explant of peritoneum with intact mesothelium. The mesothelium is labeled with monoclonal antibody to cytokeratin and stained with diaminobenzidine (*arrows*). Endometrial stromal cells are seen interposed between the endometrial glands and the mesothelium (*arrowheads*). **(A)** Low power view (original magnification: ×200; counterstain with hematoxylin). **(B)** High power view (original magnification: ×1000).

CA) at 568 nm. Rhodamine emission was detected using a 585-nm long-pass filter. Digital images of 512×512 pixels were recorded using a speed of 16 s/scan. Corresponding bright field images were also recorded. Fluorescein and rhodamine emissions were pseudocolorized with green and red, respectively. Images were processed for printing using Adobe Photoshop® (San Jose, CA) on a Dell personal

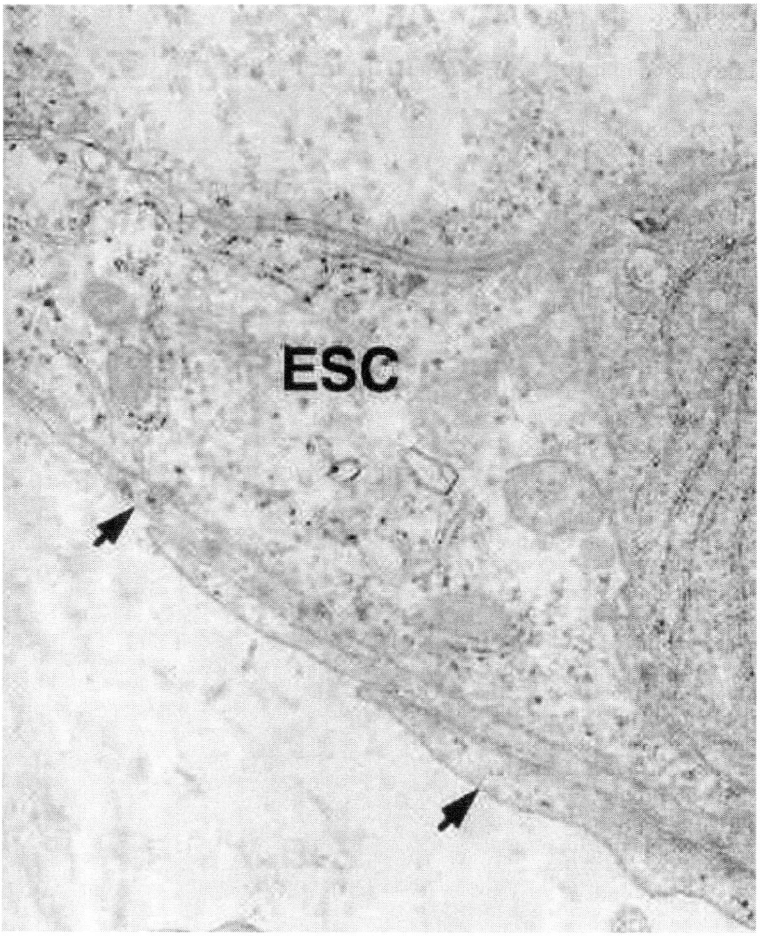

FIGURE 2. Transmission electron micrograph illustrating intact mesothelium (*arrows*) beneath an attached endometrial stromal cell (ESC). This section was taken through an endometrial implant similar to that seen in FIGURE 1. Attached cells were identified as endometrial stroma using light microscopy. Tissue was postfixed with osmium tetroxide. (Original magnification: ×15,000.)

computer (Austin, TX). Negative controls were performed by substituting nonimmune mouse immunoglobulin (Dako) for the primary antibody.

Transmission Electron Microscopy (TEM)

Sections of AP explants with ($n = 9$) and without ($n = 2$) dispersed endometrium were fixed in phosphate-buffered 4% formaldehyde/1% glutaraldehyde for 1 hour, postfixed with 1% osmium tetroxide for 30 min, and dehydrated in increasing concentrations of ethanol. The tissue was then embedded in Poly/Bed 812 Embedding

Resin (Polysciences, Inc., Warrington, PA). Ultrathin sections (70–90 nm) were examined under the transmission electron microscope.

RESULTS

Cultures (18–24 Hours)

The endometrial fragments adhered to the explants from both the AP and US. Using the dissecting microscope, endometrium could be seen attached to the mesothelial side and nonepithelial side of the AP and US. Endometrial fragments collected during the proliferative and secretory phase were found attached to the mesothelium.

Initial attempts with the dissecting microscope were made to quantitate the number of fragments attached to the mesothelium after 18–24 hours. There were no differences noted in the frequency of attachment of the endometrial fragments to the AP and US. However, this technique proved to be inaccurate in quantitating the amount of adherent endometrium. Serial sections of the explants taken at 50-μm intervals revealed a much larger number of small fragments that were not detected with the dissecting microscope. There was no obvious difference noted between the frequency of attachment of endometrium to the AP or US when collected during the proliferative or secretory phase of the cycle.

Under the majority (approximately 90%) of attached endometrial fragments, an intact layer of mesothelium could not be identified. Rather, an intact layer of mesothelium could be identified on either side of the attached fragment. However, in approximately 10% of the implants, an intact layer of mesothelium was identified beneath the endometrium. Serial 5-μm sections did not reveal a breach in the mesothelium (FIG. 1). TEM of several of these endometrial implants confirmed a continuous mesothelial layer at the site of attachment (FIG. 2).

In one implant of endometrium, an intact layer of mesothelium was identified with a single breach by an endometrial stromal cell. This was interpreted as possible invasion of the endometrial implant through the mesothelium and into the stroma of the peritoneum (FIG. 3). In all cases of attachment, endometrial stromal cells were found adherent to the AP and US. Endometrial glandular cells attached to the AP and US via intervening stromal cells. Direct attachment of endometrial glands to the mesothelium was not observed after 18–24 hours in culture.

Cultures (1 Hour)

Using H&E staining, all explants of peritoneum had endometrium attached after 1 hour of culture. In all but 3 explants, serial sections revealed endometrium that was adherent to intact mesothelium. There was no evidence of transmesothelial invasion at any site of attachment. Although there was no attempt to quantitate the number of attached endometrial fragments, there appeared to be a similar number of attached fragments from proliferative and secretory endometrium. In most cases, endometrium was adherent to mesothelium via endometrial stroma, although there were sites of endometrial epithelium-mesothelium attachment (FIG. 4).

In some areas underlying large endometrial fragments, a distinct layer of intact mesothelium was difficult to identify using H&E staining. When serial sections

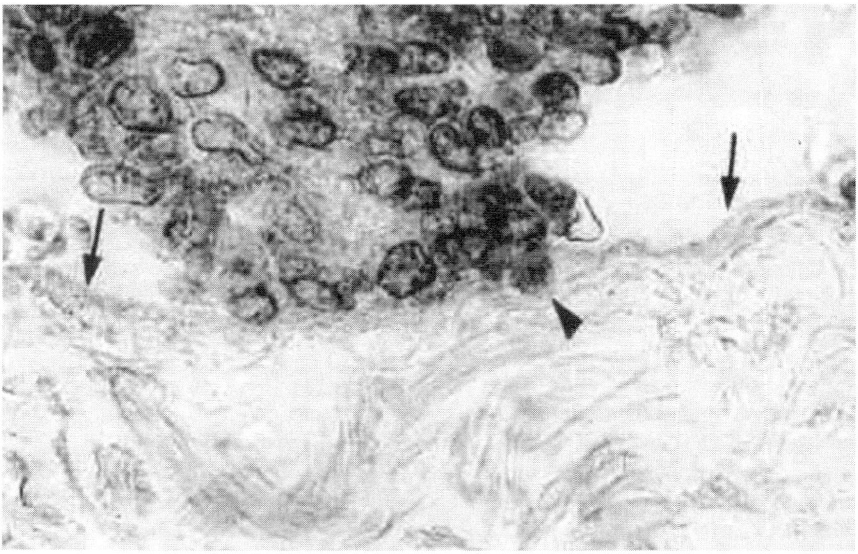

FIGURE 3. Early invasion of endometrial implant through the mesothelium. The mesothelium is labeled with monoclonal antibody to cytokeratin and stained with diaminobenzidine (*arrows*). An endometrial stromal cell (*arrowhead*) passing through the mesothelium is thought to represent the initial step of invasion into the stroma of the peritoneum. (Original magnification: ×1000; counterstain with hematoxylin.) [Figure reduced to 64%.]

were examined, the resolution of the CLSM allowed for identification of a distinct layer of cytokeratin-positive mesothelial cells underlying the site of endometrial attachment (FIG. 5A). In addition, cytokeratin labeling of epithelial cells differentiated endometrial epithelial cells (EECs) from endometrial stromal cells (ESCs) (FIG. 5B). There was no labeling of tissue when nonimmune mouse immunoglobulin was substituted for the anticytokeratin primary antibody (data not shown).

TEM demonstrated intact, viable mesothelial cells below sites of attachment. The mesothelial cell ultrastructure and the submesothelial extracellular matrix were identical to both immediately fixed and cultured control peritoneum (data not shown). FIGURE 6 illustrates attachment of EECs to intact, viable mesothelium. The endometrium appears to initially attach by binding to mesothelial cell microvillus processes.

DISCUSSION

Several *in vitro* models have been reported to study the interaction between tumor cells and endometrium with the peritoneum. Monolayer cultures of mesothelium from the rat and human have been used to evaluate the attachment of various tumor cell lines to the peritoneum.[9,10] Fresh whole sections of mouse peritoneum have been used in a similar model.[11] Monolayer cultures of human mesothelium have also been used to evaluate the effects of cytokines on the attachment of ESCs and whole endometrial fragments to mesothelium.[12,13]

In our studies, whole explants of human peritoneum and endometrium are used in a novel model of the initial attachment of endometrium to the peritoneum.[14,15] Human peritoneum was chosen for this model as there are no studies comparing the

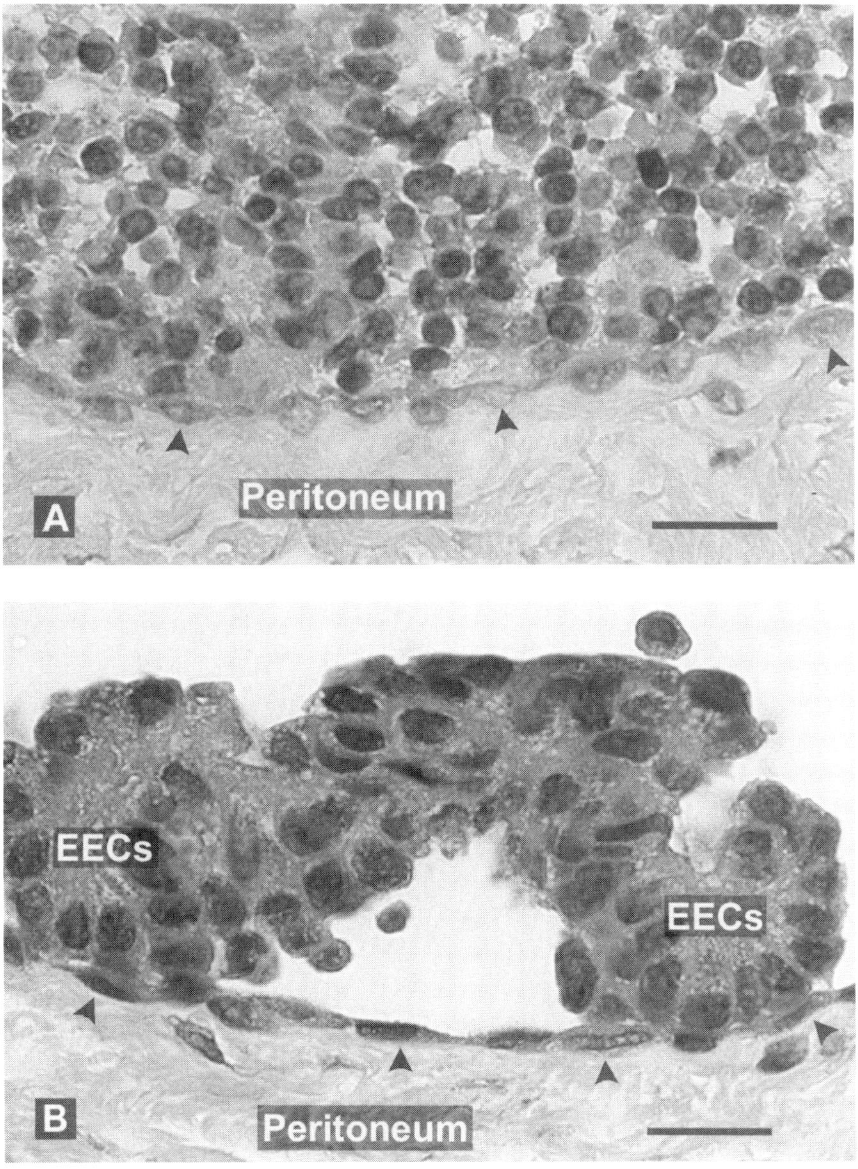

FIGURE 4. Hematoxylin and eosin stain demonstrating attachment of endometrial stroma (ESCs) **(A)** and epithelium (EECs) **(B)** to intact mesothelium (*arrowheads*). (Original magnification: ×250; bar = 20 μm.) [Figure reduced to 90%.]

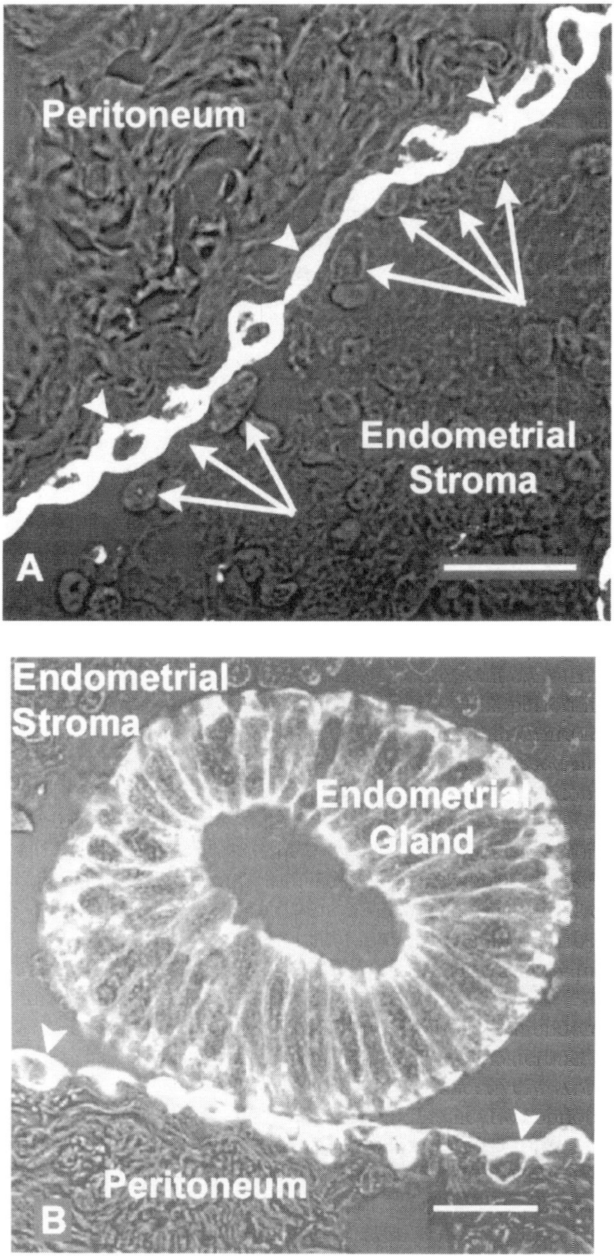

FIGURE 5. Confocal laser-scanning microscope image of **(A)** endometrial stromal cells (*white arrows*) and **(B)** an endometrial gland attached to an intact layer of mesothelial cells labeled with anticytokeratin antibody (*white arrowheads*). [(A) Original magnification: ×375; bar = 20 μm; (B) original magnification: ×300; bar = 20 μm.]

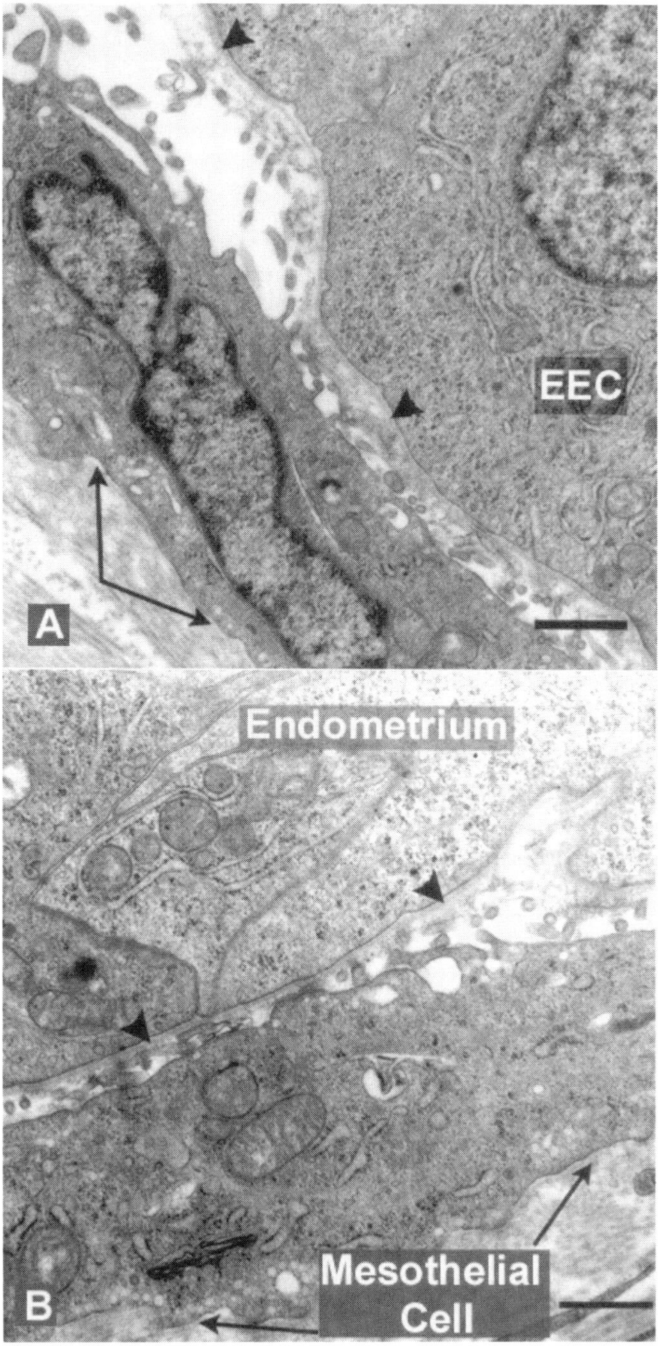

FIGURE 6. *See following page for legend.*

adhesion characteristics of animal peritoneum to human mesothelium *in vivo*. In addition, explants of peritoneum maintain mesothelial cell integrity over a normal basement membrane. This may represent a better model of attachment of endometrium than passaged mesothelial cells as previously reported.[12,13]

In our initial study using 18- to 24-hour cultures,[14] we demonstrated that mechanically dispersed endometrium could attach to the surface of the peritoneum. Serial sectioning of the endometrial implants allowed visualization of the points of attachment. Endometrium was adherent to intact mesothelium of peritoneum explants from tissue collected in both the proliferative and secretory phases. In all cases of adhesion to intact mesothelium, the endometrium was attached via stromal cells. Adhesion of endometrial epithelium to the mesothelium was not identified after 18–24 hours in culture.

These observations suggest that endometrium attaches to the peritoneum and then invades through the mesothelium in less than 18–24 hours. Using immunohistochemical staining, a break in the mesothelium was identified below the majority of the implants. In most cases, an intact layer of mesothelium could be identified running up to the edge of the endometrial implant. The earliest stage of the invasion of endometrium through the mesothelium is shown in FIGURE 3. Here, a small tongue of ESCs is invading through the mesothelium.

In contrast to our conclusions, some investigators have questioned the role of the mesothelial cell in the attachment of ectopic cells to the peritoneum. Groothuis *et al.* used light microscopy and TEM to study adhesion of proliferative-phase endometrium, from women without endometriosis, to peritoneal explants cultured for 16 hours.[16] Adhesion of endometrial fragments was observed only at locations where the mesothelium was absent or damaged and the basement was exposed. The authors concluded that intact mesothelium constitutes a defense barrier that prevents adhesion of endometrial fragments. They hypothesized that trauma to the mesothelial lining is a prerequisite for endometrial cell adhesion.[16]

Consequently, we elected to repeat our studies using a 1-hour incubation time to demonstrate that endometrium rapidly adheres to the peritoneum and to confirm our finding of endometrial attachment to intact mesothelium.[15] Using CLSM, the results clearly confirm endometrium attached to intact peritoneal mesothelium. Combined with our previous investigation of overnight peritoneal explant culture, this suggests that transmesothelial invasion of endometrium occurs between 1 and 18 hours.[14]

The 1-hour cultures also demonstrate that both ESCs and EECs, as well as stroma, can attach to mesothelium. It is unclear why we did not encounter epithelial cells attached to intact mesothelium when explants were examined following 18- to 24-hour culture. It is possible that EECs bind less firmly to mesothelial cells and later become detached.

In summary, these studies demonstrate that proliferative and secretory endometrial cells, both stroma and epithelium, adhere to intact mesothelium. It appears

---

FIGURE 6. Transmission electron microscopy demonstrating attachment of endometrial epithelium to intact mesothelial cells (*black arrows*). Interaction of mesothelial microvilli can be seen with the basement membrane (*black arrowheads*) of the endometrial epithelium. [(A) Original magnification: ×14,330; bar = 2 μm; (B) original magnification: ×28,150; bar = 1 μm.]

that endometrial attachment to the mesothelium occurs rapidly (i.e., within 1 hour) and transmesothelial invasion occurs within between 1 and 18–24 hours. We conclude that the mesothelium is not a "no-stick" surface and that molecules present at the surface of the mesothelium are likely involved in the pathogenesis of the early endometriotic lesion. We believe that investigation of mesothelial cell adhesion molecules is central to understanding the pathogenesis of endometriosis.

REFERENCES

1. Sampson, J. 1927. Peritoneal endometriosis is due to the menstrual dissemination of endometrial tissue into the peritoneal cavity. Am. J. Obstet. Gynecol. **14:** 422–469.
2. Jenkins, S., D.L. Olive & A.F. Haney. 1986. Endometriosis: pathogenic implications of the anatomic distribution. Obstet. Gynecol. **67:** 335–338.
3. Halme, J., M.G. Hammond, J.F. Hulka *et al.* 1984. Retrograde menstruation in healthy women and in patients with endometriosis. Obstet. Gynecol. **64:** 151–154.
4. Keetel, W.C. & R.J. Stein. 1951. The viability of the cast-off menstrual endometrium. Am. J. Obstet. Gynecol. **61:** 440.
5. Mungyer, G., W.N.P. Willemsen, R. Rolland *et al.* 1987. Cells of the mucous membrane of the female genital tract in culture: a comparative study with regard to the histogenesis of endometriosis. In Vitro Cell. Dev. Biol. **23:** 111–117.
6. Ridley, J.H. & I.K. Edwards. 1958. Experimental endometriosis in the human. Am. J. Obstet. Gynecol. **76:** 783.
7. van der Linden, P.J.Q., A.F. de Goeij, G.A. Dunselman *et al.* 1996. Endometrial cell adhesion in an *in vitro* model using intact amniotic membrane. Fertil. Steril. **65:** 76–80.
8. La Rocca, P. & J. Rheinwald. 1984. Coexpression of simple epithelia keratin and vimentin by human mesothelium and mesothelioma *in vivo* and in culture. Cancer Res. **44:** 2991–2995.
9. Sawada, M., J. Shii, H. Akedo & O. Tanizawa. 1994. An experimental model for ovarian tumor invasion of cultured mesothelial cell monolayer. Lab. Invest. **70:** 333–338.
10. Niedbala, M., K. Crickard & R. Bernacki. 1985. Interactions of human ovarian tumor cells with human mesothelial cells grown on extracellular matrix. Exp. Cell Res. **160:** 499–513.
11. Asao, T., S. Yazawa, S. Kudo *et al.* 1994. A novel *ex vivo* model for assaying adhesion of cancer cells to the peritoneum. Cancer Lett. **78:** 57–62.
12. Zhang, R., R.A. Wild & J.M. Ojago. 1993. Effect of tumor necrosis factor-α on adhesion of human endometrial stromal cells to peritoneal mesothelial cells: an *in vitro* system. Fertil. Steril. **59:** 1196–1201.
13. Wild, R.A., R. Zhang & D. Medders. 1994. Whole fragments form characteristics of *in vivo* endometriosis in a mesothelial cell co-culture system: an *in vitro* model of the histogenesis of endometriosis. J. Soc. Gynecol. Invest. **1:** 165–168.
14. Witz, C.A., I.A. Montoya-Rodriguez & R.S. Schenken. 1999. Whole peritoneal explants—a novel model of the early endometriosis lesion. Fertil. Steril. **71:** 56–60.
15. Witz, C.A., M.R. Thomas, I.A. Montoya-Rodriguez *et al.* 2001. Short-term culture of peritoneum explants confirms attachment of endometrium to intact peritoneal mesothelium. Fertil. Steril. **75:** 385–390.
16. Groothuis, P.G., C.A. Koks, A.F. de Goeij *et al.* 1999. Adhesion of human endometrial fragments to peritoneum *in vitro*. Fertil. Steril. **71:** 1119–1124.

A Modified Baboon Model for Endometriosis

ASGERALLY T. FAZLEABAS,[a] ALLISON BRUDNEY,[a] BILGIN GURATES,[a] DANIEL CHAI,[b] AND SERDAR BULUN[a]

[a]*Department of Obstetrics and Gynecology, University of Illinois at Chicago, Chicago, Illinois 60612, USA*

[b]*Institute for Primate Research, Nairobi, Kenya*

ABSTRACT: Endometriosis is one of the most common causes of infertility and chronic pelvic pain and affects 1 in 10 women in the reproductive-age group. Although existence of this disease has been known for over 100 years, our current knowledge of its pathogenesis, the pathophysiology of related infertility, and its spontaneous evolution is limited. Several reasons contribute to our lack of knowledge, the most critical being the difficulty in carrying out objective long-term studies in women. Thus, we and others have developed the baboon as an appropriate nonhuman primate to study the etiology of this disease. We suggested that endometriosis develops in two distinct phases. Phase I is invasive and dependent on ovarian steroids. Phase II, which is the active phase of the disease, is characterized by endogenous estrogen biosynthesis. Following inoculation with menstrual endometrial tissues in two consecutive menstrual cycles, baboons develop lesions that are similar to those seen in humans. Laparoscopy at 1, 4, and 10 months revealed a preponderance of red raised nodules at the first month, while both red lesions and reddish-blue proliferative endometriotic lesions were evident at 4 and 10 months. The presence of glandular tissue and stromal fibroblasts in these lesions was confirmed by histology. Lesions obtained at 1 and 4 months expressed estrogen receptor β (ERβ), matrix metalloproteinase-7 (MMP-7), and vascular endothelial growth factor (VEGF) predominantly. However, aromatase expression was only readily evident at 10 months, although some lesions obtained at 4 months expressed low levels of aromatase. Therefore, our preliminary data suggest that endometriosis can be artificially induced in baboons, and the role of exogenous and endogenous estradiol in proliferation, angiogenesis, and immune modulations can now be evaluated in a potentially systemic manner.

KEYWORDS: baboon; endometriosis; model; steroid receptors; gene expression

INTRODUCTION

Endometriosis is an estrogen-dependent gynecological condition that affects an estimated 5 million American women during their reproductive life span. Although multiple theories exist regarding the etiology of the disease, the implantation hypothesis of Sampson[1] is the most widely accepted. According to Sampson's theory,[1] fragments of menstrual endometrium are refluxed through the fallopian

Address for correspondence: Asgi T. Fazleabas, Ph.D., Department of Obstetrics and Gynecology, University of Illinois at Chicago, 820 South Wood Street (M/C 808), Chicago, IL 60612-7313. Voice: 312-996-0994; fax: 312-996-4238.
asgi@uic.edu

tubes into the peritoneal cavity and then attach and grow on peritoneal surfaces. However, the fundamental mechanisms by which menstrual endometrium adheres, proliferates, and establishes a functional vasculature in an ectopic site remain to be elucidated. The baboon is a valuable and clinically relevant model to study the etiology and consequences to fertility of this enigmatic disease.[2] Experimental evidence indicates that intrapelvic injections of menstrual endometrium can induce endometriosis in this primate, thereby supporting the basic tenets of Sampson's hypothesis.[1]

THE BABOON AS A MODEL

Endometriosis is defined as the presence of endometrium-like tissue outside of the uterine cavity. It is one of the most common causes of infertility and chronic pelvic pain and affects 1 in 10 women in the reproductive-age group.[3] This incidence increases up to 30% in patients with infertility and up to 45% in patients with chronic pelvic pain.[4] As other common chronic diseases such as diabetes mellitus and asthma, endometriosis is inherited in a polygenic manner with a complex and multifactorial etiology. The existence of this condition has been known for more than 100 years. However, our current knowledge of its pathogenesis, the pathophysiology of related infertility, and its spontaneous evolution is limited. Several reasons contribute to our lack of knowledge. First, at the time of diagnosis, most patients have had the disease for an extended period of time, therefore making it difficult to study etiology and progression. Second, because of individual differences in progression and symptomatology of the disease, it is difficult to carry out objective long-term studies in women. Finally, endometriosis only occurs naturally in humans and nonhuman primates. Thus, because of ethical and practical considerations that limit studies in humans, it follows that an appropriate animal model needs to be developed. Rodent models, particularly those using immunocompromised mice, have been developed and are advantageous from both a cost standpoint and the ability to study the behavior and biochemistry of the human endometrium *in vivo* due to limited graft rejection. Valuable data have been obtained with regard to the role of MMPs, secretory proteins, and cytokines on transplanted eutopic human endometrium from the proliferative and secretory stages of the menstrual cycle. In contrast, the disadvantages of rodent models employing transplantation of homologous uterine tissues are numerous. The anatomy and physiology of the rodent endometrium do not apply to the human endometrium, and rodents do not develop endometriosis. In addition, induction of endometriosis, which is performed through autotransplantation of endometrial fragments or uterine tissues, is not physiological. The types of lesions that result are quite different from those found in humans.[5–7] On the other hand, experimental endometriosis caused by intraperitoneal injections of menstrual endometrium into baboons supports Sampson's hypothesis.[8,9] This method of induction resulted in red raised and reddish-blue implants to scarred lesions with powder burn appearance that were macroscopically similar to those seen in women with spontaneous endometriosis. In this experimental model, the proportion of red lesions were also higher, supporting the concept that these lesions represent the active form of the disease.[7] In a few instances, endometrial explants lacking hemosiderin, which are white opaque lesions, were also evident.

Although more expensive than most other species, the baboon offers a clear advantage for basic studies focused on endometriosis. First, it is phylogenetically very close to humans and shares many ancestral characters.[10] Second, detailed accounts of baboon reproductive anatomy and physiology, similar to that of humans, are available, including menstrual cycle characteristics, embryo implantation, and fetal development.[11] Our group has been at the forefront of studies relating to uterine receptivity and implantation in the baboon.[12] Third, the baboon is a proven model for research in cardiovascular and endoscopic surgery, endocrinology, teratology, toxicology, testing of contraceptive agents,[13,14] and endometrial and placental development.[12,15] Fourth, the baboon is a continuous breeder that has menstrual cycles throughout the year, which continue in captivity.[14] Fifth, the baboon is a larger and stronger primate than the rhesus or cynomolgus monkey, allowing for repetitive blood sampling and complex experimental surgery.[14] Sixth, specific advantages of the baboon model in gynecologic research include the spontaneous presence of peritoneal fluid and the accessibility of the uterine cavity through the cervix, allowing endometrial sampling without hysterotomy.[8] Seventh, spontaneous endometriosis in the baboon has been found to range from minimal[16] to disseminated forms,[17] similar to the various stages of disease in women. For all these reasons, the baboon is considered to be a good model for research in reproduction and specifically for endometriosis in this context.[2]

The experimentally induced baboon endometriosis model was first established by D'Hooghe *et al.*[8] in a series of extensive studies at the Institute for Primate Research in Nairobi, Kenya.[2] Intraperitoneal injection of menstrual endometrium resulted in endometriosis as defined by incidence of endometriotic lesions, histological criteria, and cycle fecundity.[8] We have refined the original procedure described by D'Hooghe *et al.*[8] and have been successful in inducing the disease with menstrual endometrium in a total of 12 baboons at both the University of Illinois at Chicago and the Institute for Primate Research in Nairobi.

We have proposed in our experimental model that endometriosis develops in two distinct phases. Phase I is invasive and dependent on ovarian steroids. Phase II, which is the active phase of the disease, is characterized by endogenous estrogen biosynthesis as a consequence of aromatase expression in these lesions.[18]

INDUCTION OF THE DISEASE

Menstrual endometrium (0.84 ± 0.22 g) was harvested on day 2 of menses using a Unimar Pipelle just prior to laparoscopy. The peritoneal cavity and reproductive tract were visualized by laparoscopy in the minimal invasive surgical suite and the absence of any lesions or adhesions was documented by video recording. Under laparoscopic guidance, the menstrual tissue in Pipelle was deposited at three sites: the pouch of Douglas, the broad ligament adjacent to the oviducts, and the ovaries. At the subsequent menses, the animals underwent a second laparoscopy and endometrial reseeding at the same ectopic sites. Following the second seeding and the third menses, laparoscopy was performed to evaluate the extent of endometriosis. Subsequent laparoscopies were performed at 4 and 10 months following the initial inoculation as the second and third diagnostic operative laparoscopies. Initially, the peritoneal cavity was visualized, and the presence of lesions documented by video recording. Then, endometriotic lesions and portions of normal peritoneum were biopsied using a harmonic scalpel under laparoscopic guidance. During laparoscopies, eutopic endometrium was obtained by Pipelle biopsy. Portions of the tissue were snap-frozen in liquid nitrogen for RNA extraction or fixed in buffered formalin for histology. These data indicate that intraperitoneal injections of menstrual endometrium result in endometriotic lesions, thereby substantiating the Sampson hypothesis.[1]

EVALUATION OF THE LESIONS

Endometriosis can take on a variety of appearances. A wide range of lesion types that were described in humans were also evident in the baboon model. For example, red raised nodules on the superficial peritoneum or reddish-blue proliferative endometriotic nodules are most commonly encountered in the baboon. The white opaque peritoneal nodules that lack hemosiderin were also evident. The classic brownish focal adhesions were only observed at 10 months. In the baboon, the majority of lesions that resulted following inoculation of menstrual endometrium were observed on the peritoneum and uterine surface. There was no evidence of ovarian implants that are termed endometriomas, which are commonly observed in women. Previous studies in the baboon also failed to detect any evidence of endometriomas.[2] The lesions that were present on the peritoneum and uterine surface at 1 and 4 months were primarily raised red lesions or reddish-blue lesions (FIG. 1). Larger lesions obtained from the animals at 10 months postinoculation were more comparable to the "chocolate cysts" described in humans. There was also evidence of significant adhesion of the peritoneum to the ovary as the disease progressed.

Microscopic evaluation of endometriotic lesions should reveal endometrial glands and stroma, along with evidence of fibrosis and hemorrhage. Pathological confirmation of the disease traditionally requires the presence of at least two of these components. In our baboon model, we established the criteria that both endometrial glands and stroma have to be evident in lesions that were classified as being endometriosis. Based on these criteria, it is evident that baboon lesions that result following the artificial induction of the disease do have distinct endometrial glands and stroma (FIG. 2). A high degree of vascularization as evidenced by the presence of capillaries in the surrounding peritoneum was also evident (FIG. 2A).

Progression of endometriosis is dependent on ovarian steroids. Radioligand binding studies suggested that both ER and PR are present in endometriotic lesions.[19] These were later confirmed by immunocytochemical data.[20,21] However, in contrast to the normal endometrium, receptor content in endometriotic explants was heterogenous and did not undergo cyclic changes that are evident in the normal endometrium. In our baboon studies, early (at 1 and 4 months) endometriotic lesions were primarily harvested on day 10 postovulation. In a few animals, lesions were also harvested during menstruation and in the proliferative phase of the cycle. Immunocytochemical analyses for ERα, ERβ, and PR revealed that ERβ was the dominant steroid receptor present in endometriotic explants regardless of the phase of the cycle. ERα and PR were present at lower levels compared to eutopic endometrium from the same baboon and did not show the predictable cyclic changes.[22] Thus, it is evident from these studies that experimentally induced endometriosis is histologically similar to that obtained from women with spontaneous disease. Further, the presence of steroid receptors, particularly ERβ, suggests that these lesions can respond to both exogenous and endogenous estrogen at all phases of the menstrual cycle.

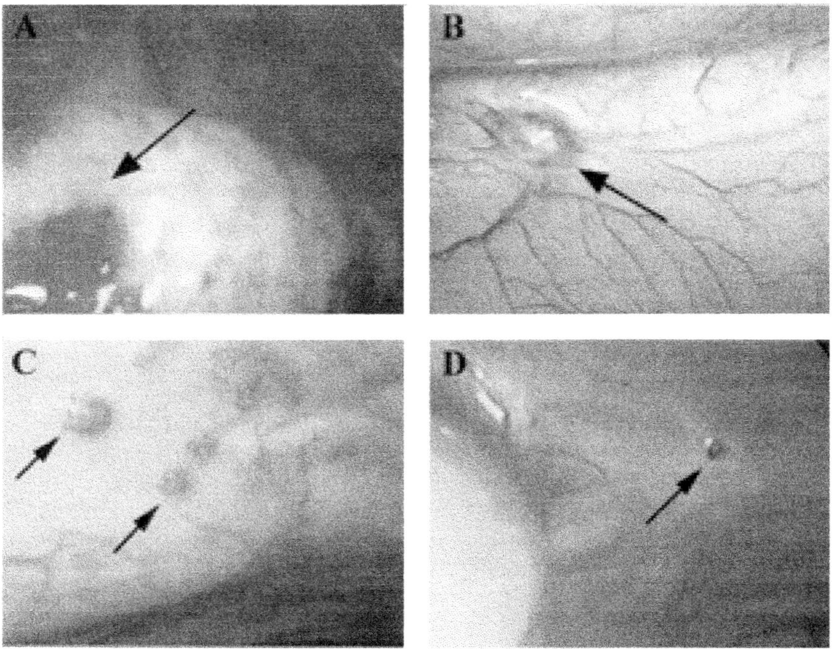

FIGURE 1. Laparoscopic evaluation of endometriotic lesions. Panels A and B are observed at 1 month postinoculation, while panels C and D are from an animal at the 4-month time point. Note that red (A, C), blue (D), and powder burn (B) lesions are all evident in the experimental baboon model.

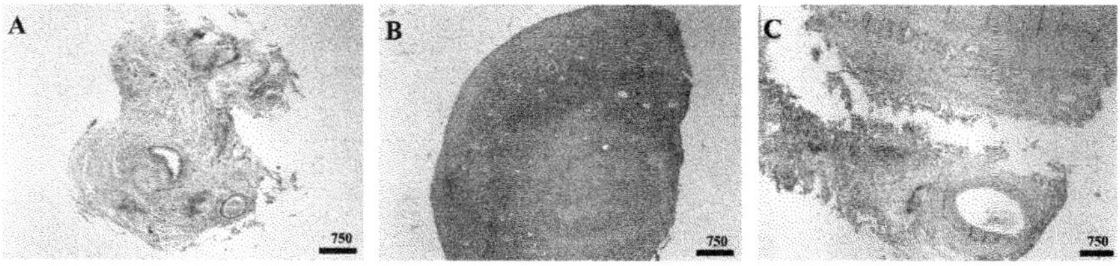

FIGURE 2. Histological evaluation of lesions. Panel A is a section through a red lesion obtained at 1 month, panel B is a section through a blue lesion obtained at 4 months, and panel C is a section through a chocolate cyst obtained at 10 months. Note that glands and stroma are evident in all sections. Hemosiderin is readily evident in panels A and C, and note also the adherence to the ovary at 10 months (C). Bar: 750 μm.

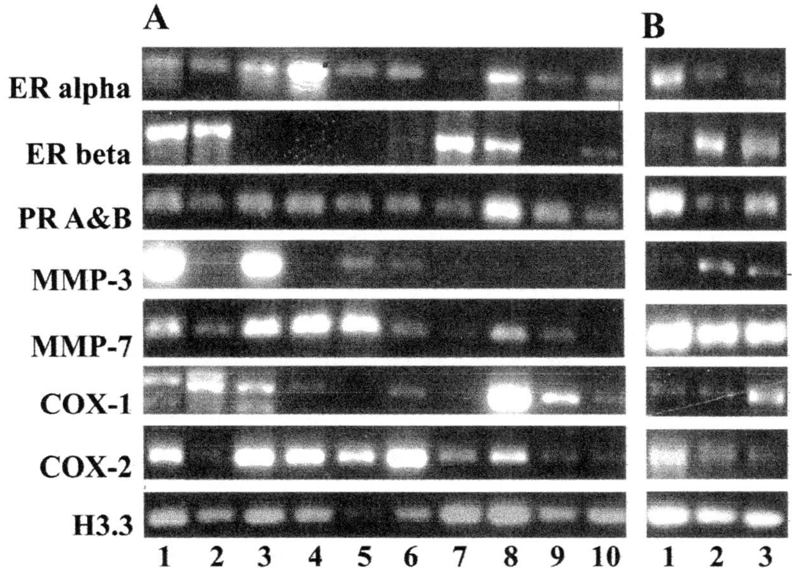

FIGURE 3. Ethidium bromide–stained RT-PCR gel from tissues obtained at 1 month (A) and 10 months (B). Each product is noted on the left side of the gel. For each primer: lane 1, specific positive control; lane 2, endometriotic cells from a human ovarian endometrium; lanes 5–10, tissues from the same animal who had experimentally induced endometriosis; lanes 3–5, baboon menstrual endometrium; lane 6, eutopic endometrium on day 10 PO; lane 7, normal peritoneum; lane 8, red endometriotic lesion (FIG. 1A); lane 9, endometriotic deep nodule; lane 10, endometriosis-associated adhesion.

MOLECULAR ANALYSIS OF ENDOMETRIOTIC LESIONS

Preliminary studies on endometriotic lesions from baboons support our overall hypothesis that the disease is established in two phases. The RT-PCR data from tissues obtained in phase I are shown in FIGURES 3A and 4A. Eutopic and ectopic tissues were harvested on day 10 postovulation (PO), following two intraperitoneal inoculations as described above (phase I of the disease). RT-PCR using specific primers that had been validated for baboon tissues[23] were used to document the expression of ERα, ERβ, PR, MMP-3, MMP-7, COX-1, and COX-2 in endometriotic lesions. The histone gene H3.3 was used as an internal standard. These expression patterns were compared with menstrual endometrium (starting inoculating material), eutopic endometrium obtained on the same day (day 10 PO) as the lesion biopsies, and stromal cells from human endometriomas.

As expected, ERα was expressed in all tissues, except for the normal peritoneum (FIG. 3A). In contrast, intense expression of ERβ, a recently identified form of the estrogen receptor,[24] was only evident in endometriotic tissues from baboons and humans (FIG. 3A; lanes 2 and 8). Interestingly, normal peritoneum also expressed ERβ (FIG. 3A; lane 7). PR A and B did not show much variability and were present

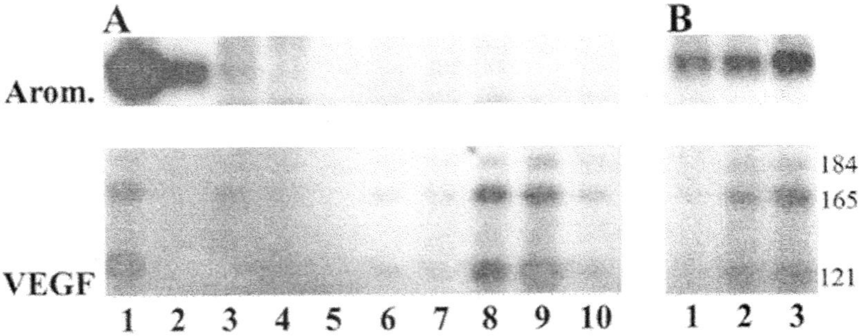

FIGURE 4. Autoradiographic film of ^{32}P-labeled RT-PCR products from the same samples shown in FIGURE 3. Each product is noted on the left side of the gel. For each primer: lane 1, specific positive control; lane 2, endometriotic cells from a human ovarian endometrium; lanes 5–10, tissues from the same animal who had experimentally induced endometriosis; lanes 3–5, baboon menstrual endometrium; lane 6, eutopic endometrium on day 10 PO; lane 7, normal peritoneum; lane 8, red endometriotic lesion (FIG. 1A); lane 9, endometriotic deep nodule; lane 10, endometriosis-associated adhesion.

at all times. In addition, PR expression was also evident in normal peritoneum, which confirms previous data from human tissues.[25]

The MMPs are thought to play a critical role in tissue remodeling and tumor invasion.[26] They have also been associated with the establishment of endometriosis, and their suppression inhibits the establishment of ectopic lesions in a nude mouse model.[27] Of the two MMPs analyzed in our study, MMP-7 was most intensely expressed in all three samples of menstrual endometrium (FIG. 3A; lanes 3–5), an observation consistent with our previous studies.[28] MMP-3, in contrast, was higher at day 2 of menses (FIG. 3A; lanes 3 and 5) compared to day 3 (FIG. 3A; lane 4). In the early lesions (phase I), MMP-7 expression was most evident (FIG. 3A; lanes 8 and 9).

Cyclooxygenases (COX) are the rate-limiting enzymes for prostaglandin (PG) biosynthesis: COX-1 expression is highest in the endometriotic lesions (FIG. 3A; lanes 8 and 9). Menstrual endometrium had a low level of expression of COX-1, but it was evident in the eutopic endometrium at day 10 PO as previously reported.[23] In contrast, COX-2 expression was evident in all samples. However, in spite of the ability of these early lesions to express both COX-1 and COX-2, aromatase was not evident during phase I of the disease (FIG. 4A; lanes 8 and 9), whereas VEGF (predominantly $VEGF_{165}$ and $VEGF_{121}$) was highly expressed in the endometriotic lesions (FIG. 4A; lanes 8 and 9). COX-2 expression and resulting PGE_2 synthesis have been postulated to be essential for aromatase expression in endometriotic stromal cells obtained from women.[18]

Collectively, these data suggest that MMP-7 is the dominant metalloproteinase during the initial establishment of the disease (phase I) and may regulate the invasive potential of the endometriotic tissue. The high expression of COX-1 and VEGF in endometriotic lesions could enhance PG-mediated vasodilation locally and could enable the ectopic tissues to utilize the VEGF-mediated angiogenesis necessary for survival.

The data shown in FIGURES 3B and 4B represent tissues obtained at 10 months (phase II) following the establishment of the disease. The tissue was obtained during the late proliferative phase. The stage of the cycle was confirmed by the high levels of expression of ER, PR, and MMP-7 in the eutopic endometrium.[22,28] Both MMP-3 and MMP-7 expression are now increased, while both COX-1 and COX-2 continue to be evident. Interestingly, however, aromatase expression now increases markedly in both eutopic and endometriotic lesions (FIG. 4B; phase II), in contrast to the lack of expression in phase I.

SUMMARY AND CONCLUSIONS

Our novel observation of ERβ expression specifically in endometriotic tissues of baboons provides a mechanism by which this estrogen-dependent disease can establish itself in the peritoneum and further supports reports in human endometriosis.[29] Taylor *et al.*[30] reported that estradiol has a rapid and direct effect on VEGF expression in endometrial stromal cells. More recent studies[26,28] have suggested that MMP-7 expression is also modulated by estradiol in the baboon and human endometrium. In addition, estradiol has also been shown to enhance IL-1-induced expression of monocyte chemotactic protein-1 in endometrial cells obtained from women with endometriosis.[31] Collectively, these data imply that estradiol could modulate three major components associated with endometriosis—that is, angiogenesis, proteolysis associated with cell migration, and macrophage infiltration.[32] Furthermore, since progesterone enhances rather than suppresses ERβ,[33] this mechanism will enable this ectopic tissue to respond to the estrogenic stimulus at all stages of the menstrual cycle. Alternatively, since endometriotic tissues have been reported to be progesterone-resistant,[34,35] low levels of ERα expression are also maintained, ensuring that the required estrogenic stimulus is not affected.

In addition, when endometriotic lesions were harvested at 10 months following menstrual seeding, aromatase expression was readily evident. This would substantiate the data in human studies in which high aromatase expression has been documented in tissues of women with severe disease.[36]

The direct and indirect roles of both exogenous and endogenous estradiol in the establishment and maintenance of endometriosis in women have been confirmed previously by the use of GnRH agonists to suppress ovarian cyclicity[37] and aromatase inhibitor treatment.[18] However, the studies with women and human tissues are prospective following diagnosis of the disease. Our baboon model, in contrast, affords the opportunity to understand both the endocrine and intracrine effects of estradiol and its ability to modulate many of the mechanisms associated with ectopic transplantation of the menstrual endometrium.

ACKNOWLEDGMENTS

This work was supported by a University of Illinois Center Seed Grant from the Vice-Chancellor for Research and by NIH Fogarty Grant No. TW01339.

REFERENCES

1. SAMPSON, J.A. 1927. Peritoneal endometriosis due to menstrual dissemination of endometrial tissue into the peritoneal cavity. Am. J. Obstet. Gynecol. **14:** 422–469.
2. D'HOOGHE, T.M. 1997. Clinical relevance of the baboon as a model for the study of endometriosis. Fertil. Steril. **68:** 613–625.
3. ESKENAZI, B. & M. WARNER. 1997. Epidemiology of endometriosis. Obstet. Gynecol. Clin. North Am. **24:** 235–258.
4. GRUPPO ITALIANO. 1994. Prevalence and anatomical distribution of endometriosis in women with selected gynecological conditions: results from a multicentric Italian study (Gruppo Italiano per lo Studio dell'Endometriosi). Hum. Reprod. **9:** 1158–1162.
5. JANSEN, R.P.S. & P. RUSSELL. 1986. Nonpigmented endometriosis: clinical, laparoscopic, and pathologic definitions. Am. J. Obstet. Gynecol. **155:** 1160–1163.
6. MARTIN, D.C., G.D. HUBERT, R. VANDER *et al.* 1989. Laparoscopic appearances of peritoneal endometriosis. Fertil. Steril. **51:** 63–67.
7. NISOLLE, M., F. CASANAS-ROUX, V. ANAF *et al.* 1993. Morphometric study of the stromal vascularization in peritoneal endometriosis. Fertil. Steril. **59:** 681–684.
8. D'HOOGHE, T.M., C.S. BAMBRA, B.M. RAEYMAEKERS *et al.* 1995. Intrapelvic injection of menstrual endometrium causes endometriosis in baboons (*Papio cynocephalus*, *Papio anubis*). Am. J. Obstet. Gynecol. **173:** 125–134.
9. D'HOOGHE, T.M., C.S. BAMBRA & J.A. HILL. 1997. A very sticky riddle [letter]. Fertil. Steril. **67:** 182–183.
10. MARKS, J. 1982. Evolutionary tempo and phylogenetic inference based on primate karyotypes. Cytogenet. Cell Genet. **34:** 261–264.
11. HENDRICKX, A.G. 1971. Reproduction methods. *In* Embryology of the Baboon, pp. 1–44. University of Chicago Press. Chicago.
12. FAZLEABAS, A.T., J.J. KIM, S. SRINIVASAN *et al.* 1999. Implantation in the baboon: endometrial responses. Semin. Reprod. Endocrinol. **17:** 257–265.
13. D'HOOGHE, T.M., C.S. BAMBRA, I.O. FARAH *et al.* 1993. High intra-abdominal pressure during laparoscopy: effects on clinical parameters and lung pathology in baboons (*Papio anubis*, *Papio cynocephalus*). Am. J. Obstet. Gynecol. **169:** 1352–1356.
14. ISAHAKIA, M.A. & C.S. BAMBRA. 1990. Primate models for research in reproduction. *In* Gamete Interaction: Prospects for Immunocontraception, pp. 487–500. Wiley-Liss. New York.
15. PIJNENBORG, R., T. D'HOOGHE, L. VERCRUYSSE *et al.* 1996. Evaluation of trophoblast invasion in placental bed biopsies of the baboon, with immunocytochemical localization of cytokeratin, fibronectin, and laminin. J. Med. Primatol. **25:** 272–281.
16. MERRILL, J.A. 1968. Spontaneous endometriosis in the Kenya baboon. Am. J. Obstet. Gynecol. **101:** 569–570.
17. FOLSE, D.S. & L.C. STOUT. 1978. Endometriosis in the baboon. Lab. Anim. Sci. **28:** 217–219.
18. BULUN, S.E., K.M. ZEITOUN, K. TAKAYAMA *et al.* 2000. Estrogen biosynthesis in endometriosis: molecular basis and clinical relevance. J. Mol. Endocrinol. **25:** 35–42.
19. JÄNNE, O., A. KAUPPILA, E. KOKKO *et al.* 1981. Estrogen and progestin receptors in endometriosis lesions: comparison with endometrial tissue. Am. J. Obstet. Gynecol. **141:** 562–566.
20. BERGQVIST, A., S. JEPPSSON & O. LJUNBERG. 1985. Histochemical demonstration of estrogen and progesterone binding in endometriotic tissue and in uterine endometrium: a comparative study. J. Histochem. Cytochem. **33:** 155–161.
21. LESSEY, B., D. METZGER, A. HANEY *et al.* 1989. Immunohistochemical analysis of estrogen and progesterone receptors in endometriosis: comparison with normal endometrium during the menstrual cycle and the effect of medical therapy. Fertil. Steril. **51:** 409–415.
22. HILD-PETITO, S., H.G. VERHAGE & A.T. FAZLEABAS. 1992. Immunocytochemical localization of estrogen and progestin receptors in the baboon (*Papio anubis*) uterus during implantation and pregnancy. Endocrinology **130:** 2343–2353.

23. KIM, J.J., J. WANG, C. BAMBRA *et al.* 1999. Expression of cyclooxygenase-1 and -2 in the baboon endometrium during the menstrual cycle and pregnancy. Endocrinology **140:** 2672–2678.
24. KUIPER, G.G.J.M., E. ENMARK, M. PELTO-HUKKO *et al.* 1996. Cloning of a novel estrogen receptor in the rat prostate. Proc. Natl. Acad. Sci. U.S.A. **93:** 5925–5930.
25. HIGUCHI, T., S. NARUKAWA, H. KANZAKI *et al.* 1995. Expression of messenger of ribonucleic acid for gonadal steroid receptors in the human pelvic peritoneum. Fertil. Steril. **63:** 52–57.
26. COX, K.E., K.L. SHARPE-TIMMS *et al.* 2000. Stromelysin-1 (MMP-3) and matrilysin (MMP-7) are differentially regulated in the baboon endometrium. J. Soc. Gynecol. Invest. **7:** 242–248.
27. MATRISIAN, L.M. 1992. The matrix degrading metalloproteinases. Bioassays **14:** 455–463.
28. BRUNNER, K.L., L.M. MATRISIAN, W.H. RODGERS *et al.* 1997. Suppression of matrix metalloproteinases inhibits establishment of ectopic lesions by human endometrium in nude mice. J. Clin. Invest. **99:** 2851–2857.
29. FUJIMOTO, J., R. HIROSE, H. SAKAGUCHI *et al.* 1999. Expression of oestrogen receptor alpha and beta in ovarian endometriomata. Mol. Hum. Reprod. **5:** 742–747.
30. SHIFREN, J., J. TSENG, C. ZALOUDEK *et al.* 1996. Ovarian steroid regulation of vascular endothelial growth factor in the human endometrium: implications for angiogenesis during the menstrual cycle and in the pathogenesis of endometriosis. J. Clin. Endocrinol. Metab. **81:** 3112–3118.
31. AKOUM, A., C. JOLICOEUR & A. BOUCHER. 2000. Estradiol amplifies IL-1 induced monocyte chemotactic protein-1 expression by ectopic endometrial cells of women with endometriosis. J. Clin. Endocrinol. Metab. **85:** 896–904.
32. TAYLOR, R.N., I.P. RYAN, E.S. MOORE *et al.* 1997. Angiogenesis and macrophage activation in endometriosis. Ann. N.Y. Acad. Sci. **828:** 194–207.
33. TESSIER, C., S. DEB, A. PRIGENT-TESSIER *et al.* 2000. Estrogen receptors alpha and beta in rat decidua cells: cell-specific expression and differential regulation by steroid hormones and prolactin. Endocrinology **141:** 3842–3851.
34. ZEITOUN, K., K. TAKAYAMA, H. SASANO *et al.* 1998. Deficient 17β-hydroxysteroid dehydrogenase type 2 expression in endometriosis: failure to metabolize 17β-estradiol. J. Clin. Endocrinol. Metab. **83:** 4474–4480.
35. ATTIA, G.R., K. ZEITOUN, D. EDWARDS *et al.* 2000. Progesterone receptor isoform A, but not B is expressed in endometriosis. J. Clin. Endocrinol. Metab. **85:** 2897–2902.
36. NOBLE, L.S., E.R. SIMPSON, A. JOHNS *et al.* 1996. Aromatase expression in endometriosis. J. Clin. Endocrinol. Metab. **81:** 174–179.
37. HURST, B.S. & J.A. ROCK. 1989. Endometriosis: pathophysiology, diagnosis, and treatment. Obstet. Gynecol. Surv. **44:** 297–304.

Using Rats as a Research Model for the Study of Endometriosis

KATHY L. SHARPE-TIMMS

Department of Obstetrics and Gynecology, University of Missouri-Columbia, Columbia, Missouri 65212, USA

ABSTRACT: Although there are disadvantages of extrapolating data across species, the rat model may be used to study events involved in the pathogenesis and pathophysiologies of endometriosis or novel therapeutic approaches for this disorder that are not accessible in humans. Rat endometriotic tissues are similar to human lesions *in vivo*, and rat endometriotic tissues and cells perform in a similar manner as human endometriotic tissues and cells in organ explant culture and isolated cell culture. The rat model permits studies of mechanisms and regulators in a controlled manner free from confounding influences such as individual patient variation and environmental influences. The primary method used for induction of endometriosis in rats has been autotransplantation of uterine squares (implants) into the peritoneal cavity. Beyond mere growth of endometrium in ectopic locations, rats with endometriosis display similar symptoms, including a reduction in fertility and fecundity, and the endometriotic implants react similarly to therapeutics as those of humans with the disease. Similar alterations in gene expression and protein production have been observed in endometriotic tissues from rats and humans that may, in part, be causative agents involved in the pathogenesis or pathophysiologies of endometriosis.

KEYWORDS: endometriosis; endometrium; pathogenesis; pathophysiology; rat model; therapeutics

CURRENT STATE OF KNOWLEDGE

In the 1920s, attempts at establishing animal models for endometriosis, in the rabbit and in the monkey, were reported.[1,2] Since this pioneering work, a variety of surgical techniques have been developed for induction of endometriosis in a variety of species.[3] The method of choice for induction of endometriosis in rats has been autotransplantation of uterine squares into the peritoneal cavity.[4] This model consists of obtaining several equal-size pieces (2×2 mm) of uterine tissue from ablation of one of the two uterine horns. Rats have a bicornuate uterus, consisting of two equal parts; thus, endometriotic implants can be compared to the remaining intact uterine tissue (the nonablated horn).[5–14] The uterine squares, called implants, are autotransplanted to the arterial cascade of the intestinal mesentery (FIG. 1). Attempts

Address for correspondence: Kathy L. Sharpe-Timms, Ph.D., HCLD, Department of Obstetrics and Gynecology, University of Missouri-Columbia, 1 Hospital Drive, Columbia, MO 65212. Voice: 573-882-7937; fax: 573-882-9010.
timmsk@health.missouri.edu

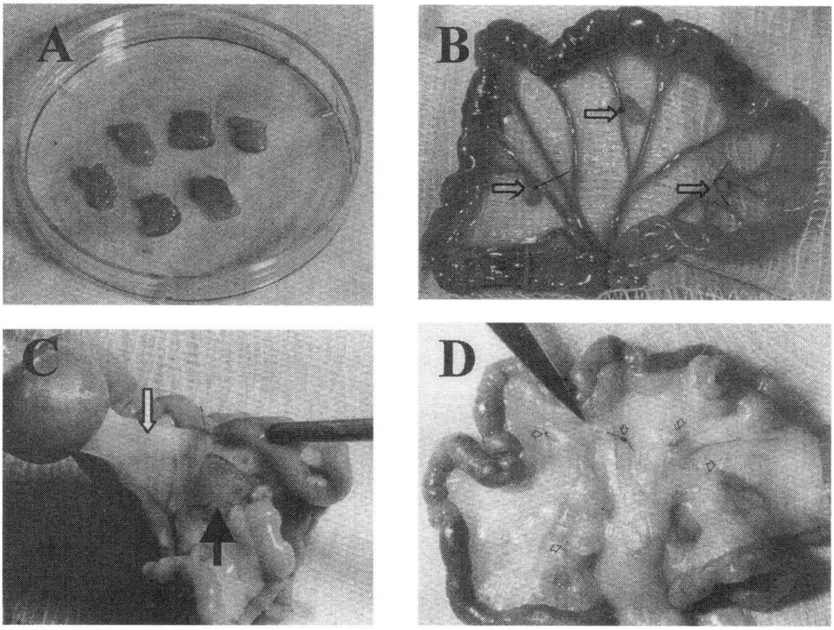

FIGURE 1. Surgically induced endometriosis in the rat and the effects of GnRH agonist therapy. **(A)** Squares (2×2 mm) of uterine tissue are obtained by ablating one of the two rat uterine horns. **(B)** The uterine squares are sutured to the arterial cascades of the small intestine with nonabsorbable suture *(open arrows)*. **(C)** At 4 weeks, endometriotic implants *(black arrow)* appear as well-vascularized, encapsulated cysts. A dense fibrous adhesion *(white arrow)* has formed and attaches the endometriotic implant to the bowel. **(D)** Preoperative GnRH agonist therapy is effective in reducing endometriotic implant growth and adhesion formation (only the sutures were visible; no endometriotic implants or adhesions were present).

at injection of endometrium into the peritoneal cavity of rats have failed to elicit ectopic endometrial tissue growth.[5] Surgically transplanted uterine tissue in the rat grows and behaves in a similar manner as human endometriotic lesions, it is responsive to steroid treatment, and histologically it contains endometrial glands and stroma.[4,5] It has been noted that rat endometriotic implants have epithelial cell regression and stromal fibroblastic transformation similar to histologic findings in human endometriotic lesions.[15]

Rationales for using rats as models for studies of endometriosis include the ethical restrictions of both repeated surgeries and use of experimental drugs in women. Furthermore, animal models permit studies of mechanisms and regulators in a controlled manner free from confounding influences such as individual patient variation in age, stage of the menstrual cycle, use of medications, dietary intake, and environmental influences. The rat model has been used to evaluate the pathogenesis and pathophysiologies of endometriosis, including fertility, pain, and adhesive disease. It allows integration of cellular and molecular techniques and an opportunity to develop novel methods of management of this disorder, including noninvasive diagnostics, classification systems, and therapeutic regimes.

As with any model system, there are both advantages and disadvantages to using the rat as a model for endometriosis. The advantages of this model have been previously reviewed.[3–5] Briefly, the laboratory rat exhibits a 4- to 5-day estrous cycle; hence, 70 to 80 reproductive cycles can be observed per year as compared to the 12 cycles per year in primates. Puberty occurs within 2 months of birth and the reproductive life span of the rat is about 2 years. The highly reproducible reproductive cycle of the rat has been well characterized and can be monitored noninvasively by vaginal lavage. The reproductive endocrine pattern of the rat follows a similar temporal sequence as the human, yet the luteal phase is shorter in the rat. Surgical induction of endometriosis in the rat is a relatively brief procedure and highly successful. Therefore, anomalies in the reproductive cycle of rats with surgically induced endometriosis can be readily characterized. Further, compared to primates, costs associated with housing and care of rats are significantly less.

The disadvantages of using the rat as a model for endometriosis include the wide phylar gap between rats and humans. The uterine endometrium of rats does not undergo tissue breakdown that results in menstruation, but their endometrium does, however, undergo proteolysis of the extracellular matrix as measured by endometrial wet weight and collagen content.[16]

As studies involving repetitive invasive surgeries in women are prohibited, the pathogenic mechanisms of endometriosis are incompletely understood. The surgical induction of endometriosis in rats provides a model to study endometrial-peritoneal interactions including tissue remodeling and lesion progression. Also, while endometrial tissues injected into the peritoneal cavity of rats do not adhere and form lesions, rat endometrial cells do adhere to rat peritoneal cells *in vitro* and elicit distinct proliferative and morphogenic changes.[9] Peritoneal mesothelial cells augment proliferation and induce cell aggregation of uterine stromal cell monolayers, and peritoneal subserosal cells amplify proliferation and induce an irregular compacted morphology of uterine epithelial cells.[9] Strikingly, at the ultrastructural level, rat peritoneal cells cocultured with endometrial cells developed numerous secretory vesicles containing electron-dense material in the cytoplasm (FIG. 2), correlating with an increase in *de novo* synthesis and secretion of a uniquely glycosylated form of haptoglobin into the cell culture media. *In vitro*, we have found that rat peritoneal cells cultured on plastic synthesize and secrete significantly more haptoglobin than cultured rat uterine cells and that a dramatic upregulation of haptoglobin production occurs with the coculture of rat uterine and peritoneal cells (FIG. 3).

We have recently documented that established rat and human endometriotic lesions express haptoglobin mRNA and protein *in vivo*.[10,13,17,18] Uniquely glycosylated haptoglobin, in association with specific disease states, has been found to have immunomodulatory and angiogenic properties.[19] Endometriotic haptoglobin binds to and interferes with macrophage phagocytic function, while increasing macrophage activation as measured by increased interleukin-6 (IL-6) production, which in turn increases endometriotic haptoglobin.[20,21] Similarly, treating cultured human endometriotic cells with IL-6 significantly increases haptoglobin production in a dose- and time-dependent manner.[22] This suggests a plausible feed-forward mechanism that exists in both rats and humans with endometriosis that is responsible for failure of peritoneal immune cells to clear ectopic endometrial tissue from the peritoneal cavity (FIG. 4).

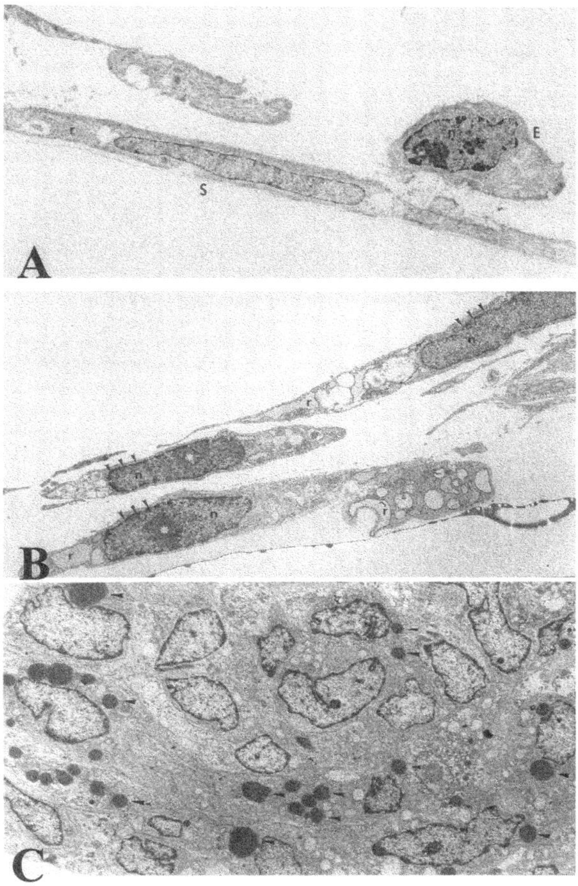

FIGURE 2. Electron micrographs of endometrial cells and peritoneal cells in culture. **(A)** Cultured endometrial epithelial cells [E] and stromal cells [S] (×11,600). Endometrial stromal cells are polymorphous in shape with microvilli [m], prominent nuclei [n] with mottled chromatin, and large mitochondria in the cytoplasm. Endometrial stromal cells are elongated with centrally located nuclei [n] occupying about one-half of the cytoplasm, and with the cytoplasm containing abundant, nondilated rough endoplasmic reticulum [r]. **(B)** Cultured peritoneal cells (×8700). Peritoneal cells are elongated and varied in shape. Their scant cytoplasm contains numerous ribosomes and rough endoplasmic reticulum [r] with dilated cisternae. Their nuclei [n] are large, occupying most of the cytoplasm, and have an even distribution of chromatin, except at their periphery where the chromatin formed a narrow, dense band on the inner aspect of the nuclear membrane (*arrows*). Prominent nucleoli are characteristic (*white asterisk*). **(C)** Coculture of endometrial and peritoneal cells (×5600). Strikingly, peritoneal cells cocultured with endometrial cells [but not isolated peritoneal cells (compare to panel B)] develop numerous secretory vesicles (*arrowheads*) containing electron-dense material in the cytoplasm.

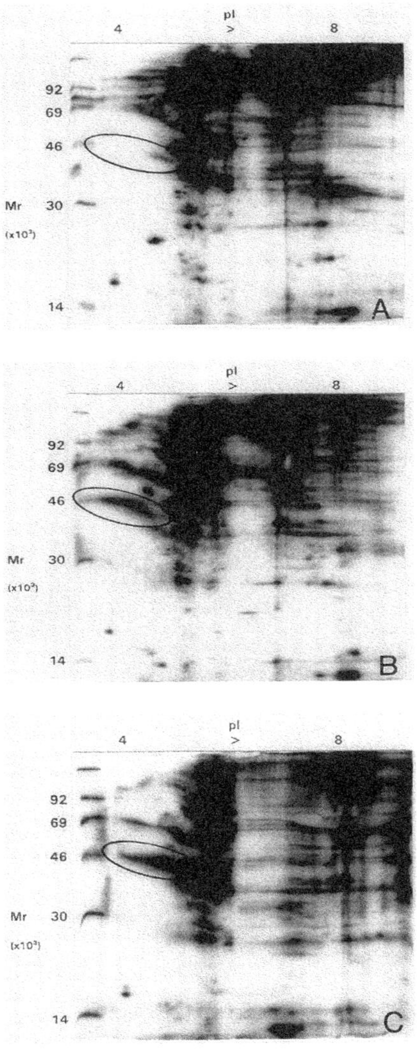

FIGURE 3. Two-dimensional SDS-PAGE fluorographs of *de novo* synthesized and secreted proteins, including endometriotic haptoglobin, by **(A)** endometrial, **(B)** peritoneal, and **(C)** cocultured endometrial and peritoneal cells. **(A)** Isolated endometrial cells produce little endometriotic haptoglobin (*oval*). **(B)** Isolated peritoneal cells synthesize and secrete endometriotic haptoglobin (M_r = 35–55 kDa; p*I* = 4.0–5.5). **(C)** Coculture of endometrial cells on a basal layer of peritoneal cells increases endometriotic haptoglobin production severalfold. We have previously confirmed that both rat and human endometriotic haptoglobin share significant cDNA sequence and protein sequence homology with hepatic haptoglobin.[13,17]

Evidence is emerging that suggests the metalloproteinase enzymes and their inhibitors that play a significant role in normal endometrial remodeling are anomalously expressed in endometriosis.[23–28] We have found that both rat and human endometriotic lesions misexpress MMP-3 and TIMP-1.[10,12,18,28,29] We have further shown that progesterone suppresses MMP-3 in cultured rat endometrial tissue explants and stromal cells, but not MMP-3 mRNA or MMP-3 protein production by cultured rat endometriotic cells (see Sharpe-Timms and Cox in this volume). This persistent MMP-3 expression in the presence of progesterone was correlated with elevated levels of IL-1α mRNA detected in the endometriotic cells and IL-1α protein in their culture media, as compared to little or no IL-1α expression by endo-

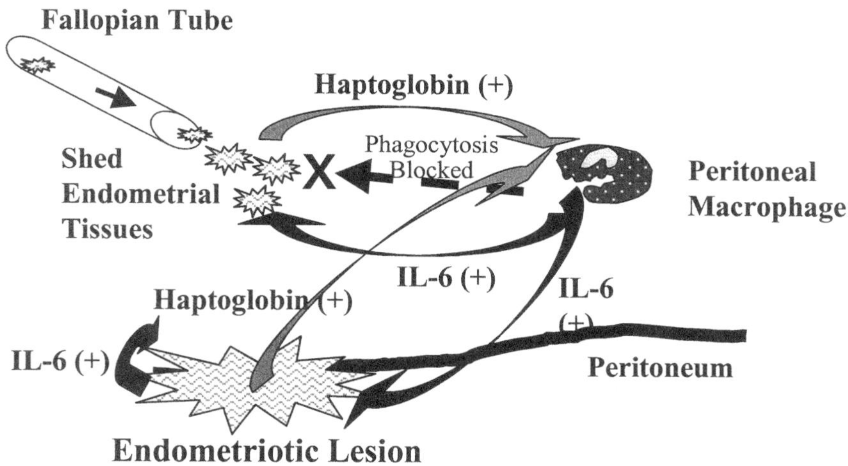

FIGURE 4. Endometriotic haptoglobin interacts with and alters peritoneal macrophage function. Retrogradely shed endometrial tissue fragments and established rat and human endometriotic lesions express haptoglobin mRNA and protein. This uniquely glycosylated haptoglobin binds to and blocks macrophage phagocytic function, while increasing macrophage activation as measured by increased IL-6. The IL-6, in turn, increases endometriotic lesion haptoglobin production in a dose- and time-dependent manner. This suggests a plausible feed-forward mechanism that exists in both rats and humans with endometriosis that is responsible for failure of peritoneal immune cells to clear ectopic endometrial tissue from the peritoneal cavity.

metrial stromal cells. The progesterone-induced loss of sensitivity to IL-1α stimulation of MMP observed in eutopic endometrial cells did not occur in the endometriotic lesion cells (see Sharpe-Timms and Cox in this volume). These preliminary data offer a plausible IL-1α-related mechanism for the perpetuation of MMP-3 production by endometriotic cells in the presence of progesterone. Hence, the rat serves as a valid model to study the mechanisms of the associated establishment and progression of the endometriotic lesion, including the biochemical and molecular nature of the lesions.

Beyond the mere growth of the endometrium in ectopic locations, rats with endometriosis display similar symptoms as primates and humans with the disease.[5,30–32] Rat endometriosis mimics human endometriosis as observed by a reduction in the animal's fertility and fecundity,[5] in part by increasing the number of luteinized unruptured ovarian follicles,[33] decreasing the implantation rate, and increasing the rate of spontaneous abortion.[34] Altered protein synthesis and secretion have been observed in both rats with endometriosis and humans and may be involved in these pathophysiologies.[3,10,29,35–37] For example, prostaglandins are suggested as one of the causative agents of the pain and infertility associated with endometriosis. Complement component C3 is also aberrantly expressed by endometriotic implants of rats with surgically induced endometriosis. The production of C3 in the peritoneal cavity may evoke some of the immunological phenomena observed in women with endometriosis.

The rat has also been used to examine the efficacy of therapeutic approaches for endometriosis.[5–8,38–42] Studies have investigated the efficacy of the steroid hormones and their antagonists, danocrine, GnRH agonists and antagonists, immune modulators, and photosensitization. The majority of these treatments elicited rapid regression of the endometriotic lesions followed by a recurrence of the disease upon cessation of the treatment. Studies using rat models have also shown that steroid add-back therapy, which has been advocated to alleviate hypogonadal side effects associated with some therapies for endometriosis, elicited a rapid recurrence of the disease in the rat.[8] Adverse side effects of some treatment have also been identified using the rat endometriosis model.[6]

As evidence has accumulated defining a link between cell-mediated immune deficiencies and endometriosis, more recent studies have evaluated the immune modulators as therapeutics for endometriosis using the rat model.[15] The compounds levamisole and loxoribine exhibit immune-enhancing properties. Loxoribine is a guanosine analogue. As a group, these analogues enhance NK cell activity, stimulate proliferation of B cells, increase antibody-dependent cell-mediated cytotoxicity, stimulate macrophage-mediated cytotoxicity, and stimulate differentiation of cytolytic T cells. Loxoribine selectively enhances IL-1α, TNF-α, TNF-β, IL-6, INF-α, and INF-γ. Levamisole is currently used as an anthelmintic drug in treatment of colorectal adenocarcinomas. Treatment with both of these immune modulators did not disrupt the reproductive cycle, but did increase the numbers of dendritic cells (derived from monocytes; exhibit low phagocytic activity; are capable of presenting antigen; produce growth factors, cytokines, and chemotactic factors) and phagocytizing macrophages in the endometriotic implants. Endometriotic implants from the loxoribine-treated group showed a marked and significant reduction of epithelial and stromal endometrial components and a depletion of NK cells in contrast to the levamisole-treated group or controls.

The rat model for endometriosis has also been used to evaluate adhesive disease and therapeutic approaches for this condition. Preoperative gonadotropin-releasing hormone agonist (GnRHa) therapy reduced adhesion formation in rats with surgically induced endometriosis, and combined pre- and postoperative GnRHa therapy (but not postoperative GnRHa therapy alone) was effective in reducing adhesion reformation after adhesiolysis (FIG. 1).[11] The mechanisms of adhesion formation and GnRHa prevention of formation were also evaluated in the rat endometriosis model.[14] Surgical manipulation of tissues in the peritoneal cavity increased peritoneal fluid matrix metalloproteinase (MMP) activity and plasminogen activator inhibitor (PAI) activity. GnRHa therapy decreased plasminogen activator (PA) and MMP activities plus increased PAI and MMP inhibitor activities. Hence, this GnRHa-induced shift to a less invasive phenotype altered fibrinolysis and extracellular matrix remodeling and was believed to play a role in the mechanism of GnRHa-induced reduction in adhesion formation.

EMERGING ISSUES AND CONTINUING GAPS IN KNOWLEDGE

Although there are disadvantages of extrapolating data across species, it is still possible to utilize animal models to study events involved in the pathogenesis and pathophysiologies of endometriosis that are not accessible in humans. Rat endometriotic tissues and cells perform in a similar manner as human endometriotic cells in organ explant culture and isolated cell culture.[9,10,29,35,36] As human endometriotic lesions must be obtained by invasive surgical procedures, rat endometriotic implants are more available. Further, the actual amount of human endometriotic lesion tissue and cells obtained is relatively small in humans, yet can be unlimited in rats.

To date, it is not known why endometrial tissues injected into the peritoneal cavity of the rat do not attach, invade, and form endometriotic lesions. While intraperitoneal injection of endometrial tissues is unsuccessful in establishment of endometriosis in rats, studies defining the mechanisms associated with the failure of attachment and invasion or immune clearance of the ectopic endometrium may provide insight into the pathogenesis of endometriosis. Several studies have demonstrated ectopic growth of both normal human endometrium and endometriotic tissue in athymic nude mice,[43,44] suggesting the failure of these tissues to establish lesions in immune-competent rats may be attributed to immune clearance of the ectopic endometrial tissues. The nude mouse as a recipient animal for human tissue has also been used as a model to examine the role that steroid-sensitive MMP expression might play in the establishment of endometriosis.[45] The results of this study indicated a direct role for MMPs in the ability of human tissue to establish ectopic lesions within the peritoneum of the recipient nude mice and suggest that steroid regulation of these enzymes is also important in the pathophysiology of endometriosis. Similar studies have not been performed in the rat.

While the rat model for endometriosis has been used to identify effects of ectopic endometrial tissue growth on ovarian function, embryo implantation, spontaneous pregnancy loss, and adhesion formation, the mechanisms eliciting these effects remain elusive. To date, these mechanisms remain undefined in humans as well. Hence, further studies utilizing the rat as a model for endometriosis may provide insight into the mechanisms of these pathologies that may lead to novel therapeutic approaches for this enigmatic disease.

REFERENCES

1. Jacobson, V.C. 1922. The autotransplantation of endometrial tissue in the rabbit. Arch. Surg. **5:** 281.
2. Jacobson, V.C. 1926. The intraperitoneal transplantation of endometrial tissue: an experimental study. Arch. Pathol. Lab. Med. **1:** 169.
3. Vernon, M.W. 1990. Experimental endometriosis in laboratory animals as a research model. *In* Current Concepts in Endometriosis, pp. 49–60. Alan R. Liss. New York.
4. Vernon, M.W. & G.D. Hodgen. 1987. Experimental endometriosis. *In* Endometriosis, pp. 207–223. Alan R. Liss. New York.
5. Vernon, M.W. & E.A. Wilson. 1985. Studies on the surgical induction of endometriosis in the rat. Fertil. Steril. **44:** 684–694.
6. Sharpe, K.L., M.C. Bertero, B.P. Lyon *et al.* 1990. Follicular atresia and infertility in rats treated with a gonadotropin-releasing hormone (GnRH) antagonist. Endocrinology **127:** 25–31.
7. Sharpe, K.L., M.C. Bertero & M.W. Vernon. 1990. Rapid regression of endometriosis by a new gonadotropin-releasing hormone antagonist in rats with surgically induced disease. *In* Current Concepts in Endometriosis, pp. 449–458. Alan R. Liss. New York.
8. Sharpe, K.L., M.C. Bertero & M.W. Vernon. 1991. Spontaneous and steroid-induced recurrence of endometriosis following suppression by a gonadotropin-releasing hormone antagonist in the rat. Am. J. Obstet. Gynecol. **164:** 187–194.

9. SHARPE, K.L., R.L. ZIMMER, R.S. KHAN & L.L. PENNEY. 1992. Proliferative and morphogenic changes induced by the co-culture of rat uterine and peritoneal cells: a cell culture model for endometriosis. Fertil. Steril. **58:** 1220–1229.
10. SHARPE, K.L. & M.W. VERNON. 1993. Polypeptides synthesized and released by rat endometriotic tissue differ from those of the uterine endometrium in culture. Biol. Reprod. **48:** 1334–1340.
11. WRIGHT, J.A. & K.L. SHARPE-TIMMS. 1995. Gonadotropin-releasing hormone agonist (GnRHa) therapy reduces postoperative adhesion formation and reformation following adhesiolysis in rat models for adhesion formation and endometriosis. Fertil. Steril. **63:** 1094–1100.
12. SHARPE-TIMMS, K.L., L.L. PENNEY, R.L. ZIMMER *et al.* 1995. Partial purification and amino acid sequence analysis of endometriosis protein-II (ENDO-II) reveal homology with tissue inhibitor of metalloproteinases-1 (TIMP-1). J. Clin. Endocrinol. Metab. **80:** 3784–3787.
13. SHARPE-TIMMS, K.L., M. PIVA, E.A. RICKE *et al.* 1998. Endometriotic lesions synthesize and secrete a haptoglobin-like protein. Biol. Reprod. **58:** 988–994.
14. SHARPE-TIMMS, K.L., R.L. ZIMMER, W.J. JOLLIFF *et al.* 1998. Gonadotropin-releasing hormone agonist (GnRHa) therapy alters activity of plasminogen activators (PA), matrix metalloproteinases (MMP), and their inhibitors (PAI and MMPI) in rat models for adhesion formation and endometriosis: potential GnRHa-regulated mechanisms reducing adhesion formation. Fertil. Steril. **69**(5)**:** 916–923.
15. KEENAN, J.A., P.K. WILLIAMS-BOYCE, P.J. MASSEY *et al.* 1999. Regression of endometrial explants in a rat model of endometriosis treated with the immune modulators loxoribine and levamisole. Fertil. Steril. **72**(10)**:** 135–141.
16. YOCHIM, J.M. & D.G. BLAHA. 1976. Effects of oestrone and progesterone on collagen and ascorbic acid content in the endometrium and myometrium of the rat. J. Reprod. Fertil. **47:** 79–82.
17. PIVA, M. & K.L. SHARPE-TIMMS. 1999. Peritoneal endometriotic lesions differentially express a haptoglobin-like gene. Mol. Hum. Reprod. **5**(1)**:** 71–78.
18. SHARPE-TIMMS, K.L., E.A. RICKE, M. PIVA & G.M. HOROWITZ. 2000. Differential *in vivo* expression and localization of endometriosis protein-I (ENDO-I), a haptoglobin homologue, in endometrium and endometriotic lesions. Hum. Reprod. **15**(10)**:** 101–105.
19. DOBRYSZYCKA, W. 1997. Biological functions of haptoglobin—new pieces to an old puzzle. Eur. J. Clin. Chem. Clin. Biochem. **35:** 647–654.
20. SHARPE-TIMMS, K.L., R.L. ZIMMER, E.A. RICKE & G.M. HOROWITZ. 2000. Aberrant adherence of peritoneal macrophages in endometriosis. O-057. Am. Soc. Reprod. Med., San Diego.
21. SHARPE-TIMMS, K.L., R.L. ZIMMER, E.A. RICKE *et al.* 2001. Haptoglobin binds to and alters peritoneal macrophage interleukin-6 production in endometriosis. P-431. Soc. Gynecol. Invest., Toronto.
22. PIVA, M., G.M. HOROWITZ & K.L. SHARPE-TIMMS. 2001. Interleukin-6 differentially stimulates haptoglobin production by peritoneal and endometriotic cells *in vitro*: a model for endometrium-peritoneum interaction in endometriosis. J. Clin. Endocrinol. Metab. **86:** 2553–2561.
23. KOKORINE, I., M. NISOLLE, J. DONNEZ *et al.* 1997. Expression of interstitial collagenase (matrix metalloproteinase-1) is related to the activity of human endometriotic lesions. Fertil. Steril. **68:** 246–251.
24. SPUIJBROEK, M.D.E.H., G.J. DUNSELMAN, P.P.C.A. MENHEERE & J.L.H. EVERS. 1992. Early endometriosis invades the extracellular matrix. Fertil. Steril. **58:** 929–933.
25. SAITO, T., H. MIZUMOTO, K. KUROKI *et al.* 1995. Expression of MMP-3 and TIMP-1 in the endometriosis and the influence of danazol. Acta Obstet. Gynaecol. Jpn. **47:** 495–496.
26. KOKS, C.A., P.G. GROOTHUIS *et al.* 2000. Matrix metalloproteinases and their tissue inhibitors in antegradely shed menstruum and peritoneal fluid. Fertil. Steril. **73**(3)**:** 604–612.
27. MARBAIX, E., J. DONNEZ, P.J. COURTOY & Y. EECKHOUT. 1992. Progesterone regulates the activity of collagenase and related gelatinases A and B in human endometrial explants. Proc. Natl. Acad. Sci. U.S.A. **89:** 11789–11793.

28. COX, K.E., M. PIVA & K.L. SHARPE-TIMMS. 2001. Differential regulation of matrix metalloproteinase-3 (MMP-3) gene expression in endometriotic lesions as compared to endometrium. Biol. Reprod. **65:** 1297–1300.
29. SHARPE, K.L., R.L. ZIMMER, W.T. GRIFFIN & L.L. PENNEY. 1993. Polypeptides synthesized and released by human endometriosis tissue differ from those of the uterine endometrium in culture. Fertil. Steril. **60:** 839–851.
30. MUSE, K.N. & E.A. WILSON. 1982. How does endometriosis cause infertility. Fertil. Steril. **38:** 145–152.
31. RANNEY, B. 1980. Endometriosis: pathogenesis, symptoms, and findings. Clin. Obstet. Gynecol. **23**(3)**:** 865–874.
32. RANNEY, B. 1980. Etiology, prevention, and inhibition of endometriosis. Clin. Obstet. Gynecol. **23**(3)**:** 875–882.
33. MOON, C.E., M.C. BERTERO, T.E. CURRY *et al.* 1993. The presence of luteinized unruptured follicle syndrome (LUFS) and altered folliculogenesis in rats with surgically induced endometriosis. Am. J. Obstet. Gynecol. **169:** 676–682.
34. BERTERO, M.C., K.L. SHARPE, C.E. MOON & M.W. VERNON. 1991. Fetal loss during early pregnancy in rats with surgically-induced endometriosis. O-079. Am. Fertil. Soc., Orlando.
35. ISAACSON, K.B., C. COUTIFARIS, C. GARCIA & C.R. LYTTLE. 1989. Production and secretion of complement component 3 by endometriotic tissue. J. Clin. Endocrinol. Metab. **69:** 1003–1009.
36. ISAACSON, K.B., Q. XU & C.R. LYTTLE. 1991. The effect of estradiol on the production and secretion of complement component 3 by the rat uterus and surgically induced endometriotic tissue. Fertil. Steril. **55:** 395–402.
37. VERNON, M.W., J.S. BEARD, K. GRAVES *et al.* 1986. Classification of endometriotic implants by morphologic appearance and capacity to synthesize prostaglandin F. Fertil. Steril. **46:** 801–806.
38. JONES, R.C. 1987. The effect of a luteinizing hormone releasing hormone (LRH) agonist, levonorgestrel, danazol, and ovariectomy on experimental endometriosis in the rat. Acta Endocrinol. **114:** 379.
39. TJADEN, B., D. GALETTO, J.D. WOODRUFF & J.A. ROCK. 1993. Time-related effects of RU486 treatment in experimentally induced endometriosis in the rat. Fertil. Steril. **59**(2)**:** 437–440.
40. STOECKMANN, K., C. HEGELE-HARTUNG & K. CHWALISZ. 1995. Effects of the progesterone antagonists onapristone (ZK 98 299) and ZK 136 799 on surgically induced endometriosis in rats. Hum. Reprod. **10:** 3264–3271.
41. YANG, J.Z., J.P. VAN DIJK-SMITH, D.A. VAN VUGT *et al.* 1996. Fluorescence and photosensitization of experimental endometriosis in the rat after systemic 5-aminolevulinic acid administration: a potential new approach to the diagnosis and treatment of endometriosis. Am. J. Obstet. Gynecol. **174**(1)**:** 154–160.
42. SCHOR, E., E.C. BARACAT, M.J. SIMONES *et al.* 1999. Effects of conjugated estrogens and progestogen in surgically induced endometriosis in oophorectomized rats. Clin. Exp. Obstet. Gynecol. **26**(3–4)**:** 158–161.
43. ZAMAH, N.M., M.G. DODSON, L.C. STEPHENS *et al.* 1984. Transplantation of normal and ectopic human endometrial tissue into athymic nude mice. Am. J. Obstet. Gynecol. **149:** 591–597.
44. BERGQVIST, A., S. JEPPSSON, S. KULLANDER & O. LJUNGBERG. 1985. Human uterine endometrium transplanted into nude mice: morphological effects of various steroid hormones. Am. J. Pathol. **121:** 337–341.
45. BRUNER, K.L., L.M. MATRISIAN, W.H. RODGERS *et al.* 1997. Suppression of matrix metalloproteinases inhibits establishment of ectopic lesions by human endometrium in nude mice. J. Clin. Invest. **99:** 2851–2857.

Experimental Endometriosis

The Nude Mouse as a Xenographic Host

KAYLON L. BRUNER-TRAN, DEBORAH WEBSTER-CLAIR, AND KEVIN G. OSTEEN

Women's Reproductive Health Research Center, Vanderbilt University School of Medicine, Nashville, Tennessee 37232, USA

ABSTRACT: Endometriosis is a complex disease that can develop as a consequence of retrograde menstruation, occurring in association with the cyclic loss of endometrial tissue in primates and humans. In addition, progression of disease parallels a woman's exposure to ovarian steroids, rarely occurring prior to menarche and generally resolving following menopause. Because of the cost of developing primate models to study endometriosis, numerous small animal models have been established to approach various elements related to the pathophysiology of this disease. Our laboratory has developed an experimental endometriosis model using nude mice as a xenographic host for human tissues. Our goal is to approach the basic cellular mechanisms of estrogen and progesterone action that link these hormones to the development or prevention of endometriosis. In our initial studies, we have sought to understand steroid-associated regulation of matrix metalloproteinases (MMPs) with regard to the development of experimental endometriosis. Using both short-term organ cultures and nude mice as xenographic hosts of human tissue, we have demonstrated a critical role of progesterone and progesterone-associated cytokines in preventing the initial establishment of experimental disease. Women with endometriosis appear to lack normal endometrial responsiveness to progesterone, resulting in altered expression of several MMPs and an enhanced ability of these tissues to establish ectopic lesions in nude mice. Developing a better understanding of the impairments in the normal endometrial physiology of women with endometriosis should aid in the development of better treatment or diagnostic strategies.

KEYWORDS: MMPs; progesterone; nude mouse/mice; cytokine action

INTRODUCTION

Endometriosis, the presence of endometrial glands and stroma at an extrauterine site, is a persistent disease with a complex and elusive etiology. Although a number of theories have been proposed that attempt to explain the development of endometriosis, it is largely accepted that most incidences of the disease result from the ectopic establishment of refluxed menstrual tissue.[1,2] Interestingly, endometriosis is classified as a benign medical condition, but can mimic a malignancy in that new

Address for correspondence: Kevin G. Osteen, Ph.D., Vanderbilt University School of Medicine, 1161 21st Avenue South, MCN B-1100, Nashville, TN 37232. Voice: 615-322-4196; fax: 615-343-7913.

kevin.osteen@mcmail.vanderbilt.edu

lesions can be established via colonization of existing lesions.[3] The disease is estimated to occur in 10% to 15% of all reproductive-age women and often results in severe pain, dysmenorrhea, and reduced fertility. As many as 40% of infertile women may have endometriosis[4] and the disease is responsible for more than 100,000 hysterectomies each year.[5] While much progress has been made in recent years toward diagnosing endometriosis, the pathophysiology of disease establishment and progression and the associated infertility are not well understood. From both a clinical and a scientific standpoint, endometriosis is a difficult disease to study. Women are rarely diagnosed in the very early stages of the disease, making it difficult to gain insight into the development and progression of ectopic lesions in a large population. For this reason, numerous experimental models of endometriosis have been developed in order to investigate both the pathophysiology and the consequences of this disease.

In order to test Sampson's theory of retrograde menstruation in the development of endometriosis, Ridley and Edwards[6,7] asked women who were scheduled to undergo laparotomy for leiomyomectomy to collect their own menstrual effluent for intraperitoneal injection. Months later, at the time of surgery, 2 of 15 women in the study (13%) were found to have developed endometriotic lesions, reflecting the natural occurrence of the disease within the American population. Although these studies provided significant support for Sampson's theory, ethical issues now prevent such experiments and thus a number of studies have been undertaken using nonhuman primates. The rhesus monkey (*Macaca mulatta*) is especially susceptible to endometriosis and has been used to assess the role of steroid hormones on the establishment and maintenance of endometriotic lesions.[8,9] Additionally, although epidemiologic data suggest a role for environmental toxins in the development of endometriosis, controlled studies to fully address this issue would not be feasible in human populations. Hence, nonhuman primates have also been used to investigate the potential effects of endocrine disruptors in the development of this disease.[10,11]

Although humans and nonhuman primates are the only mammals that spontaneously develop endometriosis, the limitations of human studies and the expense of primate studies have prompted investigators to pursue the use of small animal models. Nonprimate species used commonly for medical research do not menstruate and do not develop endometriosis; nevertheless, a number of investigators have mechanically introduced endometrial tissue into the peritoneal cavity of rabbits, rats, and mice in order to investigate multiple aspects of this disease.[12–15] However, while these types of studies have proven to be valuable for studying some aspects of the disease, surgical induction of endometriosis does not address the basic cellular mechanisms of endometrial attachment and invasion that are critical for the initial establishment of ectopic lesions in women. Therefore, investigators have attempted to develop animal models that more closely mimic the natural history of the human disease.

IMMUNOCOMPROMISED MICE AS A MODEL FOR ENDOMETRIOSIS

Immune-compromised animals, such as the athymic (nude) mouse and the severe combined immunodeficient mouse (SCID), do not reject xenographic tissue, which can be introduced subcutaneously or into the peritoneal cavity. In addition to allowing the use of human tissue, these animal models are advantageous in that tissues can be manipulated *in vitro*, and tissue response subsequently correlated to the presence and/or severity of disease. Zamah *et al.*[16] and Bergqvist *et al.*[17] were the first investigators to establish endometriosis-like growth of human endometrium and endometriosis tissues in immune-deficient nude mice, and our laboratory has adapted elements of this model to investigate the impact of steroid hormones on early invasion of ectopic lesions[18] and, more recently, neovascularization of these tissues. More recently, experimental endometriosis has also been established using similar transplantation of human tissues into SCID mice.[19] SCID mice possess a congenital deficiency of B and T lymphocytes and thus cannot efficiently trigger either cellular or humoral immunity. Although their severe immunodeficient state results in a higher percentage of successful grafts compared to nude mice, SCID animals are also highly susceptible to murine pathogens and exhibit a reduced life span due to a high incidence of thymic lymphomas. Although partial defects in B cell immunity have been observed in nude mice, these animals are much less susceptible to pathogens than are SCID mice. Additionally, since nude mice are essentially hairless, subcutaneous lesions can be visualized through the skin, making these animals especially useful for monitoring therapeutic regimens.

Relationship of Experimental Endometriosis to Steroid Exposure

Our research group has utilized the nude mouse as a human tissue recipient to examine the role of steroid-regulated MMP expression in the establishment of experimental endometriosis. Previous studies have indicated a role for MMPs in normal endometrial remodeling[20,21] and these enzymes are broadly expressed in ectopic lesions of endometriosis.[22,23] In the normal endometrium, estradiol is associated with endometrial remodeling and MMP expression, while progesterone is associated with a loss of MMP expression and endometrial differentiation. Endometriosis is a steroid-dependent disease and both estrogen and progesterone can affect its development or recurrence. For example, many of the risk factors for endometriosis, such as early menarche and nulliparity, are associated with prolonged estrogen exposure.[24] In contrast, endometriosis has been found to regress in some women in the progesterone-rich environment of pregnancy[25] or during progestin therapy in the absence of pregnancy.[26] Despite the apparent relationship between steroids and endometriosis, the precise mechanisms by which estrogen and progesterone affect the initial establishment of disease remain speculative.

To examine the role that regulation of MMPs by steroids might play in the establishment of endometriotic-like lesions in nude mice, we obtained endometrial biopsies on days 10–12 of the menstrual cycle from women with no history of endometriosis. Obtaining tissue prior to ovulation allows us to maintain the endometrial fragments for 18–24 hours in the presence of estradiol, which sustains MMP expression, or in a combination of estradiol and progesterone, which suppresses MMP expression. Following *in vitro* culture, human tissues were introduced via intraperitoneal injection into ovariectomized nude mice previously implanted with an estradiol-releasing pellet. Animals with estradiol-releasing pellets are receptive to experimental endometriosis and can be sacrificed after 5–10 days and examined for the presence of peritoneal sites of viable human tissue growth. As shown in TABLE 1, 95% of mice receiving tissues treated with estradiol develop experimental endometriosis compared to approximately 6% of mice receiving progesterone-treated

TABLE 1. Effects of steroids on the development of endometriotic-like lesions in nude mice

Tissue treatment	Animal treatment	Number of mice	Percent with lesions	Total number of lesions
E	E	30	96	71
EP	E	30	6	3

NOTE: All mice were implanted with an estradiol-releasing pellet at 24 hours prior to intraperitoneal injection of human endometrial tissues. Mice were injected with proliferative-phase endometrial tissues treated *in vitro* for 24 hours with estradiol (E = 10^{-9} M) or estradiol plus progesterone (EP: E = 10^{-9} M; P = 5×10^{-7} M). Ten days after tissue injection, mice were sacrificed and necropsied for endometriotic-like disease.

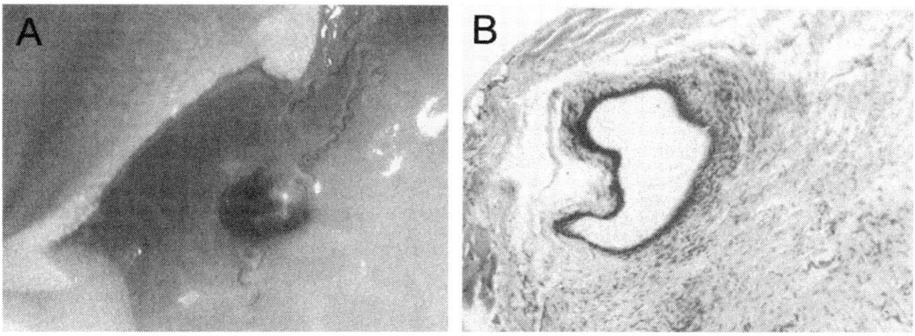

FIGURE 1. Human endometrium growing as ectopic lesions in nude mice. (**A**) Gross view of an endometriotic-like lesion. Note the developing vasculature. Magnification: ×20. (**B**) Hematoxylin and eosin stain of a lesion removed from a nude mouse. Note the distended gland and minimal supporting stroma. Magnification: ×200. [Figure reduced to 94%.]

tissues.[18,27] Following *in vitro* estradiol treatments, human tissue lesions excised from the peritoneum of mice appear similar to lesions acquired from native human endometriosis following either gross morphological or microscopic analysis (FIG. 1). Taken together, these results support the use of nude mice in investigating the initial, steroid-dependent biology of early ectopic lesion formation.

The minimal development of experimental endometriosis observed in nude mice receiving human endometrium treated *in vitro* with progesterone suggests that suppression of MMPs may be linked to the therapeutic benefits of progestin-based therapy in women with this disease. Unfortunately, clinical experience suggests that many women fail to respond significantly to progestin therapy, and a decreased sensitivity to progesterone appears to confound treatment of this disease.[28–30] For example, although MMP-11 mRNA is rapidly suppressed by postovulatory progesterone exposure in normal endometrial tissue,[21] this enzyme is persistent in both eutopic and ectopic endometrial tissues acquired from women with endometriosis (FIG. 2). Specifically, *in situ* hybridization analysis reveals intense expression of MMP-11 mRNA in both eutopic and ectopic endometrium removed during the secretory phase from a woman with endometriosis. This disruption in MMP regulation can be added to the growing body of evidence that indicates that a failure of progesterone action may be a key component in the development of endometriosis.

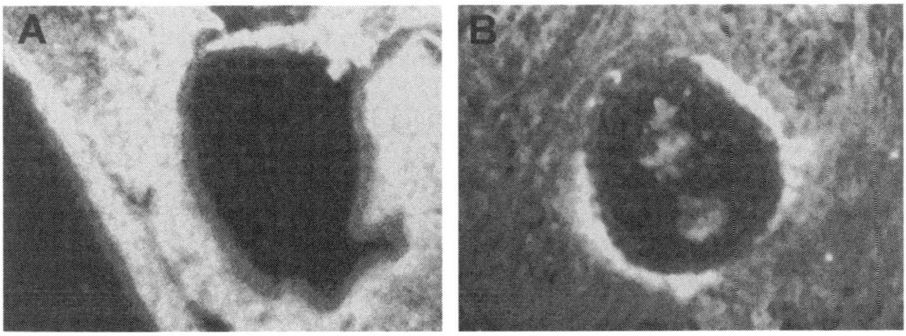

FIGURE 2. *In situ* hybridization localization of MMP-11 mRNA in (**A**) eutopic and (**B**) ectopic endometrium removed from a patient during the secretory phase. Magnification: ×200.

Relationship of Experimental Endometriosis to Growth Factors and Cytokines

Although we have linked steroid-mediated MMP expression to the establishment of experimental endometriosis, growth factors and cytokines control numerous aspects of cell-cell communication in the endometrium. Under differing biological conditions, locally produced factors may alter the normal impact of steroids on MMP expression. For example, inflammatory cytokines such as interleukin-1α (IL-1α) or tumor necrosis factor-α (TNF-α) appear to stimulate the expression of multiple endometrial MMPs during menstruation.[31] In *in vitro* models, these cytokines have been reported to interfere with progestin-induced decidualization of isolated human stromal cells.[32] Reflecting on the impact of inflammatory cytokines on MMP regulation, IL-1α treatments antagonize the ability of progesterone to suppress MMPs in organ cultures of proliferative human endometrium, thereby promoting the ability of this tissue to establish experimental endometriosis in nude mice.[33] However, the impact of inflammatory

TABLE 2. Effects of steroids and cytokines on the development of endometriotic-like lesions in nude mice

Tissue treatment	Animal treatment	Number of mice	Percent with lesions	Total number of lesions
E	E	10	100	26
EP	E	10	0	0
RA	E	10	10	1
TGF-β	E	10	100	47
EP + anti-TGF-β	E	8	100	20
RA + anti-TGF-β	E	9	70	12

NOTE: All mice were implanted with an estradiol-releasing pellet at 24 hours prior to intraperitoneal injection of human endometrial tissues. Mice were injected with proliferative-phase endometrial tissues treated *in vitro* for 24 hours with estradiol (E = 10^{-9} M), estradiol plus progesterone (EP: E = 10^{-9} M; P = 5×10^{-7} M), E plus retinoic acid (RA = 10^{-6} M), E plus 2 ng TGF-β (TGF-β), EP plus 10 μg of an antibody against TGF-β (EP + anti-TGF-β), or RA plus 10 μg of an antibody against TGF-β (RA + anti-TGF-β). Ten days after tissue injection, mice were sacrificed and necropsied for endometriotic-like disease.

cytokines on endometrial MMP expression does not completely override normal steroid control. We have shown that either *in vivo* exposure to progesterone or exposure of isolated endometrial stromal cells to progesterone for 2–4 days *in vitro* can prevent the stimulatory action of IL-1α on MMP-3 expression.[34] The ability of prior progesterone exposure to block the stimulatory impact of inflammatory cytokines on endometrial MMP expression may provide new insight into controlling the altered expression of these enzymes that appears to occur in association with endometriosis. Since local growth factors and cytokines are known to regulate MMP expression, we have examined whether local factors, produced during *in vitro* decidualization, may be required for normal progesterone-mediated suppression of MMPs. Based on our previous observations in normal endometrium, we have focused on the potential role(s) of retinoic acid and transforming growth factor-β2 (TGF-β2). These locally produced factors can impact endometrial MMP expression and have been associated with progesterone-induced stromal cell decidualization.[35,36]

In a series of *in vitro* studies, we have previously demonstrated that progesterone acts to suppress endometrial MMPs[37] and have recently demonstrated that retinoic acid has a similar effect in the absence of progesterone.[38] Additionally, treatment of human endometrial tissues *in vitro* with either progesterone or retinoic acid will prevent the establishment of endometriotic-like lesions in our nude mouse model (TABLE 2). As noted above, the expression of TGF-β is critical to endometrial MMP regulation and this growth factor is required for the inhibitory action of progesterone and retinoic acid on establishment of experimental endometriosis. More specifically, the addition of anti-TGF-β antibodies to endometrial organ cultures will block the ability of either progesterone or retinoic acid to prevent the subsequent establishment of experimental endometriosis. However, in the absence of pretreatments with retinoic acid or progesterone, this growth factor cannot independently prevent experimental disease (TABLE 2). Taken together, these observations support the existence of a highly interactive steroid- and cytokine-based regulatory system for normal control of endometrial MMP expression. By extension, the cooperative actions of both steroids and local factors would appear necessary for prevention of experimental endometriosis.

Endocrine Disruptors and Experimental Endometriosis

The environmental contaminant, 2,3,7,8-tetrachlorodibenzo-*p*-dioxin (TCDD or dioxin), has been found to have endocrine-disrupting properties and has been specifically implicated in the development of endometriosis in exposed primates.[10,11] Although direct evidence for a relationship between exposure to TCDD or other dioxin-like compounds and the development of endometriosis in women is lacking, a number of retrospective studies in accidentally exposed populations indicate a possible link.[39–42] Nevertheless, despite compelling epidemiological and experimental data, the basic cellular and molecular mechanisms linking TCDD exposure to the pathophysiology of this disease remain elusive. TCDD is classified as an antiestrogen and animal studies indicate that this toxicant can disrupt the effects of estrogen on reproduction.[43–46] However, since estrogen is a risk factor for endometriosis, logic would seem to dictate that the antiestrogen activity of TCDD should aid in the prevention of this disease rather than be associated with its development. In our experimental model, estrogen promotes the development of human tissue

TABLE 3. Effects of TCDD on the development of endometriotic-like lesions in nude mice

Tissue treatment	Animal treatment	Number of mice	Percent with lesions	Total number of lesions
E	E	10	100	27
EP	E	10	0	0
E + TCDD	E	10	100	50
EP + TCDD	E	10	100	56

NOTE: All mice were implanted with an estradiol-releasing pellet at 24 hours prior to intraperitoneal injection of human endometrial tissues. Mice were injected with proliferative-phase endometrial tissues treated *in vitro* for 24 hours with estradiol ($E = 10^{-8}$ M), estradiol plus progesterone (EP: $E = 10^{-9}$ M; $P = 5 \times 10^{-7}$ M), E plus TCDD ($E = 10^{-8}$ M; $TCDD = 10^{-9}$ M), or EP plus TCDD ($E = 10^{-9}$ M; $P = 5 \times 10^{-7}$ M; $TCDD = 10^{-9}$ M). Ten days after tissue injection, mice were sacrificed and necropsied for endometriotic-like disease.

growth in nude mice, while progesterone suppression of endometrial MMPs serves to largely prevent experimental disease.[18] Therefore, we have examined whether exposure of endometrial tissue to TCDD might interfere with progesterone-mediated MMP regulation in this organ system.[47] Using short-term organ cultures of proliferative-phase endometrium, we initially observed that *in vitro* TCDD exposure could block progesterone-mediated induction of TGF-β2, a required paracrine signal for inhibition of MMP expression. Predictably, when endometrial tissues treated with progesterone and TCDD were introduced into nude mice, progesterone failed to inhibit MMP suppression or to prevent development of disease. Indeed, experimental lesions resulting from TCDD treatments were more numerous compared to estrogen-treated control mice (TABLE 3). The ability of TCDD to interfere with the expression of a key growth factor related to the ability of either progesterone or retinoic acid to regulate endometrial MMP expression implicates this toxin in the disruption of a basic biologic pathway linked to the development of experimental endometriosis. Further studies are needed to determine whether exposure of human populations to this ubiquitous environmental toxin represents a new risk factor for developing endometriosis.

Therapeutic Testing in a Model of Experimental Endometriosis

Developing a better understanding of the cellular and molecular mechanisms linking endometrial biology to the pathophysiology of endometriosis remains an important aspect of our studies; however, another aspect of an experimental disease model is testing the effectiveness of novel therapeutic agents. For example, in addition to blocking the initial establishment of experimental endometriosis,[18] it is equally possible to establish endometriotic-like disease in nude mice in order to examine the therapeutic potential of various biological agents. To establish experimental endometriosis, normal, proliferative-phase endometrium is treated *in vitro* with estradiol and injected subcutaneously into nude mice that have been previously implanted with an estrogen-releasing pellet. After 10 days, the hairless mice can simply be visually inspected for the presence of ectopic lesions. For example, in order to test the therapeutic potential of retinoic acid, mice with experimental endo-

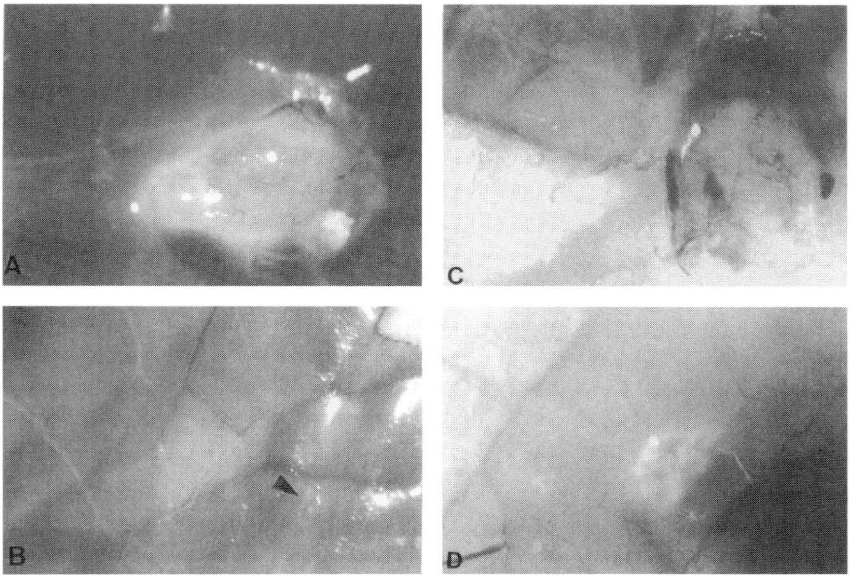

FIGURE 3. Regression of experimental endometriosis. Human endometrium was established as ectopic lesions in nude mice receiving exogenous estradiol. Ten days after introduction of tissues into mice, animals received **(A, B)** no additional treatment, **(C)** progesterone, or **(D)** retinoic acid. Mice were sacrificed after a total of 20 days. Lesions observed in mice receiving only estradiol are larger with extensive vascularization compared to lesions in mice treated with either progesterone or retinoic acid.

metriosis were divided into three groups on day 10 following injection of human tissue. Group A received no further intervention, group B was implanted with a progesterone-releasing pellet, and group C was implanted with a retinoic acid–releasing pellet. Mice were sacrificed at 10 or 20 days after receiving the second "therapeutic" pellet. Under these experimental conditions, either progesterone or retinoic acid treatments were able to mediate regression of human lesions; however, progesterone therapy was most effective in reducing lesion size (FIG. 3).

The experiments described above indicate that natural inhibitors of endometrial MMP expression, including progesterone and retinoic acid, can be effective therapeutic agents in our experimental model using normal endometrial tissue. However, clinical evidence indicates that women with endometriosis may not respond to progestin-based therapy alone, and the use of retinoic acid for treating potentially fertile women with endometriosis is not yet a practical approach. Therefore, we have also used our nude mouse model of experimental endometriosis to investigate the possible effectiveness of other potentially effective therapeutics, including anti-angiogenic factors. Angiogenesis is essential for tumor growth, and a number of natural and synthetic angiogenic-inhibiting substances are currently under investigation for use as anticancer agents.[48] Since new blood vessel formation also appears to be critical to the survival of ectopic endometrial tissues,[49,50] targeting this process will likely become an important therapeutic intervention.[51] In collaboration with Metris Therapeutic Limited (London), we found that the extensive vascularization associated with experimental disease could be inhibited by blocking VEGF activity either *in vitro* or *in vivo*. In these studies, we found that blocking the impact of VEGF on neovascularization prevented establishment of lesions, as well as causing a regression of existing lesions (Charnock-Jones, unpublished observations). The results of each of the studies noted here support the utility of using the nude mouse model of experimental endometriosis to identify potentially useful therapeutic agents in a cost-effective, small animal system.

SUMMARY

We have found that the nude mouse is a useful animal in which important aspects of endometriosis can be examined. Although no experimental model of endometriosis can precisely mimic all aspects of the disease, the establishment of human lesions in nude mice can provide important insights into disease development. Using the nude mouse model of endometriosis, we have implicated the expression of MMPs to the establishment of ectopic lesions. Moreover, our studies indicate that the nude mouse can be used to assess the possible role of environmental toxins in development of disease, which in humans can only be examined retrospectively. Finally, using the nude mouse in "preclinical" therapeutic testing allows an initial determination of efficacy, so human trials can be performed on only those agents demonstrating the most promise.

ACKNOWLEDGMENTS

We gratefully acknowledge the donors who provided endometrial samples and the physicians of our department who performed these critical biopsies. This work was supported in part through a cooperative agreement (No. U54-HD-37321) as part of the Specialized Cooperative Centers Program in Reproduction Research. Additional support was provided by grants from the United States Environmental Protection Agency (No. R826300) and The Endometriosis Association Research Program at Vanderbilt.

REFERENCES

1. Sampson, J.A. 1927. Peritoneal endometriosis due to menstrual dissemination of endometrial tissue into the peritoneal cavity. Am. J. Obstet. Gynecol. **14:** 422–469.
2. Ishimaru, T. & H. Masuzaki. 1991. Peritoneal endometriosis: endometrial tissue implantation as a primary etiologic mechanism. Am. J. Obstet. Gynecol. **165:** 210–214.
3. Mahmood, T.A. & A. Templeton. 1990. Pathophysiology of mild endometriosis: review of literature. Hum. Reprod. **5:** 765–784.
4. Cramer, D.W., E. Wilson, R.J. Stillman *et al.* 1986. The relation of endometriosis to menstrual characteristics, smoking, and exercise: J. Am. Med. Assoc. **255:** 1904–1908.
5. Carlson, K., B. Miller & F.J. Fowler. 1994. The Maine Women's Health Study: I. Outcomes of hysterectomy. Obstet. Gynecol. **83:** 556–565.
6. Ridley, J.H. & I.K. Edwards. 1958. Experimental endometriosis in the human. Am. J. Obstet. Gynecol. **76:** 783–790.
7. Ridley, J.H. 1961. The validity of Sampson's theory of endometriosis. Am. J. Obstet. Gynecol. **82:** 777–782.

8. MANN, D.R., D.C. COLLINS, M.M. MITH *et al.* 1986. Treatment of endometriosis in monkeys: effectiveness of continuous infusion of gonadotropin-releasing hormone agonist compared to treatment with progestational steroid. J. Clin. Endocrinol. Metab. **63:** 1277–1283.
9. BROSENS, I.A., P.R. KONINCKX & P.A. CORVELEYN. 1978. A study of plasma progesterone, oestradiol-17β, prolactin, and LH levels, and of the luteal phase appearance of the ovaries in patients with endometriosis and infertility. Br. J. Obstet. Gynaecol. **85:** 246–250.
10. RIER, S., D.C. MARTIN, R.E. BOWMAN *et al.* 1993. Endometriosis in rhesus monkeys (*Macaca mulatta*) following chronic exposure to 2,3,7,8-tetrachlorodibenzo-*p*-dioxin [see comments]. Fundam. Appl.Toxicol. **21:** 433–441.
11. YANG, J.Z., S.K. AGARWAL & W.G. FOSTER. 2000. Subchronic exposure to 2,3,7,8-tetrachlorodibenzo-*p*-dioxin modulates the pathophysiology of endometriosis in the cynomolgus monkey. Toxicol. Sci. **56:** 374–381.
12. JACOBSON, V.C. 1922. The autotransplantation of endometrial tissue in the rabbit. Arch. Surg. **5:** 281–300.
13. VERNON, M.W. & E.A. WILSON. 1985. Studies on the surgical induction of endometriosis in the rat. Fertil. Steril. **44:** 684–694.
14. CUMMINGS, A.M., J.L. METCALF & L. BIRNBAUM. 1996. Promotion of endometriosis by 2,3,7,8-tetrachlorodibenzo-*p*-dioxin in rats and mice: time-dose dependence and species comparison. Toxicol. Appl. Pharmacol. **138:** 131–139.
15. CUMMINGS, A.M. & J.L. METCALF. 1996. Effect of surgically induced endometriosis on pregnancy and the effect of pregnancy and lactation on endometriosis in mice. Proc. Soc. Exp. Biol. Med. **212:** 332–337.
16. ZAMAH, N.M., M.G. DODSON, L.C. STEPHENS *et al.* 1984. Transplantation of normal and ectopic human endometrial tissue into athymic nude mice. Am. J. Obstet. Gynecol. **149:** 591–597.
17. BERGQVIST, A., S. JEPPSSON, S. KULLANDER & O. LJUNGBERG. 1985. Human uterine endometrium and endometriotic tissue transplanted into nude mice: morphologic effects of various steroid hormones. Am. J. Pathol. **121:** 337–341.
18. BRUNER, K.L., L.M. MATRISIAN, W.H. RODGERS *et al.* 1997. Suppression of matrix metalloproteinases inhibits establishment of ectopic lesions by human endometrium in nude mice. J. Clin. Invest. **99:** 2851–2857.
19. AWWAD, J.T., R.A. SAYEGH, X.J. TAO *et al.* 1999. The SCID mouse: an experimental model for endometriosis. Hum. Reprod. **14:** 3107–3111.
20. RODGERS, W.H., K.G. OSTEEN, L.M. MATRISIAN *et al.* 1993. Expression and localization of matrilysin, a matrix metalloproteinase, in the human endometrium. Am. J. Obstet. Gynecol. **168:** 253–260.
21. RODGERS, W.H., L.M. MATRISIAN, L.C. GIUDICE *et al.* 1994. Patterns of matrix metalloproteinase expression in cycling endometrium imply differential functions and regulation by steroids. J. Clin. Invest. **94:** 946–953.
22. SAITO, T., H. MIZUMOTO, K. KUROKI *et al.* 1995. Expression of MMP-3 and TIMP-1 in endometriosis and the influence of danazol. Acta Obstet. Gynaecol. Jpn. **47:** 495–496.
23. OSTEEN, K.G., K.L. BRUNER & K.L. SHARPE-TIMMS. 1996. Steroid and growth factors regulation of matrix metalloproteinase expression and endometriosis. Semin. Reprod. Endocrinol. **14:** 247–255.
24. HALME, J. & D. STOVALL. 1995. Endometriosis and its medical management. *In* Reproductive Medicine and Surgery, pp. 695–710. Mosby. St. Louis.
25. RAMZY, I. 1989. Pathology. *In* Endometriosis: Contemporary Concepts and Clinical Management, pp. 60–62. Lippincott. Philadelphia.
26. OLIVE, D.L. 1989. Medical treatment: alternatives to danazol. *In* Endometriosis: Contemporary Concepts and Clinical Management, p. 192. Lippincott. Philadelphia.
27. BRUNER, K.L., E. EISENBERG, F. GORSTEIN & K.G. OSTEEN. 1999. Progesterone and transforming growth factor-β coordinately regulate suppression of endometrial matrix metalloproteinases in a model of experimental endometriosis. Steroids **64:** 648–653.
28. LESSEY, B.A., D.A. METZGER, A.F. HANEY & K.S. MCCARTY. 1989. Immunohistochemical analysis of estrogen and progesterone receptors in endometriosis:

comparison with normal endometrium during the menstrual cycle and the effect of medical therapy. Fertil. Steril. **51:** 409–415.
29. BERGQVIST, A. & M. FERNO. 1993. Oestrogen and progesterone receptors in endometriotic tissue and endometrium: comparison of different cycle phases and ages. Hum. Reprod. **8:** 2211–2217.
30. ATTIA, G.R., K. ZEITOUN, D. EDWARDS *et al.* 2000. Progesterone receptor isoform A, but not B is expressed in endometriosis. J. Clin. Endocrinol. Metab. **85:** 2897–2902.
31. SALAMONSEN, L.A. & D.E. WOOLLEY. 1996. Matrix metalloproteinases in normal menstruation. Hum. Reprod. **11:** 124–133.
32. MIZUNO, K., T. TANAKA, N. UMESAKI & S. OGITA. 1999. Inhibition of cAMP-mediated decidualization in human endometrial stromal cells by IL-1β and laminin. Horm. Metab. Res. **31:** 307–310.
33. OSTEEN, K.G., K.L. BRUNER, E. SIERRA-RIVERA & L.I. GOLD. 1997. Progesterone and transforming growth factor-β co-mediate matrix metalloproteinase expression in a model of endometriosis. *In* Endometriosis Today. Vol. 13, pp. 200–209. Parthenon. Lancaster, United Kingdom.
34. KELLER, N.R., E. SIERRA-RIVERA, E. EISENBERG & K.G. OSTEEN. 2000. Progesterone exposure prevents matrix metalloproteinase-3 (MMP-3) stimulation by interleukin-1α in human endometrial stromal cells. J. Clin. Endocrinol. Metab. **85:** 1611–1619.
35. OSTEEN, K.G., N.R. KELLER, F.A. FELTUS & M.H. MELNER. 1999. Paracrine regulation of matrix metalloproteinase expression in normal human endometrium. Obstet. Gynecol. Invest. **48:** 2–13.
36. BRUNER, K.L., W.H. RODGERS, M. KORC *et al.* 1995. Transforming growth factor-β mediates the progesterone suppression of an epithelial metalloproteinase by adjacent stroma. Proc. Natl. Acad. Sci. U.S.A. **92:** 7362–7366.
37. OSTEEN, K.G., W.H. RODGERS, M. GAIRE *et al.* 1994. Stromal-epithelial interaction mediates steroidal regulation of metalloproteinase expression in human endometrium. Proc. Natl. Acad. Sci. U.S.A. **91:** 10129–10133.
38. OSTEEN, K.G., K.L. BRUNER-TRAN, N.R. KELLER & E. EISENBERG. 1999 (September). Retinoic acid treatments can mimic the effects of progesterone therapy in an experimental model of endometriosis [abstract]. Presented at the Fifty-fifth Annual Meeting of the Society for Reproductive Medicine, Toronto.
39. KONINCKX, P.R., P. BRAET, S.H. KENNEDY & D.H. BARLOW. 1994. Dioxin pollution and endometriosis in Belgium [see comments]. Hum. Reprod. **9:** 1001–1002.
40. PAUWELS, A.A., J. BROUWER, P. WEYLER & J.C. SCHEPENS. 2000 (May). The risk of endometriosis associated with the exposure to dioxins and related compounds: a case control study [abstract]. Presented at the Seventh Biennial World Endometriosis Congress, London.
41. MAYANI, A., S. BAREL, S. SOBACK & M. ALMAGOR. 1997. Dioxin concentrations in women with endometriosis. Hum. Reprod. **12:** 373–375.
42. YOSHIDA, K., S. IKEDA & J. NAKANISHI. 2000. Assessment of human health risk of dioxins in Japan. Chemosphere **40:** 177–185.
43. WANG, W., R. SMITH III & S. SAFE. 1998. Aryl hydrocarbon receptor–mediated antiestrogenicity in MCF-7 cells: modulation of hormone-induced cell cycle enzymes. Arch. Biochem. Biophys. **356:** 239–248.
44. GIERTHY, J.F., D.W. LINCOLN II, S.J. KAMPCIK *et al.* 1988. Enhancement of 2- and 16-alpha-estradiol hydroxylation in MCF-7 human breast cancer cells by 2,3,7,8-tetrachlorodibenzo-*p*-dioxin. Biochem. Biophys. Res. Commun. **157:** 515–520.
45. GIERTHY, J.F., D.W. LINCOLN, M.B. GILLESPIE *et al.* 1987. Suppression of estrogen related extracellular tissue plasminogen activator activity of MCF-7 cells by 2,3,7,8-tetrachlorodibenzo-*p*-dioxin. Cancer Res. **47:** 6198–6203.
46. TIAN, Y., S. KE, T. THOMAS *et al.* 1998. Transcriptional regulation of estrogen receptor gene expression by TCDD. J. Steroid Biochem. Mol. Biol. **67:** 17–34.
47. BRUNER-TRAN, K., S.E. RIER, E. EISENBERG & K.G. OSTEEN. 1999. The potential role of environmental toxins in the pathophysiology of endometriosis. Gynecol. Obstet. Invest. **48:** 45–56.
48. OSTROWSKI, K. & A. KINSNER. 2001. Inhibition of angiogenesis in the treatment of tumors. Arch. Immunol. Ther. Exp. **49**(1)**:** 27–31.

49. TAYLOR, R.N., I.P. RYAN, E.S. MOORE *et al.* 1997. Angiogenesis and macrophage activation in endometriosis. Ann. N.Y. Acad. Sci. **828:** 194–207.
50. FUJIMOTO, J., H. SAKAGUCHI, R. HIROSE *et al.* 1999. Angiogenesis in endometriosis and angiogenic factors. Gynecol. Obstet. Invest. **48:** 14–20.
51. FRASER, H.M. & S.F. LUNN. 2000. Angiogenesis and its control in the female reproductive system. Br. Med. Bull. **56:** 787–797.

Panel Discussion (Part VIII)

B.A. LESSEY (*University of North Carolina, Chapel Hill, NC*): A question for Kathy Sharpe-Timms. Is the effect of haptoglobin to increase IL-6 direct, or is it indirect through induction of IL-1 or TNFα or through inhibition of retinoic acid?

K.L. SHARPE-TIMMS (*University of Missouri, Columbia, MO*): Haptoglobin directly upregulates IL-6 production by peritoneal cells. We have blocked haptoglobin-induced IL-6 upregulation with an antihaptoglobin antibody. We also have administered additional IL-6 to endometriotic lesions *in vitro* and have been able to modulate the amount of haptoglobin produced by the lesions. It is possible that other mechanisms may be involved.

J.L. MCLACHLAN (*Tulane University, New Orleans, LA*): I have a question for Dr. Bruner-Tran. You showed that human endometrium seems to be more invasive or it takes hold in the peritoneal cavity, whereas in other species, nonprimate species, this does not happen. We have thought that this is related to the regurgitating menses and the cell is available for implantation. In your model, have you ever tried applying the same technique that you use on human endometrium—in other words, doing it on rat or rabbit endometrium, putting it into a nude mouse or immunosuppressed animal, and seeing if these other species, for which there is no spontaneous endometriosis, are able to establish in the same way as happens with human endometrium?

K.L. BRUNER-TRAN (*Vanderbilt University School of Medicine, Nashville, TN*): No, we have not, but that is a great idea. We have talked about doing that actually to the nude mouse to see if tissue will be autographed. I know that Jacobson back in the 1920s had a rabbit model of endometriosis, but he actually had to sew the tissue in. However, it is a great idea to use the nude mouse to accept other types of tissue.

N. SIDELL (*Emory University, Atlanta, GA*): How did you monitor the serum levels of retinoic acid in your *in vivo* treated nude mice?

BRUNER-TRAN: We do not have a serum assay for retinoic acid. When we did the first studies, we did RIA for progesterone and estrogen and we knew that we were getting an appropriate amount released from the pellet. We have had to take on faith that the pellets that came from the same company that were the retinoic acid pellets were also working as effectively as the estrogen and progesterone. Certainly, our results would indicate that this was so, but I cannot give you a value.

SIDELL: Retinoic acid is a little tricky given *in vivo*. First of all, it induces its own catabolism; once you start getting therapeutic levels, very quickly it is reduced, so you no longer see it in the serum. That is one problem that you have to deal with. Also, I assume it is systemics, or is the pellet right near the endometriotic growth?

BRUNER-TRAN: The pellets are placed just beneath the scapula on the back and all the injections are done about the area of the umbilicus, either intraperitoneal or subcutaneous depending on our outcome.

K. CHWALISZ (*TAP Pharmaceutical Products, Lake Forest, IL*): Is it possible to induce progesterone with bleeding in your model with either antiprogestins or progesterone withdrawal?

BRUNER-TRAN: It probably is possible to use an antiprogestin, although we have not done it. I do not think it would be feasible to just do progesterone withdrawal because of the time frame that it takes to induce an effect. The tissues treated with progesterone continue to demonstrate a response to progesterone for several days. Withdrawal bleeding does not occur until 3 or 4 days and our explants will not survive that long, but it might be possible to do it with onapristone or mifepristone.

K. YOSHINAGA (*National Institute of Child Health and Human Development, National Institutes of Health, Bethesda, MD*): This is addressed to Dr. Schenken. In your *in vitro* systems, have you tried any stromal tissue other than uterine stromal tissue, such as intestinal stromal tissue?

R.S. SCHENKEN (*University of Texas Health Science Center, San Antonio, TX*): I do not have any results for you yet as this is in progress. I am smiling because we had that discussion a few weeks ago about using other tissues in this model system.

R.M. BRENNER (*Oregon Regional Primate Research Center, Beaverton, OR*): Along that line, what phases in the cycle did you select your human endometrial tissues and have you tried menstrual effluent tissue, which would be the richest in these invasive enzymes?

SCHENKEN: The studies that I have shown you initially with the explant models involved minced endometrium that was obtained in either the proliferative or the secretory phase. We failed to observe any difference with regard to whether it was proliferative or secretory. We subsequently used menstrual endometrium; after removing the blood, we repeated the experiments and it was found to do the same thing. It attaches to the intact peritoneal mesothelium during the short-term 1-hour cultures. The individual cells, the isolated endometrial epithelial cells and the endometrial stromal cells, were also taken from the proliferative and secretory phases and, at this point, although the numbers are small, we do not seem to notice any difference in attachment ability. We have not done that with separated stromal and epithelial cells from menstrual endometrium.

K. OSTEEN (*Vanderbilt University School of Medicine, Nashville, TN*): Have you tried to add inflammatory cytokines to your peritoneal interface culture system? Did it enhance the invasion or the interactions at all? Have you looked at inflammatory cytokine action relative to your model?

SCHENKEN: The problem with the explant model where we actually used the minced tissue is that it is very difficult to quantitate. Thus, we could not use that particular model to look at an effect of cytokines or any other factors. That is why we went to the adhesion assay where we use mesothelial cell monolayers. At the present time, we have very preliminary data on the effects of different cytokines on that attachment assay, but that is definitely what we hope to pursue.

C.R. LYTTLE (*Wyeth Ayerst Research, Radnor, PA*): My question is addressed to Dr. Fazleabas. Could you speculate on the role of the expression of the ERβ in these tissues?

A.T. FAZLEABAS (*University of Illinois, Chicago, IL*): I was just thinking about that too. From what Franco DeMayo was saying, one potential idea is the increased hypersensitivity of the ERβ. Perhaps, the subrogation of ERβ along with the down-regulation of PRB might make these tissues hypersensitive to estrogen and might allow them to proliferate and develop initially.

LYTTLE: Actually, I think the data need to be reversed. There must be some misunderstanding because, in the ERβ knockout, the hypothesis is that they are more sensitive. Thus, here, we have an overexpression of ERβ, so they should be considerably less sensitive.

FAZLEABAS: Oh, I see what you are saying. It is an interesting point. I am just wondering in terms of compensation since this is really new data. I have not even had a chance to think about it and digest it, but it was one thing that came to mind. However, you are right. It is the opposite of what I was thinking.

LYTTLE: I was just trying to make a role for ERβ somewhere.

F. DEMAYO (*Baylor College of Medicine, Houston, TX*): If you look at the PRA data and if PRA and ERβ are repressors, they both seem to be big players in endometriosis as opposed to PRB and ERα. Thus, maybe there is some mechanism there that is linked between the two isoforms of the receptors.

CHWALISZ: Moreover, ERβ is also associated with inflammation. Thus, it might be a secondary response to the inflammatory reaction.

S.E. BULUN (*University of Illinois, Chicago, IL*): Can I make a comment about ERβ? To my knowledge, ERβ knockout mice do not have a uterine phenotype, but the reverse experiment has not been done. In other words, ERβ has not been overexpressed in the uterus. I do not think we have an answer to that yet.

LESSEY: Soy is a target for ERβ. Now guess who has the most endometriosis in the world? The Japanese. Perhaps, there is a link here.

LYTTLE: I think you are right. However, while certain soy components are somewhat ERβ-selective, they are not truly selective. They are only about 40-fold selective. Hence, they really do stimulate both receptors.

MCLACHLAN: Let me make a quick comment. We have a paper in press looking at uterine fibroids in humans. When comparing the normal myometrium and the lyomyomatous tissue, the ratio of ERα and ERβ switches and the ERβ is much higher in the disease tissue. Whether ERβ plays some overall role as a repressor or control agent is unknown, but it shows up in uterine disease pretty much consistently.

LYTTLE: It also shows up in a number of other diseases where you have events occurring. In ischemic models, for example, in the CNS, you see an increase in ERβ expression when you have neurodegenerative events. Thus, whether it has something to do with inflammation or other systems is really not known. I was just curious that it was so overexpressed here.

Conventional Medical Therapies for Endometriosis

VALERIE MONTGOMERY RICE

Department of Obstetrics and Gynecology, University of Kansas Medical Center, Kansas City, Kansas 66160, USA

ABSTRACT: Endometriosis is a common gynecologic disorder that affects approximately 14% of all women and 30% to 50% of infertile women. Since the most common symptoms of endometriosis—progressive dysmenorrhea, dyspareunia, chronic pelvic pain, and infertility—are also symptoms of multiple disorders, a diagnosis of endometriosis can be elusive and confirmed only by visualization, that is, laparoscopy. Endometriosis is often treated surgically upon diagnosis; however, the rate of recurrence is high, suggesting that a combination of therapeutic approaches might provide better outcomes than any one option alone. The most widely utilized hormonal treatments for endometriosis are GnRH agonists and oral contraceptives; agents indicated by the Food and Drug Administration include GnRH agonists and the androgen, danazol. The majority of evidence in support of medical therapy for endometriosis is largely observational, with the exception of studies of GnRH agonists, danazol, and a few progestins. Conventional treatment approaches for the medical management of endometriosis focus on suspected endometriosis, following a diagnosis of endometriosis, following surgical treatment of endometriosis, long-term management, and retreatment. Although major advances have been made in the treatment of endometriosis in recent decades, lack of randomized clinical trials evaluating the use of agents such as oral contraceptives alone or as add-back therapy for GnRH agonists, or those that examine combined medical and surgical treatments, has hampered the ability of physicians to provide the broadest range of medical therapies for this disorder. Future trials addressing these issues are warranted.

KEYWORDS: GnRH agonists; danazol; medroxyprogesterone acetate; treatment

INTRODUCTION

The classical description of endometriosis is the presence of endometrial glands and stroma outside the uterine cavity. It affects up to 1 in 7 women and as many as 30% to 50% of all infertile women. Endometriosis can be found anywhere in the pelvis, including the broad ligaments, uterosacral ligaments, and ovaries. The diagnosis of endometriosis can be elusive since its most common symptoms—progressive dysmenorrhea, dyspareunia, chronic pelvic pain, and infertility—are also symptoms of multiple disorders.

Address for correspondence: Valerie Montgomery Rice, M.D., Associate Professor, Department of Obstetrics and Gynecology, University of Kansas Medical Center, 3 Wescoe Pavilion, 3901 Rainbow Boulevard, Kansas City, KS 66160. Voice: 913-588-6261; fax: 913-588-6271.
vmontgomery-rice@kumc.edu

TABLE 1. Agents used to treat endometriosis

Class	Drug	Dosage
Androgen	Danazol	400–800 mg/day po for 4–6 months
GnRH agonist	Leuprolide	1 mg/day sc
	Leuprolide depot	3.75 mg IM q 28 days
	Buserelin	300–400 μg tid intranasally
	Goserelin	3.6 mg sc q 28 days
	Nafarelin	400–800 μg/day intranasally
Progestin	Gestrinone	2.5–5 mg/day
	MPA	20–30 mg/day po for 6 months, followed by 100 mg IM q 2 weeks for 2 months, then 200 mg IM monthly for 4 months
Oral contraceptive	Combination estrogen/ progestin	Ethinyl estradiol 30–35 μg plus a progestin; 1 tablet/day for 4–6 months

The primary goal of suppression of ovarian function is to halt the growth and activity of endometriotic lesions. Medications used to achieve this goal include androgens (such as danazol), progestogens (medroxyprogesterone acetate [MPA], norethindrone acetate), and gonadotropin-releasing hormone (GnRH) agonists (such as leuprolide acetate, nafarelin, buserelin, and goserelin) (TABLE 1). The most widely used agents are GnRH agonists and oral contraceptives; however, the majority of evidence in support of medical therapy for endometriosis is largely observational, with the exception of studies of a few progestins, GnRH agonists, and danazol. The Food and Drug Administration has formally approved GnRH agonists and danazol for the treatment of endometriosis.

Conventional medical therapies for women with endometriosis can be divided into five approaches: medical management for suspected endometriosis; medical management following a diagnosis of endometriosis; medical management following surgical treatment of endometriosis; long-term medical management of endometriosis; and medical management/retreatment issues.

MEDICAL MANAGEMENT FOR SUSPECTED ENDOMETRIOSIS

The central dogma guiding medical management of endometriosis is the observation that sex steroid hormones are the major regulators of the growth and function of endometriotic lesions. This view is supported by both laboratory and clinical observations: most endometriotic lesions contain estradiol, progesterone, and androgen receptors. In general, estradiol promotes growth in endometriotic lesions, androgens cause atrophy, and progestins can cause complex effects, depending on the dose and progestin used (TABLE 2).

Although endometriotic lesions may have both estradiol and progesterone receptors, the responsiveness of individual implants seems to be determined by the

TABLE 2. The effects of estradiol, androgen, and progestins on endometrium and endometriotic lesions

Steroid	Physiologic concentration	Pharmacological concentration
Estradiol	Growth	Growth or atrophy
Androgen	Atrophy	Atrophy
19-Norprogestin	Secretory changes, decidual changes, or atrophy	Decidual changes or atrophy
C-21 progestin	Secretory changes or atrophy	Decidual changes

relative amount of stromal and glandular components.[1] Furthermore, endometriotic lesions do not seem to respond to the effects of estradiol and progesterone like normal endometrium. The difference in concentration of estrogen and progesterone receptors may contribute to the dyssynchrony between the endometrium and endometriotic lesions in the same woman. These differences may also explain the apparent failure of endometriosis in some women to respond to the administration of progestins.

The rationale for empiric therapy of suspected endometriosis is threefold: pelvic pain with a negative workup is usually due to endometriosis; lack of visualization of endometriosis does not preclude it as a cause of pain; and the response of endometriosis to medical therapy is excellent. In a community survey of 1318 women who underwent laparoscopy for pelvic pain, Howard[2] found that no pathology was apparent in 516 (39%), whereas endometriosis was present in 364 (28%) and adhesions in 331 (25%). Endometriosis has been visualized laparoscopically in 70% of women with pelvic pain,[3] 84% of women with pain and infertility,[3] 45% of women with no symptoms,[4] and 25% of biopsies of the normal peritoneum.[5]

Hormonal treatment of suspected endometriosis includes the use of analgesics and antiprostaglandin agents such as nonsteroidal anti-inflammatory drugs (NSAIDs); however, the physician should determine when a dose is no longer adequate and to proceed to the next line of therapy, which typically includes combination estrogen/progestin oral contraceptives, progestins, suppressors of estrogen production such as danazol, and GnRH agonists. Psychotropic drugs have also been used in the management of chronic pelvic pain; however, such use requires caution and administration by an appropriate medical specialist, as well as a workup to rule out other causes of the pain.

The first line of medical therapy for chronic pelvic pain is usually acetaminophen or aspirin. Most patients will have tried these agents prior to presenting to their physicians. The second line of therapy is NSAIDs, which inhibit prostaglandin synthesis and thus are most effective when administered prior to onset of symptoms. Failure of one NSAID to provide relief should not preclude use of others in the same class; limitations to NSAID use include over-the-counter doses that may be insufficient to relieve pain and the potential for gastrointestinal toxicity when given chronically at high doses.

Combination estrogen/progestin oral contraceptives are often used initially for women with chronic pelvic pain who have an otherwise negative evaluation. Rationale for use includes inhibition of ovulation and a decrease in overall mean gonadotropin levels; decreased menstrual flow; and decidualization of implants, including decreased production of intracellular receptors. However, there is an increased conversion of the most potent estrogen, estradiol, to the weak estrogen, estrone, which may result in stimulation of disease. There are no randomized controlled clinic trials of oral contraceptives in women suspected of endometriosis when pelvic pain is a major component of the associated symptoms. In 1993, Vessey *et al.*[6] provided some epidemiologic data supporting the concept of use of combined oral contraceptives being associated with a reduced incidence of endometriosis.[7] If the patient does not respond to oral contraceptives, surgical diagnosis and treatment or use of GnRH agonists should be considered. To date, no data have demonstrated greater benefits for cyclic versus continuous use or low-dose versus high-dose agents.

Treatment with progestins alone for endometriosis may also be used to suppress gonadotropin release, resulting in a hypoestrogenic state. Progestins have a direct effect on endometrial tissue, resulting in glandular atrophy and decidualization. The side effects of progestins include spotting and breakthrough bleeding in approximately half of all patients, depression in 5% to 10%, breast tenderness, fluid retention, and increased appetite and weight gain, which often lead to discontinuation of therapy. No randomized controlled trials have evaluated the use of progestins for suspected endometriosis.

The observation that a hyperandrogenic state could induce atrophy of endometrium led to the use of androgens in the treatment of endometriosis. One such androgen is danazol, a synthetic isoxazole derivative chemically related to 17α-ethinyltestosterone. Danazol acts to increase the concentration of free testosterone by binding to sex-hormone-binding globulin, thereby displacing testosterone. Furthermore, it also inhibits steroid production from the ovaries, resulting in a decrease in ovarian estrogen production. Danazol has also been found to interfere with follicle-stimulating hormone (FSH) and luteinizing hormone (LH) secretion by the pituitary gland, all of which contribute to an inhibition of endometrial growth within and exterior to the endometrial cavity. Multiple nonrandomized trials have shown that use of danazol resulted in an improvement in pain associated with endometriosis, ranging from 66% to 100% of the women evaluated.[8–10] Danazol also reduced the size of endometriosis lesions. The main drawback to use of danazol is its androgenic side effects. In fact, up to two-thirds of women discontinue the drug due to complaints of weight gain, breast atrophy, hot flushes, and hirsutism.[1,8,11,12] The majority of trials that have utilized danazol for the treatment of endometriosis were conducted in the late 1980s and early 1990s and there are no randomized control trials comparing danazol to no treatment. Although the literature supports its use for symptom relief, few patients are likely to use danazol over a long period of time because of its side effects. Given the paucity of randomized placebo-controlled trials, well-designed studies to investigate the overall effect of this drug may be useful.

GnRH agonists were first used in clinical trials for the treatment of endometriosis in 1981; Meldrum *et al.* reported the results of treating 5 women with D-Trp6-Pro9-Net-LHRH in 1982.[13] GnRH agonists act to decrease pituitary synthesis and secretion of gonadotropins, resulting in hypogonadism and a state of hypoestrogenemia. The effect of the GnRH agonist leuprolide acetate depot was studied in 100 women with chronic pelvic pain who were not relieved by doxycycline, NSAIDs, or oral contraceptives.[14] Prior to laparoscopy, the women were randomized to receive leuprolide acetate depot at 3.75 mg every 4 weeks or a placebo injection for 12 weeks, after which they were laparoscoped. Approximately 85% of the women were demonstrated to have endometriosis; those treated with the GnRH agonist reported greater improvement in pelvic pain, dysmenorrhea, and dyspareunia than women treated with placebo. In women with suspected endometriosis, a noninvasive diagnostic workup can identify women with chronic pelvic pain likely to have endometriosis, and these women can be treated effectively with GnRH agonists.

MEDICAL MANAGEMENT FOLLOWING A DIAGNOSIS OF ENDOMETRIOSIS

The incidence of endometriosis in patients with pelvic pain ranges from 30% to 50% of all infertile women and is 71% in those with chronic pain.[3] There is little correlation between pain and amount of disease. A diagnosis of endometriosis is initially confirmed laparoscopically.

The advantage of an oral contraceptive over other hormonal treatments is that it can be taken indefinitely. Only one trial has evaluated use of combination oral contraceptive compared with monthly subcutaneous injection of GnRH agonist in the reduction of dysmenorrhea, dyspareunia, and nonmenstrual pain in the presence of a laparoscopically confirmed diagnosis of endometriosis.[7] Of the 57 patients evaluated, no significant differences between the two treatments for any of three symptoms evaluated at the end of the 6-month follow-up were found; there was a trend, however, toward oral contraceptives being more effective in treating dysmenorrhea and the GnRH agonist being more effective for dyspareunia. Although the oral contraceptives failed to make women pain-free, they did report a reduction in pain scores from moderate-to-severe pain to mild dysmenorrhea. The implications of research in the area of use of oral contraceptives for the treatment of endometriosis are obvious because of the commonality of the disease and the widely empiric use of oral contraceptives for the implied suppression of the hormonal etiology of the endometriosis. If oral contraceptives could be shown to be at least as effective as danazol or GnRH agonists, treatment options for long-term management of the disease could be broadened. Therefore, larger randomized controlled trials are clearly needed to evaluate the ability of oral contraceptives to reduce the pain ascribed to endometriosis.

Dmowski and Cohen documented a 40% to 50% recurrence rate up to 4 years in patients with laparoscopically confirmed endometriosis treated with danazol.[15] In another study, 5-year follow-up found an overall crude recurrence rate of 33%, with 22% with minimal disease and 50% with severe disease.[12] In 15 studies comparing danazol and GnRH agonists in 1299 women, only 1 study identified a difference in posttreatment revised American Fertility Society scores: mean percent reduction in the revised endometriosis score after 24 weeks of treatment was 53% for the GnRH agonist, goserelin, compared with 33% for danazol.[16] Many clinical trials have also compared the efficacy of danazol with that of the GnRH agonist, nafarelin. Results showed nafarelin to be as effective as danazol in reducing both the growth of endometriotic implants and symptoms during the treatment phases of the trial. Nafarelin also prevented the return of symptoms during the initial 6- to 12-month follow-up after cessation of therapy.[17–19] The obvious difference between the GnRH agonist and danazol has been the profile of the side effects: the agonist has side effects associated more with a hypoestrogenic state and danazol more with an androgenic state. Other agents under investigation for the treatment of endometriosis include mifepristone and gestrinone.

MEDICAL MANAGEMENT FOLLOWING SURGICAL TREATMENT OF ENDOMETRIOSIS

At the time of a diagnostic laparoscopy, the majority of cases of endometriosis at all stages can be treated by ablative techniques (i.e., laser vaporization or electrical, thermal, or mechanical ablation) or excision. The need for medical therapy after what is considered to be complete surgical treatment has been debated. However, it is generally accepted that disease can be left behind after surgery, suggesting a benefit for medical therapy in combination with surgical ablation. Oral contraceptives, danazol, and GnRH agonist therapy have all been studied for the postoperative management of endometriosis.

Oral contraceptives may be useful in treating dysmenorrhea. However, there are potential drawbacks to the use of oral contraceptives as postoperative therapy for endometriosis. The high estrogenic milieu (EE 5 μg = 0.625 mg) may inhibit implant regression, despite the presence of progestins. Little data exist that demonstrate the benefit of oral contraceptives as either primary or secondary therapy for endometriosis. In addition, endometriotic implants appear to have fewer progesterone receptors than normal endometrium, compromising their function and significantly lessening the impact of oral contraceptives. Perhaps the greatest drawback is that the majority of patients with chronic pelvic pain have already failed an empiric course of oral contraceptives prior to surgical treatment, reducing the likelihood that it would be effective postoperatively. No studies have evaluated oral contraceptives following surgical treatment of endometriosis.

In 1999, Bianchi *et al.* evaluated the use of danazol postoperatively for 3 months in 77 women with moderate-to-severe disease and found it did not markedly improve either short-term reproductive prognosis or pelvic pain.[20] A randomized trial that compared danazol to placebo and MPA found that MPA at 100 mg/day resulted in a complete resolution of lesions in 50% of patients and a partial resolution in 13% at 12 months posttherapy, compared with 16% and 6% in the placebo group, respectively. Both MPA and danazol decreased symptom scores and pelvic pain scores.[11] In one study, 70% of patients who received ablation plus 6 months of postoperative GnRH agonist analog therapy and 60% of those treated with excision alone were pain-free at the end of 2 years, compared with 23% who received ablation alone.[21]

LONG-TERM MEDICAL MANAGEMENT OF ENDOMETRIOSIS

The limiting factor in the long-term use of a GnRH agonist is related to its induction of a hypoestrogenic state, resulting in a decrease in bone mineral density (BMD) after 6 months. This is because the effects of estradiol on target tissues are dose-related, with a hierarchy of organ tissue response; calcium metabolism is the most sensitive and endometriosis is the least sensitive. This has led to development of the estrogen threshold hypothesis, which suggests that a concentration of estradiol that will partially prevent bone loss may not stimulate endometrial growth.[22]

TABLE 3. Recommended use of add-back regimens

GnRH agonist use	Add-back	Bone density scan
<3 months	Unnecessary	Unnecessary
3–6 months	Optional	High-risk patients only
>6 months	Strongly recommended	Every 6–12 months
Retreatment	Logical, but untested	Prior to retreatment

TABLE 4. GnRH agonist add-back regimens tested for the treatment of endometriosis

Regimen	Maximal duration studied
Progestin only	
MPA	6 months
NEt	12 months
NEt Ac	12 months
Tibolone	6 months
Progestin + bisphosphonate	
NEt + sodium etidronate	48 weeks
Estrogen + progestins	
MPA + CEE	6 months
MPA + 17β-E_2	6 months
NEt + 17β-E_2	6 months
NEt Ac + CEE	12 months

TERMS: MPA = medroxyprogesterone acetate; NEt = norethindrone; NEt Ac = norethindrone acetate; CEE = conjugated equine estrogens; 17β-E_2 = 17β-estradiol.

Multiple studies have now shown that several regimens are effective as add-back therapy to minimize or eliminate the hypoestrogenic effects of the GnRH agonist while preserving its therapeutic efficacy;[23–28] the ultimate goal is to enhance compliance and potentially prolong duration of therapy. Although several regimens have been successful in reducing the adverse effects of the GnRH agonist and minimizing BMD loss, it is not possible to delineate a single add-back regimen for all patients with documented and clinically suspected endometriosis, given the dearth of large-scale clinical trials. TABLES 3 and 4 summarize the suggested use of an add-back regimen and different regimens reported in the treatment of endometriosis.

MEDICAL MANAGEMENT: RETREATMENT

Due to the lack of data on BMD changes during longer or repeated courses of GnRH agonists, the Food and Drug Administration has approved GnRH agonist use for the management of endometriosis for only one 6-month treatment period. Given that the annual recurrence rate of endometriosis is 5% to 20% and can reach 40% at 5 years posttherapy, a second treatment course of GnRH agonist therapy is desirable, especially by patients wishing to avoid additional surgery.

In an international multicenter trial to determine the safety and efficacy of GnRH agonist retreatment, 45 women with recurrent endometriotic symptoms after a 6-month course of a GnRH agonist were administered a 3-month retreatment course.[29] At least 6 months must have elapsed after the last dose of the first treatment course. No entry laparoscopy was performed. A control group of 10 healthy volunteers was included to provide comparative longitudinal data on BMD. At the end of treatment, the GnRH agonist provided a substantial and significant relief of both patient-perceived symptoms (dysmenorrhea, pelvic pain, dyspareunia) and physician-recorded signs of endometriosis (pelvic tenderness, induration). At 3 months post-treatment, symptom severity remained significantly lower than at baseline and occurred without a sustained loss of BMD, suggesting that repeated short-term GnRH agonist therapy may be feasible. Benefits of such a regimen include having a lesser impact on bone mass and fewer hypoestrogenic adverse effects.

In a similar multicenter trial, Hornstein *et al.*[30] followed 36 women whose endometriotic symptoms recurred at 3 or 6 months after a course of GnRH agonist. Each was administered a 3-month retreatment course of GnRH agonist at least 6 months after the last dose of the first course. No entry laparoscopy was performed and there was no control group. At the end of treatment, the majority of patients reported a marked decline in symptom severity; this effect was also seen at the end of the second month of treatment.

Candidates for retreatment with GnRH agonists include women with recurrent symptoms who have had a good response to a prior GnRH agonist regimen and no pelvic mass. Any changes in symptoms or physical examination require a reevaluation. At least 6 months should elapse after the last dose of the first course if no add-back therapy is administered. A pretherapy BMD evaluation should be considered; however, there is no need for laparoscopy unless there is a change in symptoms or physical examination. Unresolved questions regarding GnRH agonist retreatment include the number of courses that may be considered safe; whether the duration of the retreatment course should be 3 months, 6 months, or another time period; the ideal interval of time between courses; what should be considered appropriate monitoring (i.e., BMD lipids, etc.); and whether use of add-back therapy would alter the decision made. Currently, data from controlled studies are insufficient for developing recommendations.

The long-term effects of GnRH agonist and add-back therapy retreatment and reoperative rates have not been assessed. The implications for further research with the GnRH agonist in the area of comparative studies of the agonist with simple therapy such as oral contraceptives are desirable. There is also no literature available to compare the differences between the GnRH agonist therapy and surgical therapy. Further studies would also be required to establish the optimum add-back regimen, the ideal interval between treatment courses, the number of courses that would be safe, and what monitoring would be appropriate to determine the safety profile. Many of these issues could be addressed in an appropriately designed clinical trial; however, long-term follow-up would be desirable to assess the long-term treatment effects of an agonist beyond 1 to 2 years.

SUMMARY AND CONCLUSIONS

Although major advances have been made in the development of medical therapies for the treatment of endometriosis, the lack of randomized clinical trials evaluating the use of agents other than those indicated for its treatment prevents physicians from pursuing all available options. Future studies comparing use of oral contraceptives to GnRH agonists and danazol and as add-back therapy for GnRH agonists, and those that compare outcomes of various agents used in combination with surgical procedures, will help define the optimal regimen for the treatment of endometriosis.

REFERENCES

1. METZGER, D.A., D.L. OLIVE & A.F. HANEY. 1988. Limited hormonal responsiveness of ectopic endometrium: histologic correlation with intrauterine endometrium. Hum. Pathol. **19:** 1417–1424.
2. HOWARD, F.M. 1993. The role of laparoscopy in chronic pelvic pain: promise and pitfalls. Obstet. Gynecol. Surv. **48:** 357–387.
3. KONINCKX, P.R., C. MEULEMAN, S. DEMEYERE *et al.* 1991. Suggestive evidence that pelvic endometriosis is a progressive disease, whereas deeply infiltrating endometriosis is associated with pelvic pain. Fertil. Steril. **55:** 759–765.
4. BALASCH, J., M. CREUS, F. FABREGUES *et al.* 1996. Visible and non-visible endometriosis at laparoscopy in fertile and infertile women and in patients with chronic pelvic pain: a prospective study. Hum. Reprod. **11:** 387–391.
5. MURPHY, A.A., W.R. GREEN, D. BOBBIE *et al.* 1986. Unsuspected endometriosis documented by scanning electron microscopy in visually normal peritoneum. Fertil. Steril. **46:** 522–524.
6. VESSEY, M.P., L. VILLARD-MACKINTOSH & R. PAINTER. 1993. Epidemiology of endometriosis in women attending family planning clinics. BMJ **306:** 182–184.
7. VERCELLINI, P., L. TRESPIDI, A. COLOMBO *et al.* 1993. A gonadotropin-releasing hormone agonist versus a low-dose oral contraceptive for pelvic pain associated with endometriosis. Fertil. Steril. **60:** 75–79.
8. ORAL, E. & A. ARICI. 1996. Peritoneal growth factors and endometriosis. Semin. Reprod. Endocrinol. **14:** 257–267.
9. DMOWSKI, W.P. & M.R. COHEN. 1975. Treatment of endometriosis with an antigonadotropin, danazol: a laparoscopic and histologic evaluation. Obstet. Gynecol. **46:** 147–152.
10. BUTTRAM, V.C., JR., R.C. REITER & S. WARD. 1985. Treatment of endometriosis with danazol: report of a 6-year prospective study. Fertil. Steril. **43:** 353–360.
11. TELIMAA, S., J. PUOLAKKA & A. KAUPPILA. 1987. Placebo-controlled comparison of danazol and high dose medroxyprogesterone acetate in the treatment of endometriosis after conservative surgery. Gynecol. Endocrinol. **1:** 13–23.
12. BARBIERI, R.L., S. EVANS & R.W. KISTNER. 1982. Danazol in the treatment of endometriosis: analysis of 100 cases with a 4-year follow-up. Fertil. Steril. **37:** 737–746.
13. MELDRUM, D.R., R.J. CHANG, W. VALE *et al.* 1982. Medical oophorectomy using a long-acting GnRH agonist: a possible new approach to the treatment of endometriosis. J. Clin. Endocrinol. Metab. **54:** 1081–1083.
14. LING, F.W. 1999. Randomized controlled trial of depot leuprolide in patients with chronic pelvic pain and clinically suspected endometriosis: the Pelvic Pain Study Group. Obstet. Gynecol. **93:** 51–58.
15. DMOWSKI, W.P. & M.R. COHEN. 1978. Antigonadotropin (danazol) in the treatment of endometriosis: evaluation of posttreatment fertility and three-year follow-up data. Am. J. Obstet. Gynecol. **130:** 41–48.

16. ROCK, J.A., J.A. TRUGLIA & R.J. CAPLAN. 1993. Zoladex (goserelin acetate implant) in the treatment of endometriosis: a randomized comparison with danazol—The Zoladex Endometriosis Study Group. Obstet. Gynecol. **82:** 198–205.
17. HENZEL, M.R., S.L. CORSON, K. MOGHISSI *et al.* 1988. Administration of nasal nafarelin as compared with oral danazol for endometriosis. N. Engl. J. Med. **318:** 485–489.
18. KENNEDY, S.H., I.A. WILLIAMS, J. BRODRIBB *et al.* 1990. A comparison of nafarelin acetate and danazol in the treatment of endometriosis. Fertil. Steril. **53:** 998–1003.
19. THE NAFARELIN EUROPEAN ENDOMETRIOSIS TRIAL GROUP (NEET). 1992. Nafarelin for endometriosis: a large-scale, danazol-controlled trial of efficacy and safety, with 1-year follow-up. Fertil. Steril. **57:** 514–522.
20. BIANCHI, S., M. BUSACCA, B. AGNOLI *et al.* 1999. Effects of 3 month therapy with danazol after laparoscopic surgery for stage III/IV endometriosis: a randomized study. Hum. Reprod. **14:** 1335–1337.
21. WINKEL, C.A. 1999. Combined medical and surgical treatment of women with endometriosis. Clin. Obstet. Gynecol. **42:** 645–663.
22. BARBIERI, R.L. 1992. Hormone treatment of endometriosis: the estrogen threshold hypothesis. Am. J. Obstet. Gynecol. **166:** 740–745.
23. KIILHOLMA, P., M. KORHONEN, R. TUIMALA *et al.* 1995. Comparison of the gonadotropin-releasing hormone agonist goserelin acetate alone versus goserelin combined with estrogen-progestagen add-back therapy in the treatment of endometriosis. Fertil. Steril. **64:** 903–908.
24. BERQVIST, A., J. JACOBSON & S. HARRIS. 1997. A double-blind randomized study of the treatment of endometriosis with nafarelin or nafarelin plus norethisterone. Gynecol. Endocrinol. **11:** 187–194.
25. MAKARAINEN, L., L. RONNBERG & A. KAUPPILA. 1996. Medroxyprogesterone acetate supplementation diminishes the hypoestrogenic side effects of gonadotropin-releasing hormone agonist without changing its efficacy in endometriosis. Fertil. Steril. **65:** 29–34.
26. SURREY, E.S. & H.L. JUDD. 1992. Reduction of vasomotor symptoms and bone mineral density loss with combined norethindrone and long-acting gonadotropin-releasing hormone agonist therapy of symptomatic endometriosis: a prospective randomized trial. J. Clin. Endocrinol. Metab. **75:** 558–563.
27. SURREY, E.S., B. VOIGT, N. FOURNET *et al.* 1995. Prolonged gonadotropin-releasing hormone agonist treatment of symptomatic endometriosis: the role of cyclic sodium etidronate and low dose norethindrone "add-back" therapy. Fertil. Steril. **63:** 747–755.
28. SURREY, E.S., J.C. GAMBONE, J.K.H. LU *et al.* 1990. The effects of combining norethindrone with a gonadotropin-releasing hormone agonist in the treatment of symptomatic endometriosis. Fertil. Steril. **53:** 620–626.
29. ADAMSON, G.D., W.L. HEINRICHS, M.R. HENZEL *et al.* 1997. Therapeutic efficacy and bone mineral density response during and following a three-month re-treatment of endometriosis with nafarelin (Synarel). Am. J. Obstet. Gynecol. **177:** 1413–1428.
30. HORNSTEIN, M.D., A.A. YUZPE, K. BURRY *et al.* 1997. Retreatment with nafarelin for recurrent endometriosis symptoms: efficacy, safety, and bone mineral density. Fertil. Steril. **67:** 1013–1018.

Research Aspects of Endometriosis Surgery

DAN C. MARTIN

Department of Gynecology and Obstetrics, University of Tennessee, Memphis, Tennessee, USA

ABSTRACT: This paper asks various questions regarding endometriosis surgery. These address the research issues of the necessity of treatment, surgical technique, terminology, the definition of the rectovaginal septum, standards for research, and the impact of RBRVS/RDG.

KEYWORDS: endometriosis; symptoms; excision; surgical techniques; atypical; appearance; coagulation; rectovaginal septum; retrocervical endometriosis; recognition; RBRVS; DRG

IS TREATMENT NEEDED?

The finding of endometriosis does not necessarily mean that patients require treatment.[1] Patients are often found to have asymptomatic endometriosis that appears to be under homeostatic control. This appears to have been found in 61% of patients having surgery for myomata, 50% of patients undergoing sterilization,[2] and 25% of patients having tubal sterilization reversal.[3] Furthermore, 93% of postmenopausal patients with endometriosis are relatively asymptomatic and only 39 (29%) of 136 postmenopausal patients with endometriosis had disease that appeared to be clinically significant.[4]

Unfortunately, the occurrence of asymptomatic disease does not determine who will have progression of their disease and who may need subsequent treatment. Moen found that the odds ratio of diagnosing endometriosis in women increased to 4.5 at 10 years when compared with the first 5 years after delivery.[5] Even though these women were free of symptoms, the prevalence of the disease was increasing with length of voluntary infertility. This implies that endometriosis may be the result of infertility, whether voluntary or involuntary. Moreover, with longer follow-up, some may progress and become symptomatic.[6]

Cornillie[7] noted that the activities of superficial, intermediate, and deep lesions were 58%, 25%, and 68%, respectively. This was similar to the percent in phase with the endometrium: 57%, 38%, and 74%, respectively. The activity of superficial lesions is in agreement with Vernon,[8] Goldstein,[9] Davis,[10] Vercellini,[11] and Perper.[12] These studies suggest that superficial implants are a significant disease and they argue against the opposite conclusion by Evers[13] and Brosens.[14] The degree of activity shown by Cornillie[7] suggests that superficial and deep disease are more likely to be

Address for correspondence: Dan C. Martin, M.D., Department of Gynecology and Obstetrics, University of Tennessee, 1717 Kirby Parkway, Suite 100, Memphis, TN 38120-4331. Voice: 901-751-0300; fax: 901-751-9977.

Dan@DanMartinMD.com

symptomatic than intermediate stages. This would be compatible with the hypothesis that intermediate lesions are commonly a residual of activity by the patient's homeostatic mechanisms. These intermediate lesions are less likely to require treatment than superficial or deep lesions. Research based on staging needs to consider this possibility.

IS EXCISION SUPERIOR TO COAGULATION?

Although there are no prospective randomized trials comparing electrosurgical coagulation with sharp excision,[15] excision appears to be superior under certain circumstances. These circumstances include deep lesions, lesions close to vital organs, and lesions of uncertain pathology.

The ability to see what is cut is helpful for deep lesions. Prolonged electrosurgical coagulation has an increased risk of burning deep unseen organs or vessels. If an organ is cut during excision, it is likely to be seen.

Small (less than or equal to 2 mm) lesions are adequately destroyed by coagulation (electrosurgical, thermal, or laser), vaporization, or excision. Lesions of 3 mm to 5 mm are generally excised or vaporized. Larger lesions generally require excision.[1,6,16–19] Laparoscopy is adequate for the majority of patients.

Even if excision results in lower recurrence and/or persistence rate, this degree of surgery is associated with increased risk compared to superficial coagulation or nonsurgical treatment.[20] This risk must be weighed against any anticipated advantages. These patients may benefit by laparotomy.

IS "ATYPICAL" A REASONABLE TERM?

The term "atypical" has been applied to both the histologic appearance of premalignant lesions and the gross appearance of endometriosis.[21,22] This creates confusion about whether we are talking about malignancy or about endometriosis. "Subtle" may be a more appropriate term for the gross appearance. This is particularly true since subtle lesions occur more often (65%) than those that have commonly been called typical (60%).[3]

On the other hand, subtle appearances can also be confused with endosalpingiosis, psammoma bodies, and cancer. Subtle appearances are associated with an increased chance of atypical histology.[23–27] Terms need to be chosen with care.

DOES RECTOVAGINAL ENDOMETRIOSIS INVADE THE RECTOVAGINAL SEPTUM?

The rectovaginal (RV) pouch covers part of the vagina and rectum and its base is the upper limit of the RV septum. The RV pouch is not the RV septum.[28,29] Retroperitoneal endometriosis[30] and posterior vaginal fornix endometriosis are behind the RV pouch and not within it. The Adamyan classification[31] demonstrates the retrocervical location of this area.

The depth of the RV pouch extends to the middle one-third of the vagina in 93% of women.[32,33] The RV pouch has an average depth of 5.3 cm in nulliparous women and 5.4 cm in multiparous women. The RV septum is 2.1 cm in nulliparous women and 3.3 cm in multiparous women with otherwise normal anatomy.[32] The RV pouch can descend 11% to 89% of the length of the vagina.[34] Shortening of the RV pouch and elongation of the RV septum with RV involvement appears to be related to contraction of this area.[29,35] Illustrations of this on the web are available at www.DanMartinMD.com/rvendo.htm.

Articles often describe involvement of the RV septum where this is not present. A 1917 article by Cullen[36] has illustrations and a 1989 article by Chen[37] has an MRI of retrocervical RV pouch endometriosis with minimal or no involvement of the RV septum.

Precise identification of the area of surgery is important in research and education. Although the surgical treatment by Anaf[38] is said to be of RV endometriosis, it is similar to that for cul-de-sac endometriosis[39] and retrocervical endometriosis described by other authors.[31,40,41] Retrocervical may be a more descriptive term when used to describe RV pouch, retroperitoneal, and vaginal fornix endometriosis behind or beneath the cervix with no rectal involvement. RV is used when there is involvement of both the vaginal and rectal areas of the pouch and may include involvement of the RV septum. These distinctions are surgically important because treatment of retrocervical endometriosis is less complex than treatment of RV endometriosis.[42–46] Limiting extensive surgery to select centers is reasonable as most gynecologists will see only a few cases of deep rectal endometriosis in their careers.[35]

DO RESEARCH STUDIES NEED A GOLDEN STANDARD FOR RECOGNITION?

Recognition has always been said to be difficult due to the different sizes and colors.[3,47–51] Recognition can also be a function of the distance of observation. When specimens are observed at approximately 12 inches using 4× loop magnification, the incidence of microscopic endometriosis has been as high as 25%.[52] When observed at laparoscopy using standard techniques, this decreases to 13%.[53] This is as low as 0.5% using near-contact laparoscopy.[54,55] Near-contact laparoscopy[49] has been used to identify lesions as small as 180 to 200 μm.[3,51]

However, small lesions can be missed due to their size, while larger lesions[3,6,16,56] may be missed due to distortion by adhesions or due to a retroperitoneal position. These deep lesions are often more palpable than visual. Palpation during menses increases the chance of detecting these nodules.[6]

Although visualization is said to be the golden standard, surgical sensitivity and specificity are often low. Gynecologists may see and note only 41% to 70% of the endometriosis that they remove and send to pathology.[57,58] This sensitivity of physicians is linearly associated with the number of cases of resection of confirmed endometriosis.[57] Specificity is also low. Confirmation occurred in 64.5% at The Johns Hopkins Hospital,[58] from 57% to 99% in Memphis,[57] and from 42% to 76% at Yale.[59] A Belgian study quotes a 100% confirmation by the most experienced laparoscopist in that study.[53] This wide range leads to the conclusion that confirmation of lesions in a general practice is not essential. In a general clinical practice, biopsies and histology may be more valuable to rule out cancer versus other pathology than it is to confirm endometriosis. This appears particularly true with clear and opaque vesicles. These can be endometriosis, psammoma bodies, endosalpingiosis, or cancer.[24] However, typical appearance has also been associated with endometrioid cancer.[27] Concerns of cancer are increased in infertility patients with adhesions.[60]

Although visualization may be adequate for most endometriosis surgery, it may be inadequate for research studies. Drawing serious academic conclusions from studies with no (0%) confirmation in 66 endometriomas[61] may not be reasonable. Confirmation of ovarian endometriomas is more generally reported at 86%.[62,63] The contention by Fayez that the implants on the cyst lining can be "easily washed out"[64] was not confirmed in the pictures or photomicrographs in other articles.[62]

Treatment problems may also occur due to inadequate use of either laser vaporization or electrosurgery. Low power densities and inadequate time of exposure may inadvertently leave endometriosis behind. If laser vaporization is used, surgeons can perform excision of the area immediately after vaporization to look for residual endometriosis. If electrosurgical coagulation is used, then observations at second-look laparoscopy are needed to determine residual endometriosis. These techniques do not appear useful in clinical practice, but may be needed when determining qualifications of physicians doing surgical research in endometriosis.

WILL RBRVS AND DRG IMPACT ON SURGICAL ENDOMETRIOSIS RESEARCH?

RBRVS is an acronym for resources-based relative value scale. Although RBRVS was designed to allocate reimbursement based on time and work, it is based on a finite set of codes to describe an infinite set of combinations. This finite set is then assigned a value that represents average cases. When a case is simpler than average, reimbursement is increased per hour. When cases are difficult, reimbursement is decreased per hour. This concept works very well for primary care gynecologists who can do basic cases and who refer the more difficult cases to tertiary care. This works poorest for tertiary care physicians, who see a higher-than-average number of difficult cases that pay less per hour.

Although prolonged difficult cases have always been relatively under-reimbursed, relative under-reimbursement in 1990 at 275% of Medicare was still high enough to make most internists jealous. However, relative under-reimbursement in 1990 is generally at 80% to 130% of Medicare. Current reimbursement may not cover the overhead for providing the service. There is negative financial incentive for these cases. Although physicians wish to provide excellent care to their patients, the concern is that money will speak louder than words or philosophy.

In a similar fashion, DRGs (diagnostic-related groups) have a similar effect on surgical facilities. Simple quick cases in the same DRG pay more than complex cases. In my recent DRG report card, DRG 358 covered procedures ranging from a simple myomectomy to a procedure that included removal of bowel endometriosis, 2 ovarian chocolate cysts, peritoneal endometriosis, the appendix, 7 myomas, and a hernia. The hospital nets more money on the patient who has 1 myoma removed than on the patient who had the multistaged operation with 13 specimens. Although surgeons performing these operations may have been encouraged by their hospitals 15 years ago before DRGs, they may be discouraged by the same hospitals today.

REFERENCES

1. Martin, D. 1995. Rationale for surgical treatment of endometriosis. *In* Endometriosis: Advanced Management and Surgical Techniques. Springer-Verlag. New York/Berlin.
2. Rawson, J.M.R. 1991. Prevalence of endometriosis in asymptomatic women. J. Reprod. Med. **36:** 513–515.
3. Martin, D.C., G.D. Hubert, R. Vander Zwaag *et al.* 1989. Laparoscopic appearances of peritoneal endometriosis. Fertil. Steril. **51:** 63–67.
4. Kempers, R.D., M.B. Dockerty, A.B. Hunt *et al.* 1960. Significant postmenopausal endometriosis. Surg. Gynecol. Obstet. **111:** 348–356.
5. Moen, M.H. 1991. Is a long period without childbirth a risk factor for developing endometriosis? Hum. Reprod. **6:** 1404–1407.
6. Koninckx, P.R. & D.C Martin. 1992. Deep endometriosis: a consequence of infiltration or retraction or possibly adenomyosis externa? Fertil. Steril. **58:** 924–928.
7. Cornillie, F., J.D. Oosterlynck, J.M. Lauweryns *et al.* 1990. Deeply infiltrating pelvic endometriosis: histology and clinical significance. Fertil. Steril. **53:** 978–983.
8. Vernon, M.W., J.S. Beard, K. Graves *et al.* 1986. Classification of endometriotic implants by morphologic appearance and capacity to synthesize prostaglandin F. Fertil. Steril. **46:** 801–806.
9. Goldstein, D.P., C. De Cholnoky & S.J. Emans. 1980. Adolescent endometriosis. J. Adolesc. Health Care **1:** 37–41.
10. Davis, G.D., E. Thillet & J. Lindemann. 1993. Clinical characteristics of adolescent endometriosis. J. Adolesc. Health **14:** 362–368.
11. Vercellini, P., L. Bocciolone, N. Vendola *et al.* 1991. Peritoneal endometriosis: morphologic appearance in women with chronic pelvic pain. J. Reprod. Med. **36:** 533–536.
12. Perper, M.M., F. Nezhat, H. Goldstein *et al.* 1995. Dysmenorrhea is related to the number of implants in endometriosis patients. Fertil. Steril. **63:** 500–503.
13. Evers, J.L.H. 1994. Endometriosis does not exist; all women have endometriosis. Hum. Reprod. **9:** 2206–2209.
14. Brosens, I.A. 1994. Is mild endometriosis a progressive disease? Hum. Reprod. **9:** 2209–2211.
15. Farquhar, C. 2000. Endometriosis. *In* Clinical Evidence. BMJ Pub. London.
16. Moore, J.G., M.A. Binstock & W.A. Growdon. 1988. The clinical implications of retroperitoneal endometriosis. Am. J. Obstet. Gynecol. **158:** 1291–1298.
17. Martin, D.C. & M.P. Diamond. 1986. Operative laparoscopy: comparison of lasers with other techniques. Curr. Probl. Obstet. Gynecol. Fertil. **9:** 563–601.
18. Martin, D.C. 1991. Tissue effects of lasers. Semin. Reprod. Endocrinol. **9:** 127–137.
19. Martin, D.C. 1995. Tissue effects of lasers and electrosurgery. *In* Laparoscopic Surgery: An Atlas for General Surgeons. Lippincott. Philadelphia.
20. Koninckx, P.R., B. Timmermans, C. Meuleman *et al.* 1996. Complications of CO_2 laser endoscopic excision of deep endometriosis. Hum. Reprod. **11:** 2263–2268.
21. Moll, U.M., J.C. Chumas, E. Chalas *et al.* 1990. Ovarian carcinoma arising in atypical endometriosis. Obstet. Gynecol. **75:** 537–539.
22. Rock, J.A. 1993. Endometriosis and pelvic pain. Fertil. Steril. **60:** 950–951.
23. Martin, D.C. 1991. Laparoscopic Appearance of Endometriosis. First Revision. Color Atlas. Resurge Press. Memphis.
24. Martin, D.C., V. Khare & L. Parker. 1994. Clear and opaque vesicles: endometriosis, psammoma bodies, endosalpingiosis, or cancer. *In* Progress in the Management of Endometriosis. Parthenon. New York.

25. MARTIN, D.C., V.K. KHARE & B.E. MILLER. 1995. Association of *Chlamydia trachomatis* immunoglobulin gamma titers with dystrophic peritoneal calcification, psammoma bodies, adhesions, and hydrosalpinges. Fertil. Steril. **63:** 39–44.
26. KHARE, V.K. & D.C. MARTIN. 1995. Anecdotal association of endosalpingiosis with *Chlamydia trachomatis* IgG titers and Fitz-Hugh-Curtis adhesions. J. Am. Assoc. Gynecol. Laparosc. **2:** 143–145.
27. MARTIN, D.C. 1997. Cancer and endometriosis: do we need to be concerned? Semin. Reprod. Endocrinol. **15:** 319–324.
28. NETTER, F.H. 1965. *In* Ciba Collection of Medical Illustrations. Volume 2: Reproductive System. Ciba Pharmaceutical Company.
29. VERCELLINI, P., G. AIMI, S. PANAZZA *et al.* 2000. Deep endometriosis conundrum: evidence in favor of a peritoneal origin. Fertil. Steril. **73:** 1043–1046.
30. KONINCKX, P.R. & F.J. CORNILLIE. 1993. Infiltrating endometriosis: infiltration, retraction, or adenomyosis externa? *In* Atlas of Endometriosis. Gower Med. Pub. London.
31. ADAMYAN, L. 1993. Additional international perspectives. *In* Gynecologic and Obstetric Surgery. Mosby Year Book. St. Louis.
32. KUHN, R. & V. HOLLYOCK. 1982. Observations on the anatomy of the rectovaginal pouch and septum. Obstet. Gynecol. **59:** 445–447.
33. BATT, R.B. 1999. Abdominopelvic diagnostic laparoscopy. *In* Atlas of Female Surgery. Third edition. Mosby. St. Louis.
34. BAESSLER, K. & B. SCHUESSLER. 2000. The depth of the pouch of Douglas in nulliparous and parous women without genital prolapse and in patients with genital prolapse. Am. J. Obstet. Gynecol. **182:** 540–544.
35. MARTIN, D.C. & R.E. BATT. 2001. Retrocervical, rectovaginal pouch, and rectovaginal septum endometriosis. J. Am. Assoc. Gynecol. Laparosc. **8:** 12–17.
36. CULLEN, T.S. 1917. Adenomyoma of the recto-vaginal septum. Johns Hopkins Bull. **321:** 343–348.
37. CHEN, T.F., D.S.J. COLLIER, W.G. EVERETT *et al.* 1989. Endometriosis of the rectovaginal septum treated by anterior resection. Ann. Chir. Gynaecol. **78:** 324–326.
38. ANAF, V., P. SIMON, I. EL NAKADI *et al.* 2001. Impact of resection of rectovaginal pouch of Douglas endometriotic nodule on pelvic pain and some elements of patient's sexual life. J. Am. Assoc. Gynecol. Laparosc. **8:** 55–60
39. MARTIN, D.C. 1988. Laparoscopic and vaginal colpotomy for the excision of infiltrating cul-de-sac endometriosis. J. Reprod. Med. **33:** 806–808.
40. PERRY, C.P. & M.M. VICTORIA. 1995. Occult retrocervical endometriosis. J. Reprod. Med. **40:** 652–654.
41. DAVIS, G.D. 1997. Complications of laparoscopy and hysteroscopy. *In* Endometriosis in the Cul-de-Sac: Complications of Treatment. Second edition. Blackwell Science. Malden, MA.
42. SMITH, T. 1978. Surgical treatment of endometriosis. Clin. Obstet. Gynaecol. **5:** 557–570.
43. REICH, H., F. MCGLYNN & J. SALVAT. 1991. Laparoscopic treatment of cul-de-sac obliteration secondary to retrocervical deep fibrotic endometriosis. J. Reprod. Med. **36:** 516–522.
44. REDWINE, D.B. 1992. Laparoscopic *en bloc* resection for treatment of the obliterated cul-de-sac endometriosis. J. Reprod. Med. **37:** 695–698.
45. NEZHAT, C., F. NEZHAT & E. PENNINGTON. 1992. Laparoscopic treatment of infiltrating rectosigmoid and rectovaginal septum endometriosis by the technique of videolaparoscopy and CO_2 laser. Br. J. Obstet. Gynaecol. **99:** 664–667.
46. POSSOVER, M., H. DIEBOLDER, K. PLAUL *et al.* 2000. Laparoscopically assisted vaginal resection of rectovaginal endometriosis. Obstet. Gynecol. **96:** 304–307.
47. SAMPSON, J.A. 1924. Benign and malignant endometrial implants in the peritoneal cavity, and their relation to certain ovarian tumors. Surg. Gynecol. Obstet. **38:** 287–311.
48. KARNAKY, K.J. 1969. Theories and known observations about hormonal treatment of endometriosis *in-situ*, and endometriosis at the enzyme level. Ariz. Med. **26:** 37–41.
49. REDWINE, D.B. 1987. Age-related evolution in color appearance of endometriosis. Fertil. Steril. **48:** 1062–1063.
50. JANSEN, R.P.S. & P. RUSSELL. 1986. Nonpigmented endometriosis: clinical, laparoscopic, and pathologic definition. Am. J. Obstet. Gynecol. **155:** 1154–1159.

51. STRIPLING, M.C., D.C. MARTIN, D.L. CHATMAN *et al.* 1988. Subtle appearance of pelvic endometriosis. Fertil. Steril. **49:** 427–431.
52. MURPHY, A.A., W.R. GREEN, D. BOBBIE *et al.* 1986. Unsuspected endometriosis documented by scanning electron microscopy in visually normal peritoneum. Fertil. Steril. **46:** 522–524.
53. NISOLLE, M., B. PAINDAVEINE, A. BOURDON *et al.* 1990. Histologic study of peritoneal endometriosis in infertile women. Fertil. Steril. **53:** 984–988.
54. REDWINE, D.B. & L.B. YOCUM. 1990. A serial section study of visually normal pelvic peritoneum in patients with endometriosis. Fertil. Steril. **54:** 648–651.
55. NEZHAT, F., C.J. ALLAN, C. NEZHAT *et al.* 1991. Nonvisualized endometriosis at laparoscopy. Int. J. Fertil. **36:** 340–343.
56. NESBITT, R.E. & P.T. RIZK. 1971. Uterosacral ligament syndrome. Obstet. Gynecol. **37:** 730–733.
57. MARTIN, D.C., R. AHMIC, F.A. EL-ZEKY *et al.* 1990. Increased histologic confirmation of endometriosis. J. Gynecol. Surg. **6:** 275–279.
58. SCOTT, R.B. & R.W. TELINDE. 1950. External endometriosis—the scourge of the private patient. Ann. Surg. **131:** 697–720.
59. PARDANANI, S. & R.L. BARBIERI. 1998. The gold standard for the surgical diagnosis of endometriosis: visual findings or biopsy results? J. Gynecol. Tech. **4:** 121–124.
60. LAIS, C.W., T.J. WILLIAMS & T.A. GAFFEY. 1988. Prevalence of ovarian cancer found at the time of infertility microsurgery. Fertil. Steril. **49:** 551–553.
61. FAYEZ, J.A. & M.F. VOGEL. 1991. Comparison of different treatment methods of endometriomas by laparoscopy. Obstet. Gynecol. **78:** 660–665.
62. MARTIN, D.C. & J.D. BERRY. 1990. Histology of chocolate cysts. J. Gynecol. Surg. **6:** 43–46.
63. BATEMAN, B.G., L.A. KOLP & S. MILLS. 1994. Endoscopic versus laparotomy management of endometriomas. Fertil. Steril. **62:** 690–695.
64. FAYEZ, J.A. 1992. Comparison of different treatment methods of endometriomas by laparoscopy [letter to the editor]. Obstet. Gynecol. **79:** 315–316.

The Treatment of Endometriosis

A Review of the Evidence

DAVID L. OLIVE[a] AND ELIZABETH A. PRITTS[b]

[a]*Department of Obstetrics and Gynecology, University of Wisconsin–Madison Medical School, Madison, Wisconsin, USA*

[b]*University of California–San Francisco School of Medicine, San Francisco, California, USA*

ABSTRACT: The treatment of endometriosis focuses upon amelioration of two symptoms: pain and infertility. The treatment of endometriosis-associated pain has been well studied and all major medical therapies appear to be superior to placebo. In addition, none seems to be drastically better than another. Surgical therapy also appears to be efficacious, albeit with a relatively high rate of recurrence of symptoms following conservative surgical intervention. There are no trials comparing the relative value of medical versus surgical therapy. Combination surgery/medical therapy has several high-quality trials for evaluation, but its value remains unclear. The treatment of endometriosis-associated infertility presents a different picture: medical therapy has not been shown to be of any value and may prove detrimental to fertility. Surgical treatment does improve fertility, probably for all stages of disease. Assisted reproduction also seems to be efficacious, with both controlled ovarian hyperstimulation and intrauterine insemination as well as *in vitro* fertilization shown to be of benefit. Finally, the combination of *in vitro* fertilization and either medical or surgical therapy may be beneficial with advanced endometriosis, but further study is required.

KEYWORDS: endometriosis; pain; fertility/infertility; treatment; trials; therapy

Endometriosis is a highly enigmatic, yet common disorder in gynecology. While most practitioners encounter patients with this disease on a daily basis, appropriate treatment is elusive to many. A plethora of data presenting seemingly contradictory or inconclusive results have appeared in the medical literature in recent years, changing our concepts of how to best approach endometriosis and its associated problems.

This review will address what we do and do not know about the treatment of endometriosis. For this purpose, we will use hierarchical rules of investigation and generate recommendations based upon the best available evidence.[1]

Address for correspondence: David L. Olive, M.D., Department of Obstetrics and Gynecology, University of Wisconsin–Madison Medical School, H4/654 Clinical Science Center, 600 Highland Avenue, Madison, WI 53792-6188. Voice: 608-263-1201; fax: 608-263-0191.
lapskyboy@aol.com

EVALUATING TREATMENT TRIALS FOR ENDOMETRIOSIS

When determining the value of a treatment modality, it is important to assess appropriate outcomes. With endometriosis, two symptoms have primarily been relied upon as outcome measures: pelvic pain and infertility.

Pain from endometriosis is frequently used as an outcome measure and represents the most common symptom of the disease. Three factors are critical in evaluating pain in treatment trials: a validated pain scale, a time-dependent evaluation, and consideration of placebo or sham-surgery effect.[2] Such issues are best addressed by well-constructed, controlled trials with defined time points for follow-up.

Fertility is also used to assess the value of treatment. As objective as pregnancy may seem, it has several characteristics that make its use as an outcome variable problematic. First, multiple confounding factors often affect fertility status. In addition, pregnancy (like pain) is a time-dependent phenomenon. Finally, endometriosis rarely causes an absolute inability to conceive; thus, a background pregnancy rate in the untreated patient must be used as a source of comparison.[3] These concerns mandate trials with appropriate controls, defined follow-up, and sophisticated statistical analysis.

Given the nature of the above outcome measures, it is readily apparent that poorly constructed investigation is of limited value. To generate meaningful information, randomized clinical trials with sufficient sample size, comprehensive follow-up, and thorough analysis are imperative. This review will focus on such trials and the data that they provide; when necessary, lesser quality studies will be cited with appropriate caution. Where sample size is inadequate for even negative conclusions, this will be noted.

TREATMENT OF ENDOMETRIOSIS-ASSOCIATED PAIN

Medical Therapy

Placebo-controlled studies offer the best evidence as to the efficacy of pharmaceutical agents in the treatment of endometriosis-associated pain. Only two such high-quality studies exist. The first, by Telimaa and colleagues, evaluated the effect of medroxyprogesterone acetate (100 mg/day) or danazol (600 mg/day) for 6 months in 59 women.[4] Both medications produced a significant and substantial improvement in pain scores while patients received the medication, as well as up to 6 months following discontinuation. In fact, the relative attributable experimental effect (percent decrease in pain severity attributable solely to treatment) was 50% to 74% at the conclusion of follow-up.

Dlugi and associates enrolled women with endometriosis-associated pain into a randomized clinical trial (RCT) comparing leuprolide acetate to placebo for 6 months.[5] Three-month data suggested a similar effect as was seen in the Telimaa study, but placebo follow-up was too incomplete after this time point to draw further conclusions.

RCTs of two or more drugs also provide useful information. GnRH agonists have been shown to provide virtually identical pain relief as danazol.[6–21] Oral contraceptives have also been compared to GnRH agonists: in a study designed to have 80%

power to detect a 35% difference in effect, cyclic use of oral contraceptive proved significantly inferior to GnRH agonists for relief of dysmenorrhea, nearly as effective for relief of dyspareunia (statistically significantly different using one of two rating scales, but of questionable clinical significance), and equally efficacious in the treatment of nonspecific pelvic pain.[22]

A number of RCTs have addressed the efficacy of "add-back" therapy in conjunction with GnRH agonist during 6-month treatment courses.[23–28] Using the add-back approach, pain symptoms were relieved as efficaciously as with GnRH agonist alone. However, the addition of add-back significantly reduced side effects of GnRH agonist. Two prospective, randomized trials have assessed the role of GnRH agonist with add-back beyond 6 months of administration, with results similar to those studies of only 6-month duration.[29,30] It thus appears that, in the majority of patients, add-back therapy can be added to GnRH agonist treatment without loss of efficacy, but with a substantial amelioration of hypoestrogenic symptoms. This seems to be the case even when the add-back therapy is begun during the first month of treatment, suggesting that an "add-back-free" interval at the beginning of a treatment cycle is unnecessary.[28]

Thus, it appears that all major medical therapies are likely to be superior in the treatment of endometriosis-associated pain compared to placebo, and none seems to be drastically better than another. Further studies with additional protocols are needed to help clarify the precise roles of each of the agents in the treatment of pain symptoms.

Surgical Therapy

Only one randomized, masked, sham-controlled surgical trial has been conducted to evaluate the effect of surgery on endometriosis-associated pain. Sutton *et al.* reported a study of 74 women randomized to ablation of implants, lysis of adhesions, and LUNA versus diagnostic laparoscopy alone for stage I–III disease.[31] Sixty-three women completed 6 months of follow-up, with a significant improvement demonstrated in 62.5% of treated women and 22.6% of controls. Thus, the number of patients needed to treat (NNT) to produce one "cure" was approximately 2.5. Follow-up of those having relief of pain at 6 months after conservative surgery revealed that 90% continued to have decreased pain at 1 year.[32]

The above study by Sutton involves both conservative surgery and LUNA, but what of the value of each procedure individually? Two small studies address this issue and both suggest that LUNA adds little to surgery directed at the lesions.[33] When comparing conservative surgery plus LUNA to conservative surgery alone, Dover and associates noted comparable pain scores at baseline and at 6 months post-procedure. Vercellini *et al.* also examined conservative surgery with or without LUNA, finding no difference between groups at 9 months following surgery. A 12-month Kaplan-Meyer calculation of the cumulative probability of recurrence of moderate to severe dysmenorrhea also showed no difference, with 33.7% recurrence for the experimental group and 27.55% for controls. An intention-to-treat analysis of subject satisfaction similarly showed no difference between treatments. Therefore, there is no evidence that LUNA adds value to conservative surgery for endometriosis-associated pain.

Presacral neurectomy has been investigated in two randomized trials as an adjunctive procedure to conservative surgery.[34,35] In both studies, there was a significant and substantial decrease in midline dysmenorrheic pain, but no effect on other types of pain. Although the number of patients studied is small, these trials suggest that presacral neurectomy may be of value when endometriosis is associated with midline pain at the time of menses. In addition, small effects upon other types of pelvic pain cannot be completely excluded due to sample size considerations.

Definitive surgery has been poorly studied, with no RCTs to date. A single cohort study suggests that retention of ovaries after hysterectomy in women with endometriosis leads to an 8-fold increase in reoperation for pelvic pain.[36] In this study, the incidence of persistent/recurrent pain after ovarian extirpation was 10%. However, it is unclear that the endometriosis was actually removed at the time of hysterectomy in this study; one should be cautious about the need for ovarian removal in such patients, especially in young women.

Combination Medical/Surgical Therapy

Three randomized, placebo-controlled trials have evaluated the use of postoperative medical therapy as a means of further providing pain relief. Studies by Telimaa *et al.*[37] (danazol or medroxyprogesterone) and Hornstein *et al.*[38] (GnRH agonist) suggest a benefit for this combination approach. The former study demonstrated a significant relative decrease in pain scores attributable to combination therapy of more than 60% for each drug. The Hornstein study found that combination therapy decreased the number of patients needing retreatment within 2 years from 57% to 31%. However, no significant difference in pain scores was seen between groups. In contrast, Parazzini *et al.* found no difference in the use of 3 months of GnRH agonist postoperatively versus surgery alone, with 1-year follow-up.[39] Heterogeneity among these studies does not allow for combining them into a valid meta-analysis. These results fail to present a consistent view of the value of combination therapy; clearly, more such studies are needed to clarify the picture.

TREATMENT OF ENDOMETRIOSIS-ASSOCIATED INFERTILITY

Medical Therapy

Most of the medical therapies used to treat endometriosis-associated pain have also been instituted in an attempt to treat the subfertility seen in women with endometriosis. Four randomized trials with five treatment arms have compared a medical treatment directed at endometriosis to placebo or no treatment, with fertility as the outcome measure.[40–43] Another eight RCTs compared danazol to a second medication.[11,17,20,44–48] All have been summarized recently by a meta-analysis by Hughes *et al.*[49] (FIG. 1). Clearly, no increase in fertility can be demonstrated with these medications when compared to expectant management, nor has any medication proven superior to danazol in this regard. Frequently overlooked is the fact that not only do these medications fail to enhance fertility, they may also delay fertility in that the patient is unable to conceive while being medicated for several months. If the above data are reanalyzed with follow-up beginning at the time of diagnosis rather

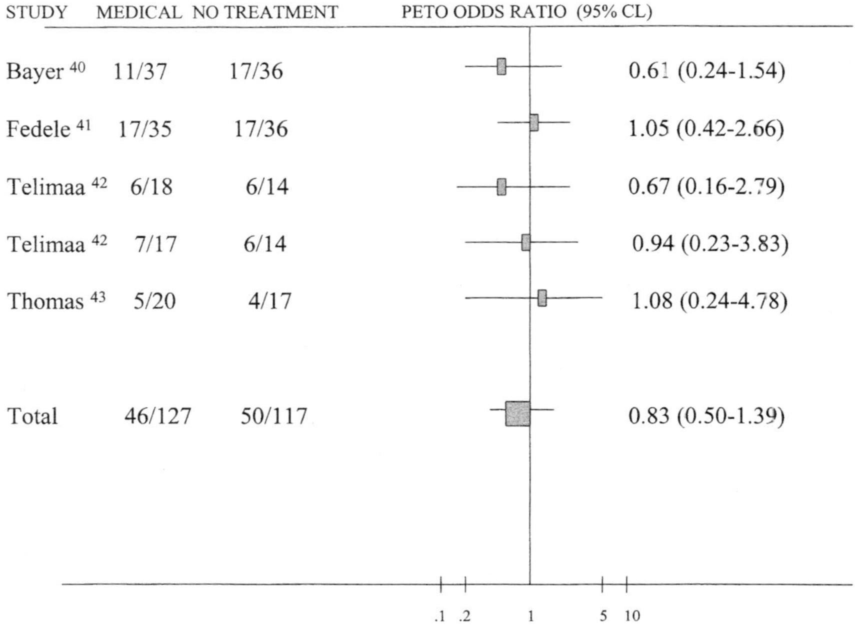

FIGURE 1. Meta-analysis of randomized trials comparing medical therapy of endometriosis-associated infertility versus placebo or expectant management. Follow-up time for all studies began at conclusion of treatment (medical therapy and placebo) or following laparoscopy (expectant management). Adapted from Hughes *et al.*[49]

than at the conclusion of therapy, medical therapy is significantly worse than no treatment, with a relative risk at 1 year of 0.60 (FIG. 2). Thus, there appears to be no role for medical therapy in the treatment of endometriosis-associated infertility.

Surgical Therapy

It is widely accepted that endometriosis of sufficient severity to cause distortion of the pelvis (stages III and IV) impairs fertility by interfering with oocyte pickup and transport. Such anatomic distortion is commonly attacked via surgery for all manners of disease, and endometriosis is no exception. For advanced endometriosis, no randomized trials exist to determine efficacy of this approach. However, a low-background pregnancy rate approaching zero in these women[50] and numerous uncontrolled trials proving that pregnancies do occur after reparative surgery suggest the value of this approach.

More controversial is the situation with early-stage (I or II) endometriosis. While an association clearly exists between even this early-stage disease and reproductive dysfunction, it has been unclear whether or not this represents a cause-effect relationship. Therefore, the value of surgical intervention in these patients is in need of evaluation.

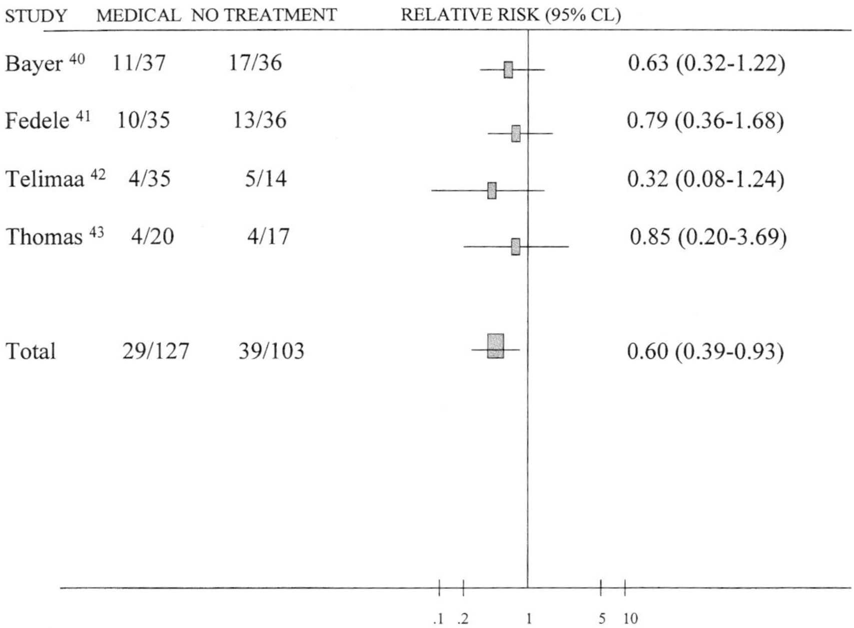

FIGURE 2. Meta-analysis of randomized trials comparing medical therapy of endometriosis-associated infertility versus placebo or expectant management. Pregnancy rates are for 12 months of follow-up following diagnosis (diagnostic laparoscopy). All medical treatment patients received 6 months of therapy and attempted to conceive for 6 months; all placebo/expectant management patients attempted conception for all 12 months. If patients were lost to follow-up prior to 12 months, they were assumed to have not conceived for the 12-month period (medical treatment: 2; no treatment: 16). Results are expressed as relative risk of conception with medical therapy (±95% confidence limits).

A meta-analysis of nonrandomized trials suggested that surgical treatment of early-stage endometriosis-associated infertility might be of value; however, there was sufficient heterogeneity among the studies to diminish confidence in such a conclusion.[51] Clearly, a large-scale RCT was needed. This was accomplished recently by Marcoux and colleagues in a Canadian collaborative trial termed ENDOCAN.[52] This study randomized 341 infertile women with stage I or II endometriosis to either diagnostic laparoscopy or surgical treatment of the disease. The women were followed for 36 weeks postoperatively and for up to 20 weeks if they conceived. The rate of pregnancy greater than 20 weeks was significantly higher in the surgically treated women (30.7% vs. 17.7%).

Shortly thereafter, however, a second multicenter study addressed this issue. The Gruppo Italiano per lo Studio dell'Endometriosi conducted a similar RCT with 101 subjects.[53] Their investigation demonstrated a live birthrate of 19.6% in the treatment group and 22.2% in the controls within 1 year of surgery. This study differed from the Canadian trial in that patients had a longer median duration of infertility

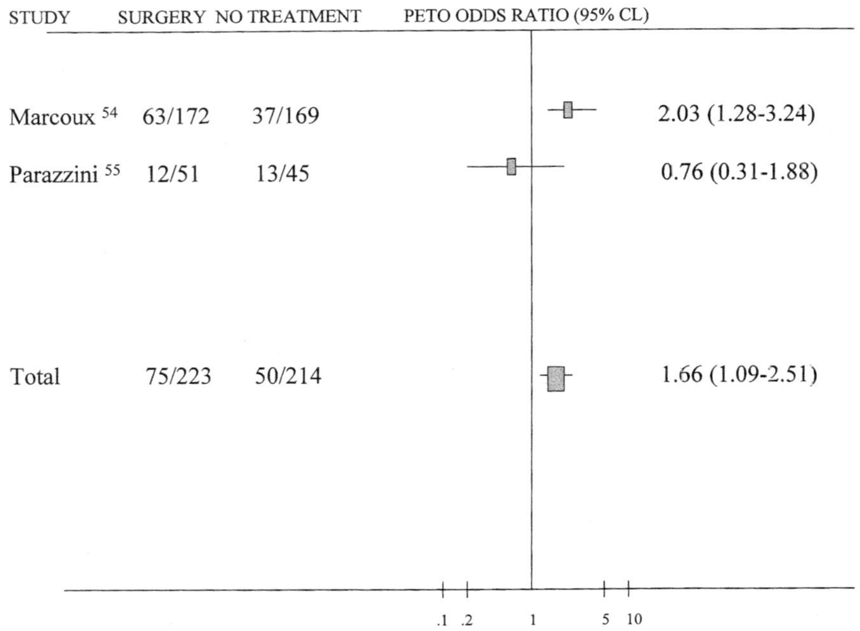

FIGURE 3. Meta-analysis of randomized trials comparing surgical therapy of early-stage endometriosis-associated infertility versus diagnostic laparoscopy (no therapy).

and slightly more extensive disease. Moreover, the small sample size was designed to detect a 2.5-fold difference in pregnancy rate; the power to detect a 13% difference (as with the Canadian trial) was only 32%. Combining the results of these two trials into a meta-analysis (FIG. 3) still favors surgical treatment, albeit by less than was seen with ENDOCAN alone (odds ratio for pregnancy = 1.7; 95% confidence limits = 1.1–2.5).

In summary, the issue of efficacy of surgery in the enhancement of early-stage endometriosis-associated infertility remains unsettled. However, it is likely that the effect is small: even if ENDOCAN is correct, the NNT for the production of one additional pregnancy is 7.7 surgeries. This figure may prove unacceptable to many clinicians, patients, and health plans.

Assisted Reproduction

Many researchers have examined the role of empiric assisted reproduction in an attempt to enhance fertility in the patient with endometriosis. Three randomized trials have addressed the value of ovulation induction, and two have combined it with intrauterine insemination.[54–56] These data can be seen in TABLE 1. From these results, it is apparent that fertility can be hastened in women with endometriosis by using these approaches.

TABLE 1. The use of superovulation in the treatment of endometriosis: comparison to expectant management by randomized trial

Author	Year	Regimen	Cycle fecundity rate	
			Experimental	Control
Fedele *et al.*[54]	1992	GnRH-a, LH/FSH	15%	4.5%
Deaton *et al.*[55]	1990	CC + IUI	9.5%	3.3%
Tummon *et al.*[56]	1997	FSH + IUI	11%	2%

TERMS: GnRH-a = gonadotropin-releasing hormone agonist; LH/FSH = combined gonadotropin preparation; CC = clomiphene citrate; IUI = intrauterine insemination; FSH = follicle-stimulating hormone.

The role of the advanced reproductive technologies such as *in vitro* fertilization (IVF) has also been addressed, albeit inadequately. Soliman, in the only available RCT comparing IVF to no treatment, investigated the effect of these therapies on infertile women with endometriosis.[57] Although the study was large, only 21 patients were noted to have endometriosis (15 for IVF, 6 for no treatment). Such small numbers make conclusions meaningless. Kodama and associates[58] examined the issue in a retrospective cohort study and were unable to demonstrate a significantly higher cumulative pregnancy rate between women undergoing IVF and untreated women over a 3-year follow-up period. While it is probably self-evident that IVF is of value in advanced disease, the value of this approach in early-stage disease is as yet unproven. In other words, while pregnancies certainly occur quite rapidly with IVF in women with endometriosis or any other diagnosis, it is unclear whether one cycle of IVF is comparable to 1 month, 6 months, 2 years, or a reproductive lifetime of attempting conception naturally. This question will need further examination in the future.

When women with endometriosis-associated infertility undergo IVF, several issues are raised relative to the interaction of the disease and the procedure:

(1) What is the effect of endometriosis on IVF outcome? No randomized trials have examined this question, but numerous cohort trials have produced conflicting results.[59] To date, this issue is unsettled.

(2) Does severity of the disease affect outcome? Investigations performed prior to 1989, when a majority of oocyte retrievals were performed laparoscopically, suggested pregnancy rates were lower with more advanced disease. However, recent studies with transvaginal retrieval have consistently shown no difference.[60–67]

(3) Do endometriomas affect the outcome of IVF? No RCTs exist to address this. Cohort trials provide conflicting information.[59]

(4) Does the medical treatment of endometriosis prior to IVF improve success rates, particularly with severe disease? This has also not been addressed adequately by an RCT. One randomized trial compared ovulation stimulation with gonadotropins alone to 6 months of GnRH agonist prior to gonadotropins, with a higher pregnancy rate achieved with the addition of

GnRH agonist.[68] However, it is clear that downregulation with GnRH agonist in any patient produces a higher pregnancy rate;[69] the issue of whether 2 weeks of downregulation is sufficient in these patients or if 6 months of treatment is required remains unresolved.

(5) Does the surgical treatment of endometriosis in conjunction with assisted reproduction improve pregnancy rates? An RCT by Surrey suggests that surgery for endometriosis at the time of a gamete intrafallopian transfer (GIFT) procedure does not affect the pregnancy rate in the treatment cycle; however, in the year following the assisted reproductive technology (ART) cycle, a significantly higher spontaneous pregnancy rate was seen in those undergoing surgery.[70]

It is evident from the above review that we urgently need numerous randomized trials to answer a number of questions regarding the treatment of endometriosis-associated infertility with ARTs. Although the technique is clearly worthwhile, its degree of value, cost-effectiveness, and optimal method of employment have not yet been satisfactorily addressed.

CONCLUSIONS

Research into the treatment of endometriosis can be summarized simply: "So many investigations, so few good studies!" Nevertheless, given the available information, a number of conclusions can be drawn:

(1) In treating pelvic pain, both medical and surgical therapies work (at least for a while). Also, all medical therapies appear roughly equivalent.
(2) The optimal surgical approach for endometriosis-associated pain has yet to be defined.
(3) No comparison of medical versus surgical therapy exists in the treatment of endometriosis-associated pain.
(4) Combination medical/surgical therapy may offer an advantage in treating pain, but the degree of advantage is unclear.
(5) For endometriosis-associated infertility, medical therapy is ineffective, while surgical therapy seems beneficial for most (if not all) forms of the disease.
(6) No comparison of assisted reproduction versus surgery exists for the initial treatment of infertile women with endometriosis; however, IVF may be a superior treatment compared to repeated surgical intervention.[71]
(7) In endometriosis-associated infertility, combination surgery/ART or medical therapy/ART may be of benefit.

Many of these conclusions are vague or tenuous at best. It is hoped that the upcoming decade will be populated by investigations of rigorous design and quality analysis that can help address the many remaining questions that we as clinicians have regarding the best way to approach this confusing disorder called endometriosis.

REFERENCES

1. OLIVE, D.L. & E.A. PRITTS. 1997. What is evidence-based medicine? J. Am. Assoc. Gynecol. Laparosc. **4:** 615–621.
2. OLIVE, D.L. 1996. A scientific appraisal of gynecologic endoscopy. *In* Endoscopic Management of Gynecologic Disease, pp. 403–413. Lippincott-Raven. Philadelphia.
3. OLIVE, D.L. 1986. Analysis of clinical fertility trials: a methodologic review. Fertil. Steril. **45:** 157–171.
4. TELIMAA, S., J. PUOLAKKA, L. RONNBERG & A. KAUPILLA. 1987. Placebo-controlled comparison of danazol and high-dose medroxyprogesterone acetate in the treatment of endometriosis. Gynecol. Endocrinol. **1:** 13–25.
5. DLUGI, A.M., J.D. MILLER & J. KNITTLE. 1990. Lupron depot (leuprolide acetate for depot suspension) in the treatment of endometriosis: a randomized, placebo-controlled, double-blind study. Fertil. Steril. **54:** 419–427.
6. ANONYMOUS. 1996. Goserelin depot versus danazol in the treatment of endometriosis: the Australian/New Zealand experience. Aust. N.Z. J. Obstet. Gynaecol. **36:** 55–60.
7. CHANG, S.P. & H.T. NG. 1996. A randomized comparative study of the effect of leuprorelin acetate depot and danazol in the treatment of endometriosis. Chin. Med. J. (Taipei) **57:** 431–437.
8. CIRKEL, U., H. OOCHS & H.P.G. SCHNEIDER. 1995. A randomized, comparative trial of triptorelin depot (D-Trp6-LHRH) and danazol in the treatment of endometriosis. Eur. J. Obstet. Gynecol. Reprod. Biol. **59:** 61–69.
9. CROSIGNANI, P.G., A. GASTALDI, P.L. LOMBARDI *et al.* 1992. Leuprorelin acetate depot versus danazol in the treatment of endometriosis: results of an open multicentre trial. Clin. Ther. **14**(suppl. A)**:** 29–36.
10. DMOWSKI, W.P., E. RADWANSKA, Z. BINOR *et al.* 1989. Ovarian suppression induced with buserelin or danazol in the management of endometriosis: a randomized, comparative study. Fertil. Steril. **51:** 395–400.
11. FRASER, I.S., R.P. SHEARMAN, R.P. JANSEN & P.D. SUTHERLAND. 1991. A comparative treatment trial of endometriosis using the gonadotropin-releasing hormone agonist, nafarelin, and the synthetic steroid, danazol. Aust. N.Z. J. Obstet. Gynaecol. **31**(2)**:** 158–163.
12. HENZL, M.R., S.L. CORSON, K. MOGHISSI *et al.* 1988. Administration of nasal nafarelin as compared with oral danazol for endometriosis: a multicenter double-blind comparative clinical trial. N. Engl. J. Med. **318:** 485–489.
13. ADAMSON, G.D., L. KWEI & R.A. EDGREN. 1994. Pain of endometriosis: effects of nafarelin and danazol therapy. Int. J. Fertil. Med. Stud. **39:** 215–217.
14. WHEELER, J.M., J.D. KNITTLE & J.D. MILLER. 1992. Depot leuprolide versus danazol in treatment of women with symptomatic endometriosis: I. Efficacy results. Am. J. Obstet. Gynecol. **167:** 1367–1371.
15. DAWOOD, M.Y., J. RAMOS & F.S. KHAN-DAWOOD. 1995. Depot leuprolide acetate versus danazol for treatment of pelvic endometriosis: changes in vertebral bone mass and serum estradiol and calcitonin. Fertil. Steril. **63:** 1177–1183.
16. THE NAFARELIN EUROPEAN ENDOMETRIOSIS TRIAL GROUP (NEET). 1992. Nafarelin for endometriosis: a large-scale, danazol-controlled trial of efficacy and safety, with 1-year follow-up. Fertil. Steril. **57:** 514–522.
17. ROLLAND, R. & P.F. VAN DER HEIJDEN. 1990. Nafarelin versus danazol in the treatment of endometriosis. Am. J. Obstet. Gynecol. **162:** 586–588.
18. KENNEDY, S.H., I.A. WILLIAMS, J. BRODRIBB *et al.* 1990. A comparison of nafarelin acetate and danazol in the treatment of endometriosis. Fertil. Steril. **53:** 998–1003.
19. ROCK, J.A. 1991. A multicenter comparison of GnRH agonist (Zoladex) and danazol in the treatment of endometriosis. Fertil. Steril. **56:** S49.
20. SHAW, R.W. 1992. An open randomized comparative study of the effect of goserelin depot and danazol in the treatment of endometriosis: Zoladex Endometriosis Study Team. Fertil. Steril. **58:** 265–272.
21. PRENTICE, A., A. DEERY, S. GOLDBECK-WOOD *et al.* 1999. Gonadotropin-releasing hormone analogues for pain associated with endometriosis. *In* The Cochrane Library, Issue 3. Update Software. Oxford.

22. VERCELLINI, P., L. TRESPIDI, A. COLOMBO *et al.* 1993. A gonadotropin-releasing hormone agonist versus a low-dose oral contraceptive for pelvic pain associated with endometriosis. Fertil. Steril. **60:** 75–79.
23. SURREY, E. & H. JUDD. 1992. Reduction of vasomotor symptoms and bone mineral density loss with combined norethindrone and long-acting gonadotropin-releasing hormone agonist therapy of symptomatic endometriosis: a prospective randomized trial. J. Clin. Endocrinol. Metab. **75:** 558–563.
24. MAKARAINEN, L., L. RONNBERG & A. KAUPPILA. 1996. Medroxyprogesterone acetate supplementation diminishes the hypoestrogenic side-effects of gonadotropin-releasing hormone agonists without changing its efficacy in endometriosis. Fertil. Steril. **65:** 29–34.
25. TABKIN, O., A.H. YAKINOGHE, S. KUCUK *et al.* 1997. Effectiveness of tibolone on hypoestrogenic symptoms induced by goserelin treatment in patients with endometriosis. Fertil. Steril. **67:** 40–45.
26. EDMONDS, D. & R. HOWELL. 1994. Can hormone replacement therapy be used during medical therapy of endometriosis? Br. J. Obstet. Gynaecol. **101:** 24–26.
27. KIIHOLMA, P., M. KORHONEN, R. TUIMALA *et al.* 1995. Comparison of the gonadotropin-releasing hormone agonist goserelin acetate alone versus goserelin combined with estrogen-progestogens add-back therapy in the treatment of endometriosis. Fertil. Steril. **64:** 903–908.
28. MOGHISSI, K.S., W.D. SCHLAFF, D.L. OLIVE *et al.* 1998. Goserelin acetate (Zoladex) with or without hormone replacement therapy for the treatment of endometriosis. Fertil. Steril. **69:** 1056–1062.
29. SURREY, E.S., B. VOIGT, N. FOURNET & H.L. JUDD. 1995. Prolonged gonadotropin-releasing hormone agonist treatment of symptomatic endometriosis: the role of cyclic sodium etidronate and low dose norethindrone "add-back" therapy. Fertil. Steril. **63:** 747–755.
30. HORNSTEIN, M.D., E.S. SURREY, G.W. WEISBERG & L.A. CASINO. 1998. Leuprolide acetate depot and hormonal add-back in endometriosis: a 12-month study—Lupron Add-Back Study Group. Obstet. Gynecol. **91:** 16–24.
31. SUTTON, C.J., S.P. EWEN, N. WHITELAW & P. HAINES. 1994. Prospective, randomized, double-blind, controlled trial of laser laparoscopy in the treatment of pelvic pain associated with minimal, mild, and moderate endometriosis. Fertil. Steril. **62:** 696–700.
32. SUTTON, C.J., A.S. POOLEY, S.P. EWEN & P. HAINES. 1997. Follow-up report on a randomized controlled trial of laser laparoscopy in the treatment of pelvic pain associated with minimal to moderate endometriosis. Fertil. Steril. **68:** 1070–1074.
33. WILSON, M.L., C.M. FARQUHAR, O.J. SINCLAIR & N.P. JOHNSON. 2000. Surgical interruption of pelvic nerve pathways for primary and secondary dysmenorrhea. *In* The Cochrane Library, Issue 1. Update Software. Oxford.
34. CANDIANI, G.B., L. FEDELE, P. VERCELLINI *et al.* 1992. Presacral neurectomy for the treatment of pelvic pain associated with endometriosis: a controlled study. Am. J. Obstet. Gynecol. **167:** 100–103.
35. TJADEN, B., W.D. SCHLAFF, A. KIMBALL & J.A. ROCK. 1990. The efficacy of presacral neurectomy for the relief of midline dysmenorrhea. Obstet. Gynecol. **76:** 89.
36. NAMNOUM, A.B., T.M. HICKMAN, A.B. GOODMAN *et al.* 1995. Incidence of symptom recurrence after hysterectomy for endometriosis. Fertil. Steril. **64:** 898–902.
37. TELIMAA, S., L. RONNBERG & A. KAUPPILA. 1987. Placebo-controlled comparison of danazol and high dose medroxyprogesterone acetate in the treatment of endometriosis after conservative surgery. Gynaecol. Endocrinol. **1:** 363–371.
38. HORNSTEIN, M.D., R. HEMMINGS, A.A. YUZPE & W.L. HEINRICHS. 1997. Use of nafarelin versus placebo after reductive laparoscopic surgery for endometriosis. Fertil. Steril. **68:** 860–864.
39. PARAZZINI, F., L. FEDELE, M. BUSACCA *et al.* 1994. Postsurgical medical treatment of advanced endometriosis: results of a randomized clinical trial. Am. J. Obstet. Gynecol. **171:** 1205–1207.
40. BAYER, S.R., M.M. SEIBEL, D.S. SAFFAN *et al.* 1988. Efficacy of danazol treatment for minimal endometriosis in infertile women: a prospective, randomized study. J. Reprod. Med. **33:** 179–183.

41. FEDELE, L., F. PARAZZINI, E. RADICI *et al.* 1992. Buserelin acetate versus expectant management in the treatment of infertility associated with minimal or mild endometriosis: a randomized clinical trial. Am. J. Obstet. Gynecol. **166:** 1345–1350.
42. TELIMAA, S. 1988. Danazol and medroxyprogesterone acetate inefficacious in the treatment of infertility in endometriosis. Fertil. Steril. **50:** 872–875.
43. THOMAS, E. & I. COOKE. 1987. Successful treatment of asymptomatic endometriosis: does it benefit infertile women? BMJ **294:** 1117–1119.
44. DMOWSKI, W.P., I. TUMMON, P. PEPPING *et al.* 1989. Ovarian suppression induced with buserelin or danazol in the management of endometriosis: a randomized comparative study. Fertil. Steril. **51:** 395–400.
45. FEDELE, L., S. BIANCHI, L. ARCAINI *et al.* 1989. Buserelin versus danazol in the treatment of endometriosis-associated infertility. Am. J. Obstet. Gynecol. **161:** 871–876.
46. FEDELE, L., S. BIANCHI, T. VIEZZOLI *et al.* 1989. Gestrinone versus danazol in the treatment of endometriosis. Fertil. Steril. **51:** 781–785.
47. HENZL, M., S.L. CORSON, K. MOGHISSI *et al.* 1998. Administration of nasal nafarelin as compared with oral danazol for endometriosis: a multicenter double-blind comparative clinical trial. N. Engl. J. Med. **384:** 485.
48. NOBLE, A.D. & A.T. LETCHWORTH. 1979. Medical treatment of endometriosis: a comparative trial. Postgrad. Med. J. **55:** 37–39.
49. HUGHES, E., D. FEDORKOW, J. COLLINS & P. VANDEKERCKHONE. 2000. Ovulation suppression for endometriosis. *In* The Cochrane Library, Issue 1. Update Software. Oxford.
50. OLIVE, D.L. & K.L. LEE. 1986. Analysis of sequential treatment protocols for endometriosis-associated infertility. Am. J. Obstet. Gynecol. **154:** 613–619.
51. HUGHES, E.G., D.M. FEDORKOW & J.A. COLLINS. 1993. A quantitative overview of controlled trials in endometriosis-associated infertility. Fertil. Steril. **59:** 963.
52. MARCOUX, S., R. MAHEUX & S. BERUBE. 1997. Laparoscopic surgery in infertile women with minimal or mild endometriosis: Canadian Collaborative Group in Endometriosis. N. Engl. J. Med. **337:** 217–222.
53. PARAZZINI, F. 1999. Ablation of lesions or no treatment in minimal-mild endometriosis in infertile women: a randomized trial—Gruppo Italiano per lo Studio dell'Endometriosi. Hum. Reprod. **14:** 1332–1334.
54. FEDELE, L., S. BIANCHI, M. MARCHINI *et al.* 1992. Superovulation with human menopausal gonadotropins in the treatment of infertility associated with minimal or mild endometriosis: a controlled randomized study. Fertil. Steril. **58:** 28–31.
55. DEATON, J.L., M. GIBSON, K.M. BLACKMER *et al.* 1990. A randomized, controlled trial of clomiphene citrate and intrauterine insemination in couples with unexplained infertility or surgically corrected endometriosis. Fertil. Steril. **54:** 1083–1088.
56. TUMMON, I.S., L.J. ASHER, J.S. MARTIN & T. TULANDI. 1997. Randomized controlled trial of superovulation and insemination for infertility associated with minimal or mild endometriosis. Fertil. Steril. **68:** 8–12.
57. SOLIMAN, S., S. DAYA, J. COLLINS & J. JARRELL. 1993. A randomized trial of *in vitro* fertilization versus conventional treatment for infertility. Fertil. Steril. **59:** 1239–1244.
58. KODAMA, H., J. FUKUDA, H. KARUBE *et al.* 1996. Benefit of *in vitro* fertilization treatment for endometriosis-associated infertility. Fertil. Steril. **66:** 974–979.
59. DOKRAS, A. & D.L. OLIVE. 1999. Endometriosis and assisted reproductive technologies. Clin. Obstet. Gynecol. **42:** 687–698.
60. CHILLIK, C.F., A.A. ACOSTA, J.E. GARCIA *et al.* 1985. The role of *in vitro* fertilization in infertile patients with endometriosis. Fertil. Steril. **44:** 56–61.
61. MATSON, P.L. & J.L. YOVICH. 1986. The treatment of infertility associated with endometriosis by *in vitro* fertilization. Fertil. Steril. **46:** 432–434.
62. OEHRINGER, S., A.A. ACOSTA, D. KREINER *et al.* 1988. *In vitro* fertilization and embryo transfer (IVF/ET): an established and successful therapy for endometriosis. JIVFET **5:** 249–256.
63. INOUE, M., Y. KOBAYASHI, I. HONDA *et al.* 1992. The impact of endometriosis on the reproductive outcome of infertile patients. Am. J. Obstet. Gynecol. **167:** 278–282.
64. OLIVENNES, F., D. FELDBERG, H.C. LIU *et al.* 1995. Endometriosis: a stage-by-stage analysis—the role of *in vitro* fertilization. Fertil. Steril. **64:** 392–398.

65. GEBER, S., T. PARASCHOS, G. ATKINSON *et al.* 1995. Results of IVF in patients with endometriosis: the severity of the disease does not affect outcome or the incidence of miscarriage. Hum. Reprod. **10:** 1507–1511.
66. DMOWSKI, W.P., N. RANA, J. MICHALOWSKA *et al.* 1995. The effect of endometriosis, its stage and activity, and of autoantibodies on *in vitro* fertilization and embryo transfer success rates. Fertil. Steril. **63:** 555–562.
67. ARICI, A., E. ORAL, O. BUKULMEZ *et al.* 1995. The effect of endometriosis on implantation: results from the Yale University *in vitro* fertilization and embryo transfer program. Fertil. Steril. **65:** 603–607.
68. DICKER, D., J.A. GOLDMAN, T. LEVY *et al.* 1992. The impact of long-term gonadotropin-releasing hormone analogue treatment on preclinical abortions in patients with severe endometriosis undergoing *in vitro* fertilization–embryo transfer. Fertil. Steril. **57:** 597–600.
69. HUGHES, E.G., D.M. FEDORKOW, S. DAYA *et al.* 1992. The routine use of gonadotropin-releasing hormone agonists prior to *in vitro* fertilization and gamete intrafallopian transfer: a meta-analysis of randomized controlled trials. Fertil. Steril. **58:** 888–896.
70. SURREY, M.W. & D.L. HILL. 1994. Treatment of endometriosis by carbon dioxide laser during intrafallopian transfer. J. Am. Coll. Surg. **179:** 440–442.
71. PAGIDAS, K., T. FALCONE, R. HEMMINGS & P. MIRON. 1996. Comparison of re-operation for moderate (stage III) and severe (stage IV) endometriosis-related infertility with an *in vitro* fertilization–embryo transfer. Fertil. Steril. **65:** 791–795.

Selective Progesterone Receptor Modulators (SPRMs)

A Novel Therapeutic Concept in Endometriosis

KRISTOF CHWALISZ,[a] RAMESH GARG,[a] ROBERT M. BRENNER,[b] GERD SCHUBERT,[c] AND WALTER ELGER[d]

[a]*TAP Pharmaceutical Products Incorporated, Lake Forest, Illinois, USA*

[b]*Oregon Regional Primate Center, Beaverton, Oregon, USA*

[c]*Jenapharm GmbH and Co. K.G., Jena, Germany*

[d]*EnTec GmbH, Jena, Germany*

Abstract: Endometriosis, the presence of endometrial tissue outside the uterus, is a progressive, estrogen-dependent disease and occurs nearly exclusively in menstruating women of reproductive age. Pain syndrome, however, represents the major clinical problem of this disease, manifested as dysmenorrhea, pelvic pain, lower abdominal pain, and dyspareunia. The manifestation of the disease, that is, the pain syndrome, rather than the disease itself currently represents the major indication for both the medical and surgical therapies of endometriosis. The major drawbacks of current medical therapies of endometriosis are sometimes severe side effects. In this review, selective progesterone receptor modulators (SPRMs, mesoprogestins) as a potential therapeutic concept in endometriosis are discussed. Due to endometrial selectivity and favorable pharmacological profile, SPRMs may have advantages over the current medical treatments of this disease. Other emerging therapeutic approaches for this disease are also mentioned.

Keywords: endometriosis; SPRMs; ovulation; therapeutic; treatment

INTRODUCTION

Endometriosis, the presence of endometrial tissue outside the uterus, is a progressive, estrogen-dependent disease, which occurs nearly exclusively in menstruating women of reproductive age. The ectopic endometrium usually responds to changes in ovarian steroids, estrogen and progesterone, in terms of proliferation, differentiation, and bleeding. Increased angiogenesis and local inflammatory reaction are typical morphological changes in the endometriotic lesions.[1] Patients with endometriosis may present many different symptoms. Pain syndrome, however, represents the major clinical problem of this disease, manifested as dysmenorrhea, pelvic pain, lower abdominal pain, and dyspareunia.[2] In some women, the ectopic endo-

Address for correspondence: Kristof Chwalisz, M.D., Ph.D., TAP Pharmaceutical Products Incorporated, 675 North Field Drive, Lake Forest, IL 60045. Voice: 847-582-6283; fax: 847-582-6499.

Kristof.Chwalisz@TAP.com

metrium becomes highly invasive and forms so-called deep lesions, which often cause severe pain,[3] but the exact mechanism of pain in endometriosis is still unclear. It is believed that endometriosis-associated pain is caused by a local inflammatory reaction, which exacerbates during the perimenstrual period.[4] Since nonsteroidal anti-inflammatory drugs are effective in the treatment of endometriosis symptoms,[5] prostaglandins may play an important role in the pathogenesis of endometriosis-associated pain.

The manifestation of the disease, that is, the pain syndrome, rather than the disease itself currently represents the major indication for both the medical and surgical therapies of endometriosis. The major goal of the current medical treatment of endometriosis is to create an acyclic, hypoestrogenic environment by blocking ovarian estrogen secretion (GnRH agonists and antagonists; GnRH-a), by inducing pseudopregnancy, or by locally inhibiting estrogenic stimulation of the ectopic endometrium (progestins, androgenic progestins). Although all major therapies are effective for the treatment of pain, no single treatment seems to be superior in terms of efficacy.[5] The major drawbacks of the current medical therapies of endometriosis are sometimes severe side effects. The side effects of GnRH-a are due to an induced hypoestrogenic state, which adversely affects the skeletal and urogenital systems, while producing vasomotor symptoms at the same time. The major side effects of chronically administered progestins include breakthrough bleeding, bloating, breast tenderness, and mood changes. Chronic treatment with androgenic progestins such as danazol and gestrinone is often accompanied by seborrhea, acne, hirsutism, and negative changes in lipid profiles. Some androgenic side effects of danazol and gestrinone such as deepening of the voice, hirsutism, and clitoral hypertrophy are potentially irreversible. Hence, improvement of the profile of side effects should be considered a chief objective of new therapies of endometriosis.

In this brief review, we discuss the selective progesterone receptor modulators (SPRMs, mesoprogestins) as a potential therapeutic concept in endometriosis. Due to endometrial selectivity and favorable pharmacological profile, SPRMs may have advantages over the current medical treatments of this disease. We also comment on other emerging therapeutic approaches for this disease.

SELECTIVE PROGESTERONE RECEPTOR MODULATORS (SPRMs, MESOPROGESTINS)

SPRMs are defined as a new class of progesterone receptor (PR) ligands, which exhibit both progesterone agonistic and antagonistic activities *in vivo*.[6] FIGURE 1 shows the chemical structures of the best-known SPRMs, J867, J956, J912, and J1042, synthesized and characterized at Jenapharm GmbH and Co. K.G. (Jena, Germany).

Like progestins and progesterone antagonists (antiprogestins), SPRMs show high-binding affinity to PR (TABLE 1). When compared to either progestins or progesterone antagonists (antiprogestins), the SPRMs, however, exert markedly different effects in various animal models. In the absence of progesterone, the SPRMs act like weak progestins. In the presence of progesterone, they may also show weak antiprogestagenic properties in some tissues, particularly in the endometrium. In marked contrast to progesterone antagonists, SPRMs show only a slight labor-inducing activity in pregnant animals (TABLE 1). FIGURE 2 schematically shows the graded

TABLE 1. Studies of relative binding affinities (RBA) and ED_{50} of labor-inducing activity of SPRMs in pregnant guinea pigs

Compound	RBA (%) PR	RBA (%) GR	Labor-inducing activity (ED_{50}) (mg/animal/day)
RU 486	506	685	3.8
Onapristone	22	39	~3.0
J867	302	78	>100
J956	345	154	20
J912	162	76	>100
J1042	164	42	≫100

NOTE: The guinea pigs were treated sc on pregnancy days 43–44; autopsy pregnancy, day 50. PR (rabbit uterus): progesterone = 100%. GR (rat thymus): dexamethasone = 100%. Modified from reference 6, with permission from *Steroids* (one typing error corrected).

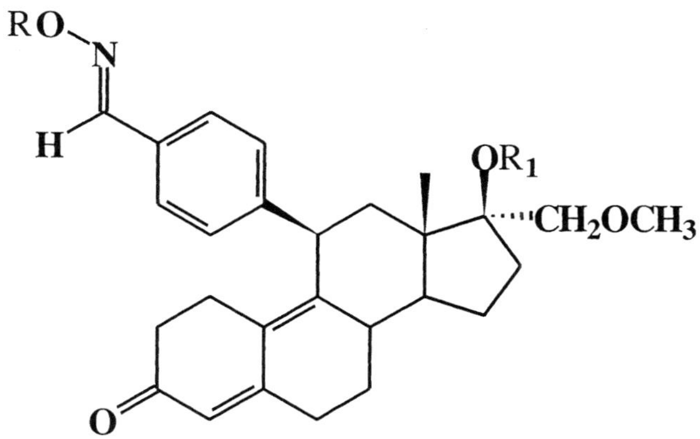

compound	R	R_1	
J 867	H	CH_3	oxime
J 912	H	H	17ß-hydroxy oxime
J 956	$CONHC_2H_5$	CH_3	oxime (ethyl carbamate)
J 1042	$COSC_2H_5$	CH_3	oxime (ethyl thiol carbonate)

FIGURE 1. Chemistry of progesterone receptor modulators (SPRMs, mesoprogestins). These compounds are 11β-benzaldoxime-estra-4,9-diene derivatives.

progesterone agonistic and antagonistic activities in various animal models discussed below. The "pure" progesterone antagonists, onapristone and ZK 230 211,[7] are presented on the left side of this scale. These compounds do not show any progesterone agonistic activity. Progesterone and the pure synthetic progestin, R 5020, represent PR agonists with maximum progestagenic effects *in vivo*. Although some agonistic activities of RU 486 have been previously described,[8,9] this compound acts predominantly as a progesterone antagonist *in vivo*, particularly during pregnancy.[10,11]

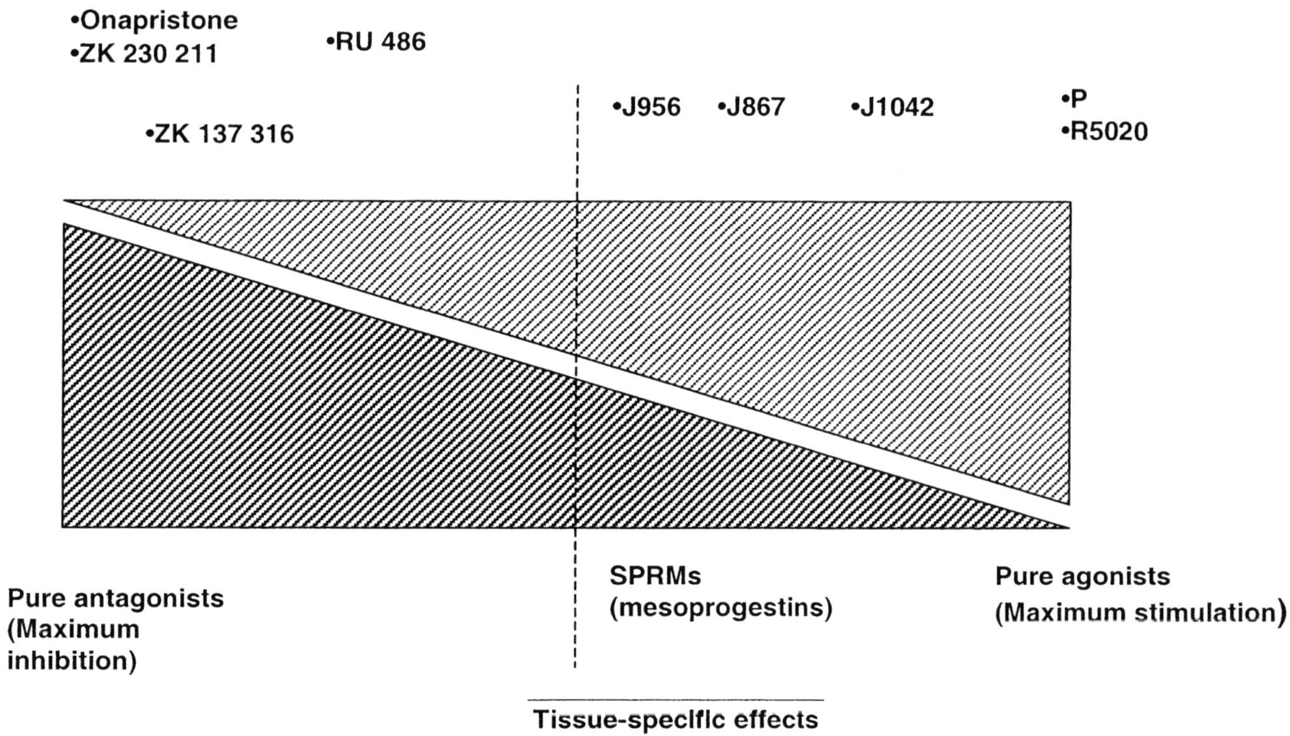

FIGURE 2. Spectrum of antagonistic and agonistic activities of PR ligands in *in vivo* animal models (guinea pigs, rabbits, rats).

The SPRMs are placed in the middle of this scale. J1042 is the strongest PR agonist of all J-compounds evaluated to date.[6]

Other hormonal activities: The SPRMs presented in FIGURE 1 exhibit a reduced binding affinity to glucocorticoid receptors (GR) compared to RU 486 (TABLE 1), which corresponds to marginal antiglucocorticoid effects of these compounds *in vivo*. They virtually do not bind to estrogen receptors (ER) and have no estrogenic activity *in vivo*.[6] At high doses, they show some mixed androgenic/antiandrogenic activities in rats.[6]

Effects of SPRMs on the Rabbit Uterus

The mixed progesterone agonistic/antagonistic activities of SPRMs are clearly evident in the juvenile, estrogen-primed rabbit uterus. This classical bioassay (McPhail test) has been frequently used to characterize both progestagenic and antiprogestagenic activities (FIG. 3, panels a and b).

In the rabbit uterus, progesterone stimulates proliferation and differentiation of epithelial endometrial cells, an effect that can be semiquantitatively assessed with a McPhail score. By definition, progesterone induces maximum stimulatory effects in this model (McPhail score 4). In the absence of progesterone, the SPRMs show a pronounced agonistic activity in the rabbit uterus (FIG. 3a). The stimulatory effects of SPRMs, however, are weaker than those of progesterone. Importantly, increasing the dose cannot enhance these effects. In the presence of progesterone, SPRMs exhibit some antagonistic activity (FIG. 3b). This activity, however, is significantly less than that of various progesterone antagonists such as mifepristone and other compounds such as onapristone, lilopristone, ZK 137 316, and ZK 230 211, which completely antagonize progesterone effects in this model (not shown). In analogy to the agonistic activity, increasing the dose does not enhance SPRM antagonistic effects. Importantly, RU 486 acts in this model as a "pure" progesterone antagonist, showing no agonistic activity at all. Similarly, other potent progesterone antagonists such as onapristone and ZK 137 316 do not exhibit progesterone agonistic activity in the rabbit uterus (not shown). The dose-response curves for both agonistic and antagonistic activities indicate that SPRMs stabilize the function of PR at an intermediate activity level in the rabbit uterus.

Effects of SPRMs in Pregnancy Models

The tissue selectivity of SPRMs is clearly evident in pregnancy models. SPRMs fail to maintain pregnancy in ovariectomized pregnant rodents such as mice and rats due to the fact that they have only partial progesterone agonistic activity. Yet, in rats and guinea pigs, the SPRMs inhibit both endometrial receptivity and implantation acting, in a manner similar to progesterone antagonists.[6] During early pregnancy, SPRMs act predominantly on the endometrium by inhibiting the decidual reaction and (most likely) other PR-dependent events.[6]

During advanced pregnancy, when the myometrium and cervix are the major target tissues for progesterone action, the SPRMs show only marginal effects in terms of induction of parturition or cervical ripening. The dissociation between endometrial and myometrial/cervical effects was most clearly observed in pregnant guinea pigs. Pregnant guinea pigs are considered a relevant animal model of human abortion and parturition.[12,13] The similarities between the guinea pig model and

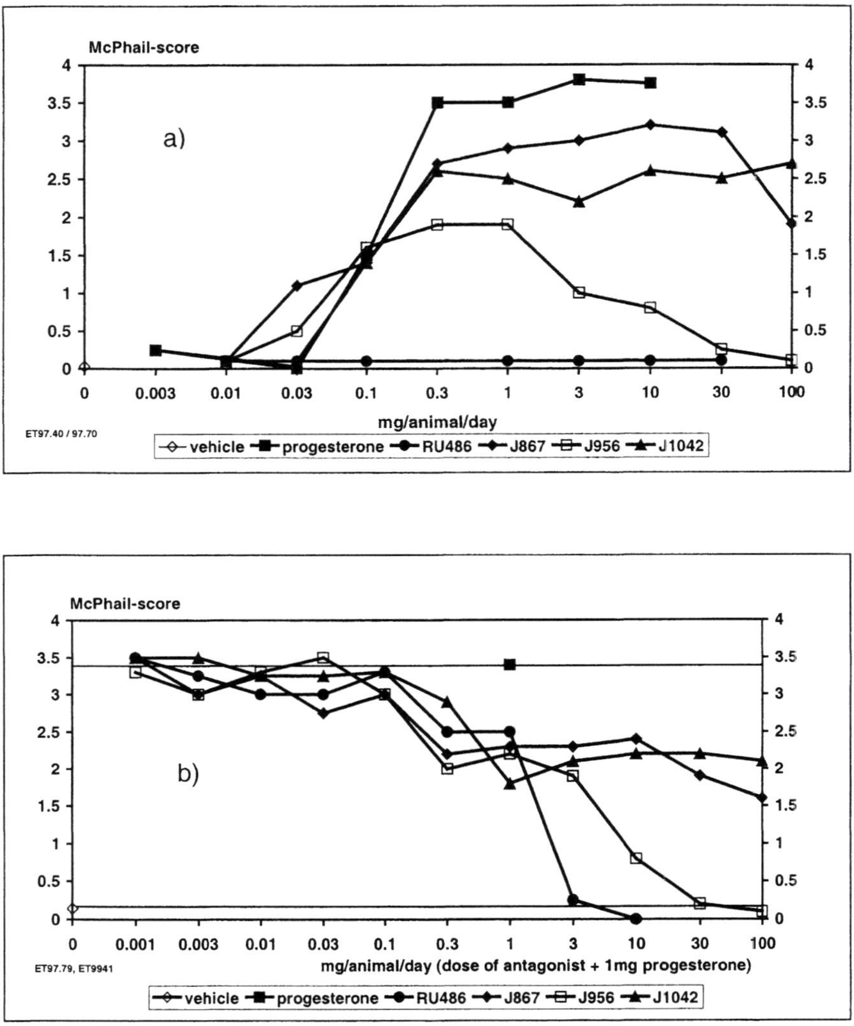

FIGURE 3. The PR agonistic (**a**) and antagonistic (**b**) activities of selective progesterone receptor modulators (SPRMs, mesoprogestins) in infantile estrogen-primed rabbits (modified McPhail assay). The juvenile rabbits were primed for 6 consecutive days with estradiol benzoate (5 μg/animal/day, sc). The PR ligands were then administered sc for 7 consecutive days. At 24 hours after the last injection, the uteri were collected for morphological evaluation. The assessment of stimulatory/inhibitory effects was performed according to the McPhail score (0 = no progestagenic activity; 4 = maximum progestagenic activity). (**a**) Agonistic activity of SPRMs. In this experiment, the animals were treated with the SPRMs only. (**b**) Antagonistic activity of SPRMs. The rabbits were treated with SPRMs in the presence of progesterone (1 mg/animal/day). Note that the threshold for agonistic activity of some of the antagonists is below that of progesterone. (From reference 6, with permission from *Steroids*.)

human pregnancy were also extensively discussed by Van Look and Bygdeman.[10] In this model, the progesterone antagonists such as mifepristone, onapristone, and lilopristone are very potent in inducing abortion or preterm parturition, which is brought about by both induction of labor and cervical ripening.[12–14] In marked contrast to these progesterone antagonists, both J867 and J956 have only marginal labor-inducing (abortifacient) activity in this model, irrespective of the dose.[6] Another structurally similar mesoprogestin, J1042, is in fact unable to terminate pregnancy in both guinea pigs and rats.[6] SPRMs exert only marginal effects on cervical ripening in guinea pigs during late pregnancy (K. Chwalisz, unpublished data). Collectively, these data strongly suggest that the SPRMs would not be suitable to terminate pregnancy in primates.

Effects of SPRMs on Ovulation and Ovarian Steroid Secretion

Comparative ovulation inhibition studies with progesterone antagonists and SPRMs in rats, guinea pigs, and primates show species-specific differences in the mechanism of progesterone action.[6,14,15] The macaque model seems to be the most suitable one to predict effects of SPRMs and antiprogestins on the ovarian and menstrual cycle. Paradoxically, both progestins and progesterone antagonists can inhibit ovulation in primates, acting most likely at different regulatory levels. Significantly, in primates, neither progesterone antagonists[17] nor SPRMs[16] suppress ovarian estrogen production, suggesting that these compounds do not impair the early stages of folliculogenesis. Our studies in cynomolgus monkeys with J1042 suggest that, in comparison with pure antiprogestins, SPRMs show stronger effects on the endometrium than on the hypophyseo-ovarian axis. In nonhuman primates, the antiovulatory activity of SPRMs is somewhat variable, which is in contrast to pure progesterone antagonists showing high inhibitory effects on ovulation.[15,16,18]

EFFECTS OF SPRMs ON THE PRIMATE ENDOMETRIUM

The primate endometrium represents a unique tissue with regard to vascular changes during the cycle and differs in this respect from that of other species such as rodents. If implantation does not occur, the upper part of the endometrium, the functionalis, is shed during menstruation in response to progesterone withdrawal at the end of the luteal phase. This effect is induced by the contraction of endometrial spiral arteries unique to primates. Cyclic changes of the endometrial blood vessels such as their damage during menstruation, neovascularization, and an increase in the growth and number of blood vessels occur within a single month. In humans, maximum growth and coiling of spiral arteries are observed during the secretory phase, an effect that is accompanied by an increased angiogenic activity.[19] Since similar cyclic changes are observed in the macaque endometrium,[20] studies in menstruating old-world monkeys such as cynomolgus or rhesus monkeys seem to be most relevant to humans.

The Endometrial Antiproliferative Effect of SPRMs and Progesterone Antagonists

Data from studies in nonhuman primates demonstrate that both SPRMs and progesterone antagonists are capable of suppressing endometrial growth at high

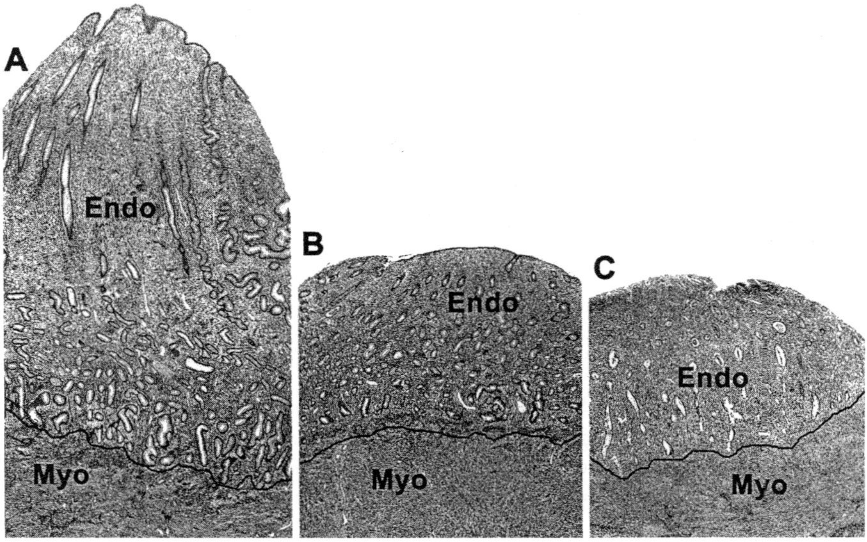

FIGURE 4a. Low-power micrographs of paraffin-embedded, hematoxylin/eosin-stained endometrial sections from cynomolgus macaques treated with vehicle (A), J1042 (B), or ZK 230 211 (C). Naturally cycling animals were treated on cycle days 2–22, and endometria were removed on day 23. Vehicle-treated monkeys revealed a typical progestational state marked by stromal expansion and glandular sacculation (A), while monkeys treated with the SPRM (B) and antiprogestin (C) showed a striking reduction in endometrial thickness with compacted stroma. Original magnification: 25×. [Figure reduced to 75%.]

estradiol blood concentrations. The suppression of endometrial growth was first observed after treatment with RU 486 at relatively high doses.[21–23] This unexpected effect was initially termed "noncompetitive antiestrogenic effect".[21,22] Since the inhibitory effects of progesterone antagonists and SPRMs are specific to the endometrium, we therefore prefer the term "endometrial antiproliferative effects". More recent studies in nonhuman primates show that newer antiprogestins such as ZK 137 316 and ZK 230 211 are capable of inducing endometrial antiproliferative effects at very low doses.[15,17,18] In monkeys, progesterone antagonists typically reduced endometrial thickness, induced degeneration of endometrial glands, inhibited mitotic activity in the endometrial epithelium, and induced stromal compaction. Paradoxically, these effects were accompanied by increased endometrial expression of ER and PR, which indicates that not all estrogenic responses in the primate endometrium were inhibited by this treatment.[17]

Our recent study shows that SPRMs can also exert endometrial antiproliferative effects on the primate endometrium.[16] This study compared the treatment effects of the progesterone antagonists ZK 230 211 and ZK 137 316 with those of the most-agonistic SPRM, J1042, in intact cynomolgus monkeys. All three compounds exhibited a similar profound inhibitory effect on endometrial growth, characterized by low endometrial thickness and the absence of mitotic activity, and induced a distinct stromal compaction (FIG. 4a) (also see FIG. 4b). In summary, the studies reviewed above demonstrate that both SPRMs and progesterone antagonists are capable of suppressing estrogen-induced endometrial growth. Within the reproductive tract, this effect seems to be endometrium-specific since no inhibition of estrogen responses could be observed in other organs such as the vagina and oviducts.[15]

More recently, inhibitory effects of SPRMs on mammary gland development could also be observed in a 39-week toxicological study with J867 in female cynomolgus monkeys after oral administration (R. Garg, unpublished data). FIGURE 5 shows the mammary gland morphology of a representative female monkey treated with J867. These effects were consistently observed in all animals exposed to J867 doses, producing an AUC (area under the curve) of 16.81 μg × h/mL or higher. This observation indicates that SPRMs have the potential to suppress both the endometrium and the mammary gland. It remains to be investigated whether this effect (1) is due to the inhibition of estrogen or progesterone effects in the mammary gland and (2) occurs at lower doses. It is well established that both progesterone and estrogen exhibit mitogenic activity on the primate mammary gland.

The exact mechanism of the endometrial antiproliferative effect is still unknown. At least four mechanisms are currently under consideration: (i) blockade of progesterone action on growth and function of spiral arteries;[15] (ii) suppression of the proliferative estrogen effects, specifically the mitotic activity of the endometrial glands via reduction of endometrial blood supply (vascular hypothesis);[15] (iii) down-regulation of stromal growth factors; and (iv) induction of androgen receptor (AR) expression in the endometrium.[24]

Major progress in understanding the mechanism of action of both antiprogestins and SPRMs on the primate endometrium could be achieved by including full-thickness endometrial biopsies in the morphological evaluation.[17] These studies demonstrated profound inhibitory effects of progesterone antagonists on spiral arteries, which showed either perivascular degeneration or inhibition of growth depending on the dose and duration of treatment. After treatment with the reference SPRM, J1042, however, the endometrial glands were not degenerated and showed residual secretory activity suggestive of partial agonistic activity. Interestingly, the number of spiral arteries and their diameter were similarly reduced after treatment with both antiprogestins (ZK 137 316, ZK 230 211) and J1042 (FIG. 4b).[16] The perivascular hyalinization and degenerative changes were only observed, though, in animals treated with antiprogestins. Hence, compared to the pure antiprogestins, J1042 seems to exhibit "milder" inhibitory effects on the endometrium, an effect that can be explained by the presence of mixed agonistic/antagonistic activities at PR.

Based on these results, we proposed that the endometrial antiproliferative effect of progesterone antagonists and SPRMs might be primarily due to the degeneration (pure progesterone antagonists) or inhibition (SPRMs) of spiral arteries. In addition, both of these classes of PR ligands may inhibit endometrial angiogenesis (FIG. 6).[15] This hypothesis would explain why both amenorrhea and endometrial atrophy can occur, even though there is an increased expression of some estrogen molecular markers in the functionalis—for example, ER and PR. The exact mechanisms underlying the degenerative changes in spiral arteries following treatment with progesterone antagonists and inhibitory effects on their function and growth by SPRMs are still unknown. There is evidence from studies in baboons that progesterone antagonists inhibit the expression of the inducible nitric oxide synthase isoform (iNOS) in the luteal phase endometrium, particularly in the stromal cells around the spiral

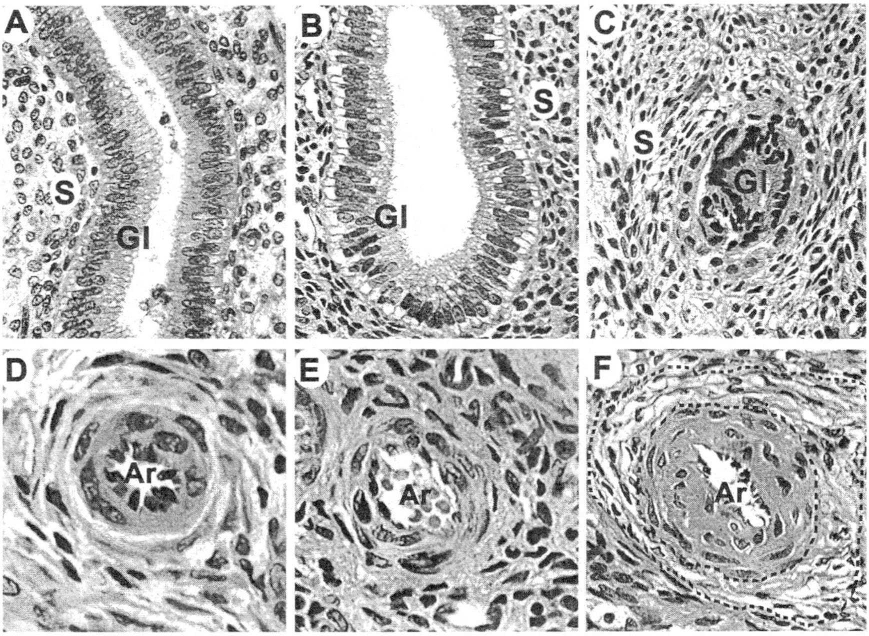

FIGURE 4b. High-power micrographs of paraffin-embedded, hematoxylin/eosin-stained endometrial sections. The vehicle-treated endometrium (panels A and D) revealed typical midluteal phase endometrial histology as evidenced by an expanded stroma (S), columnar glandular epithelium (Gl), and normal spiral arteries (Ar). Monkeys treated with J1042 (panels B and E) showed stromal compaction; however, glandular epithelium was columnar and secretory, and there were no marked degenerative changes in spiral arteries. ZK 230 211 treatments caused severe stromal compaction (panel C), pronounced degenerative changes in the glands (panel C), and signs of periarteriolar degeneration (panel F; periarteriolar zone within the two dotted lines). Original magnification: panels A–C, 312×; panels D–F, 937×. [Figure reduced to 75%.]

arteries.[25] Moreover, progesterone antagonists may alter endometrial vascular endothelial growth factor (VEGF) synthesis and other angiogenic factors, thus inhibiting angiogenesis.

Very recently, a new mechanism of endometrial antiproliferative effects of antiprogestins has been proposed based on studies of AR expression in the monkey and human endometrium exposed to antiprogestin treatment.[24] This study shows that various progesterone antagonists can dramatically induce AR expression in endometrial glands and can enhance its expression in endometrial stroma. Physiologically, AR is weakly expressed in stromal cells of the primate endometrium. Since there is substantial evidence that exogenous androgens can have inhibitory effects on the female reproductive system, including the induction of endometrial atrophy,[26–28] this mechanism may contribute to the endometrial antiproliferative effects of progesterone antagonists and SPRMs. The effects of SPRMs on AR expression still remain to be studied.

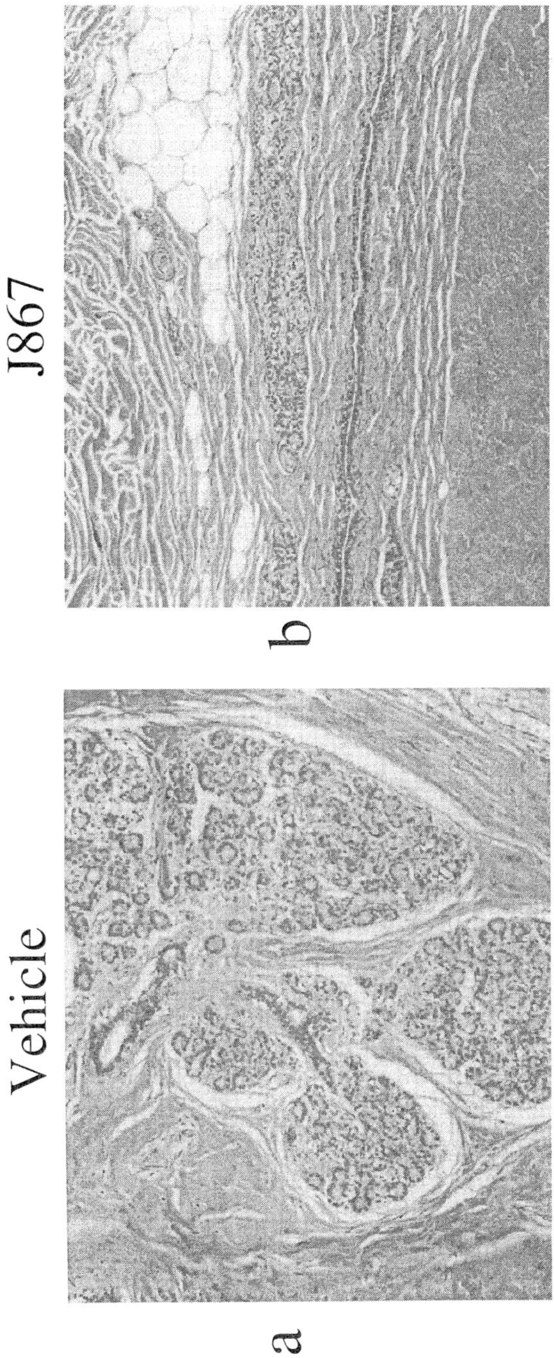

FIGURE 5. Micrograph of paraffin-embedded, hematoxylin/eosin-stained representative mammary gland section from cynomolgus macaques orally treated with high-dose J867 for 39 weeks: **(a)** vehicle control; **(b)** J867 treatment. Original magnification: 150×. [Figure reduced to 85%.]

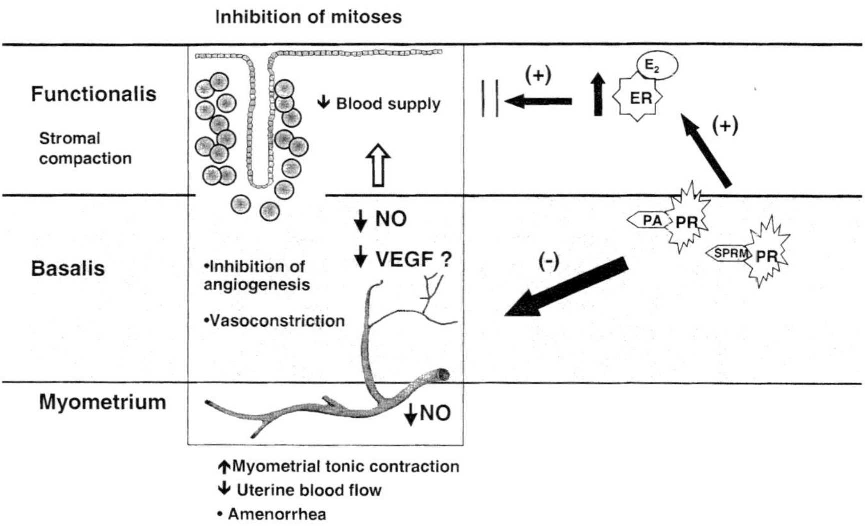

FIGURE 6. Proposed model of action of SPRMs and PAs on the primate endometrium. Inhibition or damage of spiral arteries in the basalis seems to be the primary effect of PAs and SPRMs. This effect may be due to several factors, including the downregulation of NOS leading to local NO deficiency and vasoconstriction, the inhibition of VEGF synthesis in epithelial and stromal compartments, and the general suppression of endometrial stroma. Terms: PA, progesterone antagonist; SPRM, selective progesterone receptor modulator; VEGF, vascular endothelial growth factor; NO, nitric oxide; E_2, estradiol. (Modified from reference 6, with permission from *Steroids*.)

Effects on Uterine Bleeding

The SPRMs have a potential to reversibly induce amenorrhea by selectively targeting the endometrium even in the presence of ovulation. Such an effect cannot be achieved with progestins since they inevitably produce breakthrough bleeding. The pure progesterone antagonists can also suppress menstruation in nonhuman primates.[15,18] However, the progesterone antagonist doses inhibiting ovulation and suppressing menstruation are very similar. Therefore, these compounds are not dissociated with regard to endometrial and central/ovarian effects. The presence of agonistic activity results in dissociation of these effects.

SPRMs AND UTERINE PROSTAGLANDINS

The effects of SPRMs on uterine prostaglandins may be clinically meaningful since these proinflammatory mediators are implicated in dysmenorrhea and the control of uterine blood flow. The first evidence that PR ligands directly control uterine prostaglandins came from studies in cycling guinea pigs.[12,14] It is well established in guinea pigs and some other species such as rabbits that the uterine prostaglandins are responsible for luteolysis. Hysterectomy prevents luteolysis, which results in the prolongation of the corpus luteum life span in these species. Surprisingly, treatment with progesterone antagonists prevented luteolysis in guinea pigs. This effect could be blocked with the pure progestin, R 5020.[6,14] Importantly, a prolongation of the duration of luteal phase was accompanied by a complete inhibition of uterine PGF2α secretion. Based on these experiments, it was proposed that progesterone is the major stimulator of uterine prostaglandins in the nonpregnant uterus, an effect that can be blocked at the uterine level by antiprogestins.[14] During pregnancy, the control of uterine prostaglandins seems to be more complex, with placental factors playing most likely the dominant role. More recently, the inhibition of luteolysis test in cycling guinea pigs was used to quantify the agonistic and antagonistic activities of SPRMs.[6]

The luteolysis in primates is not controlled by uterine factors. Some fundamental mechanisms related to progesterone regulation of uterine prostaglandin secretion may, however, be similar in guinea pigs and primates. The uterine cyclooxygenase isoforms (COX), the rate-limiting enzymes that catalyze the initial step in the formation of PGs from arachidonic acid, may represent a target for PR ligands. Other recent studies with the progesterone antagonist, ZK 137 316, performed in cycling and early pregnant baboons show that the constitutive isoform COX-1 is primarily regulated by progesterone, whereas regulation of the inducible isoform COX-2 may involve additional factors of embryonic origin.[29] Treatment of cycling baboons with ZK 137 316 during the luteal phase dramatically inhibited COX-1 expression in the endometrial epithelium, whereas it induced COX-2 expression in the stromal cells. With the onset of pregnancy, COX-1 expression in epithelial cells decreased dramatically, while COX-2 continued to be detected.

The effects of SPRMs on the uterine COX expression still have to be studied in the primate uterus. However, in view of the similarities between SPRMs and progesterone antagonists with regard to endometrial effects, SPRMs have a potential to inhibit uterine prostaglandins and perhaps to suppress perimenstrual pain.

CONCLUDING REMARKS AND CLINICAL IMPLICATIONS

The studies in macaques reviewed above indicate that, unlike progestins, the SPRMs have the potential to selectively suppress estrogen-dependent endometrial growth and to induce a reversible amenorrhea without adverse systemic effects of estrogen deprivation. These properties provide the rational basis for the treatment of endometriosis. Our studies indicate that the spiral arteries, which are unique to the primate endometrium, are the primary targets damaged or functionally inhibited by antiprogestins and SPRMs, respectively. The inhibitory effects of SPRMs on these unique vessels may underlie the paradoxical, endometrium-specific antiproliferative effects of these compounds. The stabilization (prevention of unscheduled bleeding) of the endometrial vessels may represent one of the major advantages of SPRMs compared to progestins. It is well known that chronic progestin treatment increases the fragility of endometrial blood vessels, leading to breakthrough bleeding. In addition, SPRMs have a potential of alleviating painful symptoms, the major clinical problem in endometriosis. Furthermore, SPRMs have a potential of controlling the progression of the disease by acting directly on the lesions. Since the ovarian estrogen production is maintained during SPRM treatment, the vasomotor symptoms and skeletal side effects related to estrogen deficiency may not occur (TABLE 2).

TABLE 2. Rationale for using SPRMs in the treatment of endometriosis

Pharmacodynamic effects
Reversible suppression of menstruation (endometrial bleeding) via a direct effect on endometrial blood vessels.
Selective inhibition of endometrial proliferation without systemic effects of estrogen deprivation.
Inhibition of uterine prostaglandins and potential pain relief.
Inhibition of ovarian progesterone secretion in the absence of estrogen deprivation.
No stimulatory effects on the mammary gland.

Other emerging technologies for the treatment of endometriosis such as selective estrogen receptor modulators (SERMs) and aromatase inhibitors are emerging. The goal of these treatments is to inhibit estrogen effects in the ectopic endometrium (SERMs) or to reduce ovarian and local estrogen production (aromatase inhibitors). The SERM raloxifene was reported to be effective in both a surgically prepared rat uterine explant model and in rhesus macaques with spontaneous endometriosis.[30] A rationale for the treatment of this condition with aromatase inhibitors is provided by recent clinical studies demonstrating that aromatase, a key enzyme of estrogen biosynthesis, is aberrantly overexpressed in endometriosis and by a casuistic observation reporting the efficacy of the aromatase inhibitor anastrozole.[31] The aromatase inhibitors may require add-back therapy to protect bones, whereas the currently available SERMs are known to stimulate gonadotropins and thereby may stimulate ovarian estrogen production. SPRMs may have some advantages over both SERMs and aromatase inhibitors since they show a high degree of endometrial selectivity in reducing estrogenic responses. Unfortunately, causative treatments of endometriosis are not yet available. As knowledge of endometriosis advances through the use of techniques from molecular biology, new concepts toward a causative therapy of endometriosis based on novel therapeutic targets may be developed in the future.

In conclusion, SPRMs represent a new opportunity in the treatment of endometriosis and other gynecological disorders. The discovery that SPRMs with either reduced or absent abortifacient activity exert inhibitory effects on the primate endometrium in terms of growth suppression, creation of reversible amenorrhea, and potential to control pain is exciting and deserves clinical study. It remains to be established in clinical trials whether SPRM therapy is superior to the current medical treatment strategies of endometriosis, which still remains, for both physician and patient, one of the most frustrating of women's diseases.

REFERENCES

1. HEALY, D.L., P.A. ROGERS, L. HII & M. WINGFIELD. 1998. Angiogenesis: a new theory of endometriosis. Hum. Reprod. Update **4:** 736–740.
2. MARTIN, D.C. & F.W. LING. 1999. Endometriosis and pain. Clin. Obstet. Gynecol. **42:** 664–686.
3. KONINCKX, P.R., D. OOSTERLYNCK, T. D'HOOGHE & C. MEULEMAN. 1994. Deeply infiltrating endometriosis is a disease, whereas mild endometriosis could be considered a non-disease. Ann. N.Y. Acad. Sci. **734:** 333–341.

4. BROSENS, I. 1997. Endometriosis—a disease because it is characterized by bleeding. Am. J. Obstet. Gynecol. **176:** 263–267.
5. OLIVE, D.L. & E.A. PRITTS. 2001. Drug therapy: treatment of endometriosis. N. Engl. J. Med. **354:** 266–275.
6. ELGER, W., J. BARTLEY, B. SCHNEIDER *et al.* 2000. Endocrine-pharmacological characterization of progesterone antagonists and progesterone receptor modulators (PRMs) with respect to PR-agonistic and antagonistic activity. Steroids **65:** 713–723.
7. FUHRMANN, U., H. HESS-STUMPP, A. CLEVE *et al.* 2000. Synthesis and biological activity of a novel, highly potent progesterone antagonist. J. Med. Chem. **43:** 5010–5016.
8. GRAVANIS, A., G. SCHAISON, M. GEORGE *et al.* 1985. Endometrial and pituitary responses to the steroidal antiprogestin RU 486 in postmenopausal women. J. Clin. Endocrinol. Metab. **60:** 156–163.
9. CHWALISZ, K., K. STÖCKEMANN, K.H. FRITZEMEIER & U. FUHRMANN. 1989. Modulation of estrogenic effects by progesterone antagonists in the rat uterus. Hum. Reprod. Update **4:** 570–583.
10. VAN LOOK, P. & M. BYGDEMAN. 1989. Antiprogestational steroids: a new dimension in human fertility regulation. Oxf. Rev. Reprod. Biol. **11:** 2–60.
11. SPITZ, I. & C.W. BARDIN. 1993. Clinical pharmacology of RU 486—an antiprogestin and antiglucocorticoid. Contraception **48:** 403–444.
12. ELGER, W., M. FÄHNRICH, S. BEIER *et al.* 1986. Mechanism of action of progesterone antagonists in pregnant guinea pigs. Contraception **6:** 47–62.
13. CHWALISZ, K. 1994. The use of progesterone antagonists for cervical ripening and as an adjunct to labour and delivery. Hum. Reprod. **9**(suppl. 1)**:** 131–162.
14. ELGER, W., M. FÄHNRICH, S. BEIER *et al.* 1987. Endometrial and myometrial effects of progesterone antagonists in pregnant guinea pigs. Am. J. Obstet. Gynecol. **157:** 1065–1074.
15. CHWALISZ, K., R.M. BRENNER, U. FUHRMANN *et al.* 2000. Antiproliferative effects of progesterone antagonists and progesterone receptor modulators on the endometrium. Steroids **65:** 741–751.
16. CHWALISZ, K., R.M. BRENNER, N. NAYAK *et al.* 2000. A comparison of the endometrial antiproliferative effects of a mesoprogestin (J1042) with the antiprogestins ZK 137 316 and ZK 230 211 in cynomolgus monkeys. J. Soc. Gynecol. Invest. **7:** 221A.
17. SLAYDEN, O.D., M.B. ZELINSKI-WOOTEN, K. CHWALISZ *et al.* 1998. Chronic treatment of cycling rhesus monkeys with low doses of the antiprogestin ZK 137 316: morphometric assessment of the uterus and oviduct. Hum. Reprod. **13:** 269–277.
18. SLAYDEN, O.D., K. CHWALISZ & R.M. BRENNER. 2001. Reversible suppression of menstruation with progesterone antagonists in rhesus macaques. Hum. Reprod. **16:** 1562–1574.
19. MAAS, J.W.M., P.G. GROOTHUIS, G.A.J. DUNSELMAN *et al.* 2001. Endometrial angiogenesis throughout the human menstrual cycle. Hum. Reprod. **16:** 1557–1561.
20. BRENNER, R.M. & O.D. SLAYDEN. 1994. Cyclic changes in the primate oviduct and endometrium. *In* The Physiology of Reproduction. Chapter 10, pp. 541–569. Raven Press. New York.
21. WOLF, J.P., J.G. HSIU, T.L. ANDERSON *et al.* 1989. Noncompetitive antiestrogenic effect of RU 486 in blocking the estrogen-stimulated luteinizing hormone surge and the proliferative action of estradiol on endometrium in castrate monkeys. Fertil. Steril. **52:** 1055–1060.
22. VAN UEM, J.F.H.M., J.G. HSIU, C.F. CHILIK *et al.* 1989. Contraceptive potential of RU 486 by ovulation inhibition: I. Pituitary versus ovarian action with blockade of estrogen-induced endometrial proliferation. Contraception **40:** 171–184.
23. SLAYDEN, O.D. & R.M. BRENNER. 1994. RU 486 action after estrogen priming in the endometrium and oviducts of rhesus monkeys (*Macaca mulatta*). J. Clin. Endocrinol. Metab. **78:** 440–448.
24. SLAYDEN, O.D., N.R. NAYAK, K.A. BURTON *et al.* 2001. Progesterone antagonists increase androgen receptor expression in the rhesus macaque and human endometrium. J. Clin. Endocrinol. Metab. **86:** 2668–2679.
25. PURCELL, T.L., A.T. FAZLEABAS, R. GIVEN *et al.* 2000. Changes in nitric oxide synthase are down-regulated by antiprogesterone in the stimulated-pregnant baboon uterus. J. Soc. Invest. **7**(suppl.)**:** 87A.

26. MILLER, N., Y.C. BEDARD, N.B. COOTER & D.L. SHAUL. 1986. Histological changes in the genital tract in transsexual women following androgen therapy. Histopathology **10:** 661–669.
27. FUTTERWEIT, W. & L. DELIGDISCH. 1986. Histopathological effects of exogenously administered testosterone in 19 female to male transsexuals. J. Clin. Endocrinol. Metab. **62:** 16–21.
28. LOESER, A.A. 1938. The action of testosterone propionate on the uterus and breast. Lancet **12:** 373–374.
29. KIM, J.J., J. WANG, C. BAMBRA *et al.* 1999. Expression of cyclooxygenase-1 and -2 in the baboon endometrium during the menstrual cycle and pregnancy. Endocrinology **140:** 26872–26878.
30. BUELKE-SAM, J., H.U. BRYANT & P.C. FRANCIS. 1998. The selective receptor modulator, raloxifene: an overview on nonclinical pharmacology and reproductive and developmental testing. Reprod. Toxicol. **12:** 217–221.
31. BULUN, S.E., K.M. ZEITOUN, K. TAKAYAMA & H. SASANO. 2000. Molecular basis of treating endometriosis with aromatase inhibitors. Hum. Reprod. Update **6**(5)**:** 413–418.

Panel Discussion (Part IX)

S.E. BULUN (*University of Illinois, Chicago, IL*): I have a question for Kris Chwalisz. A number of years ago, Kate Horwitz's group demonstrated that increased intracytoplasmic cyclic AMP would convert RU486 from an inhibitor to an agonist. Have you tried the function of your compounds in the presence or absence of cyclic AMP in any cell type?

K. CHWALISZ (*TAP Pharmaceutical Products, Lake Forest, IL*): Thank you very much for this important question. Indeed, RU486 and also the J compounds are agonists in the presence of cyclic AMP. This is probably the reason why the J compounds and to some extent RU486 are poorly effective in inducing labor compared to pure antiprogestins. The pregnant myometrium contains high amounts of cyclic AMP. In contrast, the pure antagonists, onapristone and ZK 230 211, which cannot be converted to progestins in the presence of cyclic AMP, are very potent labor inducers. Therefore, we are dealing on the one hand with compounds that act both *in vitro* and *in vivo* as progesterone receptor antagonists (left side of the graph presented during my talk) and on the other hand with a variety of compounds with various degrees of agonistic activity (middle and right side of this graph).

O. MUNEYYIRCI-DELALE (*SUNY Downstate Medical Center, Brooklyn, NY*): I have three questions: (1) Regarding nitric oxide, do you have any study on peripheral artery effects? (2) What is the recurrence rate after discontinued medication since the endometrial tissue did not become completely atrophic? (3) What are the long-term glucocorticoid effects?

CHWALISZ: First, I would like to answer the question related to the effects of SPRMs on peripheral arteries. The endometrial spiral arteries are unique arteries, which respond to progesterone withdrawal. Other arteries do not respond to changes in progesterone in this way. The observed effects are probably not related to the effects of these compounds on the endothelium. These effects may be mediated by other cells—for example, the perivascular cells. Uterine fibroblasts, NK cells, or other immune cells control the function of spiral arteries. Hence, the spiral arteries are unique with regard to progesterone dependency. The presence of progesterone receptors in the endothelium is still in dispute. We believe, therefore, that the vascular effects of SPRMs or antiprogestins are specific to the endometrium. Thus far, we have not observed comparable effects in other vascular beds.

The second question relates to the potential growth-inhibitory effects of SPRMs on the ectopic and eutopic endometrium. Do we really need a complete endometrial suppression (i.e., endometrial atrophy) for strategies such as the treatment of dysfunctional uterine bleeding? Unfortunately, we do not have any data from monkey endometriosis models, so we do not know what happens with the lesions. With regard to the eutopic endometrium, the SPRMs typically induce a "resting-type" endometrium without any bleeding, but they need not necessarily produce endometrial atrophy. Your point, however, is well taken. We will have to await the results of laparoscopy studies in patients to see if these compounds are able to reduce the endometriotic lesions. These studies have not been done yet. The FDA is primarily interested in pain reduction, but we need to initiate these types of studies to explore the effects of these compounds on the lesions. I guess Ana Murphy could comment on this question too. There are studies with RU486 that showed an effect on pain, but little effect on lesions.

A.A. MURPHY (*Emory University, Atlanta, GA*): Yes, I can comment on that. The study that did not have any effect on the lesions, but that did have an effect on pain, was the 3-month study. The only reason that we used it for 3 months is because that is all the FDA would allow us to do. Once we had that study, we then looked at a lower dose for 6 months and found a reduction not only in pain, but also in lesions.

CHWALISZ: We probably will be able to answer some of these questions by the end of this year.

MURPHY: RU486 is a very interesting compound because it really is not a very clean biologic probe, which is what we were hoping that it would be—that is, a pure antiprogestin. It has antiglucocorticoid activity. It has antiestrogenic effect. It is an antioxidant. Thus, it looks like the J compounds are a little bit better at looking at the antiprogestigenic effects. What are some of the other ones? You commented on AR and GR.

CHWALISZ: I mentioned during my talk that these compounds are quite selective to the progesterone receptor, particularly with regard to the interference with the glucocorticoid receptor (GR). We do not see any antiglucocorticoid activity. They show a mixed agonistic/antagonistic activity at the androgen receptor (AR) and no interaction with estrogen receptors. Thus, concerning the receptor selectivity, we are pretty fortunate with these compounds, which show little interaction with other steroid receptors. With regard to the antioxidant properties, we have no idea. We have not studied these effects. Definitely, though, the antiglucocorticoid activity of J compounds does not seem to be a problem at all.

MURPHY: What do you think the effects are going to be on the endometrium? With RU486, our data at 25–50 mg showed endometrial hyperplasia basically.

CHWALISZ: I agree.

MURPHY: Hold on. If you look at the monkey data, the data show atrophy, very significant atrophy. Obviously, there are some questions in terms of the two different models, humans versus primates, in the fact that humans have orosomucoid, which binds RU, whereas the primates do not. Also, the models were different because the monkeys were oophorectomized and thus there is no CNS effect.

CHWALISZ: This is one of the most important issues of the whole project: What are we going to see after chronic studies in the human endometrium? I agree with you that the monkey endometrium might be different to some extent. For example, we saw a dramatic effect of this type of compound in monkeys after 28 days of treatment and we could not confirm such a suppressive effect on endometrial growth with antiprogestin, which has been tested clinically in humans. The human endometrium may show a different level of sensitivity to progesterone and progestin treatments. We should also be aware of the fact that progesterone levels in monkeys during pregnancy are quite low. Thus, the monkey endometrium may show a lower threshold to SPRM/antiprogestin treatment. What we see in preliminary human data are similar trends in terms of stromal compaction, and the reduction of mitotic activity, but again I would like to avoid a strong statement about the endometrial effect of SPRMs in humans because the results of chronic clinical studies are not available yet. I agree with you that the effects of these compounds on the endometrium represent the key issue of the whole concept. We are well aware of this.

J.A. McLachlan (*Tulane University, New Orleans, LA*): What is known about the ethnic or racial prevalence of endometriosis? Uterine fibroids are very high in Japanese women in Japan. They are higher in African-American women than Caucasian women in the United States. Has any such study been done in terms of prevalence of endometriosis?

D.L. Olive (*University of Wisconsin, Madison, WI*): First of all, it is hard to do epidemiologic studies of endometriosis. Although we would like to go take 100 random women and laparoscope them, they tend to object and kick and scream. We do not have any good markers. Hence, what we are dealing with is either hospital-based evidence or presumptive endometriosis in most of the studies. In fact, the vast majority of the studies have failed to show any epidemiologic difference between races or between specific locations that cannot be attributed to different diagnostic criteria or different patterns of health care delivery. The one exception might be Japan, where a higher risk of endometriosis is seen in a pretty well designed epidemiologic study. However, it has not been duplicated in subsequent studies, so I just do not know if Asians or anybody else has any higher or lower rate.

McLachlan: Is this then an important point in terms of sorting out gene versus environment kinds of background?

Olive: Oh, yes. Absolutely.

V. Montgomery Rice (*University of Kansas Medical Center, Kansas City, KS*): The difficulty that comes in again is in practice patterns. If you look at hospital admissions for pelvic pain, you see a decrease. Even when women of color are admitted to the hospital for pelvic pain, they are about three times less likely to undergo a laparoscopy for their pelvic pain. They are assumed to have PID and are treated with antibiotics before going to laparoscopy. Thus, there are some practice issues that we have to address.

Olive: It goes even beyond the issue that you raise. Epidemiologists are quite frustrated by the inability to do any studies without any good markers. We have been frustrated by trying to study any type of environmental impact upon the disease simply because of the inability to diagnose it easily and noninvasively.

K. Osteen (*Vanderbilt University, Nashville, TN*): Just a comment in terms of the racial disparity. It is sort of the other end of the spectrum with premature rupture of the membranes. There is a racial disparity and it is about twice as high among African-Americans. The mechanisms of MMP regulation or inflammatory cytokines, etc., would be similar as well in that particular medical situation. Thus, we probably do not really know what we are looking at in terms of racial disparities.

McLachlan: One quick point. The National Institute of Environmental Health Sciences and Donna Baird, who is the head epidemiologist on this project, are looking at the prevalence of fibroids and they are doing sonograms on every woman walking into George Washington University Hospital. Now what Donna reported in a meeting last year is that, remarkably, African-American women always have more fibroids than white women of the same age and background, and that the prevalence reaches close to 72% in older African-American women. Do you know of any marker in fibroids, in this database, that would be useful in probing or finding out anything about endometriosis? I am not sure what sonography would mean in terms of endometriosis, but the data certainly comprise an available data set. I just cannot think what you would do with it.

OLIVE: I am not sure if it would be of much value. If they did a complete gynecological ultrasound, then we would have some information perhaps on endometriomas and that might be of some limited value, although I do not know what the numbers are for the study. We have some similar studies from Europe, particularly the Seveso Women's Health Study. This study looked at 1000 women and was able to assess these types of parameters. However, the incidence of things like endometriomas is so low that it is difficult to make any hard-core conclusions. Fibroids, as you mentioned, are highly prevalent and thus you can get some significant data for not nearly as much money as other diseases.

J. SEGARS (*National Institute of Child Health and Human Development, National Institutes of Health, Bethesda, MD*): Since there is not enough controversy on this panel, I thought that I would just take the prerogative as a surgeon to ask a question among the panel. Dr. Martin or Dr. Olive, what is the feeling regarding your diagnostic criteria. As Robert Barbieri outlined at the beginning of the conference, the majority of participants felt as if we should have a surgical biopsy–proven diagnosis. Now, Dr. Martin, you have spent specific time going over the errors that could exist at the time of surgery with a diagnosis of this disease. Therefore, is it really suitable to think about the possibility of a serum marker for this disease and would that be something that a surgeon would find acceptable?

D.C. MARTIN (*University of Tennessee, Memphis, TN*): Acceptable at what level?

SEGARS: That is my point.

MARTIN: If I had a patient with a 5-cm endometrioma coming out of the rectovaginal septum, which is stopping her from having sex, a serum marker is not going to help me. The tumor needs to be removed. You cannot rely on a serum marker to cure her pain. If you are looking for an epidemiologic marker to decide who has endometriosis and who does not in order to avoid surgery, and if we have a cure that will treat it, then a marker may be fine. We have to use a marker for something other than epidemiology. Markers are good for epidemiology, but I am not sure if you can treat endometriosis with them unless you find a therapy other than surgery that will get rid of it effectively. Most of the endometriosis that I observe is deep and not superficial. If the markers can determine superficial endometriosis, then medical therapy may be effective.

OLIVE: Let me take a slightly different approach to that question. One of the problems is that we do not design studies to answer clinical questions. The studies that I have shown are the studies that we have on endometriosis-associated symptoms. All make the assumption that you first visually diagnose endometriosis and then you go from there, but that is not really how we practice medicine. We practice clinically by seeing a patient who has a symptom and treating her symptom or by seeing a patient who has a laboratory test that is positive and treating the laboratory test. What we showed you were data on visualized or palpable and visualized endometriosis. Perhaps we should do studies on CA125-elevated associated pain or integrin-absent associated pain and stop calling it endometriosis. However, whatever it is, we need to associate something with pain that is utilizable clinically and do the study to see if intervention improves it. Only then will we have made some real headway.

MURPHY: Dr. Olive has a very valid point and that is that endometriosis is a heterogeneous disease. Moreover, until we can find a marker to distinguish these subpopulations, then we do not need to have that diagnosis at all. If you believe that oxidative stress is important and if you have evidence that this woman has a lot of oxidative stress versus one who does not, then that may predict who may or may not respond to therapy.

OLIVE: Also keep in mind that visualizable endometriosis is a subpopulation and that biopsy-demonstrated endometriosis is a subpopulation.

MONTGOMERY RICE: When I think of pelvic pain associated with endometriosis, I think of quality-of-life issues for women. When you think about a marker, then you are thinking about something that the marker can identify that will enable you to induce the therapy again that is going to improve that quality of life. Now, quality of life for some women may be reduction in pain, whereas for others it may be avoiding surgery. It may be different things. When we design our studies, we have to keep those issues in mind, particularly as it relates to pain as well as to infertility.

MARTIN: One last thing to follow up on what Dr. Olive said: that is, if something cures pain, then it does not mean it cures endometriosis. Pain that responds to GnRH is not necessarily because GnRH corrects endometriosis. It will stop pain even if endometriosis is not there. If somebody gets breast tenderness from fibrocystic breast disease, they are put on GnRH and their breasts are not tender anymore—not because the breast did not have endometriosis, but because it had an estrogen-sensitive problem. We have estrogen-sensitive headaches. We have estrogen-sensitive breast tenderness. We probably have estrogen-sensitive conditions in the pelvis that are not endometriosis, such as myomas, etc.

Summary of Future Research Directions and Recommendations

KOJI YOSHINAGA AND ESTELLA C. PARROTT

National Institute of Child Health and Human Development, National Institutes of Health, Bethesda, Maryland, USA

The foregoing papers and panel discussions transmit vividly the atmosphere of the meeting and the enthusiasm of the audience. Listed below are the future research directions and recommendations.

Basic Research

- Examine the cellular biology of endometrial cells.
- Assess the mechanisms of establishing endometrial implants.
- Characterize peritoneal-endometrial interactions, cell-cell communications, and epithelial-stromal communications.
- Clarify the impact of endometriosis on fertility.
- Determine the effects of endometriosis on eutopic endometrium.
- Develop endometriosis-derived cell lines for research.
- Identify epidemiology and risk factors of endometriosis.

Clinical Research

- Formulate pain-assessment tools and improve measurement scales for the disease.
- Clarify basic mechanisms that relate endometriosis and pelvic pain.
- Practice evidence-based medicine.
- Enhance availability of human tissues for research.
- Focus on clinical trials that compare different therapies.
- Establish useful biomarkers that identify those patients with endometriosis.
- Initiate clear guidelines for clinical studies.
- Study the effects of oral contraceptive pills on endometriosis.
- Develop orally active GnRH antagonists for the treatment of endometriosis.
- Understand the heterogeneity of endometriosis.

Address for correspondence: Koji Yoshinaga, Program Director, Reproductive Endocrinology, Reproductive Sciences Branch, Center for Population Research, National Institute of Child Health and Human Development, National Institutes of Health, 6100 Executive Boulevard, Room 8B-01, Bethesda, MD 20892-7510. Voice: 301-496-6515; fax: 301-480-2389.
ky6o@nih.gov

- Develop nonhormonal drug therapies such as inhibitors of matrix metalloproteinases.
- Focus on early disease.

Overall

- Explore multidisciplinary and international collaborations.
- Develop a website on endometriosis.
- Continue cross talk between basic researchers and clinical researchers.

Panel Discussion (Part X)

K. YOSHINAGA (*National Institute of Child Health and Human Development, National Institutes of Health, Bethesda, MD*): There are two major aspects of research on endometriosis: basic and clinical. On these two aspects, the experts in this area have updated our knowledge and identified the gaps in our knowledge. This final session summarizes them and underscores the research needed. Linda Giudice and Kevin Osteen have kindly agreed to lead the discussion.

L.C. GIUDICE (*Stanford University, Stanford, CA*): The scope of this meeting has been quite large and it was purposefully designed that way to capture nearly every aspect of endometriosis and research related to it. We have examined epidemiology, environmental effects on endometriosis, risk factors, long-term health, and potential relationships to cancers and therapies.

There was much information about the establishment of the disease, the role of enzymes and matrix degradation, and some of the intracellular pathways. However, there is no information as to why these events are happening. We really do not have a good handle as to what happens upstream leading to disease development and endometrial abnormalities. These likely involve genetics, the immune system, and the environment. Also, we do not understand why a subset of women will develop this disease and if it is all due to retrograde menstruation.

As to basic research, we discussed steroid hormone actions, steroid hormone receptors, receptor isoforms, isotypes, some of the players, and the different pathways involved. This is an extraordinarily important part of the pathogenesis of endometriosis and likely will be involved in how we are going to screen women who have a genetic predisposition for the disease or who are at higher risk because they live in an area of the country or the world where there are endocrine disrupters or other risk factors.

In terms of abnormal eutopic endometrium, does this play a role in the mechanisms of establishing the implants in the pelvic cavity and on the ovary? What are the mechanisms underlying infertility? We are just scratching the surface here, but we are making some headway. What are the effects of endometriosis and of endometriomas on oocyte complement and oocyte competence? What is the real fertility potential of women with endometriosis? Also, is a uterine factor the only one or is there a real compromise in terms of oocyte competence? There are some questions that remain unanswered, especially clinically. In terms of clinical research, we have heard a lot about the paucity of good quality randomized clinical trials. One of the things that came to my mind is that there is abundant research on OCPs, GnRH agonists, danazol, and surgical therapies. Does one merely need to spend the money to show that one is better than another for women who respond to those therapies? Perhaps the women who do not respond to those therapies are really the women for whom, if resources are limited, the strategies of new therapies may be most beneficial. Dr. Chwalisz touched on a few of those and I am sure that, as the basic research develops, the clinical translation will also develop.

We all appreciate that epidemiologic studies are extraordinarily difficult to do. That is probably not the subject of this sort of think-tank discussion. However, this is important from a clinical perspective because, as a clinician, when we see patients with endometriosis, we rarely talk about such things as this is your diagnosis and this is what may happen in terms of association with breast cancer, or association with malignant melanoma. Some of these things have been talked about by Dr. Swiersz.

As to risk factors from the disease per se and risk factors from current therapies, I believe that Dr. Parthasarathy's comments were very well taken. For example, what is happening with the lipid profiles? What about osteoporosis and some of the other side effects that women experience due to some of the current therapies?

As for pregnancy outcomes, we did not touch upon this topic, but the literature contains controversies over whether or not there is an increase in the miscarriage rate or an increase in luteal-phase deficiency in women with endometriosis. Also, let's not forget the patient. I think that it is extraordinarily important that some members of The Endometriosis Association are here today. Communication between the community of women who have this disease and the funding bodies to fund research for this disease is extremely important.

I would now like to open the discussion, Kevin, unless you have some additional thoughts. I may not have left you much room here!

K.G. OSTEEN (*Vanderbilt University, Nashville, TN*): I think that is a very appropriate platform on which to launch discussions. I want to remind the audience that the agencies are here to listen and they basically would rather respond to you than to provide the stimulus. This is our opportunity as a group of scientists and physicians who are interested in endometriosis to say what we think about new areas that we should pursue. Perhaps it would be appropriate, realizing the time constraints, that we limit our discussions on each area and try to distribute our time about half on basic research and about half on clinical research. Let's start with clinical.

V. MONTGOMERY RICE (*University of Kansas Medical Center, Kansas City, KS*): One good point is that we do have a lot of new therapies coming out and perhaps we should evaluate those in the patient who is not responsive to some of the other medications that we currently have. However, we also have to consider the way in which physicians practice. For example, it is a common practice for physicians to try patients on oral contraceptive pills and have then moved on to surgery. They then go back and put that patient on oral contraceptive pills again because that is what patients are comfortable with and they see it as the least invasive or the medical therapy that is going to have the least amount of side effects. We definitely need trials to evaluate truly what that level of effectiveness is with oral contraceptive pills after surgery because perhaps we are not putting the patient on the most appropriate therapy in order to increase her pain-free interval. We need to practice evidence-based medicine to ensure that we are using the best medical therapeutic option postsurgically, particularly as it relates to oral contraceptive pills.

S.E. BULUN (*University of Illinois, Chicago, IL*): I would like to address another specific area, which concerns both basic and clinical research. That is the availability of human tissues for basic research. This is a major limiting factor for endometriosis research. If we would like to continue our studies with respect to their relevance to human tissues, we have to have availability of both extraovarian endometriosis and ovarian endometriomas. For example, we were able to conduct most of our research on aromatase and progesterone receptors because I worked with two excellent laparoscopic surgeons in Dallas, Alan Johns and Michael Putman. We need to think of ways to increase tissue availability to investigators.

QUESTION: Earlier, I saw presentations that described unique tissue-tissue interactions that I had never thought of before. The peritoneal-endometrial interactions appear to be key to the establishment of this disease. We see that interaction can induce growth of endometrial tissue that hitherto has been difficult or impossible to do, indicating that there is a unique situation. Dr. Schenken's work seems to be the first to look at the adhesion between these two things. It seems to be a key event in the disease and this unique situation needs to be examined fully.

F. HOWARD (*University of Rochester, Rochester, NY*): Missing from your list of basic mechanisms are the basic mechanisms that relate to endometriosis and pelvic pain, which certainly carry the same importance clinically as the relationship to infertility. Hence, this needs to be a major focus in basic science. Additionally, this obviously leads to studying the relevance of both new therapies as well as what we do for patients who do not respond to our current therapies. I agree that we do, in fact, still need to look at our current therapies and compare them really in an effective and reliable way because, currently, the way we practice is not as scientific as it should be. That is why we would be remiss if we did not do clinical trials to compare our therapies.

G. ALTMAN (*University of Washington, Seattle, WA*): One thing with this is the outcome measurements. Most of the studies on pain have used a 10-point BAS scale on one single indicator on one day. However, we need better outcome measurements of all these studies looking at quality of life, looking at pain scales, looking at some of the mood scales that have been developed, or looking at depression scales. To just have pain as the indication is very limited and I would like to see us developing a much more quantifiable type of measurement.

A.A. MURPHY (*Emory University, Atlanta, GA*): I want to make some comments that basically tie this together. Pelvic pain patients are a heterogeneous population and part of the problem when we study some of the pain endpoints is that we are not specifically looking at these different types of populations. For instance, if we look at rectovaginal disease specifically, this subset of patients will respond quite well to surgery, as opposed to some of the other entities that make up pelvic pain. That population needs to be studied as a group apart from "generic" pelvic pain, which may have diverse origins. Endometriosis is a heterogeneous disease and, until we do studies that are much more specific in terms of disease type, location, and symptoms in conjunction with, say, a panel of serum markers (yet to be identified), we are not likely to be able to target our therapies as well as we should be targeting them.

GIUDICE: I just want to make a comment about adding this to the list. The list was not meant to exclude that. In fact, mechanisms and establishment of disease really do bear on both of these. One of the least understood parts of endometriosis, besides its etiology, is why do women have the pain.

K. CHWALISZ (*TAP Pharmaceutical Products, Lake Forest, IL*): I would like to stress as a representative of the pharmaceutical industry the importance of clear guidelines for the testing of new approaches in endometriosis. There are no FDA guidelines regarding clinical trials in endometriosis. The FDA is interested in pain reduction, but it is unclear how to assess pain—whether to use a 4-point or 10-point scale, for example. What about quality of life? There are many questions related to future studies that sometimes are very difficult to answer, particularly with regard to phase III studies. In my opinion, there is a need to develop clear guidelines of how to test new approaches in endometriosis. The other issue is related to different forms of endometriosis. For example, should deeply infiltrated endometriosis, often characterized by severe pain, be included in our studies or should this group of patients with deep lesions be evaluated separately? These are examples of questions that are highly relevant to clinical development of new therapies for endometriosis.

QUESTION: As Dr. Olive pointed out, all of us have different endpoints and look at data in different ways. What we need is some kind of guidance so that we can do analysis to obtain meaningful data.

B.A. LESSEY (*University of North Carolina, Chapel Hill, NC*): I would like to stress the need for biomarkers that can identify those patients with endometriosis before we start the study. Whenever we pick a population to study, we often select out those with endometriosis who do not have pelvic pain. A lot of those patients actually have endometriosis, but never get diagnosed laparoscopically, and thus we underappreciate the effect of endometriosis in areas such as infertility.

O. MUNEYYIRCI-DELALE (*SUNY Downstate Medical Center, Brooklyn, NY*): Some patients have developed a coping mechanism for pain. When we do laparoscopy or other surgery, we find extensive endometriosis. Since the patients did not come complaining of pain, we question them about having pain now or as teenagers. They state that they had a lot of pain as teenagers and could not go to school. When we treat them medically, they then realize that they were suffering and had learned how to live with the pain. When the medication is stopped and disease recurs, then the patients really have extensive pain because they lost the coping mechanism.

E. MCGEE (*University of Pittsburgh, Pittsburgh, PA*): One thing that has not been discussed much is prevention, which may be a reflection of the fact that the field has not matured enough to the point where we know who needs preventive measures and what that might entail. It seems to me that endometriosis is kind of like a polycystic ovary in that it has its roots in adolescence long before we see lesions and tissue damage. It may be that there could be some things that are fairly simple that could be done for adolescents who are at high risk for developing endometriosis, such as putting them on continuous contraceptive pills. Perhaps, we can develop biomarkers so that we can test adolescents and know who needs treatment and who does not, and prevent some of these debilitating anatomic problems that manifest later.

J.A. MCLACHLAN (*Tulane University, New Orleans, LA*): Along that same line and sort of following up with biomarkers, a strategy to understand the etiology is critical in terms of both prevention and treatment. This is a whole area of exciting new research. However, it is worth considering whether there are benign uterine disease syndromes. Is it always the case that endometriosis happens in the absence of myosis and in the absence of fibroids? Do fibroids and endometriosis often occur together? Can one type be in one place and another in some other place? As a nonclinician, it would be interesting to know if this would be another approach to see whether one disorder or one disease arises earlier. Are there different genetic components or different environment components?

N. BRACERO (*The Johns Hopkins University, Baltimore, MD*): As we review our patient populations, there is a group of patients who come in more often. This type of patient is a woman in her 40s with a recurrent endometrioma. She has completed her fertility attempts and she is concerned with developing either a clear cell or endometrioid carcinoma in that recurrent endometrioma. As more markers come up, it is going to be tougher to orient these patients. We need either guidelines or some sort of orientation for our patients and to counsel these patients.

L.M. SWIERSZ (*Stanford University, Stanford, CA*): During the session on the models of endometriosis, Dr. Schenken gave a wonderful model showing how endometriosis may invade, but unfortunately this technique is not available to everyone. The other models, primates or animal models, are expensive and they may not mimic human endometriosis. If we can develop cell lines that are derived from endometriosis instead of using stromal cells or cancer cell lines, we may be able to genetically manipulate these cells and look at them on a molecular level, and then take that knowledge to an animal model. Cancer research has been very successful with using that type of approach. It would be a useful tool. There are a few endometriosis-derived cell lines—not in the United States, not widely available—that are found in Europe and they would be useful.

S. KENNEDY (*University of Oxford, Oxford, United Kingdom*): Can I make some observations as a foreigner? The literature contains vast numbers of bits of research. If there is one thing I have learned in the last eight years in trying to pursue the research for susceptibility genes, it is that there is a crying need for collaborative research and I do not mean just a couple of centers working together. I mean large numbers of research teams working together. This is the most developed country in the world and the largest country in the world. There is a need for the NIH to start a network of centers throughout the United States that are prepared to collaborate together to collect tissues, serum, and clinical data that could be shared among all researchers in this field to avoid these small studies. Furthermore, it is incredibly embarrassing for me as an Englishman to come over here and tell a group of Americans about an NIH-sponsored group of primate centers. However, the fact is that you are sitting on the most incredible resource for the study of the epidemiology of endometriosis and the NIH is already funding that work with millions of dollars per year. That resource definitely needs to be utilized better.

M.L. BALLWEG (*The Endometriosis Association, Milwaukee, WI*): Concerning collaboration, we need collaboration across specialty lines. I am surprised how often I am called by specialists from other areas where they have something very valuable for our field, but we do not know about it, and we probably have very many valuable things for them. This is difficult in our modern environment, but we need to find ways to cross-link our common areas of interest in gynecology, immunology, and toxicology; then, at the clinical level, we need to do the same thing. We need to be working much more with pediatricians. We are struggling to help girls as young as nine with diagnosed endometriosis. Also, oncologists and pain specialists need to be included. We need to bring the strengths of each of these different groups to bear. A lot of our answers are probably out there, but it is hard to get all the pieces together.

OSTEEN: I wish to add a comment from a recent symposium held in Japan. We were all reminded that the world is getting much smaller in terms of environmental influences that have impact on disease. One of the things that became apparent is that we have all these wildlife population studies that have linked environmental exposures to various reproductive failures. Often, those individuals do not talk to people studying human diseases and thus do not share their perspectives and their findings. There is a huge amount of information. For example, I was astounded to see a sea lion exposure to PCBs that mimicked most of the uterine anomalies that we have seen in endometriosis and I really was not aware of the data. Thus, data are out there that people in human health have not really tapped into. Perhaps collaborations with those individuals as well as collaborations with groups in other countries would be very fruitful for us.

McLachlan: I would like to make a suggestion of developing a virtual center in uterine disease. We have a website for environmental hormones (E.HORMONE) and, in addition to having preprints of papers that people in the field are looking at, we have authors who are willing to put in their papers that are published. What I ask them to do is to put in a paragraph or two of why this paper is important to the field of environmental endocrinology. This will be very important in the future. We put things that come out in the news. We have a conference kiosk where the different meetings are. People download their slides there too. I often have people come and give talks at Tulane and show my slides that they have picked up off the Internet, or they do it in Japan.

What we are starting to do is get people to inventory and post what they are willing to share: antibodies, cDNAs, animal models, cell lines, critiques of different cell lines, different models, etc. You could run something like this with some funding out of Vanderbilt or somewhere else. It could be the kind of place where people would put something in saying that PCBs cause leiomyoma in sea lions and that would be interesting. The idea is a great one. One way to get at it would be to create some collegial center over the Internet where people can take advantage of it and share ideas, reagents, publications, and findings.

S. Young (*University of Missouri, Columbia, MO*): We could extend that even further if we posted things like gene array data or gene cluster analysis for candidate genes. A lot of people are probably doing arrays or will be shortly. We could also make it even more friendly for mining by putting it in a standard format that could be searchable and linked to other resources on the Web. That could be a great resource for the endometrial community.

Giudice: I wanted to just make a comment for Dr. Kennedy so that he realizes that we are, indeed, a civilized country. There is a mechanism called the Reproductive Medicine Network sponsored through the NIH. Your comments have been heard by Dr. Phyllis Leppert, who heads that program. That is probably not a venue that would be funded through this mechanism with the Reproductive Sciences Branch, but potentially could be accommodated through the Reproductive Medicine Network. With regard to the primate centers, my understanding is that they are funded through the National Center for Research Resources (NCRR), from the NIH. As much as we love to have you here, perhaps at the next meeting we can invite some of your collaborators so that they can meet investigators here with similar research interests.

P. Leppert (*National Institute of Child Health and Human Development, National Institutes of Health, Bethesda, MD*): The centers mentioned during this meeting are part of SCCPRR, which stands for Specialized Cooperative Centers Program in Reproduction Research. There are several primate centers that are members of that group, Oregon and Pittsburgh. There is a real effort within the Reproductive Science Branch to foster this research. Your comments are going to help us a lot in pushing this agenda forward, especially the comments about Internet data banks and so forth. We have funded the Ovarian Kaleidoscope Database, but we really need to have the community support us in this effort. I was really delighted to hear those comments.

GIUDICE: Perhaps we should shift gears just a little and hear from basic research investigators. Can we have some comments from interested parties?

LESSEY: We have heard a great deal of information regarding the differences between eutopic endometrium from women with and without endometriosis. It would be helpful to figure out the question of which comes first—the chicken or the egg question. Do the abnormalities in the eutopic endometrium arise first or do they come later in response to the endometriosis? I think that is a fundamental question that we need to answer.

MCLACHLAN: My comment is not really a basic science comment. It is to make a plea as a former NIH employee to NICHD and to NIEHS to look at this whole field of benign uterine diseases, endometriosis in particular, as one of the top priorities for your institute. All this research that you are hearing about is often bootlegged on reproductive biology grants and things. I am just making a case that this should move up the food chain of interest for NIH generally and NICHD and NIEHS in particular.

R.N. TAYLOR (*University of California, San Francisco, CA*): I want to follow up on both of these comments. From a hypothesis-driven approach, the way that we will find new biomarkers that may actually lead to some reasonable clinical studies is through basic investigation, through understanding the cellular physiology. For me as a clinician, the most frustrating things are what we have called "tried and true" therapies (and I am glad that we put those words in quotation marks). It is incredibly disappointing that many patients do not benefit very much from our current treatments. The reason is that those therapies are not as rationally designed as we have thought and, in fact, we really need to understand the underlying cellular biology before we can move towards developing new therapies. Hence, while there might be value in comparing one of our "tried and true" therapies versus another in a large clinical trial, I would encourage people, before spending a lot of money, to seriously ask the following: what is the real underlying pathophysiology?

MCLACHLAN: A basic science question at the heart of many of these benign uterine diseases is the following: how do cells develop uncontrolled growth or how do you immortalize epithelial cells to the point of neoplastic transformation so that you do not get tumors or cancers? They are called tumors if they are fibroids because they are growths. In this case with endometriosis, you have nests of cells that grow and grow and sort of invade, but are not neoplasms in the sense that they are not malignant, nor are fibroids malignant. When you look back at some of the work that has been done on trophoblastic diseases and invasiveness of normal trophoblasts and choriocarcinomas, there is a tremendous amount to learn about the basic biology of cell proliferation and cell migration. I think that those fundamental kinds of studies would go a long way to understanding the ways to control endometriosis.

OSTEEN: I had a similar comment since funding generates lots of data and lots of interest in the pharmaceutical industry. As reproductive biologists, we often take therapies developed in the cancer field to see if they will work in endometriosis. However, the endometrium is so rich in information that we should actually be sending information back to the cancer field. We need to start exporting a little bit of our perspective on endometrial biology—the wonders of control that exist in normal implantation—and start thinking as a group that has a lot of information to share with the broader community, instead of waiting for it to flow back to us.

GIUDICE: I want to make a comment about cell-cell interactions and cell-cell communication. There is a tremendous amount of cross talk between the epithelium and the stroma. When you look at some of the mouse knockout models of particular genes, not only do you get an implantation defect because embryos do not attach, but you usually get a decidualization defect. I think Bob Schenken's model is attractive, and certainly others have been thinking about this in terms of cell-cell interactions between endometrium and peritoneum or mesothelium. In a brief conversation with Kris Chwalisz about myometrial-endometrial interactions, we discussed that one of the most enigmatic disorders and one that has quite a bit of morbidity associated with it is adenomyosis. This disorder is very understudied, but I imagine that one could establish models for cell-cell interactions for the development of this disorder, which begins to infiltrate into the myometrium.

D. VOGEL (*National Cancer Institute, National Institutes of Health, Bethesda, MD*): With respect to the multidisciplinary nature of the research that needs to be conducted, I would like to remind everybody that one of the cosponsors of this meeting is the Office of Research on Women's Health (ORWH). Although Dr. Pinn had to leave, Dr. Parrott and myself are both serving leadership roles in the career and research subcommittees for ORWH, respectively. I mention this because endometriosis has been and will continue to be one of the explicit priorities of ORWH. While in the past they have tended to work through the individual institutes in research areas that are specific to the missions of individual institutes, their thinking is trending more recently towards coordinating and, indeed, spearheading multidisciplinary research that crosses missions of the institutes that have an interest. In this case, NICHD and ORWH can certainly be expected to be participants in this kind of thinking and in the kind of actions that will help the agenda move forward.

CHWALISZ: As a follow-up to Dr. McLachlan's comment on uterine fibroids, I would like to stress again the importance of clear guidelines for clinical studies. I mentioned earlier the problems related to endometriosis. This type of problem is even more pronounced in the case of uterine fibroids. In this indication, it is unclear which endpoints are important for clinical studies. Is the fibroid size important? What about the clinical symptoms? Should the delay of surgery be a primary endpoint? We know that there are so many local differences with regard to surgical treatments of fibroids. Thus, there is an urgent need to define how to conduct clinical studies in women with benign uterine disorders, not only for endometriosis, but also for conditions such as adenomyosis and uterine fibroids.

BALLWEG: Dr. Bulun was asking about tissue samples, so I'll pass this along. Patrice Hugo from Procrea was sharing last night at our table that they have endometrial tissue, serum, and some other tissues from 3000 women. I cannot remember the proportion who had endometriosis, but they are willing to share that tissue and they would like to see it used.

MCLACHLAN: This stimulates me again to mention a website where this kind of information can be, plus how you get in touch with them, who is getting it, whether there is an advisory group, etc. It would save a lot of time and energy, and the first thing that the NIH should do is to assign a website grant to get this thing up and running and hire a couple of people. We already have 11 websites.

GIUDICE: How about other universities, too?

OSTEEN: In terms of tissue acquisition, there is an opportunity for some partnerships here, and it always comes down to three things: money, money, and money. While there are well-meaning people out there, their pressures are such that it is very difficult for some of these small biotech or pharmaceutical companies to really be the Good Samaritan without some sort of a resource. Maybe we should think about what sort of partnership could be formed between the NIH and the pharmaceutical industry to help provide the tissue resources that would then stimulate research in this area and thus benefit everybody.

BULUN: The quality of research tissues is imperative. I learned this the hard way. Once I conducted a study with a private company who provided me with the tissues. When we finished the study, I found out that the tissues were obtained from women undergoing bilateral tubal ligation. You can all appreciate the chances of finding meaningful endometriosis in women who are going through bilateral tubal ligation. Thus, if you would try to do this in a very well coordinated effort, we should work with capable clinicians and surgeons who are well trained in the field of endometriosis. These clinicians can identify the patients with endometriosis and can remove tissues using appropriate techniques. NIH may wish to take a leading role in this.

TAYLOR: The website mechanism would actually be an inexpensive and very powerful way of developing clinical protocols to get around some of the issues that Dr. Olive raised. If we had an evolving clinical protocol site on the Web, everyone could give their input into what parameters and long-term outcomes people want to look at. It would be a much more efficient way than convening a conference like this, to try to bang out the details. This would be another benefit of a networking scheme.

D. BLITHE (*National Institute of Child Health and Human Development, National Institutes of Health, Bethesda, MD*): I want to follow up on Kevin Osteen's comment about pharmaceutical companies. Back in late January and early February, we had a workshop on GnRH antagonists and we had a lot of pharmaceutical representation there. In particular, Praecis and Amgen are collaborating to put Abarelex Depo on the market and they are currently in phase II trials on endometriosis. Ferring also has a long-acting GnRH antagonist different from Abarelex that they are intending to market for endometriosis as well as various types of cancers. Could anyone in the audience comment on the use or potential of GnRH antagonists as a therapy? GnRH agonists have been mentioned a lot in this meeting. I have not heard anything about antagonists in particular. Does anyone have any encouraging or discouraging feedback on that?

GIUDICE: The period for the agonist is fairly limited. It is only about 7 or 8 days, or a maximum of 10 days. Thus, it is unlikely that this is really going to exacerbate symptoms, although it may. I am surprised that clinical trials still go on where agonists or antagonists are given, the hypoestrogenic state is arrived at, and people are still looking at bone mineral density. We probably can get beyond that and start to add back some bisphosphonates or other agents. However, your point is very well taken about adjuncts to therapy and we likely will be seeing more and more clinical trials with GnRH antagonists since a number of companies are coming out with those products.

TAYLOR: This is an example of how we are not taking advantage of the forward movements that have potential. Antagonists are another way of attacking a pathway that we all understand quite well. However, to me, conceptually, the steps that we have made from agonists to superagonists to antagonists do not warrant the amount of investment that has been made in these agents. That is my personal opinion.

GIUDICE: I want to make one other comment. When clinical studies are done with newer therapies, it is imperative that they are well designed with appropriate controls so that we do not end up with more studies where the outcomes are not comparable.

CHWALISZ: I agree concerning the value of GnRH antagonists. However, there might still be room for new strategies based on oral application forms. There is definitely a need for an orally active GnRH agonist or antagonist—for example, for a short-term GnRH antagonist therapy. This is an area where I see future potential, but the side effects of GnRH antagonists will be probably very similar to those of the agonists, particularly during long-term use.

GIUDICE: Thank you. Are there any other recommendations? That is really our goal here this afternoon.

M. NORCUM (*University of Missouri, Columbia, MO*): I am sort of here in disguise as a representative of The Endometriosis Association because I am also a biochemist. I have heard much exciting new information about the basic cell biology of what is going on. However, when the discussion comes to testing new therapies, even though there are some beginning to be developed in the newer fields (e.g., MMP inhibitors, aromatase inhibitors), it brings to mind Linda's comment of "let's not forget the patient". There still seems to be this divide where we are focused on hormonally based therapies, which we know do not work in a significant percentage of women. They are also associated with significant side effects. I would like to see a push towards really bringing these two sides together. As is common in any association between basic science and clinical science in any medical center and in regard to just about any disease, there is not a whole lot of cross talk. One of the real values of this workshop is bringing together clinicians and basic scientists. I would like to see more and encourage more of that interaction.

Another thing is that there is a clear acknowledgment of heterogeneity of populations and from the patient perspective as well as the treatment perspective. Until we understand the etiology and can totally prevent endometriosis, there needs to be a focus on early disease and again how to recognize it as surgically confirmed endometriosis. Treatments for stage I and stage II clearly are going to be different and the focus needs to be different than for more advanced disease.

The other thing to note is that we are faced with treating developing disease. If the model is correct that much of endometriosis is due to retrograde menstruation, then you are going to have developing disease again since that is happening every month and when you pull women off a drug. Long-term therapies also need to be a focus. The basic biology is moving forward, but it is going to be a long time before the genetic, environmental, and other etiological information all come together.

J. HUTCHISON (*R.W. Johnson Pharmaceutical Research Institute, Raritan, NJ*): I would like to suggest some more clarification of the idea that endometriosis is a precondition for various types of cancer. From a drug development perspective, this could be very important. If endometriosis is a precondition for cancer, then unmet medical need is expanded beyond treatment of symptoms and infertility attributed to endometriosis. Further, there is a rationale for diagnosing and treating asymptomatic endometriosis, which usually does not get treated.

GIUDICE: I want to thank all of you for your suggestions.

E.C. PARROTT (*National Institute of Child Health and Human Development, National Institutes of Health, Bethesda, MD*): We want to thank the speakers and the planning committee for their time and effort. This was a very stimulating meeting and we want to thank the audience for coming and spending your time here with us. We thank our cosponsors, the NIEHS and the NIH Office of Research on Women's Health, for their support. We also thank our other supporters, the pharmaceutical companies, and The Endometriosis Association.

YOSHINAGA: I join with Dr. Parrott in thanking all of you.

Index of Contributors